New

Dimensions

in Women's Health Seventh Edition

Linda Lewis Alexander, PhD, FAAN
Vice President
Health and Global Advocacy
QIAGEN, Inc.

Judith H. LaRosa, PhD, RN, FAAN
Vice Dean and Professor
Graduate Program in Public Health
SUNY Downstate Medical Center

Helaine Bader, MPH
Director
Health and Global Advocacy
QIAGEN, Inc.

Susan Garfield, DrPH
Principal
EY

William James Alexander, MA
Director of Communications
Department of Neurology
Duke School of Medicine

JONES & BARTLETT
L E A R N I N G

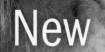

World Headquarters
Jones & Bartlett Learning
5 Wall Street
Burlington, MA 01803
978-443-5000
info@jblearning.com
www.jblearning.com

Jones & Bartlett Learning books and products are available through most bookstores and online booksellers. To contact Jones & Bartlett Learning directly, call 800-832-0034, fax 978-443-8000, or visit our website, www.jblearning.com.

Substantial discounts on bulk quantities of Jones & Bartlett Learning publications are available to corporations, professional associations, and other qualified organizations. For details and specific discount information, contact the special sales department at Jones & Bartlett Learning via the above contact information or send an email to specialsales@jblearning.com.

09142-7

Production Credits
VP, Executive Publisher: David D. Cella
Publisher: Cathy L. Esperti
Editorial Assistant: Carter McAllister
Associate Director of Production: Julie C. Bolduc
Senior Production Editor: Leah Corrigan
Director of Marketing: Andrea DeFronzo
VP, Manufacturing and Inventory Control: Therese Connell
Composition: Cenveo Publisher Services
Cover Design: Scott Moden

Rights & Media Specialist: Jamey O'Quinn
Media Development Editor: Troy Liston
Cover Images: (main photo) © NinaMalyna/Shutterstock; (side photos top to bottom) © Nadino/Shutterstock, © arek_malang/Shutterstock, © pkchai/Shutterstock, © Diego Cervo/Shutterstock, © Patrick Foto/Shutterstock, © Chad Zuber/Shutterstock, © BestPhotoStudio/Shutterstock
Printing and Binding: RR Donnelley
Cover Printing: RR Donnelley

Library of Congress Cataloging-in-Publication Data
Names: Alexander, Linda Lewis, author. | LaRosa, Judith H., author. | Bader, Helaine, author. | Garfield, Susan, author. | Alexander, William James, author.
Title: New dimensions in women's health / Linda Lewis Alexander, Judith H. LaRosa, Helaine Bader, Susan Garfield, William James Alexander.
Description: Seventh edition. | Burlington, Massachusetts : Jones & Bartlett Learning, [2016] | Preceded by New dimensions in women's health / Linda Lewis Alexander ... [et al.]. 6th ed. 2014. | Includes bibliographical references and index.
Identifiers: LCCN 2016015811 | ISBN 9781284088434 (alk. paper)
Subjects: | MESH: Women's Health | United States
Classification: LCC RA778 | NLM WA 309 AA1 | DDC 613/.04244--dc23
LC record available at https://lccn.loc.gov/2016015811

6048

Printed in the United States of America
20 19 18 17 16   10 9 8 7 6 5 4 3 2 1

BRIEF CONTENTS

CONTENTS

PREFACE

The seventh edition of *New Dimensions in Women's Health* discusses health issues that affect all women: women of all racial and ethnic groups, of all ages, of different sexual orientations, and with various degrees of physical ability. The text presents unbiased, accurate information free from any specific political agenda while allowing its readers to appreciate the range of perspectives that influence how women in the United States and around the world think about health and make decisions that affect their well-being. Each chapter presents in-depth coverage of an important aspect of women's health and examines the contributing epidemiological, historical, psychological, cultural, ethical, legal, political, and economic influences. This book is written for women, recognizing their outstanding contributions as daughters, sisters, mothers, nurses, doctors, scientists, laborers, advocates, and much more.

Organization of the Book

This book is organized into four parts, each of which covers a different dimension of women's health.

PART ONE, Foundations of Women's Health, takes a population-based approach. It introduces students to the concepts of women's health, public health, health economics, and issues of health across the lifespan.

Chapter 1 provides a brief history of the women's health movement and the political climate around women's health.

Chapter 2 focuses on the economics of health, including the payer system in the United States, various insurance plans, healthcare reform, and the impact on the aging population.

Chapter 3 introduces the concepts of health promotion and disease prevention and discusses how these efforts benefit women through the different stages of life.

PART TWO, Sexual and Reproductive Dimensions of Women's Health, addresses issues regarding sexual health and sexuality, as well as sexual violence as a public health problem.

Chapter 4 defines sexual health and discusses the cultural, economic, and biological factors that influence women's sexual health.

Chapter 5 discusses contraceptive methods and abortion, and provides information that will help inform a woman's decision around reproduction.

Building on this, **Chapter 6** covers pregnancy, childbirth, breastfeeding, and infertility.

Chapter 7 is devoted to the clinical, sociological, and epidemiological dimensions of sexually transmitted infections, including HIV/AIDS prevention, transmission, and treatment.

Chapter 8 explores menopause as a biological and cultural phenomenon, including the benefits, drawbacks, and effects of hormone therapy.

PART THREE, Physical and Life Span Dimensions of Women's Health, comprises Chapters 9 through 12.

Chapter 9 discusses exercise, nutrition, and weight management at the individual and national level, as well as ways women can improve their diet, physical activity, and weight maintenance.

Chapter 10 examines how cardiovascular disease and cancer affect women as well as how these diseases progress and can be prevented, treated, and managed.

Chapter 11 discusses other chronic diseases important to women's health, including osteoporosis, arthritis, diabetes, autoimmune diseases, and Alzheimer's disease.

Chapter 12 offers definitions of mental health and mental illness, explores the reasons why good mental health is essential, and provides information on various mental disorders.

PART FOUR, Interpersonal and Social Dimensions of Women's Health, contains Chapters 13 through 15.

Chapter 13 discusses the political, personal, economic, and cultural dimensions of drug use and abuse.

Chapter 14 provides different perspectives on violence, abuse, and harassment.

Chapter 15 discusses current trends and issues for women in the workforce.

New to This Edition

The seventh edition of *New Dimensions in Women's Health* has been extensively expanded, updated, and revised to include the most accurate and relevant women's health information in an organized, engaging manner. It includes new developments in women's health as well as practical ways women can improve their own health.
Highlights include:

NEW material discussing health care reform and its implications for individual women and the country as a whole (Chapter 1)

NEW discussion of the growing gray area and cultural influence of marijuana (Chapter 13)

NEW section on electronic cigarettes and vaping and their implications for public health (Chapter 13)

NEW sections offering practical tips and strategies for individuals who wish to quit smoking, reduce problem drinking, or quit illicit drug use (Chapter 13)

NEW section on abuse/misuse of prescription and over-the-counter drugs (Chapter 13)

NEW section on dissociative disorders, including common forms of these disorders, how they occur, and their effects on the psyche (Chapter 12)

NEW "Critical thinking" cases that involve detailed discussions of women dealing with issues discussed in relevant chapters, including smoking, sexually transmitted infections, and mental illness. Each of these case studies includes discussion questions and answers. (All chapters)

NEW Explanation of the endocrine system (Chapter 11)

EXPANDED discussions of women's health from a global perspective, with discussions of how women's health issues in developing countries, Canada, and Europe compare to those in the United States (Chapter 1)

EXPANDED discussion of menopause as a natural part of a woman's life cycle, the "medicalization" of menopause, and how hormone therapy works (Chapter 8)

EXPANDED section on stress, including the biology of the stress response, the health effects of short-term and long-term stress, sources of stress, and how to cope in a healthful manner (Chapter 12)

EXPANDED discussion of STI risk for LGBT populations and how to reduce risk (Chapter 7)

EXPANDED discussion regarding gender identity, transgender, and gender neutral (Chapter 4)

EXPANDED practical, detailed information about HPV, including information about vaccinations, Pap smears, and HPV testing, the advantages and disadvantages of each of these, and how to evaluate one's own risk for HPV and other STIs (Chapter 7)

UPDATED legal perspective on marriage for same-sex couples (Chapter 4)

UPDATED to reflect the latest developments in the HIV/AIDS epidemic in the United States and around the world, as well as the latest efforts to reduce transmission and increase treatment (Chapter 7)

UPDATED section on global tobacco use and the health effects of smoking around the world (Chapter 13)

UPDATED information on mental illnesses to discuss new DSM-V (Chapter 12)

UPDATED section on suicide, including an expanded discussion of suicide as a global public health problem (Chapter 12)

PEDAGOGY

Special features distributed throughout each chapter highlight and summarize important concepts and promote healthy lifestyle choices.

It's Your Health highlights key facts that help students improve their own health, such as disease symptoms, screening recommendations, and benefits of healthy behaviors.

Informed Decision Making provides students with detailed information for making appropriate decisions regarding their health and well-being.

It's Your Health

Equal Rights Amendment

The Equal Rights Amendment was written in 1921 by **suffragist** Alice Paul. Although it passed both houses of Congress in 1972, it was not ratified by enough state legislatures to be added to the Constitution.

Section 1. Equality of Rights under the law shall not be denied or abridged by the United States or any state on account of sex.

Section 2. The Congress shall have the power to enforce, by appropriate legislation, the provisions of this article.

Section 3. This amendment shall take effect two years after the date of ratification.

Courtesy of the National Park Service.

INFORMED DECISION MAKING

Women can reduce their risk of cardiovascular disease and cancer in several ways. For most women, prevention and taking good care of their daily and long-term health are critical actions. The old adage "An ounce of prevention is worth a pound of cure" is still correct. It is much more effective to reduce your risk of suffering a life-threatening or disabling heart attack at 55 by never smoking, eating a prudent diet, and exercising—all behaviors that should begin in childhood. Although it is better to begin these lifesaving behaviors in childhood, changing as one ages can still reduce one's risk.

Self-Assessments provide exercises to help students determine their risk of disease and need for modifying behaviors.

Self-Assessment 8.1
Strategies for Hormone Therapy Decision Making

The decision to use hormone therapy is a personal and private one.

Women should consider several factors when making the decision:

1. Personal and family medical history
   - History of breast cancer
   - Blood clots in the legs, lungs, or eyes
   - Abnormal vaginal bleeding
   - Preexisting cardiovascular conditions, such as blood clots, stroke, or uncontrolled high blood pressure
   - Liver, gallbladder, or pancreatic disease
2. Menopausal symptoms and their severity
   - Hot flashes
   - Vaginal irritation and discomfort
   - Urinary tract problems
   - Emotional and mood changes
3. Review risks and benefits
4. Reevaluate decision periodically

Contraception

Historically, contraceptive options have been largely for women. This may be due in part to the reality that women, not men, get pregnant, or the fact that family planning research and contraceptive services have focused disproportionately on women. The female reproductive system has been extensively studied for centuries. Studies on male contraceptives have been seriously limited. Today, options for the male range from mildly effective (withdrawal) to highly effective (vasectomy). It could be argued that the remarkable effectiveness of modern hormonal contraceptives for women has given women high levels of protection, but that it has absolved men from participating in contraceptive protection and decision making. Men are often silent partners in preventing pregnancies.

Several factors contribute to the dominant role women play in contraceptive decision making and the availability of services for them. Modern medical care services provide ready access to contraceptive information and options for women. Women are taught and encouraged to see a gynecologist regularly in their teens; there is not a parallel system of routine health care for men. Society educates girls and young women early that the penalty of unprotected sex will be an unwanted pregnancy, personal and family shame, and economic hardships. The educational message to boys and young men is not the same, although legal issues surrounding paternity and child support in recent years have introduced the penalty concept to an unwanted pregnancy.

Multicultural surveys demonstrate that men are willing to participate in contraception, and their female partners trust them to do so.[52] Male contraceptive research includes hormonal and nonhormonal methods. Today the most significant barriers for expanded use include limited delivery methods and perceived regulatory obstacles. Promising options include products that target sperm motility, decrease or eliminate semen emission, or interrupt sperm maturation. These products vary in delivery method and include pills, gels, ultrasound technology, and injection. Although considerable progress has been made in clinical research on male contraception, no new product is currently available.

Gender Dimensions discuss how specific health issues, ranging from breast cancer to obesity, vary between genders.

CASE STUDY

Jill, who is 32 years old, is hoping to become pregnant. She has recently stopped using birth control pills and has been having unprotected sex with her partner for the past 3 months.

Questions

1. What are some lifestyle behaviors and medical interventions that Jill may want to consider during this time?

2. What considerations should Jill be thinking about when it comes to preparing for childbirth?

Critical thinking **Case Studies** provide students with thought provoking, practical applications relevant to their personal lives on a daily basis.

Quotes offer experiences, opinions, and thoughts from women of all ages, races, and cultures.

I've made a real effort to incorporate exercise into my daily routine this semester. On Mondays, Wednesdays, and Fridays I go straight to the gym after class, and I go running Tuesdays, Thursdays, and Saturdays, taking Sunday off. It's funny, because I never really thought about exercise much until this year, but now it's a normal part of my life.

—**20-year-old student**

Michelle Obama (1964–)

Michelle Obama is a lawyer, community activist, a mother of two, and the husband of the 44th U.S. President, Barack Obama. Since becoming the First Lady of the United States in 2008, she has been a strong advocate for a balanced diet and physical fitness. In 2010, she launched a national initiative called *Let's Move!* to reduce and prevent childhood obesity and improve the health of American children. The *Let's Move!* program improves access to nutritious, affordable foods; increases children's physical activity; provides balanced meals in school; and educates and empowers parents and guardians to improve their children's physical activity.

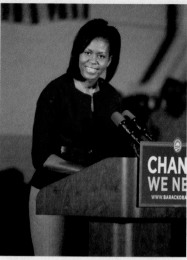

© spirit of america/Shutterstock

Mrs. Obama was born and raised in Chicago as the second of two children of Marian and Fraser Robinson. She was an excellent student and went on to study sociology at Princeton University and then law at Harvard Law School. She joined Sidley Austin, a Chicago law firm and met her future husband when she was assigned to be his mentor. Mrs. Obama left Sidley Austin in 1991 to work for the government of Chicago and to direct a Chicago nonprofit that encouraged young people to become socially active and participate in public service. Mr. and Mrs. Obama were married in 1992.

From 1996 to 2002, Mrs. Obama worked for the University of Chicago, where she helped build the university's community service center. She later worked for the University of Chicago hospitals and the University of Chicago Medical Center. Mrs. Obama continued to work part-time while she raised their two daughters, Sasha and Malia, and helped with her husband's Senate, and later, presidential campaigns.

In addition to working to improve children's physical fitness, Mrs. Obama works to help support military families, promote national service, help women balance career goals and family aspirations, and encourage education in the arts.

Profiles of Remarkable Women highlight individuals who contributed to the health and well-being of all women. These profiles showcase women as champions of health across all ages and life spans.

▮ Topics for Discussion

1. What type of ethical issues may arise with testing for genetic predisposition for various chronic diseases?

2. Have you, a close friend, or a family member ever been diagnosed with a chronic disease? How has that diagnosis changed your or his or her life?

3. How can lifestyle changes affect chronic disease management?

4. What differences exist between chronic diseases that occur early in life versus those that manifest later in life?

5. In what ways does early diagnosis help a woman and her family to cope with her disease?

Topics for Discussion at the end of each chapter encourage students to consider their own opinions on a topic and to explore the philosophical dimensions surrounding issues of women's health.

LEARNING AND TEACHING TOOLS

New Dimensions in Women's Health, Seventh Edition includes learning tools for students and teaching tools for instructors.

For the Student

Each new book comes complete with a dynamic technology solution. Navigate 2 Advantage Access provides an interactive eBook, student activities and assessments, knowledge checks, learning analytics reporting tools, as well as 17 informative animations:

- External genital differentiation — male and female
- External female sexual anatomy
- Internal female sexual anatomy
- Selection of condoms
- The three stages of labor (a–d)
- The female breast
- Three trimesters of pregnancy
- Economic benefits of breastfeeding
- Rates of different STIs
- Map indicating rates of HIV by country
- Complex carbohydrates are a good source of minerals, vitamins, and fiber
- Stroke mortality rates
- Smoking prevalence
- Clogged arteries
- Angioplasty
- Arterial splint
- Complications from chronic alcohol consumption
- How alcohol is absorbed in the body
- The principal control centers of the brain affected by alcohol consumption

Instructor Resources

For instructors teaching this course, resources include:
- Test Bank
- Slides in PowerPoint format
- Instructor's Manual

Navigate 2 also provides a dashboard that reports actionable assessment data.

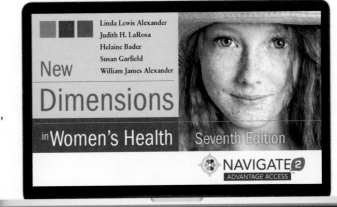

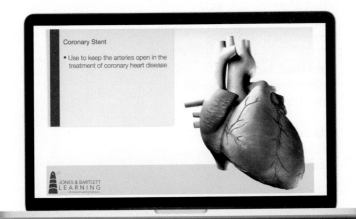

ACKNOWLEDGMENTS

This seventh edition of *New Dimensions in Women's Health* builds on the success of all previous editions. The authors remain indebted to family and friends for their support, guidance, patience, and sacrifices as we dissected and reconstructed the entire text again. Lastly, we'd like to acknowledge and remember the following remarkable women: Elizabeth Bennett, EdD, RN (1926–1998), Gail Addlestone, MD (1969–2007), and Lucille Dorey Lewis (1915–1993).

We also thank the reviewers of the sixth and seventh editions for their valuable suggestions.

Reviewers of the *Sixth Edition*

Andrea Hope, EdD
Assistant Professor
Monmouth University

Julie Williams Merten, MSH, MCHES
University of North Florida

Kim A. Sleder, MPH
Long Beach City College

Patricia Kelley RN, MSN, BC
Clinical Instructor, Nursing,
North Carolina A&T State University

Reviewers of the *Seventh Edition*

Sarah Brock, MS in Biology
Instructor
Tulane University

Cara A. Busenhart, MSN, CNM, APRN
Program Director, Nurse-Midwifery Education
University of Kansas School of Nursing

Deborah Burch, MSN, RN
Assistant Professor of Nursing
Thomas University

Erika Collazo, PhD(c), MPH
Associate Instructor
Indiana University Bloomington

Milan Motroni, MA, EdD
Professor
Modesto Junior College

Tami Ford, MA
College Assistant Professor
New Mexico State University

Luis Enrique Espinoza, MS
Instructor
Texas Woman's University

Linda Lewis Alexander, PhD, FAAN

Linda Alexander recently retired as VP, Women's Health and Global Advocacy at QIAGEN Corporation. Her previous professional positions included VP, Women's Health at Digene Corporation, President/CEO of the American Social Health Association, and VP at United Information Systems. She is also a retired lieutenant colonel, with the U.S. Army Nurse Corps and has held faculty positions at the Uniformed Services University of Health Sciences and the University of Maryland. She currently serves as Chair, Board of Directors, for Women Deliver, an international NGO dedicated to resolving the disparity in health needs among women throughout the world.

Dr. Alexander is nationally known for her leadership in women's health advocacy and has published extensively on women's health issues. Her many honors include appointments to national advisory panels on infectious diseases and women's health; she is also a fellow in the American Academy of Nursing. Dr. Alexander holds a baccalaureate degree in nursing, master's degrees in education/counseling and community health, and a doctoral degree in health education.

Judith H. LaRosa, PhD, RN, FAAN

Dr. Judith LaRosa's career has spanned education, research, clinical practice, and administration. Her present position is Vice Dean and Distinguished Service Professor, State University of New York (SUNY) Downstate School of Public Health, where her current research focus is on cultural perceptions of health and disease. She is currently on the editorial board of the *Journal of Community Health* and she serves on the board of the Bedford Stuyvesant Family Health Center—a federally qualified health center.

Before this, Dr. LaRosa served as Professor and Chair, Department of Community Health Sciences, Tulane University School of Public Health and Tropical Medicine, and Director, Tulane Xavier National Center of Excellence in Women's Health. From 1991 to 1994, she served as the first Deputy Director of the Office of Research on Women's Health, National Institutes of Health (NIH). She is a co-author of the legislatively mandated 1994 Guidelines on the Inclusion of Women and Minorities as Subjects in Clinical Research. From 1978 to 1991, Dr. LaRosa served at the NIH's National Heart, Lung, and Blood Institute (NHLBI) as the first coordinator of the NHLBI Workplace Initiative in cardiovascular disease risk factor reduction.

Dr. LaRosa has served on the Institute of Medicine's Committee on Understanding the Biology of Sex and Gender as well as the Committee on Assessing the Medical Risks of Human Oocyte Donation for Stem Cell Research; the National Institute for Nursing Research Advisory Council; the Armed Forces Epidemiological Board; and the National Science Foundation/Institute of Medicine Committee on Defense Women's Health Research. Dr. LaRosa received her Bachelor of Science degree in nursing and her Master of Nursing Education degree from the University of Pittsburgh and her PhD in health education from the University of Maryland.

Helaine Bader, MPH

Helaine Bader is a health educator and advocacy strategist, with expertise in women's health and public-private partnerships. Ms. Bader has more than 20 years of experience in women's health research, health communications, and health education. She has worked on multimedia and Web-based health campaigns in both the public and private sectors and has developed, implemented, and evaluated health education projects for various issues affecting women and children.

In her current position as a health educator and advocacy strategy consultant, Ms. Bader works with nonprofit organizations, corporations, academic institutions, and individuals to develop, implement, and evaluate health education and advocacy initiatives. Previously, Ms. Bader was responsible for corporate relations at a global maternal health organization, where she helped bring the private sector into the conversation around the Millennium Development Goals. In her prior position as Director, Women's Health and Global Advocacy at QIAGEN, Inc., she developed and implemented partnerships and educational initiatives with the NGO community. She also worked on increasing access to cervical cancer screening in low-income countries.

Ms. Bader received her baccalaureate degree in English with a minor in premedical sciences from the University of Pennsylvania and her master's degree in public health from University of Pittsburgh.

Susan Garfield, DrPH

Susan Garfield is a market access, reimbursement, and economics strategist, with an expertise in demand creation and advocacy. For eighteen years, her professional career has focused on innovations in healthcare, the economics of practice change, and the role of reimbursement and policy to the adoption of new technologies. Dr. Garfield's work has included economic modeling, coding analyses and applications, payer coverage campaigns, market strategies for innovative technologies, health policy development, government relations, and creating partnerships between industry and advocacy groups.

Currently, she is Principal at EY, running their Market Access practice. Previously, she was Executive Vice President at GfK, a market leading health care consultancy focusing on the market access needs of biotech, medical device, diagnostic, specialty, and pharmaceutical clients where she ran the U.S. consultancy practice. Prior to joining GfK, Dr. Garfield was the Director, Global Reimbursement, Policy and Economic Strategy at QIAGEN Corporation (formally Digene Corporation). In this role, she planned and executed a reimbursement strategy that resulted in near universal coverage for the company's leading cancer diagnostic product. In addition, she directed global economic and pricing analyses for the company's clinical diagnostic portfolio.

Dr. Garfield received her Bachelor of Art in English and Women's Studies from the University of Pennsylvania, a Master's of Science in Population and Development from the London School of Economics, and a Master's of Science in Health Policy and Management from Harvard University, School of Public Health, and her Doctorate of Public Health from Boston University.

William Alexander, MA

William Alexander, MA, is a writer and communications specialist focusing on medicine, global public health, and women's health. He is currently the director of communications for the Department of Neurology at the Duke School of Medicine.

Before joining Duke University, Mr. Alexander worked at TCL Institute, a private medical education company. He also worked at Ipas, an international nonprofit organization dealing with women's reproductive health, and MEASURE Evaluation, a global organization that helps USAID-funded countries improve their systems to confront disease, population issues, and poverty. He has also written for the North Carolina Department of Health and Human Services, Escapist Magazine, the Embassy of Kazakhstan, the American Social Health Association and other organizations.

Mr. Alexander received his baccalaureate degree in English from St. Mary's College of Maryland and his master's degree in medical and science journalism from UNC-Chapel Hill.

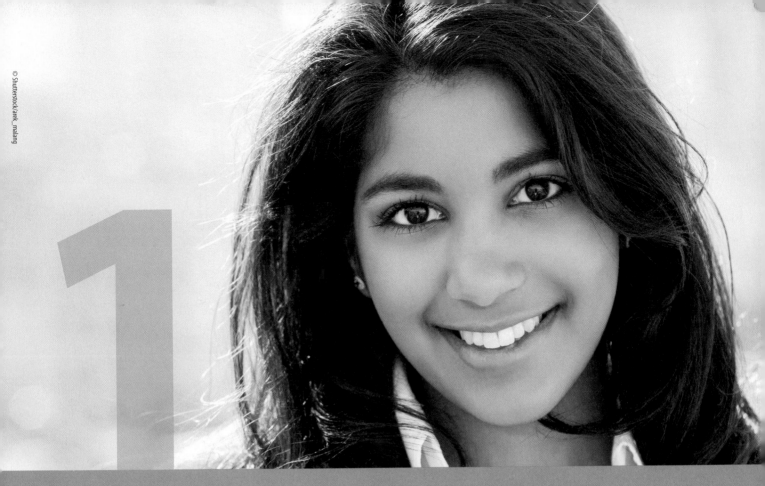

PART ONE

Foundations of Women's Health

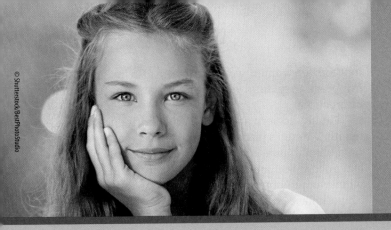

CHAPTER 1

Introduction to Women's Health

Learning Objectives

On completion of this chapter, the student should be able to discuss:

1. Major ways of thinking about and defining women's health.

2. How the women's health movement has grown and changed over the past 200 years.

3. The government's role in protecting and promoting the health of the public.

4. The responsibilities of the National Institutes of Health and the Office of Research on Women's Health.

5. The federal government's role in funding and conducting research on women's health.

6. The importance of investing in biomedical research and the inclusion of women and minorities in research studies.

7. The concept of gender-based research and basic health differences between women and men.

8. Reproductive rights, the global gag rule, and the effects that restricting abortion has on global health.

9. How lack of access to health care, lack of health insurance, cultural insensitivity, and other obstacles affect the health of women.

10. The need to train health professionals about women's health and cultural sensitivity.

11. Global efforts to support women's health and gender equity.

INTRODUCTION

Women's health is a fascinatingly complex area of study. Thousands, even millions, of factors affect the ways women develop, get sick, get well, interact with others, reproduce, age, and receive health care. Some books on women's health attempt to provide a deep but narrow level of detail by focusing on a few of these factors. This book, however, attempts to explore, or at least introduce, the significant facets of women's health from many different angles. The following sections describe areas of concern and ways of thinking about women's health and well-being that are explored in the chapters of this text.

Women's health includes the study of the whole body. Women's health examines biological characteristics unique to women, the most obvious being the reproductive organs, but also differences in body structure, childhood development, hormones, and brain chemistry. Yet women's health is also concerned with factors that affect both genders, including the common cold, heart disease, depression, and the benefits of regular physical exercise. Women's health includes the study of disease, but it also examines factors that affect a woman's physical and mental well-being.

Women's health can study populations or an individual woman. Women's health benefits from examining patterns of health and disease in populations—for example, whether women who are exposed to secondhand cigarette smoke have a greater risk for developing lung cancer than women who are not. But women's health also includes the study of how diseases affect individuals, such as ways a woman can reduce her personal risk of getting cancer; what the signs, effects, and treatments of cancer are for an individual woman who has it; how that woman's unique body acts and reacts to disease; and how a woman copes after being diagnosed.

The entire spectrum of research and social sciences can provide insight into women's health. A full understanding of women's sexual and reproductive health requires biological, cultural, historical, psychological, and political perspectives. The physical components of the reproductive system influence a woman's sexual response, but so do cultural mores and traditions that dictate when and how women are supposed to enjoy and think about their sexuality. Women's health includes reproductive health, defined as the well-being of a person's reproductive system, including their ability to decide if and when to have children.[1] Studying reproductive health requires examining the laws, practices, and cultural beliefs that influence when and where women learn about childbirth, family planning, and birth control, and their legal options for ending a pregnancy. Because women's unequal treatment affects their well-being and lives in many ways, feminism—the idea that women should have the same political, economic, and social rights and opportunities as men—is also an important part of women's health. Not all women become mothers, but because all mothers are women, women's health also includes studying pregnancy, fetal development, and mother–infant interactions.

Finally, society and culture also influence women's health. Women's place in society affects if and how often rape, sexual harassment, and other forms of sexual violence occur. Sociocultural factors also influence where and when women can enter the workforce as well as what sort of workplace they encounter. Women's health includes women's ability to obtain and benefit from health care. The study of access to health care has increased dramatically over the past 20 years. Access to health care includes not only whether women can physically get to a doctor or healthcare provider but also whether they trust that provider, whether they have insurance or some other way to pay for health care, and whether they know if and when something is wrong. Access to health care and healthcare decision making are especially important for women's health, because women are more likely than men to make decisions regarding health care for their relatives and families.

HISTORICAL DIMENSIONS: THE WOMEN'S HEALTH MOVEMENT

The past 200 years have seen enormous improvements in women's health, political and economic rights, and place in society. The following section provides a brief history of the women's health movement and advances in women's health in the United States.

Reductions in morbidity and mortality—or injuries and deaths resulting from pregnancy and childbirth—are one of the most important human achievements over the past 200 years. Until the late 1800s, rates of maternal death in the United States and Europe ranged from 25/1000 to 85/1000.[2] This means women had a 2.5% to 8.5% chance of dying every time they gave birth. Without access to family planning, the large family sizes that were often the norm made childbirth a major cause of death for women.

Today, the maternal mortality rate in the United States is about 28/100,000, less than half what it was in the 19th century.[3] Maternal mortality rates are even lower throughout most of Western Europe. Rates of infant mortality have fallen even more dramatically. In the late 1800s, anywhere between 10% and 25% of infants died either during or shortly after childbirth in Europe and the United States.[4] Today, just 0.6% of U.S. infants die during or shortly after childbirth.[5] The medical advances that allowed these changes include the knowledge of germ theory, which helped reduce infections during childbirth; improved birthing assistance techniques from doctors and midwives; access to basic medical care during childbirth; and access to family planning services. Women's political and economic rights have also grown enormously since the 1800s. In the early 19th century, women had no right to vote and were legally restricted to a small number of professions, most of them low paying and menial in nature. Women could not legally attend college and rarely had the opportunity to complete a high school education. Methods of birth control such as condoms and diaphragms existed, but they were illegal and difficult to obtain. The legal system also limited how and when women could own property, the circumstances under which they could marry and get divorced, and many other areas of women's legal life. Although there are still opportunities for improving women's health and for ending existing sources of discrimination, women today can be grateful for the advances made by previous generations of women (and men) to advance women's health.

1830s and 1840s: The Health Movement

Many historians believe the women's health movement began in the 1830s and 1840s, when small groups of women began advocating taking an active role in preventing disease and staying healthy rather than relying on formally trained physicians for treatment. This first wave of advocacy focused on eating a proper diet, the elimination of the **corset**, and periodic sexual abstinence in marriage to control family size. For the first time, a few middle-class women who became interested in their own health sought entry into the medical profession. Elizabeth Blackwell, for example, entered medical school in 1847 and prompted the opening of several medical schools for women. In 1848, the first women's rights convention was held in Seneca Falls, New York; the convention marked the official beginning of the women's rights movement.

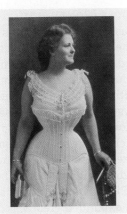
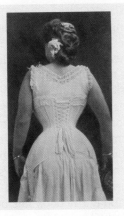

During the Popular Health Movement, women were encouraged to eliminate the corset. Corsets were worn as an undergarment or outer garment to support and shape the waistline, hips, and breasts.
© Index Stock/age fotostock

1861–1865: The Civil War

The Civil War prompted many women to volunteer as doctors and nurses; some women even disguised themselves as men to tend to wounded soldiers on the battlefield. Dorothea Dix and Clara Barton led a national effort to organize a nursing corps to care for the war's wounded and sick.

Women's participation in the war led to the opening of the first training schools for nurses in 1873; by 1890, 35 such schools existed. Although this trend represented advancement for women, the relationship between male doctors and female nurses mirrored the domestic sexual division of labor, with males as the authority figures and females as the subordinates.

Mid- to Late 1800s: The Women's Medical Movement

After the Civil War, educational and employment opportunities, though still severely limited, increased for women. The women's medical movement emerged from the growing numbers of women attending medical schools, their struggles to achieve equal status within the profession, and the popularity of challenging historical notions regarding women's fragility.

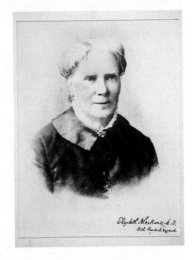

Elizabeth Blackwell was responsible for the opening of several medical schools for women in the mid-1800s.
© National Library of Medicine

> *My grandmother was a physician at a time when all of her peers were men. I have always admired her but now that I have reached the same age as she was when she started her practice, I have a better understanding of the challenges she must have faced at my age in her time.*
>
> **—24-year-old woman**

1890s–1920s: The Progressive Era

The women's medical movement gave way to the Progressive Era, which advanced the roles of women and women's rights as well as women's health. In 1920, the 19th Amendment to the U.S. Constitution, which guaranteed women the right to vote, was ratified. A few years later, the National Women's Party, formed in 1917, proposed the Equal Rights Amendment, which to this day remains unratified (see **It's Your Health**).

During this time, Margaret Sanger and other activists pushed to legalize birth control. In 1916, Sanger opened the nation's first birth control clinic in Brooklyn and was arrested shortly afterward for violating a federal ban on contraception. Sanger was found guilty and sentenced to 30 days of labor; however, in an appeal, a judge legalized contraception—but only for married couples with a doctor's prescription. Other progressives worked to promote healthy motherhood through prenatal care and child health services. The Sheppard–Towner Act of 1921 greatly increased the availability of prenatal and child health care, especially in rural areas where care was scarce. This legislation provided federal funding for programs that opened clinics for women and children, educated women about pregnancy and childbirth, and trained midwives and physicians about childbirth. The Act lasted until 1929, when a conservative Congress refused to continue its funding.

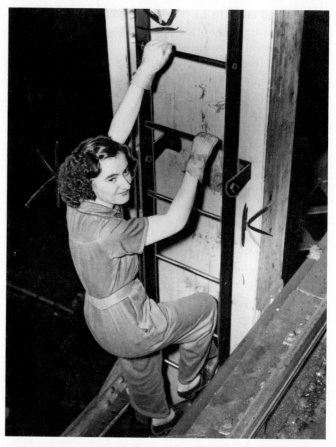

The number of women employed in the United States increased by 50% during World War II. Many of these women were forced to leave their jobs when the war ended.
© Courtesy of the National Park Service

It's Your Health

Equal Rights Amendment

The Equal Rights Amendment was written in 1921 by **suffragist** Alice Paul. Although it passed both houses of Congress in 1972, it was not ratified by enough state legislatures to be added to the Constitution.

Section 1. Equality of Rights under the law shall not be denied or abridged by the United States or any state on account of sex.

Section 2. The Congress shall have the power to enforce, by appropriate legislation, the provisions of this article.

Section 3. This amendment shall take effect two years after the date of ratification.

Courtesy of the National Park Service.

1930s–1950s: World War II and Postwar Years

The United States dramatically increased its production during World War II while millions of male workers were leaving to join the military. Women made a vital contribution to this effort. Twelve million women were working when the United States entered the war; by the time the war ended, 18 million women were employed.[6] Women began receiving more pay and worked in a greater variety of positions, though they were rarely, if ever, employed in skilled labor or managerial positions. When the war ended, women were pressured to leave their jobs and return to being homemakers.

Although many women were using birth control by the 1950s, popular culture still reinforced the idea that sexuality was simply a means for married couples to produce children. The Kinsey reports on human sexuality, issued in 1953, started to dispel this idea by revealing that, for many men and women, marriage was not a prerequisite for sex.

1960s–1970s: The Grassroots Movement

During the 1960s and 1970s, grassroots organizations challenged medical authority in the delivery of health care to women. These groups believed that the overwhelmingly male medical community excluded women from making decisions about their own health care, and they addressed issues such as unnecessary hysterectomies and cesarean sections, postpartum depression, abortion, and childbirth reform from a feminist perspective. The self-help manual *Our Bodies, Ourselves* epitomized this effort. This health book and guide to women's bodies, originally published in 1970, was written and self-published by 12 feminist activists. Today the book has been expanded greatly, is in its 13th edition, and has sold millions of copies worldwide.

Legal reforms during this time gave greater rights to women. The Food and Drug Administration (FDA) approved the birth control pill in 1960. In 1964, Congress passed the Civil Rights Act, including Title VII, which protected women against employment discrimination. In 1972, Congress passed the Equal Rights Amendment, though this amendment fell short of the 38 states needed to ratify it and add it to the Constitution. Also in 1972, legislation known as Title IX forced schools to provide equal funding for men and women in athletic programs.

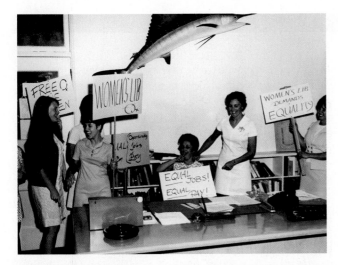

During the 1960s and 1970s, women challenged the authorities on many issues regarding gender equality.
© Creatas

For decades, the women's health movement had been composed mostly of middle-class White women. During the 1960s and 1970s, this movement began to be more inclusive. Organizations such as the National Black Women's Health Project (now called the Black Women's Health Imperative), the National Latina Women's Health Organization, the National Asian Women's Health Organization, and the Native American Women's Health Education and Resource Center were developed to focus on issues and diseases that disproportionately affect women of color.

> *Before I came to college, I thought that you had to be pretty radical and a little "anti-man" to be a feminist. Now I understand that feminists simply want women to have the same chances to make a name for themselves, have their voices heard, and live a good life as men do. I guess I've always been a feminist, but I just didn't know it.*
>
> **—19-year-old student**

> *I have an inherited condition that affects most of the women in my family. I don't know what we would have done without the support of an advocacy organization that is focused on our condition.*
>
> **—21-year-old woman**

1980s: Changing Public Policy

In the 1980s, the U.S. Public Health Service's Task Force on Women's Health Issues formed to assess the status of women's health. The Task Force issued recommendations to increase gender equity in **biomedical research** and establish guidelines for the inclusion of women in federally sponsored studies. In 1990, the National Institutes of Health (NIH) strengthened its guidelines and established the Office of Research on Women's Health (ORWH). The

ORWH ensures women's participation in clinical trials, strengthens research on diseases affecting women, and promotes the career advancement of women in science. The Women's Health Equity Act also was passed, allocating money to fund health research on particular areas of concern to women, including contraception, infertility, breast cancer, ovarian cancer, HIV/AIDS, and osteoporosis.

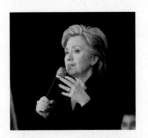
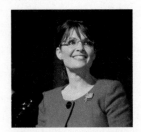
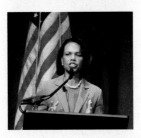
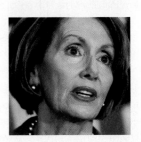

The past 20 years have seen the first major female candidate for president of the United States (Hillary Clinton), the first female vice presidential candidate for the Republican party (Sarah Palin), the first African American woman as secretary of state (Condoleeza Rice), the second female Secretary of State (Hillary Clinton), and the first female Speaker of the House of Representatives (Nancy Pelosi).
(top left) © Jose Gil/Dreamstime.com; (top right) © mistydawnphoto/ShutterStock, Inc.; (bottom left) © Susan Montgomery/ShutterStock, Inc.; (bottom right) © Chip Somodevilla/iStockphoto.com

1990s: Women's Health at the Forefront

The 1990s brought together government, healthcare institutions, academia, and advocacy organizations to analyze and promote women's health and well-being. New women's health offices in federal agencies and in regional public health service offices opened throughout the country. Existing centers broadened their scope beyond reproductive issues to take a more comprehensive look at health and disease among women.

In the 1993 NIH Revitalization Act, Congress required that women and minorities be included as subjects in all human subject research funded by NIH. This decision was a bold and innovative step. The inclusion of women in research has broadened the scientific knowledge base necessary for developing sex-specific diagnostic techniques, preventive measures, and effective treatments for diseases and conditions affecting women throughout their life span. The Family and Medical Leave Act, also introduced in 1993, gives employees unpaid medical leave for themselves or for the care of a family member or a newborn or adopted infant. In 1994, the Violence Against Women Act mandated a unified judicial response to sexual crimes committed against women.

It's Your Health

Feminism

Feminism is the idea that women should have the same political, economic, and social rights and opportunities as men. Feminism has achieved great advances for women over the past 100 years. Feminism has evolved to help different generations of women, and it will continue to evolve as women face new challenges and opportunities.

The first wave of feminism began in the late-19th and early-20th centuries, when suffragists and abolitionists worked to secure basic rights for women such as the rights to vote, own property, and inherit property.

The second wave of feminism occurred in the 1960s and 1970s. It fought against specific injustices, such as the lack of reproductive freedom, the lack of equal pay for equal work, and women's inability to receive equal access to jobs and education. The second wave of feminism attempted to highlight ways that society legally and professionally subjugated women, and thus turned women's personal struggles into political action.

The third wave of feminism began in the late 1980s and early 1990s. This new movement addressed domestic violence, access to safe and legal abortions, and sexual harassment. It also ensured equal status of women in educational, work, athletic, and social environments. The first two waves of feminism had largely come from a White, middle-class perspective. In this third movement, activists attempted to broaden the scope of feminism to include perspectives of women of color and different social classes. The third feminist wave also looked at all aspects of society, art, and science through a feminist lens. This perspective provided insights into where inequality persists and how women often contribute to supporting the status quo instead of actively fighting for change. Additionally, the third wave has focused on practical ways to help women achieve equality, such as by promoting flexible work scheduling, demanding the availability of child care, and making time off available for maternity leave and caring for sick family members.

Today, many young women are living the dreams of the women who started the feminist movement. Millions of women pursue careers and family, are equal partners in their relationships, and support feminist political agendas. Although the current generation of women may appreciate advances that feminism has made possible, they do not always feel the same personal connection with the feminist movement that women from earlier generations felt (and feel).

Women in the United States enjoy more power and opportunities than they ever have before. Women's wages have risen, and women now constitute a majority of college and university students. The past 2 decades have seen the first African American woman as secretary of state, the first female Speaker of the House of Representatives, the first major female candidate for president of the United States, and the first female vice-presidential candidate for the Republican party. However, women continue to face discrimination at home, in public, and at the workplace because of their gender; and progress on issues from rape and sexual assault to access to reproductive health care has stalled in many ways over the past 20 years.

Today, feminism is exploring many aspects of women's lives. Modern feminism acknowledges that gender differences exist even while working to eliminate gender-based favoritism and bias. Feminism also acknowledges that women may not all want to focus on their careers or even have careers (though they continue to be grateful for the opportunity). Feminists come from both genders, and different political and cultural backgrounds, ages, ethnicities, and sexual orientations; in short, they are as diverse a group as women themselves. HeForShe, a global network of male and female individuals and leaders fighting for gender equality, which is sponsored by UN Women, is a great example of this.

The 21st Century

The new millennium has brought many contributions to improving the health of the public—for example, the identification of the **human genome**, improvements in HIV/AIDS medications, public health programs targeting behavior-related health problems, the inclusion of children in **clinical trials**, and the Patient Protection and Affordable Care Act, which has extended health insurance to millions of women, men, and children. Nevertheless, women still face many difficulties in the healthcare arena. There has been a rollback of many of the advances made in the 1990s. Funding for reproductive health initiatives fell both domestically and internationally for the first decade of the 21st century. In 2012, a record number of women were elected to Congress, with 20 women serving in the Senate and more than 80 women serving in the House of Representatives. However, women remain underrepresented in national, local, and state governments. Women are living longer but not necessarily with better quality of life; and women across the United States and the world continue to be victims of individual and societal violence and discrimination.

POLITICAL DIMENSIONS OF WOMEN'S HEALTH

Government plays an important role in protecting and promoting women's health and is involved in six main areas that relate to women's health:

1. Policymaking
2. Financing
3. Protecting the health of the public

4. Collecting and disseminating information about health and healthcare delivery systems

5. Capacity building for population health

6. Managing of health services

The government directly and indirectly influences many of the areas affecting women's health. The federal government ensures that the food supply is safe, provides highway funding for states that adopt a legal drinking age, and regulates businesses that provide medications to the public.

During the 1990s, the government established many organizations and agencies devoted to women's health. The Department of Health and Human Services' Office on Women's Health (DHHS-OWH) serves as the coordinating agency for women's health initiatives throughout the agencies and offices of the U.S. DHHS, including the NIH, FDA, Centers for Disease Control and Prevention (CDC), and other agencies and departments. The Office on Women's Health finds and addresses inequities in research, healthcare services, and education that have placed the health of women at risk.

The Office of Research on Women's Health (ORWH) within NIH is the government's focal point for women's biomedical research.

- It advises the NIH director and staff on women's health research.

- It strengthens and enhances research related to diseases, disorders, and conditions affecting women.

- It ensures that NIH research addresses issues regarding women's health.

- It develops opportunities for and supports recruitment, retention, reentry, and advancement of women in biomedical careers.

- It ensures that biomedical and behavioral research studies supported by NIH represent women and women's health issues.

- It supports research on women's health issues.

The ORWH has been instrumental in national and international efforts to make women's health research part of the scientific and educational infrastructure. The ORWH works with scientists, practitioners, legislators, and lay advocates to identify research priorities and set a comprehensive research agenda. The ORWH also encourages research that examines the biological differences between the sexes—that is, gender-based biology—to more fully understand each and thereby enhance knowledge and practice.

The Healthy People initiative joined U.S. DHHS with other federal agencies, nonprofit organizations, and members of various medical industries to educate women and provide them with the knowledge needed to live long and healthy lives. Every 10 years, this initiative creates goals and objectives to guide health promotion and disease prevention efforts on a national scale. By identifying diseases that affect women the most, scientists can set future directions and goals for research. The current iteration of this initiative, Healthy People 2020, will track and analyze almost 600 public health objectives that are important to women.

U.S. DHHS also works to provide family planning services, prevent sexually transmitted infections, and reduce unintended pregnancies. The Title X program provides funding to millions of people for reproductive health and family planning services. Funding has also increased for research and programs aimed at improving the health of older women. The Administration on Aging has launched a resource center to educate older women about issues such as income security, housing, and caregiving. The Administration on Aging has also increased support for community nutrition services to combat nutrition-related illnesses in the elderly.

> *The reasons for excluding women from clinical investigations are less obvious than one might expect. In spite of a significant body of opinion to the contrary, the reasons have very little to do with male chauvinism or the gender of the investigating scientist—until the 1990s, female scientists were every bit as likely as men to exclude females from clinical protocols. Even at the most sophisticated academic medical centers, senior investigators taught young scientists that data obtained from male subjects could be extrapolated to women without modification. They assumed that women were essentially small men—identical in all respects except for their reproductive physiology. It is astonishing that in a scientific system that prides itself on its critical sense and accepts no hypothesis as true until it has been rigorously tested, we have tolerated such a leap of faith for so long.[7]*
>
> **—Marianne Legato, founder and director of the Partnership for Gender-Specific Medicine**

Investment in Biomedical Research

The federal government plays a critical role in funding biomedical research. The NIH is the main federal agency responsible for distributing money to private and public institutions and organizations for conducting medical and health research. Along with the CDC and other agencies, it advances basic research to discover new and better methods of treatment and prevention of numerous health conditions. Funding also comes from the private sector, philanthropic organizations, universities, and voluntary health agencies.

Pharmaceutical companies and private corporations also invest millions of dollars each year to research and develop new drugs, vaccines, and technologies. Investment in biomedical research and new technologies has led to increased **life expectancy**, improved health throughout the life span, and, in many cases, decreased cost of illness.

However, newer medicines, technologies, and equipment are not the only way to improve health. About one-half of the deaths in the United States are directly or indirectly caused by people's behavior choices.[8] Research can also find better ways to educate people about basic health measures, such as preventing disease; eating a healthful, balanced diet; exercising; and avoiding tobacco and other drugs, offering the potential to improve the health of millions of Americans. Promoting healthful behaviors and preventing disease are usually cheaper, more effective methods than intervening after a disease or harmful event occurs. Unfortunately, these types of programs typically receive little funding compared to pharmaceutical drugs or technologies promising the next "miracle cure" (or, for shareholders, the next revenue source).

Research on women's health has seen unprecedented growth over the past 35 years, especially with the push to include women in clinical trials. By demanding that women are included in health research, women as well as men become the studied models for the conditions that affect them and the drugs used to treat these conditions. This trend has led to the integration of women-specific data into clinical practice and the formulation of new questions in regard to women and specific diseases.

Another approach to improving women's health relies on gender-based research—studies that examine the similarities and differences between men and women to learn more about the causes of disease and responses to medication in these populations. Gender-based studies identify and investigate the biological and physiological differences between men and women. Males and females can manifest different symptoms of a disease, experience the course of a disease differently, or respond in distinct ways to pharmaceuticals. Identifying and studying gender-based differences offer remarkable potential for understanding disease epidemiology and health outcomes in both men and women. The **Gender Dimensions** box discusses several areas of women's health research that have benefited from increased funding and attention. These topics are discussed in greater detail in later chapters of this book.

Fat and body water content, steroidal sex hormone levels, and **genetic phenotype** all affect drug metabolism through pharmacokinetics (concentration of the drug) and pharmacodynamics (ability to metabolize the drug).[9] Medical literature has documented significant differences in the ways that men and women process aspirin, acetaminophen (Tylenol), lidocaine, and other commonly prescribed medications.[10] Differences such as age, hormonal status, race and ethnicity, and socioeconomic status can also affect how women metabolize drugs. The extent to which these differences prevail among the range of drugs used to prevent and treat disease is still not fully known or understood.

FDA guidelines urge drug investigators to account for gender differences in drug metabolism throughout the development process and to include women of

Table 1.1   Phases of a Clinical Trial
■ Phase I: A new drug is tested in a small group (20–80) of healthy volunteers to evaluate its safety, determine a safe dosage range, and identify side effects.
■ Phase II: The study drug is given to a larger group (100–300) of people to further evaluate its safety and effectiveness.
■ Phase III: The study drug is given to large groups (1000–3000) in clinics and hospitals to confirm its effectiveness, monitor side effects, and compare it with other treatments.
■ Phase IV: The study done after the drug is marketed to continue collecting information regarding the drug's effects in various populations.

childbearing age in both Phase I and Phase II clinical trials (**Table 1.1**). The FDA once excluded women of childbearing potential from clinical trials but has revised its guidelines to call for gender-specific analyses of safety and effectiveness in new drugs. The FDA also changed its policy of excluding women of childbearing potential from early drug studies. These measures have helped the FDA acquire better information on drug effects in women.[11]

Gender-based research has posed challenges as well as opportunities for pharmaceutical manufacturers. If research shows that a drug is effective for only one gender, the potential market for that drug could be limited, which would diminish the company's profits. However, targeting drugs for women or other specific populations can also allow researchers and pharmaceutical companies to create much more effective products.

Even with advances toward inclusion of women and minority groups in research studies, one major barrier to women's participation in biomedical research still exists. Many women are unable to take part in clinical trials because of they lack health insurance. For insured women, some states have passed legislation requiring health plans to pay for routine medical care that a person may receive as a participant in a clinical trial. In 2000, **Medicare** began covering **beneficiaries'** patient care costs in clinical trials. Clinical trials still are considered experimental by some insurance companies, however, and therefore are not covered under all standard health policies.

Including women in clinical studies may pose challenges, but leaving them out courts disaster through ignorance. Using women, particularly women of childbearing age, presents challenges to the investigation because the researchers must consider the effect of hormonal cycling on the hypothesis being tested. Furthermore, the potential for pregnancy and possible **teratogenic** effects in the fetus must be considered. These factors weigh heavily in designing and conducting any study.

Reproductive Rights

The history and politics surrounding women's decisions to control when and whether to have children are long

GENDER DIMENSIONS: Health Differences Between Men and Women

Differences between men and women are not just limited to the reproductive organs. Women and men react differently to certain medications, have distinct reactions and vulnerabilities to disease, and may show disease in different ways.

The following 10 examples show some of the ways that diseases affect men and women differently.

Heart Disease. Heart disease is the leading cause of death for women in the United States, killing 292,188 women in 2009—that's *1 in every 4* female deaths.[12] Heart disease also strikes women, on average, 10 years later than men. Compared to men, women are also more likely to have a second heart attack within a year of the first one. Symptoms of a heart attack tend to be less obvious and easier to overlook in women than in men.

Depression. Depression is two to three times more likely to affect women than men, in part because women's brains make less of the neurotransmitter serotonin, which regulates emotions.

Drug Reactions. Many common drugs, like antihistamines and antibiotics, cause different reactions and side effects in women than in men.

Autoimmune Diseases. Three out of four people suffering from autoimmune diseases, such as multiple sclerosis, rheumatoid arthritis, and lupus, are women.

Osteoporosis. Women have a higher rate of bone loss than men. Four out of five people suffering from osteoporosis are women.

Smoking. Smoking causes more cardiovascular damage in women than in men. Women have stronger withdrawal symptoms of smoking and are less likely to be able to successfully quit smoking.

Sexually Transmitted Infections. If exposed to a sexually transmitted infection, women are twice as likely as men to become infected.

Anesthesia. Women, on average, wake up from anesthesia after 7 minutes, whereas men, on average, wake up after 11 minutes.

Alcohol. Women produce less of the gastric enzyme that breaks down ethanol (alcohol) in the stomach. Therefore, even after allowing for size differences, women will have a higher blood alcohol content after drinking.

Pain. Some pain medications, such as kappa-opiates, are far more effective in relieving pain in women than in men.

Data from Society for Women's Health Research. www.women-shealthresearch.org

---

and complex. For nearly 100 years, abortion was illegal in the United States. On January 22, 1973, the landmark Supreme Court decision *Roe v. Wade* legalized abortion. However, since then, the battle has shifted to the state level; many states with socially conservative governments impose restrictions that limit where, when, and under what conditions women may receive abortions.

Roe v. Wade has also not prevented the federal government from imposing abortion restrictions in countries that receive U.S. funding. In 1984, President Reagan imposed the Mexico City policy, or "global gag rule." This rule has been particularly contentious, having been eliminated by President Bill Clinton in 1993, reimposed by President George W. Bush in 2001, and removed once more by President Barack Obama in 2009. This policy withheld U.S. assistance from foreign family planning agencies if they provided the following services, even if U.S. funds were not used for these services:

- Performing abortions in cases of pregnancy that are not life-threatening to the woman or the result of rape or incest

- Providing counseling and referral for abortions

- Lobbying to legalize abortion or increase its availability in the country in which the nongovernmental organization (NGO) is operating[13]

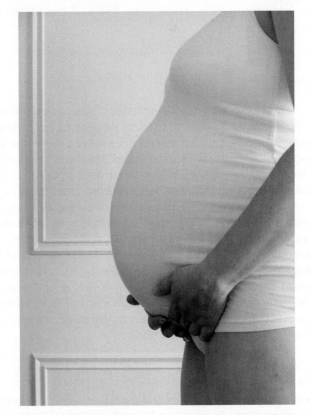

The potential for pregnancy and possible teratogenic effects in the fetus must be considered in clinical trials.
© Terry Walsh/ShutterStock, Inc.

It's Your Health

Research Studies

Epidemiologists (scientists who study trends of disease and health in populations) conduct many types of studies. Each type of study has its own advantages and disadvantages. Most of these studies are either descriptive or analytic in nature.

Descriptive studies attempt to describe or examine a disease in a population or populations as well as how that disease or phenomenon relates to variables such as race, age, or gender. Descriptive studies can find correlations between the disease and variables but cannot say if one causes the other. A descriptive cross-sectional survey might find that people who work in factories (variable) are more likely than other people to develop cancer (disease), but it could not say that working in a factory causes disease—there could be some other common factor involved, such as an environmental contaminant that affects people living near the factory. Descriptive studies include population studies, case-report studies, and cross-sectional studies.

Analytic studies compare people who are exposed to a certain variable to people who are not exposed to see whether that variable influences their chances of developing a disease. Unlike descriptive studies, analytic studies can find a cause-and-effect ratio, though they are generally more difficult to perform. Studies that have followed otherwise equal groups of smokers and nonsmokers over time and found that smokers were more likely to develop lung cancer were responsible for linking the variable of smoking to the disease of lung cancer. Analytic studies include case-control studies, cohort studies, intervention studies, and clinical trials.

The global gag rule's restrictions have had serious effects on women's health in many developing countries. Under this rule, developing countries faced a dilemma: If they agreed to the rule and accepted U.S. family planning assistance, they risked seeing death and injuries from unsafe abortions increase because women who cannot obtain safe and legal abortions may visit unqualified practitioners in secret to end their pregnancies. But if these countries rejected U.S. assistance, they lost funding for all areas of family planning, including reducing unplanned pregnancy, preventing HIV, and reducing maternal and infant deaths. This increase in unplanned pregnancies and reduction in the number of safe medical services for pregnant women may have encouraged more women in these countries to seek abortions.

Access to Healthcare Providers, Services, and Health Information

Advances in public health and medicine have improved the prevention, diagnosis, and treatment of disease. Many people are living longer and healthier lives as a result. Over the years, women have learned to seek out medical information on their own, thereby becoming informed consumers of medicine.

Unfortunately, healthcare promotion and disease prevention are not simple. Many factors prevent women from receiving adequate health care, including:

- Poverty or insufficient income to pay for care
- Lack of health insurance
- Lack of access to healthcare facilities
- Inability to understand medical personnel because of language barriers or illiteracy
- Unfair treatment by medical personnel because of race, ethnicity, or sexual orientation
- Inability to pay for the costs of medications needed for treatment
- Declined coverage for healthcare costs that are deemed unnecessary or experimental
- Fear of doctors and avoidance of seeking health care altogether

Lack of adequate access to healthcare services and information is a serious issue in the United States, with a lack of health insurance being one of the most formidable barriers. In 2010, 19 million women between the ages of 19 and 64 had no health insurance; another 17 million were underinsured, meaning their health insurance had limitations that prevented them from receiving necessary services.[14] The Patient Protection and Affordable Care Act, passed in 2010, sought to address these issues in part. Since its passage, the uninsured rate has dropped significantly, with people gaining coverage either within the expanded Medicaid programs or by leveraging private insurance made possible by state exchanges. Each woman with health insurance, however, does not enjoy the same level of coverage.

Premiums for private health insurance are extremely expensive and, therefore, many people opt to take a chance and remain uninsured when an employer does not sponsor them. When choosing between plans, many women find that affordable policies may not cover serious illnesses or extended hospital stays or may require holders to pay large copayments or deductibles for health services. When costs for health care are high, lack of insurance or underinsurance can make healthcare utilization a driver of financial instability. In many cases this causes people to make trade-offs between healthcare utilization and its related expenses and other life essentials.

A lack of cultural and gender sensitivity, as well as a lack of knowledge about specific health concerns of women, also seriously affects women's health. The health needs of women are different from those of men. Additionally, health needs vary from woman to woman, depending on many factors, including age, ethnicity/race, and sexual orientation. Several steps are being taken to make healthcare providers aware of these specific needs.

The ORWH has developed coursework for medical students to make them more sensitive toward and aware of women's health issues. Dental, nursing, and pharmacy programs, as well as **osteopathic** and **allopathic schools**, also are developing similar coursework. Healthcare providers who receive this training are better equipped to care for the diverse population of women in the United States.

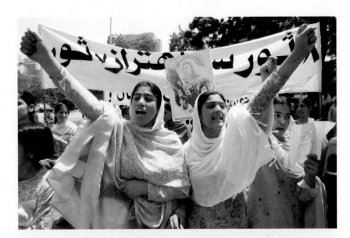

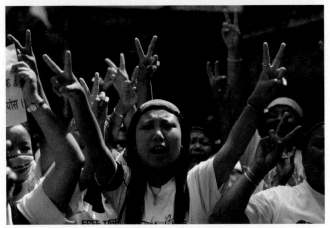

Around the world, women are working to improve their lives and make their voices heard.
(top) © Reuters/Faisal Mahmood/Landov; (bottom) © Reuters/Gopal Chitrakar/Landov

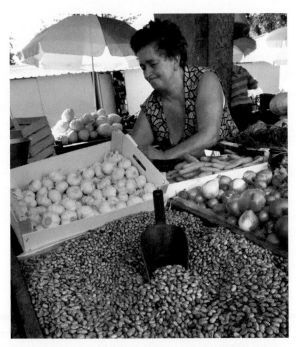

Millions of Americans work but do not have access to health care.
© PhotoCreate/ShutterStock, Inc.

Global Perspective on Women's Health

Around the world, women continue to be less likely than men to receive adequate health care, to have opportunities for economic advancement, and to have political representation. Women who live in the developing world (most countries outside of Western Europe, the United States, Canada, and Japan) are also much more likely than women in industrialized countries to die or be injured from a variety of illnesses, injuries, and diseases. Global threats to women's health include poverty, underweight and malnutrition, HIV/AIDS, violence, and **maternal morbidity and mortality** (disability, disease, or death related to pregnancy or childbirth). Women are burdened by disease and by violations of their human rights that directly affect their health. These problems include domestic violence, **female genital mutilation**, **honor killings**, **trafficking**, and barriers to reproductive health services.

Access to clean water, nutritious food, and medical care, as well as protection from violence and poor working conditions, are basic, inexpensive factors that could greatly improve global health; unfortunately, hundreds of millions of women lack these basic human rights. Social inequalities, such as lack of education, money, and decision-making freedom, pose a greater threat to women than to men; women consequently have a disproportionately higher burden of disease and poverty. In addition, women are often the primary caregivers for their children and families.

The United Nations (U.N.) has worked to advance the status of women and achieve equity in the treatment, opportunities, and status of both genders for the past 35 years. In 1979, the U.N. adopted the Convention on the Elimination of All Forms of Discrimination (CEDAW), also referred to as the international bill of rights for women.

CEDAW legally binds 165 U.N. member states to take steps to promote women's equality and to report on the steps they have taken. However, even if a country legally recognized women's rights, women in that country were not always able to exercise them. Many factors contribute to this discrepancy. Sexist attitudes often persist in popular culture and among those with political and economic power. In addition, educational opportunities for women may be limited, there are often insufficient childcare support systems for women, and men may be indifferent or even hostile toward improving women's place in society.[15] In 1995, the U.N. identified 12 critical obstacles to women's advancement (**Table 1.2**). Five years later, at the "Women 2000: Gender Equality, Development and

Profiles of Remarkable Women

Susan F. Wood, PhD (1959–)

Dr. Susan F. Wood has dedicated her career to advancing women's health, both by using scientific evidence to make better decisions about health policy and by taking a principled stand against political interference in the scientific process.

Wood studied biology and psychology and graduated with a Bachelor of Science degree from Southwestern at Memphis in 1980; she earned a PhD in biology at Boston University in 1989 and received research fellowship training in neuroscience from Johns Hopkins School of Medicine in 1990. Wood has studied the biochemistry of smells, researched how medications affect women during pregnancy, and advocated for women's participation in clinical trial research.

Wood joined the FDA in 2000. She later became the assistant commissioner for women's health, the top agency official for women's health issues. In 2005, Wood resigned from the FDA to protest the agency's continued delays on ruling about the emergency birth control pill known as Plan B. Wood believed that decisions to delay the contraceptive were politically motivated.

The FDA's independent, scientific expert advisory committees had recommended that Plan B be approved in 2003, but leadership in the FDA, appointed by President George W. Bush, refused to approve the contraceptive. Before Wood resigned, the FDA regulatory staff, an advisory committee, and the head of the FDA drug center had all found Plan B to be safe and effective and had recommended that the drug be approved for over-the-counter use. Lester M. Crawford, the head of the FDA during this time, overruled these recommendations and said the decision would be "indefinitely delayed." Wood and many other scientists believed that Crawford's decision amounted to political interference from the Bush administration over a scientific decision.

"I can no longer serve as staff when scientific and clinical evidence, fully evaluated and recommended for approval by the professional staff here, has been overruled," she wrote in an email explaining her decision.*

Wood's decision brought immediate national attention to the FDA approval process. In August 2006, less than a year later, the FDA made Plan B available without a prescription to women 18 years of age or older. Wood is currently a research professor in George Washington University's School of Public Health.

*FDA official quits over delay on Plan B, *Washington Post*, September 1, 2005.

Peace for the 21st Century" conference, held in New York, the U.N. evaluated the achievements of different governments and new action plans. Today the Beijing+20 initiative is still working to advance many of the same goals, according to the U.N.

In the early 2000s, the U.N. developed eight Millennium Development Goals (MDGs). The MDGs set global goals toward lowering global poverty, improving health,

> *"Twenty years later the Platform for Action envisioned gender equality in all dimensions of life—and no country has yet finished this agenda. Today, women earn less than men and are more likely to work in poor-quality jobs. A third suffer physical or sexual violence in their lifetime. Gaps in reproductive rights and health care leave 800 women dying in childbirth each day. The 20th anniversary of Beijing opens new opportunities to reconnect, regenerate commitment, charge up political will and mobilize the public. Everyone has a role to play—for our common good. The evidence is increasingly in, that empowering women empowers humanity. Economies grow faster, for example, and families are healthier and better-educated. The Beijing Platform for Action, still forward-looking at 20, offers important focus in rallying people around gender equality and women's empowerment. Its promises are necessarily ambitious. But over time, and with the accumulating energy of new generations, they are within reach."[16]*

Table 1.2	U.N. Conference in Beijing: Twelve Critical Areas of Concern for Women's Health

- Women and poverty
- Education and training of women
- Women and health
- Violence against women
- Women and armed conflict
- Women and the economy
- Women in power and decision making
- Institutional mechanisms for the advancement of women
- Human rights of women
- Women and the media
- Women and the environment
- The girl child

Source: United Nations WomenWatch. (2000). *The four global women's conferences, 1975–1995: Historical perspective.* United Nations Department of Public Information: DPI/2035/M

reaching environmental sustainability, and other issues to be reached by 2015. Two of the eight MDGs—improving maternal health and reaching gender equality—directly deal with women's health, while several others, such as ending poverty and hunger and providing universal education, are issues that affect women more than men. The U.N. estimates progress toward the MDGs through measures such as the ratio of boys to girls in school; the ratio of literate women to literate men; the percentage

Profiles of Remarkable Women

Gloria Steinem (1934–)

Gloria Steinem, a well-known feminist leader, activist, and journalist, is the daughter of a newspaperwoman and the granddaughter of the noted suffragette Pauline Steinem. Steinem studied in India for 2 years, an experience that made her aware of the extent of human suffering in the world. Steinem returned from India strongly motivated to fight social injustice and decided to begin her career as a journalist.

In 1960, Steinem moved to New York and began working as a freelance writer for popular magazines. One of her first major assignments in investigative journalism was a two-part series for *Show* magazine on the working conditions of Playboy bunnies. Steinem worked as a Playboy bunny for 3 weeks to prepare for the article. The articles she wrote exposed the poor working conditions and meager wages of the Playboy bunnies and the discrimination and sexual harassment that occurred at New York's Playboy Club.

In 1968, Steinem joined the staff of *New York* magazine as a contributing editor and political columnist. During these years Steinem moved into politics, covering everything from the assassination of Martin Luther King, Jr. to demonstrations of United Farm Workers led by Cesar Chavez. She also worked for various Democratic candidates. Steinem's shift to the women's liberation movement and feminism began when she started attending abortion hearings. She found herself deeply moved by the stories she heard and realized that society oppressed women in many ways.

By the late 1960s, Steinem had positioned herself as a leader of the women's liberation movement through her research, writing, and activism. In 1971, she joined Bella Abzug, Shirley Chisholm, and Betty Friedan to form the National Women's Political Caucus, encouraging women's participation in the 1972 election.

Steinem became friendly with Dorothy Pitman Hughes, an African American childcare pioneer. Steinem and Hughes spoke together publicly throughout the United States to promote women's rights, civil rights, and children's rights. In 1971 they formed the Women's Action Alliance to develop women's educational programs. Although the alliance folded in 1997, its offshoot, WISE (Women Initiating Self Empowerment), continues.

In 1972, Steinem gained funding for the first mass-circulation feminist magazine, *Ms*. The preview issue sold out, and within 5 years *Ms*. had a circulation of 500,000. As editor of the magazine, Steinem became an influential spokesperson for women's rights issues while continuing her active political life. In 1975, she helped plan the women's agenda for the Democratic National Convention, and she continued to exert pressure on liberal politicians on behalf of women's concerns. In 1977, Steinem participated in the National Conference of Women in Houston, Texas. The conference—the first of its kind—drew attention to feminist issues and women's rights leaders.

As a writer and an activist, Gloria Steinem continues to be a leader in the women's rights movement. Steinem's books include *Outrageous Acts and Everyday Rebellions* (1983), *Marilyn: Norma Jean* (1986), *Revolution from Within: A Book of Self-Esteem* (1992), *Moving Beyond Words* (1994), and *Doing Sixty and Seventy* (2006).

of women with waged employment; the proportion of seats in parliament held by women; and the percentage of births attended by a skilled health professional. Despite gains around the world in women's life spans, quality of health, and political opportunities, women still face discrimination, violence, and marginalization around the world, and women account for the majority of the world's poor.[17] The United Nations has created a set of common objectives aimed at building equity and fair treatment for everyone and has started progress toward meeting these goals. Women and men around the world will need to work together to make this goal a reality.

INFORMED DECISION MAKING: TAKE ACTION

There are many ways to advocate for women's health. Women's health organizations encourage donating, getting involved by sending letters to legislators and helping to organize events, and educating oneself on women's health issues. Visiting the Internet can be a good first step in learning about organizations and deciding where to focus personal interest and commitment. The websites section of this chapter lists several organizations that offer ways to become involved in promoting women's health.

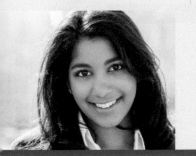
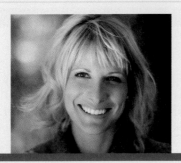
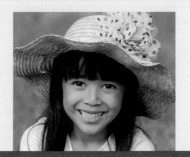
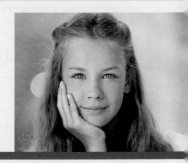

CASE STUDY

Shannon was choosing a college major but did not know which direction she was going to take. She was a strong writer and had loved her English and psychology courses so far. But something was nagging at her. She wanted to be able to do something meaningful with her degree upon graduation. She had always seen health care as an area that impacted everyone in different ways throughout their lives. She had been personally impacted by healthcare issues over the last several years, watching her mom cope with a diagnosis of breast cancer and fight to survive throughout treatment. Shannon thought about all the ways that her mom and her whole family were impacted by the different dimensions of health care—from how it gets paid for, to the role of doctors and nurses in care pathways, to the caregiving responsibilities that fell on her shoulders, to the genetic implications of the disease for her and her sister. Beyond the disease, there was so much to understand and navigate. Shannon imagined that a lot of other people went through a similar personal experience but wondered how she could apply this to her career after college. She began to look into majors that were more healthcare focused. She realized she was particularly interested in women's health and began to explore different aspects of how her education could prepare her to explore this area.

Questions

1. Should Shannon pursue a major that would prepare for a career in health care generally or women's health specifically? Are there pathways beyond being a doctor or a nurse that would fulfill her needs?

2. What types of classes would be useful to prepare someone for a career in women's health? Can you think of five different departments that might have applicable courses?

3. How can people take their own life experiences and use them to inform academic or professional life choices? How is this relevant to women's health specifically?

■ Summary

Women's health is a wide area of study that examines the biology of the female body, human development throughout the life span, the health of individuals and entire populations, factors that contribute to mental and physical health, women's place in society, and other factors. Over the past 200 years, many organizations and individuals have worked to improve women's health, rights, and status. Women's health is now recognized as a national priority, and tremendous progress has been achieved in expanding the scope and depth of women's health research. Continued success in the women's health movement depends on political commitment; sufficient funds; educated and interested scientific and lay communities; advocacy by professionals, patients, and the public; and involvement of women, men, and communities in working for equality and recognizing gender differences. These factors have driven the explosion in women's health research and are responsible for advances in developed countries and throughout the world. Findings from biological, behavioral, and social sciences all provide insights and important data that can improve women's health and well-being.

■ Topics for Discussion

1. What are some of the different ways of envisioning women's health? What do you think are the most important aspects of women's health?

2. How has the definition of feminism changed over the past 100 years? What elements have remained the same? Do you consider yourself a feminist? Can a person have socially conservative views about women's health and rights and still be a feminist?

3. What are some of the major differences in how men and women react to medications?

4. Why is it important for women to be included in clinical trials? What is gender-based research, and what areas of health could benefit from further gender-based research?

5. Why should we continue to pursue the Beijing+20 platform? How does that impact lives here in the United States versus in other countries?

6. Discuss the ways the government is involved in the following areas in relation to health:

   - Policymaking
   - Financing
   - Protecting the health of the public
   - Conducting research
   - Influencing how and where people receive health care

■ Key Terms

Allopathic school

Beneficiary

Biomedical research

Clinical trial

Corset

Female genital mutilation

Feminism

Genetic phenotype

Honor killings

Human genome

Life expectancy

Maternal morbidity and mortality

Medicare

Osteopathic school

Premium

Suffragist

Teratogenic

Trafficking

■ References

1. World Health Organization. (2012). *Reproductive health.* Available at: http://www.who.int/topics/reproductive_health/en/

2. Chamberlain, G. (2006). British maternal mortality in the 19th and early 20th centuries. *Journal of the Royal Society of Medicine* 99(11): 559–563.

3. WHO, UNICEF, UNFPA, the World Bank, and the United Nations Population Division. (2014). *Trends in maternal mortality: 1990 to 2013.* Geneva: World Health Organization. Catalog sources world development indicators. Available at: http://data.worldbank.org/indicator/SH.STA.MMRT

4. Corsini, C., & Viazzo, P. (1993). *The decline of infant mortality in Europe, 1800–1950: Four national case studies.* UNICEF Innocenti Research Centre. Available at: http://ideas.repec.org/p/ucf/hisper/hisper93-3.html#biblio

5. UNICEF, WHO, the World Bank, UN DESA Population Division. (n.d.). *Estimates developed by the UN Inter-agency Group for Child Mortality Estimation.* Available at http://www.childmortality.org; accessed at: http://data.worldbank.org/indicator/SP.DYN.IMRT.IN

6. Sorensen, A. (2004). *Rosie the riveter: Women working during World War II.* National Park Service. Available at: http://www.nps.gov/pwro/collection/website/rosie.htm

7. Legato, M. J. (1998). Belling the cat: Clinical investigation in vulnerable populations (a good idea, but who's going to volunteer?). *Journal of Gender-Specific Medicine* 1(1): 18–22.

8. Steen, J. (2007). *The primacy of public health.* American Public Health Association: Community Health Planning and Policy Development. Available at: http://www.apha.org/membergroups/newsletters/section-newsletters/comm/spring07/primacyph.htm

9. Owens, N. J., & Hume, A. L. (1994). Pharmacotherapy in women: Do clinically important gender-related issues exist? *Rhode Island Medicine* 77: 412–416.

10. Merkatz, R. B., Temple, R., Subel, S., et al. (1993). Women in clinical trials of new drugs: A change in the FDA. *New England Journal of Medicine* 329: 292–296.

11. U.S. Food and Drug Administration (FDA). (2012). *About the Office of Women's Health.* Available at: http://www.fda.gov/womens/programs.html

12. Kochanek, K. D., Xu, J. Q., Murphy, S. L., et al. (2011). Deaths: Final data for 2009 [PDF-2M]. *National Vital Statistics Reports* 60(3). Available at: http://www.cdc.gov/nchs/data/nvsr/nvsr60/nvsr60_03.pdf

13. Center for Reproductive Rights. (2009). *Myths and realities: Debunking USAID's analysis of the Global Gag Rule.* Available at: http://reproductiverights.org/en/document/myths-and-realities-debunking-usaid%E2%80%99s-analysis-of-the-global-gag-rule

14. Robertson, R., Squires, D., Garber, T., et al. (2012). *Realizing health reform's potential.* Washington, DC: The Commonwealth Fund. Available at: http://www.commonwealthfund.org/~/media/Files/Publications/Issue%20Brief/2012/Jul/1606_Robertson_oceans_apart_reform_brief.pdf

15. Murthy, P., & Smith, C. (2010). *Women's global health and human rights.* Sudbury, MA: Jones and Bartlett.

16. UNWomen. (n.d.). *The Beijing Platform for Action turns 20.* Available at: http://beijing20.unwomen.org/en/about

17. World Health Organization (WHO). (2009). *Women and health: Today's evidence, tomorrow's agenda.* Available at: http://www.who.int/gender/documents/9789241563857/en/index.html

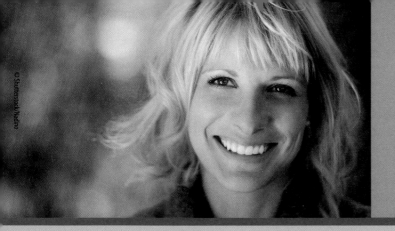

CHAPTER 2

The Economics of Women's Health

Learning Objectives

On completion of this chapter, the student should be able to discuss:

1. The third-party payer system.

2. The fee-for-service model versus managed care.

3. Factors to consider when choosing an insurance plan.

4. Types of public health insurance, including Medicare and Medicaid.

5. The substantial risks associated with being uninsured.

6. Ways that women as healthcare consumers affect demand within the healthcare system.

7. Healthcare reform and the arguments for and against a universal health system.

8. The financial burden of aging and how it disproportionately affects women.

9. Long-term care and its associated costs.

INTRODUCTION

Medical knowledge is not the only factor affecting women's health. Money also influences almost every aspect of health care, from when and where people go to get medical care, to the behaviors that they perform, to who pays for health care. Around the world, various systems of health insurance have evolved. Health insurance is a policy that pays for medical care (or part of medical care) when a person gets sick or injured. Most industrialized countries have a system of universal health insurance, or insurance provided by the government, financed through taxes, and offered to every individual. In the United States, a unique multi-payer system exists, with some Americans receiving insurance through their employer, some Americans receiving insurance through a variety of government agencies, some individuals purchasing private insurance, and many Americans going uninsured. As a result, patients, the government, hospitals and the healthcare system, employers, and the public all pay for health care.

The details surrounding health insurance—including whether health insurance should be mandatory, how much it should cost, and who it should cover—has been one of the most controversial and most discussed political topics in the United States for decades. Most people with private insurance share the cost of medical care with insurers via premiums, deductibles, copays, and coinsurance in addition to the negotiated fee schedule some providers have with insurers. People without insurance who receive care must pay for it "out-of-pocket," or with their own funds. The government provides both insurance and some free health care via public health clinics and other venues.

Different participants in the healthcare system all shape the direction of health care. Major healthcare stakeholders include providers (such as physicians, nurses, and social workers), patients, hospitals, health insurers, policymakers, health education firms, and medical manufacturers such as pharmaceutical, medical device, and diagnostic companies. Each has a different perspective on healthcare delivery and funding.

Increasingly, health care has become a consumer- or patient-oriented industry. Manufacturers, pharmaceutical companies, hospitals, and private doctors' offices develop goods and services to court consumers and drive demand for specific services. Patients are playing a more active role in shopping around for healthcare providers, demanding a wider range of services, and may have a growing willingness to pursue litigation in cases of perceived substandard care. These factors change the dynamics of how healthcare service is offered and how patients engage with providers.

Understanding the effects of women's growing economic power on women's health and the persistent limitations that marginalized women face in accessing quality women's health care is critical. Other important issues include the economics of aging and the effects of an aging population on women's health, public policy that influences the economics of health care, and the roles that women as caregivers have in the delivery of health care.

PAYING FOR HEALTH CARE

Since World War II, the amount of money Americans spend on health care has continued to grow, both in terms of dollars spent and as a percentage of the gross domestic product (GDP: the total value of all goods and services produced in the United States in 1 year). This growth has accelerated over the past 30 years, slowing only after the national economy contracted after the economic recession in 2008. In 1950, Americans spent 4.6% of the GDP on health care; this number increased to 9.2% in 1980, 12.5% in 1990, 13.8% in 2000, and 17.9% in 2012.[1,2,2a] This rapid growth has led politicians, employers, healthcare providers, individual tax payers, and others to call for healthcare reform to curb the growth in expenditures, protect individuals from healthcare-related costs, and protect access to services. Before understanding how healthcare reform policies were developed and the debates surrounding their merit, an understanding of current funding structures is needed.

In the United States, health care does not function like a traditional market setting. Unlike other markets (such as real estate or retail sales) all individuals need health care at one stage or another of their lives, often at unpredictable times or levels. People do not have control over their need for health care in the same way that they do when deciding whether to purchase a television. If a woman has heart disease and needs to go to a cardiologist, she has very little choice except to purchase the services needed or go without care. In addition, a patient must trust her physician to tell her which goods and services she needs instead of making that decision on her own. From an economic perspective, the necessity of health care and an individual's inability to have full information to make purchasing choices make health care a unique market.

Additionally, in the United States, the healthcare system is based on a **third-party payer system**, in which most individuals do not pay directly for the delivery of care (**Figure 2.1**).

Instead, many have health insurance, which, in return for a monthly or yearly payment called a premium plus

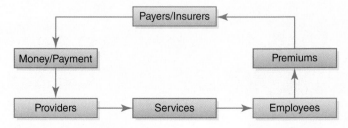

Figure 2.1 The third-party payer system.

a per-doctor's encounter fee called a copayment and/or deductible, provides coverage for health-related goods and services. Health insurance in the United States is provided through private insurers to individuals, employer-sponsored private insurance, or via public insurance programs like Medicare and Medicaid.

Before third-party payers became a mainstay of the U.S. system, patients would pay out-of-pocket for health care, either to their doctor or to hospitals. Medical care was purchased and delivered like most other commodities. If an individual became sick or was injured on the job, the financial repercussions of paying for medical care could be extreme. Private health insurance was introduced in the early 1930s as a method to lower the economic risk associated with hospital care costs. Health insurance was developed and based on an **indemnity** or **fee-for-service** system. Through this system, insurers reimbursed hospitals based on a list of charges for services rendered. Individuals paid insurers a flat fee regardless of whether they had encounters with the healthcare system. As the third-party payer system matured, it grew to include fee-for-service payments to physicians and other outpatient providers of health care (**Table 2.1**).

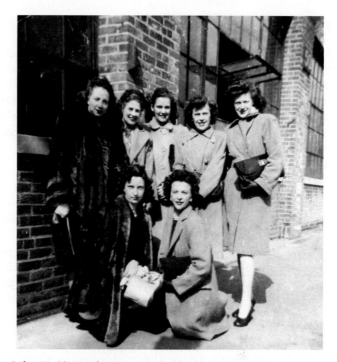

Before World War II, few Americans had health insurance.
Courtesy of Christine McKeen

Table 2.1	**Paying for Health Care Timeline**

1900s
- American Medical Association (AMA) becomes a powerful national force.
- In 1901, AMA reorganizes as the national organization of state and local associations. Membership increases from about 8,000 physicians in 1900 to 70,000 in 1910—half the physicians in the country. This period is the beginning of "organized medicine."
- Doctors are no longer expected to provide free services to all hospital patients.
- The United States lags behind European countries in offering health insurance.
- Railroads are the leading industry to develop extensive employee medical programs.

1910s
- U.S. hospitals become modern scientific institutions, valuing antiseptics and cleanliness and using medications for the relief of pain.
- American Association for Labor Legislation (AALL) organizes first national conference on "social insurance."
- Progressive reformers argue for health insurance and seem to be gaining support.
- Opposition from physicians and other interest groups, plus the entry of the United States into the war in 1917, undermines the reform effort.

1920s
- Consistent with the general mood of political complacency, there is no strong effort to change health insurance.
- Reformers now emphasize the cost of medical care instead of wages lost to sickness. The relatively higher cost of medical care is a new and dramatic development, especially for the middle class.
- The cultural influence of the medical profession grows—physicians' incomes are higher and prestige is established.
- General Motors signs a contract with Metropolitan Life to insure 180,000 workers.
- Penicillin is discovered. However, it will be 20 years before this antibiotic is used to combat infection and disease.

1930s
- The Depression changes priorities, with greater emphasis being placed on unemployment insurance and "old age" benefits.
- The Social Security Act is passed, omitting health insurance.
- There is a push for health insurance within the Roosevelt administration, but internal government conflicts over priorities undermine this effort.
- Against the advice of insurance professionals, Blue Cross begins offering private coverage for hospital care in dozens of states.

1940s
- Prepaid group health care begins; it is seen as radical.
- During World War II, wage and price controls are placed on U.S. employers. To compete for workers, companies begin to offer health benefits, giving rise to the employer-based system in place today.
- President Roosevelt asks Congress for an "economic bill of rights," including the right to adequate medical care.
- President Truman offers a national health program plan, proposing a single system that would include all of U.S. society.
- Truman's plan is denounced by the AMA and is called a Communist plot by a House subcommittee.

(continues)

Table 2.1 Paying for Health Care Timeline (continued)

1950s
- At the start of the decade, national healthcare expenditures are 4.5% of the gross national product.
- Attention turns to the Korean War and away from health reform.
- Federal responsibility for the sick poor is firmly established.
- Many legislative proposals are made to offer hospital insurance, but none succeeds.
- Many more medications are available to treat a range of diseases, including infections, glaucoma, and arthritis. New vaccines become available that prevent dreaded childhood diseases, including polio. The first successful organ transplant is performed.

1960s
- In the 1950s, the price of hospital care doubled. In the early 1960s, those outside the workplace, and especially the elderly, have difficulty affording insurance.
- More than 700 insurance companies sell health insurance.
- Concern about a "doctor shortage" and the need for more "health manpower" leads to federal measures to expand education in the health professions.
- Major medical insurance endorses high-cost medicine.
- President Lyndon Johnson signs Medicare and Medicaid into law.
- "Compulsory health insurance" advocates are no longer optimistic.
- The number of doctors reporting themselves to be full-time specialists grows from 55% in 1960 to 69% by 1969.

1970s
- President Richard Nixon renames prepaid group healthcare plans as health maintenance organizations (HMOs), with legislation providing federal endorsement, certification, and assistance.
- Healthcare costs escalate rapidly, partly due to unexpectedly high Medicare expenditures, rapid inflation in the economy, expansion of hospital expenses and profits, and changes in medical care, including greater use of technology, medications, and conservative approaches to treatment. U.S. medicine is now seen as in crisis.
- Liberals and labor unions reject President Nixon's plan for national health insurance, but his "War on Cancer" centralizes research at the National Institutes of Health (NIH).
- The number of women entering the medical profession rises dramatically. In 1970, 9% of medical students are women; by the end of the decade, the proportion exceeds 25%.

1980s
- Corporations begin to integrate the hospital system (previously a decentralized structure), enter many other healthcare-related businesses, and consolidate control. Overall, there is a shift toward privatization and corporatization of health care.
- Under President Reagan, Medicare shifts to payment by diagnosis (DRG) instead of by treatment. Private plans quickly follow suit.
- Insurance companies voice complaints that the traditional fee-for-service method of payment to doctors is being exploited.
- "Capitation" payments to doctors become more common.

1990s
- Healthcare costs rise at double the rate of inflation.
- Expansion of managed care helps to moderate increases in healthcare costs.
- Federal healthcare reform legislation fails again to pass in the U.S. Congress.
- By the end of the decade, 44 million Americans, 16% of the nation, have no health insurance at all.
- The Human Genome Project to identify all of the more than 100,000 genes in human DNA gets under way.
- By June 1990, 139,765 people in the United States have HIV/AIDS, with a 60% mortality rate.

2000s
- Healthcare costs continue to rise.
- Medicare is viewed by some as unsustainable under the present structure and must be "rescued."
- Changing demographics of the workplace lead many to believe the employer-based system of insurance cannot last.
- The Human Genome Project is completed 2 years ahead of schedule, in 2003.
- Direct-to-consumer advertising for pharmaceuticals and medical devices increases.
- Medicare expands to include a prescription drug benefit in 2006.
- Employers continue to cut health insurance benefits in an attempt to address persistent increases in costs.
- Medical savings accounts become common.
- President George W. Bush unsuccessfully tries to privatize Social Security.
- Congress passes a major expansion to State Children's Health Insurance Program (SCHIP), which will provide insurance for an additional 4 million low-income children, in 2009.

Table 2.1 Paying for Health Care Timeline (continued)		

2010s ■ The Patient Protection and Affordable Care Art (PPACA) is passed in 2010; among other features, the Supreme Court upholds the vast majority of the Act in 2012. The PPACA includes a patient's bill of rights, increases cost-free preventive services, and reduces brand-name drug prices for people with Medicare. Additional provisions of the PPACA include:

   ○ Providing small business health insurance tax credits

   ○ Relief for 4 million seniors who hit the Medicare prescription drug "donut hole"

   ○ Cutting down on healthcare fraud

   ○ Providing access to insurance for uninsured Americans with preexisting conditions

   ○ Extending coverage for young adults (up to age 26)

Data from *Healthcare Crisis: Who's At Risk?* Healthcare Timeline, PBS. Produced by Issues TV, 2000. Reprinted with permission of Issues TV. *"What's Changing and When"*. www.healthcare.gov. Reprinted with permission of the United States Department of Health and Human Services.

In 2013, just over half (54%) of Americans were covered by private health insurance, either provided by their employer or purchased individually.[3,3a] Many private health insurance plans are now structured within a managed care plan. **Managed care** was introduced as a method to control costs by changing how the delivery of care is coordinated and how health care is reimbursed. In contrast to a fee-for-service model, managed care requires patients to go to specific providers and have access to care only when certain criteria are met. In some cases, physicians receive a predetermined lump sum for all care delivered as opposed to a fee for each service rendered.

Managed care has been perceived both as a form of reform (by keeping costs down and providing broad access to services) and as a barrier to care (by placing limits on access to care). Managed care is blamed for decreased access to care by shortening physician office visits, increasing copayments, and placing more restrictions on which doctors patients can see. Managed care is continually evolving to meet the changing needs and demands of patients, employers, and providers.

The limitations on access that led patients and physicians to vilify managed care resulted in slowing the rate at which health-related expenditures grew in the United States in the 1990s (see **Figure 2.2**). Managed care

It's Your Health

Employment-based health benefit programs have existed in the United States for more than 100 years. In the 1870s, for example, railroad, mining, and other industries began to provide the services of company doctors to workers. In 1910, Montgomery Ward entered into one of the earliest group insurance contracts. Before World War II, few Americans had health insurance, and most policies covered only hospital room, board, and ancillary services. During World War II, the number of persons with employment-based health insurance coverage started to increase for several reasons. When wages were frozen by the National War Labor Board and a shortage of workers occurred, employers sought ways to get around the wage controls to attract scarce workers. Health insurance was an attractive means to recruit and retain workers during a labor shortage for two reasons: unions supported employment-based health insurance, and workers' health benefits were not subject to income tax or Social Security payroll taxes, as were cash wages. Under the current tax code, health insurance premiums paid by employers are deductible for employers as a business expense, and are excluded, without limit, from workers' taxable income.

It's Your Health

Drive-Through Deliveries

In the 1990s, HMOs and other managed care plans shortened average maternity stays for normal births. Such programs were dubbed "drive-through deliveries." Because women were being discharged from hospitals only 24 to 48 hours after giving birth, many lawmakers, alarmed that the practice would endanger newborns, adopted laws to require insurance coverage for at least 48 hours of care after delivery.

In a study conducted at Harvard Medical School, researchers found that newborns needed the same number of later emergency room visits and hospital readmissions regardless of whether they had longer initial stays or shorter ones. In essence, the shorter stays were not adding risk to the newborns, even though the "common sense" of many women and legislators suggested that it would. The study looked at 20,366 normal deliveries in the 1990s. During the period studied, newborn visits to emergency rooms kept steady at an average of about 1% every 3 months. Hospital readmissions hovered around 1.5%. The same pattern held for a more vulnerable group of young, lower-income mothers with less education.

Larry Akey, a spokesman for the Health Insurance Association of America, said that short-stay programs were designed "not entirely as cost-saving measures, but an opportunity for the mother to get home" faster. The debate continues among women's advocacy groups, health insurers, and hospitals.

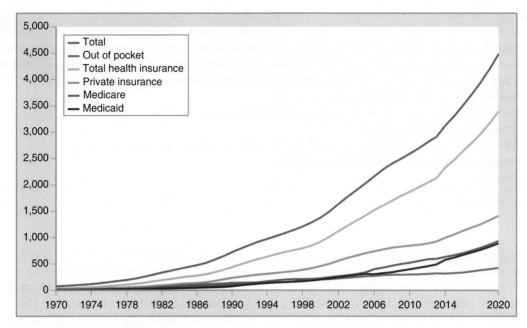

Figure 2.2   **National health expenditures, 1970–2020 (projected).**

Data from Centers for Medicare and Medicare Services, Office of the Actuary. National Health Expenditures data. Released January 2011.

limited expenditure growth by asking for stringent proof of medical necessity before services are paid for. For example, health insurers often require physicians to get prior authorizations from the payer before certain care is rendered—thereby restricting access to certain prescriptions, procedures, or referrals to only those patients they see as appropriate or medically indicated.

Another method for cost containment has been to allow members to get care only from a specific network of physicians who have contracted with insurance companies to offer lower-cost care and to make patients pay higher copayments if they see doctors who are not members of the designated network. By controlling the supply of healthcare resources, managed care organizations have been able to provide patients with a wider range of services, such as pharmaceuticals and rehabilitation services. Some health insurers also own the physician and hospital networks where participants are served. These are called Integrated Delivery Networks (IDNs) or Integrated Health Networks (IHNs). Large IDNs and IHNs include Kaiser Permanente, Geisinger Health System, and Intermountain Health.

Managed care plans differ based on how much they control the services patients receive. Types of managed care plans include preferred provider organizations (PPOs), health maintenance organizations (HMOs), and point-of-service (POS) plans. **Table 2.2** describes the various types of managed care plans. Almost all health insurers today offer some form of managed care products or include elements of managed care products, such as physician networks or tiered copayments, in their existing product lines. The least expensive option typically has the highest deductible and greatest degree of management (such as limitations on providers and requirements for prior authorization for expensive procedures).

Insurance companies decide which types of services they will cover (see **Figure 2.3**). As patient demand evolves,

It's Your Health

Global Implications

Although health insurance is provided by the government or by employers for many women in the United States, there is variability in how health care is paid in countries around the world. In the United Kingdom, there is a socialized healthcare system whereby all citizens have access to government insurance and health care provided by the National Health System (NHS). The NHS is both a provider of care and an insurer. Socialized systems like those in the UK, France, and Sweden ensure that health care is available and affordable for all citizens. In other countries, like Brazil, there is a mix of publicly available health insurance for poorer citizens and privately available care for self-pay or via private insurance. The public and private systems work alongside each other with opportunities for people with more resources to get access to higher quality care or more technology-driven care. In many developing countries there is no system of national insurance, and women pay for healthcare services on a fee-for-service self-pay basis. Some have access to affordable community care options or free care through nonprofits or aid agencies, while others have to forgo care when they do not have the money to pay for it.

Table 2.2   **Managed Care Plans**

Health Maintenance Organizations (HMO): An HMO is a managed care plan that offers a full range of services for a fixed, prepaid fee rather than charging patients for each service provided. Patients normally pay a small copayment for care. With some plans and for some services, patients also have to satisfy a deductible. Usually, patients do not have to file claims.

HMO plans typically fall into one of two categories:

- Staff Model: A staff model HMO has salaried physicians who provide services only to plan members. They offer care at a hospital, clinic, or health center in the community.
- Independent Practice Association (IPA): An IPA maintains contracts with a number of physicians and/or physician group practices. These physicians see patients in their own offices.

Point-of-Service (POS) Plan: POS plans function much like IPAs. Patients select a primary care physician who coordinates all care within the participating provider network, including specialist referrals.

Preferred Provider Organization (PPO): A PPO plan functions much like a POS plan, but it eliminates the primary care physician. As with the POS plan, patients can use a healthcare provider outside of the preferred provider network for an additional cost. Patients can usually see any participating provider—whether a primary care physician or a specialist—without a referral, at no additional cost. PPO plans often cost slightly more than HMOs.

High Deductible Health Plan (HDHP) with a Health Savings Account (HSA) or a Health Reimbursement Arrangement (HRA): An HDHP/HSA or HRA provides traditional medical coverage and a tax-free way to build savings for future medical expenses. It gives patients flexibility and discretion over how healthcare benefits are used. The HDHP features higher annual deductibles than other plans (usually $1000 to $2000) and usually has some upper limit on out-of-pocket liability. However, HDHPs make consumers share the financial burden of healthcare utilization. Most plans' coverage does not kick in until a large deductible is met, though many plans will pay for routine preventive care before the deductible is met.

some health insurance companies are beginning to cover complementary, alternative therapies and preventive care services, such as massage, acupuncture, and chiropractic care.[4]

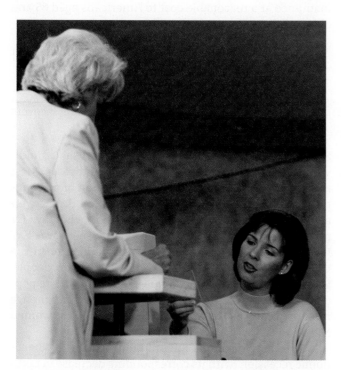

A copay is money that a patient must pay to receive healthcare services; copays are either a fixed amount of money or a percentage of the overall charge for a given service.
© Ryan McVay/Photodisc/Getty Images

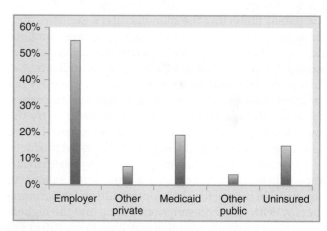

Figure 2.3   **Health insurance coverage of nonelderly Americans by source of coverage, 2014.**

Data from Kaiser Family Foundation estimates based on the Census Bureau's March 2014 Current Population Survey (CPS: Annual Social and Economic Supplements).

CHOOSING AN INSURANCE PLAN

When people choose between different insurance options, their choices are often influenced by which services are covered or what percentage of the total cost the insurer will pay. If a woman thinks that she is unlikely to use many services, as a 24-year-old woman without any existing medical conditions might, she may opt for a less expensive insurance program like an HMO. In doing so, she is making the compromise to have more restricted coverage at a lower cost rather than pay more for broader coverage. Regardless of the insurance program selected, an individual is at considerable financial risk if her insurance does not cover or only partially covers the services she uses. The inability to pay for health care beyond insurance premiums leads many people to avoid going to the doctor when necessary or to cut short therapy if it becomes too expensive.

As a method to manage rising costs, employers and health insurance companies are increasingly requiring patients to pay out of pocket for a portion of their health care. A **copayment** (or **copay**) is the amount of money a patient is responsible for paying to receive healthcare services. Copays can be either a fixed amount of money, like a $10 or $20 copay for a routine office visit, or a percentage of the overall charge for a given service (referred to as coinsurance). Insurance plans may often pay 80% or 90% of a patient's bill, with the patient responsible for the remaining amount.

With prescription drugs, many payers use a tiered copay system, which requires different payment levels for different types of medications. Most tiered copays reward patients for purchasing lower-cost generic drugs by requiring no or very low copays for these drugs and higher copays for more expensive brand-name drugs. **Generic drugs** are the chemical equivalents of brand-name drugs, but are far less expensive; they become available when the patent protecting the manufacturer's exclusive ability to market the drug expires, enabling greater competition in the marketplace. Within a tiered copay system, for example, a woman may pay $5 for a generic antibiotic, $25 for a preferred brand-name drug, and $50 or more for the premium-cost brand-name drug. In addition to copays, some health insurance plans require patients to try the lower cost generics and document treatment failure before agreeing to cover the higher-cost branded products.

Women pay more than men under many health insurance policies. Insurance policies often force women to pay sizeable copays for birth control pills or for hormone therapy, with many prescriptions falling into the highest copay tier. As a result, a woman may have to pay $20 to $40 per month to control her fertility and manage her transition into menopause. Health insurers have lists of drugs for which they provide reimbursement (i.e., **formularies**), which describe to patients and doctors which drugs are covered, into which tier each drug falls, and how much each drug will cost the patient. Out-of-pocket costs often prevent women from receiving appropriate care and from properly taking medication. A report by the Kaiser Family Foundation found that one in five (21%) nonelderly women did not fill a prescription because of the cost, compared with 13% of men.[5]

Types of Health Insurance

Employer-sponsored health insurance, as well as health insurance purchased by individuals, is considered **private health insurance**. Employers purchase and subsidize most private health insurance in the United States. When an individual has a full-time job, health insurance is often

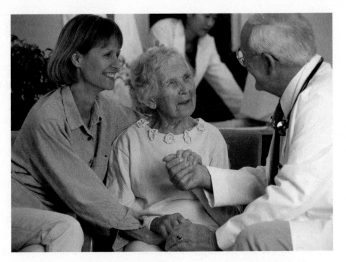

Due to the aging population and the fact that women live longer than men, an increasing majority of Medicare beneficiaries are women.
© Creatas/Jupiterimages

an integral benefit. Employer-sponsored health insurance can often be extended to cover the family of the insured individual. The government is also a major provider of health insurance, with 33% of Americans receiving some form of government-sponsored health insurance (also known as **public health insurance**).[3a,6] The federal government is the largest health insurer in the United States through its Medicare, Medicaid, Veterans Administration, Department of Defense, and Bureau of Indian Affairs insurance programs (see **Figure 2.4**). Medicare is the result of a bill enacted by Congress in 1965 to provide health insurance at a reasonable cost to Americans aged 65 and older. Medicare is provided in three parts:

- Part A is provided to all enrollees and covers inpatient hospitalization.

- Part B is optional and covers outpatient services.

- Part D was instituted in 2006 and is optional; it covers a portion of prescription drug costs.

Since 1965, Medicare has grown to cover disabled individuals and patients with end-stage renal disease. Most recently, it has expanded to include a portion of prescription drug coverage. Medicare's prescription drug coverage has already had substantial effects on who pays for prescription drugs in the United States (see **Figure 2.5**). In 2014, Medicare was the largest single insurer in the United States, covering more than 49.4 million people, 55% of whom are women.[7,7a] Due to the aging of the population and the fact that women live longer than men, a majority of the eldest Medicare beneficiaries are women (**Figure 2.6**).

The aging of the U.S. population and the 2008 economic recession (with its corresponding decrease in taxes received due to declining incomes) threatens the solvency of the Medicare system; healthcare reform implemented through the PPACA may reduce some Medicare costs, but these costs will likely continue to rise.[7]

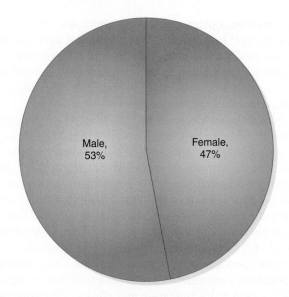

Figure 2.4 **Percentage of total uninsured by gender.**

Data from Kaiser Family Foundation estimates, based on the Census Bureau's March 2014 Current Population Survey (CPS: Annual Social and Economic Supplements).

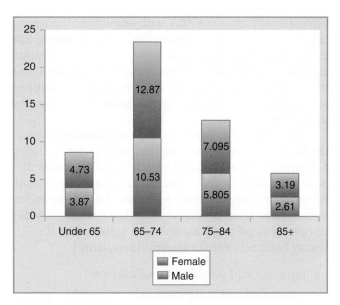

Figure 2.6 **Medicare population by age.**

Medicaid is a program jointly administered by federal and state governments that provides health insurance to low-income Americans. Whereas Medicare is a federally controlled health system, Medicaid is largely run at the state level. In some states, such as California and Tennessee, Medicaid has a state-specific name, such as MediCal or TennCare, respectively. The vast majority of Medicaid recipients are low-income women and their children; the children are covered through SCHIPs.

Medicaid and the benefits it provides are fundamental parts of providing health care to economically disadvantaged women and children in the United States. In 2009, legislation expanded SCHIP to provide coverage to an additional 4 million low-income children. Funded by an increased federal cigarette tax, the new SCHIP now insures 11 million low-income children.

In the 2014 census, Medicaid covered 68 million people, 58% of whom are women.[3a] Medicaid was significantly

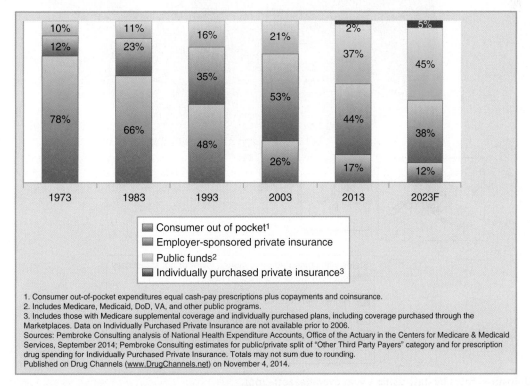

Figure 2.5 **Prescription drug spending by payer (2023 projected).**

expanded as part of the ACA, with enrollment increasing close to 17% after the bill went into effect. However, due to a landmark Supreme Court decision, state participation in the Medicaid expansion was optional. As a result, states that opted out of expansion did not see the reductions of uninsured at the same rates as those that expanded their programs.

Individuals qualify for Medicare based on income status, level of disability, need for long-term care, or by being a dependent of a Medicaid recipient. All hospitals and most physicians accept Medicaid as a form of payment, but some private physicians refuse Medicaid patients due to the lower reimbursement rates the system provides compared to private insurance. All states cover the following basic services for Medicaid recipients:

- Inpatient and outpatient medical care
- Laboratory and X-ray services
- Chronic care facilities for persons older than 21 years
- Home health care for those eligible for nursing facility services
- Services provided by a physician or nurse practitioner
- Necessary transportation

States may cover some additional services, such as prescription drugs, case management, dental care, prosthetic devices, medical transportation, intermediate care facilities, optometry, and tuberculosis-related services. Federal law requires the delivery of services that are "medically necessary." However, states exercise substantial independence in determining the amount and duration of services covered by establishing criteria for medical necessity and utilization control.

In addition to Medicare and Medicaid, the federal government provides health insurance to veterans through the Veterans Administration (VA), active service military personnel through the Department of Defense (DOD), government workers through the government's own health insurance program (Federal Employees Health Benefits Program), and Native Americans through the Indian Health Services. These programs are all separately administered and have different organizational structures. For example, the VA is a payer for health care and a network of providers. Veterans covered within this system are eligible for care at VA hospitals and clinics. This approach is similar to how the DOD provides health insurance and healthcare services to active-duty military personnel.

Uninsured Americans

In addition to those people with private insurance and those with public insurance, approximately 37 million Americans were uninsured in 2014, the lowest level in the last 20 years (**Figure 2.7**). The 25% drop in the rate of uninsured people in 2014 is due to the PPACA. One of the greatest impacts of the bill has been on people 19 to

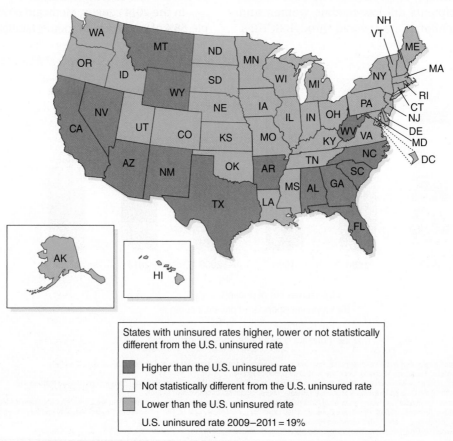

States with uninsured rates higher, lower or not statistically different from the U.S. uninsured rate

- ■ Higher than the U.S. uninsured rate
- □ Not statistically different from the U.S. uninsured rate
- ■ Lower than the U.S. uninsured rate

U.S. uninsured rate 2009–2011 = 19%

Figure 2.7   Uninsured rates by state using 3-year average, 2011–2014.

Source: Kaiser Family Foundation estimates based on the Census Bureau's March 2014 Current Population Survey (CPS: Annual Social and Economic Supplements).

25 years of age whose rates of being uninsured dropped from 34% prior to the law to 21%. This equates to approximately 4 million additional young adults being insured due to the bill's provision that allows them to remain on their parents' health insurance until age 26. A larger number of Americans are uninsured for a portion of the year (such as seasonal workers who only have health insurance for the portion of the year for which they are employed). One study found that close to one in three Americans were uninsured for all or part of the period studied. Two-thirds of these partially uninsured Americans were uninsured for 6 months or longer.[8]

The uninsured are men, women, and children, though today, men are less likely to have health insurance than women. Uninsured individuals are more likely to be sick or injured, to have a more difficult time accessing care, and to die prematurely than people with insurance. Nearly one in five families have at least one uninsured member. Most uninsured individuals are younger than age 30. In fact, 9.8% of children under 18 are uninsured, and 15.4% of children in poverty (and therefore by definition eligible for Medicaid).[7] These numbers are expected to fall under the PPACA, which will both offer insurance to a greater number of Americans and financially penalize individuals who choose to go without health insurance.

People without health insurance are at significant financial risk if they get sick or have an accident requiring emergency medical care. Because the uninsured must pay for medical services such as doctors' office visits or prescription drugs themselves, they often avoid preventive care or proper follow-up care because of cost concerns. In addition, the uninsured pay more for medical care because they are not eligible for the discounted pricing structures that health insurance companies negotiate with hospitals and doctors. As a result, the cost of care often strains family finances, jeopardizing families'

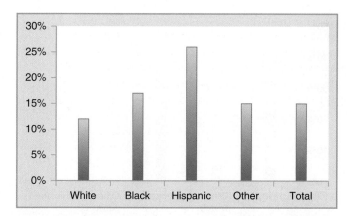

Figure 2.8   **Percentage uninsured among the nonelderly population by race, 2013.**

Data from Kaiser Family Foundation estimates based on the Census Bureau's March 2014 Current Population Survey (CPS: Annual Social and Economic Supplements). Available at: http://kff.org/uninsured/state-indicator/rate-by-raceethnicity/

physical, emotional, and economic health.[9] Long-term implications from being uninsured may include lack of preventive care, worsening of health status due to lack of appropriate care, and not being accurately monitored by a physician, leading to suboptimal care. African Americans and Hispanic Americans are less likely to have insurance than White or Asian Americans (see **Figure 2.8**).

Being eligible for some government sponsored or subsidized health programs depends on an individual or family's income. **Table 2.3** shows the 2014 income eligibility requirements for certain health insurance assistance.

Unemployment has increased significantly because of a weakening economy and rising healthcare costs for employers; as a result, many individuals who were formerly covered by their employers have suddenly lost their health insurance. A decline in coverage through employer-based

Table 2.3	Federal Poverty Guidelines for Health Insurance Support by Household Size and Income				
Persons in Household	2014 Federal Poverty Level (100% FPL)	Medicaid Eligibility* (138% of FPL)	Cost Sharing Reduction and Premium Cap Guideline (150% FPL)	Cost Sharing Reduction Subsidy Threshold (250% FPL)	Premium Subsidy Threshold (400% of FPL)
1	$11,670	$16,105	$17,505	$29,175	$46,680
2	$15,730	$21,707	$23,595	$39,325	$62,920
3	$19,790	$27,310	$29,685	$49,475	$79,160
4	$23,850	$32,913	$35,775	$59,625	$95,400
5	$27,910	$38,516	$41,865	$69,775	$111,640
6	$31,970	$44,119	$47,955	$79,925	$127,880
7	$36,030	$49,721	$54,045	$90,075	$144,120
8	$40,090	$55,324	$60,135	$100,225	$160,360
Location	Under 100%	100–199%	200–399%	400%+	Total

Data from Department of Health and Human Services.

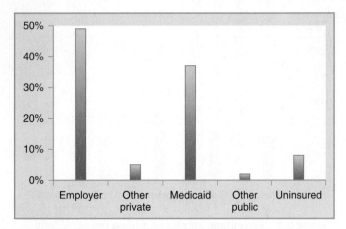

Figure 2.9 Insurance status for children aged 0 to 18 years by type of insurance.

Data from Kaiser Family Foundation estimates based on the Census Bureau's March 2014 Current Population Survey (CPS: Annual Social and Economic Supplements).

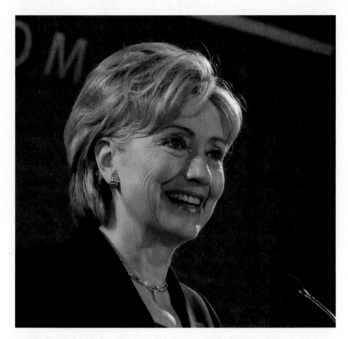

Healthcare reform is a major political topic in the United States.
© Albert H. Teich/Shutterstock

health plans, rising out-of-pocket costs associated with these plans, and skyrocketing costs for insurance premiums are seen as major drivers of this trend.

Lack of health insurance affects access to health services and contributes to poorer health, higher hospitalization rates, and more advanced disease states by the time health services are finally received. The 2009 expansion of Medicaid and the SCHIP has reduced the number of uninsured children, though close to 1 in 10 children still lack health coverage. The likelihood that a child is uninsured fell from 13.9% in 1998 to 10.5% in 2004 to 8% in 2014 (**Figure 2.9**).[7] SCHIP expansions and the PPACA are responsible for reducing this number, but these changes will likely take years for their full effects to be felt. Health insurance is particularly important for children. Uninsured children are more likely than insured children to lack a usual source of health care, to go without needed care, and to become sick, injured, or unhealthy.[10]

HEALTHCARE REFORM

In most industrialized countries, such as Canada and the United Kingdom, the government provides health insurance to all citizens through a system of **universal health insurance**. Universal healthcare systems attempt to make sure that all citizens have access to basic levels of medical care. Individuals are often allowed to purchase supplementary insurance to pay for items not covered under their national health systems. Proponents of universal health insurance systems argue that health care is a right, not a privilege, and should therefore be available to all citizens.

Their opponents counter that universal health insurance is an overly costly approach and prefer that the private sector manages and funds health care through a free-market approach. In the early 1990s, President Bill Clinton led a major drive to establish universal health

insurance in the United States. Although those efforts ultimately failed, healthcare reform has remained a major political topic. (See **It's Your Health** for more information.) In 2010, President Barack Obama signed into law the Patient

It's Your Health

Universal Health Care

Lack of health insurance harms individuals, their families, and the community at large. Because of the high costs of health care, uninsured individuals and their families have difficulties getting quality health care when they are sick. They tend to delay treatments until their illnesses become serious, and they are less likely to seek routine preventive health services that can avert or detect major illnesses early on. As a result, they tend to die sooner than people who have health insurance.

The lack of health insurance also aggravates the financial burden placed on the community as a whole. Because the uninsured tend to delay necessary treatment, they are often sicker and therefore more expensive to treat when they finally seek care. Uninsured people frequently turn to the nearest hospital emergency room, which is an expensive and inefficient way to get care. Furthermore, the primary providers of care to the uninsured—such as public hospitals, teaching hospitals, academic health centers, and nonprofit community hospitals—incur heavy losses from high rates of uncompensated care. In turn, these providers are forced to cut back on their services to all patients or even close their facilities.

Data from *Universal health care*. American Public Health Association. Available at: http://www.apha.org/advocacy/reports/facts /advocacyfacthealthcare.htm; Related APHA policy: *Public health's critical role in health reform in the United States*. 2009, 2011. Available at: http:// www.apha.org/advocacy/policy/policysearch/default.htm?id=1386

Protection and Affordable Care Act. The law's main goal was to expand coverage to uninsured Americans, provide coverage to previously uninsurable individuals like those with preexisting conditions, and make insurance more affordable for small businesses and individuals. Litigation brought the PPACA before the Supreme Court in 2012; a 5 to 4 majority ruled the vast majority of the PPACA as constitutional, allowing it to stay in effect.

Some of the changes became effective immediately, such as tax credits to small businesses to provide health benefits to workers and matching grants to states to expand their Medicaid programs to more individuals and families. Others, such as increasing Medicaid payments to primary care doctors and establishing affordable insurance exchanges, will be instituted between 2014 and 2020. One of the bill's main tenets requires individuals to have health insurance and for states to expand coverage to uninsured low-income individuals provided by Medicaid programs. Millions of people, many of whom are women and families, will gain insurance as a result of the bill. The PPACA also requires health insurers to accept patients with preexisting conditions. Before the bill's passage, a new insurer could deny coverage to women who had cervical cancer, diabetes, or other conditions based on her health history.

The bill also allows the government to explore novel ways to encourage more cost-effective care. This includes funding comparative effective research that considers the clinical and economic benefits of new technologies compared to the standard of care. This type of research is helpful in understanding the real world impact of new products and helping payers to fund technologies likely to have the greatest impact. An example in the women's health space includes research on the most effective diagnosis and treatment for osteoporosis in aging women.

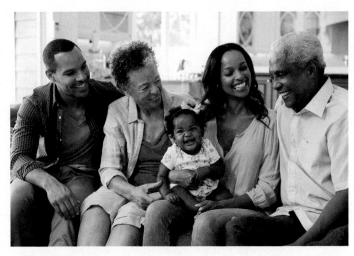

Many women are "sandwiched" with requirements for elder care and child care.
© Monkey Business Images/Shutterstock

Healthcare reform also began federal funding of Accountable Care Organizations (ACOs). ACOs are provider groups like hospitals or physicians' group practices who take complete responsibility for the care of a patient rather than just providing isolated services. ACOs receive a fixed fee for the broader provision of care and are rewarded if patients' health improves. The theory is that by shifting the financial risk to providers—if providers are no longer paid for each medical encounter but are instead paid for overall care and quality—that care will be more appropriate and effective. Some ACOs are implementing pilot programs for the care of chronic diseases like diabetes, while others are delivering more comprehensive care. These ACOs are attempting to provide a more cohesive and rational delivery of preventive services, disease management, and acute care. The influence ACOs have on the costs and quality of care will take several years to evaluate.

GENDER DIMENSIONS: Health Differences Between Men and Women

The population of the United States is getting older as disease prevention, health promotion, and innovative treatments prevent or delay disease and prolong life. In 2012, the average life expectancy for all Americans was 78 years of age: 76 years for White men and 70 years for Black men, and 81 years for White women and 77 years for Black women. On average, women now live 6 years longer than men. In 2000, there were only 70 men per 100 women over age 65, and 41 men per 100 women age 85 or older (see **Figure 2.10**). Note, however, that these figures are an aggregate of all U.S. women. When examined by race and ethnicity, life expectancy varies among both women and men.

As a result, most of the burden of aging rests on women, and increasingly women are aging into their oldest years without the support or help of a spouse.[8] The aging trends have enormous economic

ramifications. As women age, they become more likely to suffer from chronic diseases such as heart disease, cancer, and arthritis. These illnesses create significant morbidity as well as costs to affected individuals.[9] Currently, Medicare provides health insurance for all Americans over the age of 65, ensuring that all older Americans have at least some access to health care. Because Medicare covers only 80% of costs, however, a significant financial burden is often imposed on older patients when seeking care.[10]

The economic realities faced by elderly women also affect women's health. As women age, they are likely to need increased access to prescription drugs, perhaps specialty medical assistance, durable medical equipment (such as walkers and orthopedic beds), and other expensive goods and services.

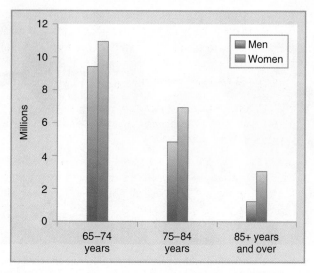

Figure 2.10   **Population 65 years and over by age and gender, 2010.**

Data from U.S. Census Bureau, 2010 Census Summary File 1.

The research and development of new technologies will influence both the types of medical care available as well as how it is delivered. Major advances in women's health will arise from research into genetic engineering, stem cell research, microscopic surgical techniques, and personalized medicine. Paying for these advancements and making them accessible to the majority of people will remain a policy challenge.

PREVENTIVE CARE AND A FOCUS ON WOMEN'S HEALTH

Preventive care is medical or health care designed to prevent or reduce the effects of disease or injury. Preventive care can improve quality of life and often save money by eliminating the need for expensive procedures. A positive outcome of this trend has been widespread support for many preventive services, such as mammograms, cervical cancer screening, and smoking cessation programs. The old saying that "an ounce of prevention is worth a pound of cure" has been proven true in most studies. Investing in preventive services and education leads to members with fewer major medical problems, such as heart disease, and the ability to diagnose diseases, such as breast cancer, at an earlier stage.

Preventive services and health education are the cornerstones of effective women's health care. As awareness and support of these and other women-specific health issues has grown, many payers have established whole departments dedicated to women's health. These departments educate patients and physicians about best practices and new treatments for women; they also analyze the benefits of new technologies. Women's health departments within payer organizations have prioritized

women's health issues by supporting prenatal checkups and strict monitoring regimens for pregnant women, promoting women's cardiac health, and ensuring universal coverage of gynecological exams. Under the PPACA, women do not have to pay copays for core preventive care like mammograms, vaccinations, and cervical cancer screening. The list of preventive services covered without cost sharing includes:

1. Well-women visits
2. Gestational diabetes screening
3. Human papillomavirus (HPV) testing
4. Counseling for sexually transmitted diseases
5. HIV testing and counseling
6. Contraceptive methods and counseling
7. Breastfeeding support, supplies, and counseling
8. Domestic violence screening and counseling

WOMEN AS HEALTHCARE CONSUMERS

Women make most of the decisions regarding health care, both for themselves and their families: one large survey found that women make 90% of their families' health-related decisions.[11] As a group, women have seen their economic power and ability to affect the overall demand within the healthcare system increase substantially. In 2012, 57.7% of women were in the labor force, with median weekly earnings of $691.[11a] According to a study by the Commonwealth Institute, more than 68% of women, compared to 55% of men, say they manage the bills in their household. Women's growing economic power has made them increasingly important in the eyes of pharmaceutical, medical device, and diagnostics manufacturers. More research and development dollars are being poured into discovering both necessary and voluntary treatments for women. In addition, women are taking a more active role in their own health care, by learning more about their health status, taking part in preventive health care, and articulating their needs to providers, payers, manufacturers, and legislatures. Together, these factors have raised awareness of women's health issues and made women's health a priority within the healthcare industry.

Despite advances over the past 40 years, however, health care is lacking for many women, especially for women who need it the most. These women are often living under or just above the poverty line. Whether due to being unemployed or underemployed, not having adequate childcare support, lacking education, being in poor health, lacking access to resources, or just not having adequate support, these women often lack the decision-making freedom of women with additional resources. Today, lower-income women are disproportionately more likely than other women to be in poor health. Thus, women with the least resources often carry the largest burden of healthcare costs, disability, and responsibility in caring for others. Women with health problems may have difficulties obtaining care because of coverage restrictions, high costs, and logistical barriers, such as transportation. For many women, coverage and access to care are unstable. Health coverage, involvement with health plans, and relationships with doctors are often short lived, resulting in spotty and fragmented care. A survey by the Kaiser Family Foundation found that almost one-quarter (24%) of nonelderly women, compared with 16% of nonelderly men, delayed or went without care in the past year because they could not afford it.[5]

LONG-TERM CARE AND WOMEN AS CAREGIVERS

Women are more likely than men to be responsible for taking care of friends and relatives who need care and to make decisions about long-term care or assisted living communities that care for elderly or disabled persons. Additionally, because women generally live longer than men, the vast majority of residents in these facilities are women.

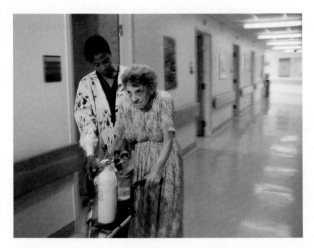

Most older women in nursing homes spend down their life savings to pay for services until Medicaid begins to cover the remaining costs of care.
© Photodisc/Getty Images

Long-term facilities provide ongoing care for people who need lengthy or even lifelong assistance with daily living due to an illness, injury, or severe cognitive impairment (such as Alzheimer's disease). Care can be provided either in a nursing home, in an assisted living facility, or at the patient's home. The national average annual cost for care in a nursing home exceeds $75,190 for a private and $52,000 for a semiprivate room.[12] Costs of long-term care and long-term care insurance are expected to continue to increase dramatically, with a semiprivate room costing $190,600 by 2030.[13] Paying for long-term care is an open-ended proposition, as some people may live in an assisted care facility and then move on to a nursing home

and live for 20 or more years in a facility; actuarial calculations on the costs have driven insurance prices up and, in 2010, forced the largest long-term care insurer (MetLife) from accepting new policies. Two insurance options are available to cover these expenses:

- Private long-term care insurance programs are very expensive and are predominantly purchased by wealthier Americans.

- Medicaid covers Americans in long-term care facilities once they have exhausted all other resources. Most older women in nursing homes spend their life savings to pay for services until Medicaid begins to cover the remaining costs of care.

With the U.S. population aging and the average life span increasing, informal caregiving by family members in the home has become a vital part of the healthcare delivery system. One national study estimates the value of unpaid caregiving at approximately $450 billion per year, twice as much as is spent on home care and nursing home services.[13] Women provide most of this care, even though most working-age women now participate in the labor force. As a result of shouldering the stress and burden for elder caregiving, women caregivers tend to suffer more adverse health events than noncaregivers.[14] According to the Commonwealth Fund, one-fourth (25%) of women caring for a sick or disabled family member rate their own health as fair or poor, compared with one-sixth (17%) of other women.[15] More than half (54%) of women caregivers have one or more chronic health conditions, compared with two-fifths (41%) of other women. In addition, one-half (51%) of all caregivers exhibit high depressive symptoms and sleeplessness.[16]

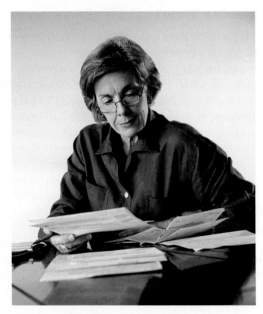

Choosing a health insurance plan is often a baffling undertaking; there are many important factors to consider other than simply the monthly premium.
© Thinkstock/Creatas

INFORMED DECISION MAKING

Choosing health insurance is often a baffling undertaking. Many options may mean little to the individual other than being associated with different monthly premiums. Most people receive their health insurance through their employers, so they usually have either a single option or a small menu of plans to choose from.

When choosing a health insurance plan, it is important to consider the following:

- **Deductibles:** Deductibles are set amounts that individuals must pay out of pocket before the benefit kicks in. For example, if a woman has a $500 deductible on her insurance plan, she must pay for the first $500 worth of healthcare services she receives before the insurance plan begins to pick up the cost. Usually, the less expensive the plan, the higher the deductible. Deductibles are common in all types of insurance programs.

- **Benefits:** The different benefits insurance provides vary from plan to plan. Look closely at the list of covered services. For example, does the insurance plan cover prescription drugs? Does it cover open access to relevant specialists or provide medical equipment needed for specific health problems?

- **Network:** Consider the implications of a restrictive network to the costs of care and access to care. Does the insurance plan restrict access to a specific network of physicians? Is your preferred doctor a member of that network? If not, what are the costs for going to a doctor out of the network? Are the major local hospitals part of the health plan's network?

- **Coinsurance:** Many plans require patients to pay a set percentage of charges, often 10–20%. While coinsurance can keep premiums affordable, patient costs can be very high if hospitalization or long-term care is required. Consumers should inquire whether their insurance plan has a maximum amount that a patient is required to pay if a hospitalization or other high-cost event occurs.

- **Emergency Services:** Often health insurance programs have restrictive criteria for use of emergency services. What is the process for receiving emergency services? Is prior authorization needed before going to the emergency room?

- **Copayments:** Copayments are fixed amounts of money a patient must pay to receive health-related goods or services. Copays usually have to be paid out of pocket, either at the doctor's office, pharmacy, or hospital.

By considering these factors when choosing health insurance, a woman is more likely to get a package that is right for her and her family.

Profiles of Remarkable Women

Katherine Swartz (1950–)

Professor Swartz's current research interests focus on implementation issues related to the PPACA, aging issues, and reasons for and ways to control episodes of care that involve extremely high expenditures. Her research related to the PPACA centers on two implementation issues: how the insurance exchanges will work with current state regulations of the sale of health insurance and how lower-income people with fluctuating income will obtain Medicaid or premium subsidies for purchasing coverage in the exchanges. She is the author of *Reinsuring Health: Why More Middle-Class People Are Uninsured and What Government Can Do*. In the book, she describes who does not have insurance today and why the middle-class are more likely to be uninsured today than 30 years ago, how insurance companies compete in the individual and small group insurance markets, and why government-sponsored reinsurance for people with very-high expenditures would make small group and individual insurance more accessible and affordable for many of the uninsured. Her proposal about reinsurance is part of the PPACA and the exchanges. Swartz also is increasingly engaged in policy issues related to the aging of the population, particularly how to develop greater efficiency in providing community long-term care services and housing options to enable more people to age in place.

Swartz was elected to the Institute of Medicine in 2007. She was the 1991 recipient of the David Kershaw Award from the Association for Public Policy Analysis and Management for research done before the age of 40 that has had a significant impact on public policy. She was also a visiting scholar at the Russell Sage Foundation between September 2000 and June 2001.

Swartz was the president of the Association for Public Policy Analysis and Management in 2009. Between November 1995 and June 2007, Swartz was the editor of *Inquiry*, a journal that focuses on health care organization, provision, and financing. Since 2005, she has been the director of the Robert Wood Johnson Foundation Scholars in Health Policy Research Program at Harvard University.

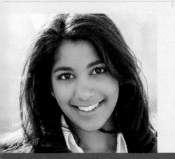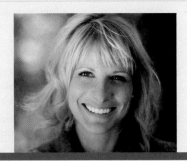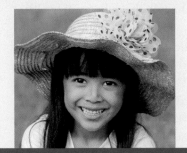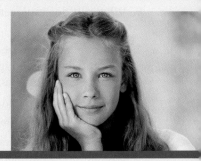

CASE STUDY

Dr. Janice Beekley is the medical director of one of the largest health insurance companies in America. It is her job to review new medical technologies and determine which ones will be covered by the health plan and which will not. To decide this, she and the committee of experts she works with review new products to see whether they have significant clinical value and what the cost of covering them would be. When products are not as effective as the current standard of care, they are usually not covered. When they are as effective but more expensive, they also may not be covered. When products are more effective but very costly, the insurance plan usually reimburses for their use—but may create access barriers to them so that physicians and patients have to demonstrate they absolutely need something prior to having access to the service.

Examples of this include CT scans for assessing back injuries. Dr. Beekley and her colleagues recently reviewed all the published evidence about CT scans to assess back injuries and came to the conclusion that they were being overused. Additionally, CT scans are very expensive and were costing the health insurer millions of dollars every year. Dr. Beekley created a specific policy that outlined when CT scans can and cannot be used. If patients get a CT scan for one of the unapproved reasons, they will have to pay for that imaging test out of their own pocket. This could cost them close to $1000. As a result, another initiative Dr. Beekley is working on is helping people to understand what is covered and what is not, and how to look up that information as part of the routine healthcare process.

Dr. Beekley's task for today is to evaluate whether or not the health insurance company should cover and pay for a new test for cervical cancer screening. It is a more expensive test, but because it is more effective than the current standard, it might save money in the long term.

Questions

1. What type of information should Dr. Beekley and her colleagues collect about the new test when assessing whether or not to cover it?

2. Who might she consult when reviewing whether or not the test has value?

3. What is more important, the efficacy or the cost of the test? Why?

4. Should health insurance plans be able to decide what products and services are covered or not?

■ Summary

Health care is one of the top expenses in modern American life. In the United States, both public and private health insurance exists to help individuals afford health care. However, millions of Americans are currently uninsured or underinsured. The Patient Protection and Affordable Care Act, enacted in 2010, will reduce but not eliminate the number of people without insurance. Lacking health insurance has many negative effects on health: People without insurance are less likely than people with insurance to be able to afford regular medical care and are more likely to be sick, injured, or unhealthy. Different health insurance plans affect the amount individuals have to pay for healthcare goods, such as prescription drugs, and services, such as physicians' office visits.

Among the elderly population, issues of access to and payment for healthcare goods and services continue to be a major problem. Although most are covered by Medicare and Medicaid, the elderly, who are predominantly women, face a unique set of economic challenges in managing their health.

■ Topics for Discussion

1. How can a person's health insurance status affect his or her health status?

2. Should everyone have access to health insurance, even if he or she cannot afford it?

3. Is access to health care a right or a privilege?

4. How will the expansion of coverage enabled by healthcare reform impact women?

5. What are some common health-related items that often are not covered by health insurance?

6. What role do employers have in the delivery of health care?

7. What are potential implications of Medicare becoming more like a managed care program and less of a fee-for-service program?

8. How can health insurance status be affected by women's different stages of life?

9. What are some central issues related to the elderly population's healthcare needs?

■ Key Terms

Copayment/copay

Fee-for-service

Formulary

Generic drug

Indemnity

Long-term facility

Managed care

Medicaid

Private health insurance

Public health insurance

Third-party payer system

Universal health insurance

■ References

1. Fuchs, V. (2012). Major trends in the U.S. health economy since 1950. *New England Journal of Medicine* 366: 973–977.

2. Martin, A., Lassman, D., Washington, B., et al. (2012). The National Health Expenditure Accounts Team. Growth in U.S. health spending remained slow in 2010; health share of gross domestic product was unchanged from 2009. *Health Affairs* 31(1): 208–219.

2a. World Health Organization National Health Account database. (n.d.). Available at: http://data.worldbank.org/indicator/SH.XPD .TOTL.ZS. Updates available at: http://apps.who.int/nha /database/DataExplorerRegime.aspx

3. DeNavas-Walt, C., Proctor, B., & Smith, J. (2011). *U.S. Census Bureau, Current Population Reports, P60-239, Income, poverty, and health insurance coverage in the United States: 2010.* U.S. Government Printing Office, Washington, DC. Available at: http://www .census.gov/prod/2011pubs/p60-239.pdf

3a. Kaiser Commission on Medicaid and the Uninsured and Urban Institute. (n.d.). Available at: http://kff.org/medicaid/state -indicator/medicaid-enrollment-by-gender/ Note: Estimates based on data from FY 2011 MSIS. Because 2011 data were unavailable, 2010 data was used for Florida, Kansas, Maine, Maryland, Montana, New Mexico, New Jersey, Oklahoma, Texas, and Utah.

4. Tait, E., Laditka, S., Laditka. J., et al. (2012). Use of complementary and alternative medicine for physical performance, energy, immune function, and general health among older women and men in the United States. *Journal of Women & Aging* 24(1): 23–43.

5. Kaiser Family Foundation. (2011). *Key findings from the Kaiser Women's Health Survey.* Available at: http://www.kff.org /womenshealth/upload/8164.pdf

6. EBRI Databook on Employee Benefits. Accessed at: http://www .ebri.org/publications/books/?fa=databook

7. U.S. Department of Health and Human Services. (August 5, 2010). *Trustees announce solvency of Medicare trust fund extended by 12 Years to 2029.* Available at: http://www.hhs.gov/news /press/2010pres/08/20100805d.html

7a. Urban Institute and Kaiser Commission on Medicaid and the Uninsured. (n.d.). *CPS: Annual social and economic supplements.* Available at: http://kff.org/medicare/state-indicator/medicare -beneficiaries-by-gender/ Note: Estimates based on the U.S. Census Bureau's March 2012 and 2013 Current Population Survey.

8. Fronstin, P. (2011). Sources of health insurance and characteristics of the uninsured: Analysis of the March 2012 Current Population Survey. *EBRI Issue Brief* 376: 1–35.

9. Auerbach, D. I., & Kellermann, A. L. (2011). A decade of health care cost growth has wiped out real income gains for an average US family. *Health Affairs* 30(9): 1630–1636.

10. O'Donnell, H. C., et al. (2011). Healthcare consumers' attitudes towards physician and personal use of health information exchange. *Journal of General Internal Medicine* 26(9): 1019–1026.

11. Fronstin, P. (2012). Findings from the 2012 EBRI/MGA consumer engagement in health care survey. *EBRI Issue Brief* 379.

11a. Bureau of Labor Statistics. (2014). *Women in the labor force: A databook.* Report 1049. Available at: http://www.bls.gov/cps/wlf -databook-2013.pdf

12. U.S. Bureau of Labor Statistics. (2011). *Women's earnings and employment by industry, 2009.* Available at: http://www.bls.gov /opub/ted/2011/ted_20110216.htm

13. U.S. Department of Health and Human Services. (2012). *The Federal Long Term Care Insurance Program on-line calculator.* Available at: http://www.healthcare.gov/law/timeline/index.html

14. Coughlin, J. (2010). *Estimating the impact of caregiving and employment on well-being. Outcomes & Insights in Health Management.* Available at: http://www.well-beingindex.com/files/20100513 _CHR_CareGiving.pdf

15. Kim, H., et al. (2012). Predictors of caregiver burden in caregivers of individuals with dementia. *Journal of Advanced Nursing* 68(4): 846–855.

16. Casado, B. L., van Vulpen, K. S., & Davis, S. L. (2011). Unmet needs for home and community-based services among frail older Americans and their caregivers. *Journal of Aging and Health* 23(3): 529–553.

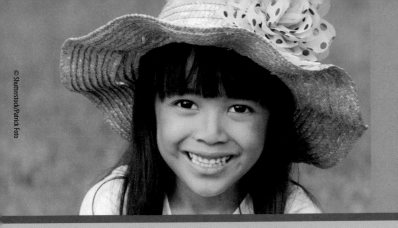

CHAPTER 3

Health Promotion and Disease Prevention

Learning Objectives

On completion of this chapter, the student should be able to discuss:

1. Health promotion and disease prevention at the individual and population levels.

2. Concepts of epidemiology, incidence, prevalence, morbidity, and mortality, and why they are important.

3. Primary, secondary, and tertiary levels of prevention.

4. How race, ethnicity, age, sexual orientation, and other factors influence public health.

5. Barriers to healthcare access experienced by different groups of women.

6. Major health concerns in the developing world, and how these concerns compare to those in developed countries.

7. How life expectancy differs by gender and race.

8. Healthcare concerns and preventive measures for adolescents.

9. Healthcare concerns and preventive measures for young adults.

10. Healthcare concerns and preventive measures for women in midlife.

11. Healthcare concerns and preventive measures for senior women.

12. Taking responsibility for one's own health.

INTRODUCTION

Health is more than the absence of disease. Health depends on many positive factors as well, including what people eat, how often they are physically active, how they interact with their environment, and what kinds of relationships they have. Fully one-half of the deaths in the United States are due to people's behavioral choices.[1] Health promotion is the act of encouraging people to improve their health and maintain a healthy lifestyle.

A specific type of health promotion called disease prevention attempts to improve public health by preventing diseases. Heart disease, stroke, cancer, and many other chronic diseases lack simple cures, but diet, physical activity, and other lifestyle choices can often either prevent them from occurring or help manage the conditions after they develop. In addition, many diseases or conditions can be prevented, partially mitigated, or treated more easily if they are found and treated early.

At an individual level, health promotion can consist of efforts to learn about one's own health and to develop and maintain healthful behaviors. At the population level, health promotion often consists of major public health campaigns run by government entities, nongovernmental organizations, universities, and other organizations. These campaigns may seek to change a law, encourage a healthful behavior, educate a group of people, or improve the areas where people live. A health promotion campaign could be as broad as a national cigarette tax or speed limit or as narrow as an effort to increase knowledge of birth defects of teenage Latina women living in a specific Chicago neighborhood.

At both the individual and population levels, effective health promotion depends on knowledge of the target audience. The population of women can be examined in many ways, including by race, ethnicity, age, geography, sexual orientation, body type, and psychological temperament.

Recognizing this diversity, and how it influences causes, diagnoses, progression, and treatment of disease, is important for women's health. These differences create a need for tailoring the delivery of health education and healthcare services. The health needs of a White, 54-year-old single actress living in New York City may differ sharply from those of a Black, married, 24-year-old homemaker in rural Alabama, but the needs of both women are equally important.

Political Dimensions

There are many players in the health system, including government agencies, advocacy groups, national health education associations, hospitals, and volunteer groups. The federal health infrastructure starts with the Department of Health and Human Services (DHHS), part of the U.S. cabinet. Led by the Secretary of Health and Human Services, this department provides basic human services and protects the health of all Americans. As the U.S. government's principal health agency, the DHHS includes more than 300 programs. DHHS works with state, local, and tribal governments and funds some local services. Eleven DHHS operation divisions—eight agencies in the U.S. Public Health Service and three human service agencies (**Figure 3.1**)—administer the DHHS's programs.

Within the DHHS and under the Secretary of Health and Human Services is the Surgeon General, who acts as the country's leading spokesperson about public health. Nicknamed "America's doctor," the Surgeon General advises the president and provides the public with information on how to improve health and lower the chances of disease and injury. The Surgeon General publishes reports and publications on topics such as smoking, nutrition, mental health, violence, overweight and obesity, suicide, and sexual health. One of these initiatives, Healthy People, aims to identify national health improvement priorities, increase awareness of public health issues, and improve the health of all Americans. The current phase of the initiative, Healthy People 2020, offers a set of national disease prevention and health promotion objectives for the United States. These objectives range from reducing obesity and lowering the number of infections acquired in hospitals and clinics to improving sleep and reducing racial and ethnic disparities in health care.

The eight agencies of the U.S. Public Health Service have different mandates:

- **National Institutes of Health (NIH):** The world's premier medical research organization, NIH supports more than 35,000 research projects nationwide studying diseases such as cancer, Alzheimer's disease, diabetes, arthritis, cardiovascular disease, and AIDS.

- **Food and Drug Administration (FDA):** The FDA ensures the safety of foods and cosmetics and the safety and efficacy of pharmaceuticals, biological products, and medical devices.

- **Centers for Disease Control and Prevention (CDC):** Working with states and other partners, CDC provides health surveillance to monitor and prevent disease outbreaks, implement disease prevention strategies, and maintain national health statistics.

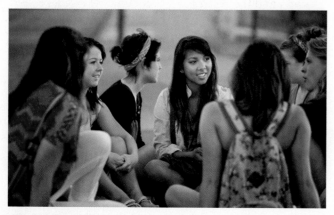
Women are not a homogenous population.
© CREATISTA/Shutterstock

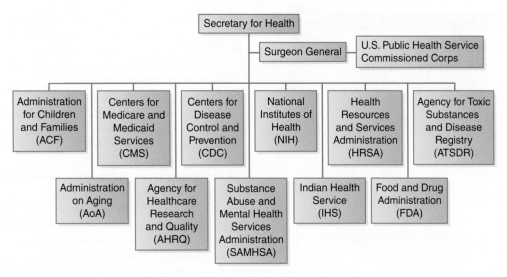

Figure 3.1   The U.S. Department of Health and Human Services (DHHS).

■ **Agency for Toxic Substances and Disease Registry (ATSDR):** ATSDR helps prevent exposure to hazardous substances from waste sites on the U.S. Environmental Protection Agency's National Priorities List, and it develops toxicological profiles of chemicals found at these sites.

■ **Indian Health Service (IHS):** The IHS provides health services to the 1.9 million American Indians and Alaska Natives of 564 federally recognized tribes in 35 states.

■ **Health Resources and Services Administration (HRSA):** HRSA provides access to essential health services for people who are poor, uninsured, or live in rural and urban neighborhoods where health care is scarce. Working with state and community organizations, HRSA also helps insure healthy mothers and children, increase the number and diversity of healthcare professionals in underserved communities, and support people fighting human immunodeficiency virus (HIV) infection and acquired immune deficiency syndrome (AIDS) through the Ryan White Care Act.

■ **Substance Abuse and Mental Health Services Administration (SAMHSA):** SAMHSA funds and collects information on substance abuse prevention, addiction treatment, and mental health services. This agency provides federal block grants to the states to support and maintain substance abuse and mental health services.

■ **Agency for Healthcare Research and Quality (AHRQ):** AHRQ supports research designed to improve the quality of health care, reduce its cost, improve patient safety, address medical errors, and broaden access to essential services. It provides evidence-based information on healthcare outcomes; quality; and cost, use, and access.

The Assistant Secretary for Health oversees these eight health agency divisions of DHHS as well as the Commissioned Corps, a uniformed service of more than 6000 health professionals who serve at DHHS and other federal agencies.

The DHHS also includes three human service agencies:

■ **Centers for Medicare and Medicaid Services (CMS):** CMS administers the Medicare and Medicaid programs, which provide health care to approximately one in four Americans. Medicare provides health insurance for more than 48 million elderly and disabled Americans. Medicaid, a joint federal–state program, provides health coverage for about 50 million low-income individuals, as well as nursing home coverage for low-income elderly people. The State Children's Health Insurance Program (SCHIP), expanded in 2009, now covers more than 11 million children.

■ **Administration for Children and Families (ACF):** This agency administers the state–federal welfare program, the national child support enforcement system, and the Head Start program. The ACF oversees some 60 programs that promote the economic and social well-being of families, children, individuals, and communities.

■ **Administration on Aging (AoA):** AoA is the federal agency in charge of the interests and concerns of the elderly and their caregivers. Among other duties, the AoA provides services to the elderly, such as home meal delivery and transportation services, that enable them to remain independent.

Economic Dimensions

Public health policies, health-promotion efforts, and prevention campaigns can help people make healthier decisions and reduce the burden of illness, enhance quality of

It's Your Health

Cost Benefits of Prevention Programs

Investing in disease prevention programs has been shown to save both lives and dollars. Some examples from the National Center for Chronic Disease Prevention and Health Promotion show the cost benefits of prevention programs:

- One quality-adjusted year of life is saved for the cost of a smoking cessation program ($1109 to $4542).

- For each $1 spent on school HIV, other sexually transmitted infection (STI), and pregnancy prevention programs, roughly $2.65 is saved on medical and social costs.

- For every $1 spent on preconception care programs for women with diabetes, $1.86 can be saved by preventing birth defects among their offspring.

- A mammogram every 2 years for women ages 50–69 years costs only about $9000 per year of life saved.

- For the cost of 100 Papanicolaou (Pap) tests for low-income elderly women, about $5907 and 3.7 years of life are saved.

Source: U.S. Department of Health and Human Services, Centers for Disease Control and Prevention, National Center for Chronic Disease Prevention and Health Promotion. Available at: http://www.cdc.gov/nccdphp/index.htm

---

Table 3.1   Leading Behavior-Related Causes of Death in the United States

- Smoking: 467,000
- High blood pressure: 395,000
- Overweight/obesity: 216,000
- Inadequate physical activity and inactivity: 191,000
- High blood sugar: 190,000
- High LDL cholesterol: 113,000
- High dietary salt: 102,000
- Low dietary omega-3 fatty acids (seafood): 84,000
- High dietary trans fatty acids: 82,000
- Alcohol use: 64,000 (alcohol use averted a balance of 26,000 deaths from heart disease, stroke, and diabetes, because moderate drinking reduces risk of these diseases. But these deaths were outweighed by 90,000 alcohol-related deaths from traffic and other injuries, violence, cancers, and a range of other diseases).
- Low intake of fruits and vegetables: 58,000
- Low dietary polyunsaturated fatty acids: 15,000

Source: Goodarz, D., Ding, E. L., Mozaffarian, D., et al. (2009). The preventable causes of death in the United States: Comparative risk assessment of dietary, lifestyle, and metabolic risk factors. *PLoS Medicine* 6(4).

---

life, and increase the life span. Additionally, public health efforts that focus on changing behavior are usually much less expensive than later medical intervention.

Unfortunately, these types of programs are critically underfunded. In 2012, total per capita health expenditure came out to approximately $8900 per person, yet only $60 per person was spent on public health efforts.[1,1a] **Table 3.1** lists the major behavior-related causes of death in the United States.

The growing number of people who are overweight or obese is a major public health concern. An estimate of the direct medical costs of treating obesity and overweight in the United States found these costs came to more than $147 billion per year.[2] The indirect costs are also great: Obesity may cost U.S. employers more than $45 billion a year in lost productivity and health expenditures.[3] By changing their behaviors, such as modifying diet and increasing exercise, individuals can improve their own health and greatly reduce healthcare costs down the road. But education efforts and policies that promote healthy behaviors are also important to promote health. Requiring that school lunches meet basic nutritional requirements or helping to fund local farmer's markets so that people can purchase fresh fruits and vegetables, for example, are two ways to encourage healthful decision making.

Total costs associated with diseases are often significantly lower for people who take part in preventive care measures. For example, let's consider cervical cancer, which is frequently caught in its early stages by widespread Pap- and HPV-test-based screening programs. According to the American Cancer Society, the 5-year survival rate for cervical cancers detected at the earliest invasive stage is 93%; the 5-year survival rate for cancers detected at the latest stages is only 15%.[3a] The costs and associated morbidity of treating women with early cellular changes, or minor cervical cancers, are significantly lower than that associated with treating women for invasive disease once cervical cancer has spread. Early detection can reduce both the financial cost and the human costs counted in pain, suffering, and anxiety.

Some health insurers and employers have grown to understand the economic value of health promotion and preventive care, and they recognize their importance by covering these services. Some insurers and employers now offer incentives for joining a health club or provide partial payment or reimbursement for alternative therapy services such as massage or chiropractic adjustments.

Epidemiology

Health promotion and disease prevention depend on epidemiology, the study of patterns of disease in the population. Although many people think of health and disease as issues relating to individuals, epidemiologists examine the health of communities, specific populations, and entire countries. Epidemiology examines the frequency and types of diseases in groups of people and the factors that influence the distribution of disease. Epidemiologists use the following terms to describe conditions or diseases within a population:

- **Incidence:** new cases of a condition that occur during a specified period of time.
- **Prevalence:** the total number of people affected by a given condition at a point in time or during a period of time.
- **Mortality rate:** the incidence of death in a given population during a particular time period. It is calculated by dividing the number of deaths in a population by the total population.
- **Morbidity rate:** the incidence of illness in a given population during a particular time period. Morbidity rate is calculated in a similar manner to mortality rate.

Incidence and prevalence rates allow epidemiologists to examine how diseases or conditions progress. A condition with a high prevalence and a low incidence (a common condition with few new cases), for example, might eventually stabilize or drop within a population, whereas a condition with a low prevalence but a high incidence (a rare condition with many new cases) may indicate a new and dangerous outbreak. Morbidity and mortality rates can be calculated across the entire population or within a specific subpopulation, such as age, gender, or race, to show relevant variations across those groups.

It's Your Health

Important Epidemiological Terms

Measures of morbidity (illness):

Incidence—number of new cases of a disease during a given period of time/total population at risk

Prevalence—number of existing cases of a disease at a given point in time/total population at risk

Measures of mortality (death):

Mortality rate—number of deaths in a population in a given period of time/total population

Within the field of epidemiology, health education and health promotion are two important public health concepts. Health education consists of efforts to improve people's knowledge and awareness about health. Health education can focus on teaching individuals, communities, or entire populations. Health education can cover any health-related topic, including prenatal care, improving physical fitness, or recognizing signs of stroke. Health promotion focuses on getting people to change their behavior. Health promotion includes health education as well as policies designed to improve the public health. (New York City's ban of trans fats in foods in restaurants is one such policy.) Health promotion deals primarily with lifestyle and chronic disease factors, such as smoking, drinking, use of primary care facilities, and sexual activity.

Many diseases and conditions are a result of lifestyle factors, such as poor nutrition or smoking, and are therefore preventable. Health promotion efforts attempt to allow individuals and populations to make informed decisions regarding lifestyle behaviors and disease prevention practices.

Prevention is practiced at three different levels—primary, secondary, and tertiary.

- **Primary prevention** involves reducing exposure to a risk factor that may lead to disease or injury. Primary preventive measures include healthful diet, regular physical activity, cessation of smoking, and safe sexual practices.
- **Secondary prevention** refers to early detection and prompt treatment of disease. Secondary prevention includes screening tools such as mammography and cervical cancer screening tests that detect disease before it spreads, thereby preventing further complications or disease progression. Secondary prevention also includes the use of medications and lifestyle behaviors to control chronic diseases that cannot be prevented.
- **Tertiary prevention**, which takes place once a disease has advanced, involves alleviating pain, providing comfort, halting progression of an illness, and limiting disability that may result from disease. It consists of rehabilitation in situations where a person can work on restoring certain functions, such as those lost after suffering a stroke.

Primary prevention is largely the responsibility of the individual. Secondary prevention requires both the guidance of the healthcare provider and the compliance of the individual. Tertiary prevention remains a goal of both healthcare providers and caregivers.

WOMEN AS A POPULATION

The population of the United States is always evolving. As this population changes, its health needs also change. Some of these developments are along racial and ethnic lines, such as the growth of the Hispanic and Asian American sectors of the population, as well as in the increased numbers of people of mixed racial backgrounds. By 2030, one in five American women will be of Hispanic heritage, and one in 14 will be Asian (**Figure 3.2**). Significant diversity exists among women based on age as well. By 2030, one in four American women will be over the age of 65.[4] Because a majority of the elderly population in the United States is female, the needs of the elderly represent a significant women's health issue.

Women's increased educational attainment adds to the diversity of the population. Educated women tend to be more knowledgeable in their decisions about health care. Differing education levels creates heterogeneity

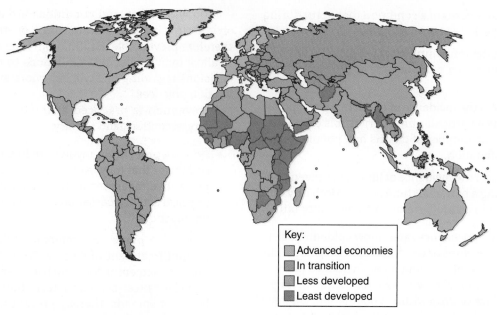

Figure 3.2 **World map: developed and developing countries.**
Data from The World Bank.

among women, because women with little or no education and women with advanced education may have different health and health education needs. The increased number of women in the workforce has presented new opportunities and challenges in women's health. Women work in a variety of settings, creating differences in their healthcare needs. For example, women working at home, in factories, in offices, in agriculture, and in retail will encounter different work-related health issues.

Another difference in the female population relates to the ways and stages of life in which women become mothers. Many women are delaying marriage and family to focus on careers, and thus are having children at a later age than they were one or two generations ago. This trend creates new issues surrounding childbirth, fertility, and parenting that impact women in their thirties, forties, and fifties as opposed to primarily young women in their teens and twenties. Other women are having children at younger ages, becoming teenage mothers. Many of these women are either raising their children alone or having their parents take a leadership role in childrearing responsibilities. Some women choose not to have children, instead pursuing careers and other opportunities.

Health needs of women also differ by sexual orientation. Health concerns specific to lesbians are often overlooked, leaving many women without proper guidance and medical attention. When lesbians share health concerns and risks with heterosexual women, misconceptions about the health needs of lesbians by healthcare providers and lesbians themselves may create barriers to receiving adequate care. Both lesbians and healthcare providers often believe that women who have sex with women do not need cervical cancer screening, routine gynecological care, or information about sexually transmitted infections (STIs), including HIV/AIDS. Other barriers to health care may include homophobia among providers and lack of health insurance coverage, because many lesbians are unable to share their partner's benefits or are eligible for less-complete benefit coverage than a spouse of the opposite gender would be.[5]

Incarcerated women face special health-related challenges. Many have unmet medical needs that relate to drug addiction, mental health, and reproductive health. Women in prison often lack access to regular gynecological visits, breast exams, and basic medical care. Many women in prison are survivors of physical and sexual abuse, putting them at increased risk for high-risk pregnancies, HIV/AIDS, hepatitis C, and cervical cancer. Pregnant incarcerated women face challenges to their health and to the health of their developing fetuses.

I had a bad experience with a former gynecologist after she found out I was a lesbian. She went from being friendly and chatty to stiff and formal. I felt so uncomfortable I started missing appointments. I'm glad I have a better provider now.

—31-year-old woman

Women with disabilities face unique challenges to their health. Physical barriers, such as facilities or examination equipment that are inaccessible or difficult to access, present major problems for these women in obtaining adequate health care. Communication barriers may pose a problem if a patient has visual, hearing, or verbal disabilities. Women with disabilities, as well as uninformed healthcare professionals, may believe that they are not at risk for sexually transmitted infections or other diseases. Many times, healthcare providers focus on the woman's

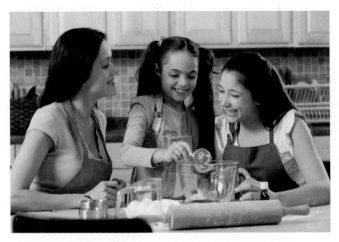

By 2030, one in five American women will be of Hispanic heritage.
© Jupiterimages/Cornstock/Thinkstock

disability and associated issues, rather than on basic routine healthcare needs.[6] Whether a woman's disability is a mobility, vision, hearing, speech, or cognitive challenge, greater levels of research, support, and compassion are needed to adequately address her health concerns.

GLOBAL HEALTH ISSUES FOR WOMEN

Standards of living vary greatly around the world. Traditionally, experts have distinguished between developed and developing countries (see **Figure 3.3**). Developed countries (Western Europe, the United States, Russia, Canada, Japan, South Korea, Australia, and New Zealand) have economies, health infrastructure, and standards of living that are significantly higher and more developed than those in developing countries (Latin America and the Caribbean, Eastern Europe, Africa, Latin America, and most of Asia and Oceania). In practice these generalizations do not always hold (countries like Mexico, Brazil,

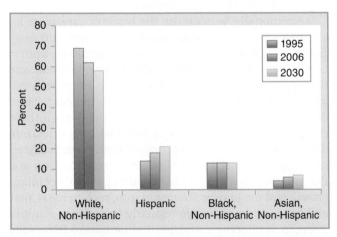

Figure 3.3   **Projected U.S. population by race and Hispanic origin, 1995–2030.**

Data from U.S Census Bureau.

and China have seen rapid growth and development, and standards of living may vary widely within a country), but as a broad tool, these terms are useful.

In developing countries, the health needs of women are extensive and often differ from the needs of U.S. women. The World Health Organization (WHO) lists 10 factors that account for more than 40% of the disease burden worldwide[6] (**Figure 3.4**). Major behavioral and environmental risk factors that contribute to death and disease worldwide include the following:

- Underweight
- Unsafe sex
- High blood pressure
- Tobacco consumption
- Alcohol consumption
- Unsafe water, sanitation, and hygiene
- Iron deficiency
- Indoor smoke from solid fuels
- High cholesterol
- Obesity

All ages are at risk for **underweight** (living below a healthy weight), but this condition is most common among children younger than 5 years of age. Unsafe sex closely follows underweight as a risk factor and is the major factor in the spread of HIV/AIDS. HIV/AIDS is now the world's fourth leading cause of death. It is estimated that 35 million people are living with HIV, 3.2 million of whom are children and over 15 million of whom are women. Two-thirds of women with HIV live in sub-Saharan Africa. Each year, about 2.1 million people are newly infected with HIV, and 1.5 million people will die from AIDS.[7] AIDS is a devastating disease. It primarily infects the adolescent and young adult sectors of the population—people who are parents, caregivers, and primary breadwinners. AIDS is wreaking havoc on already fragile health systems in many of the countries most dramatically affected. Over the past decade, the global community has organized an unprecedented campaign to fight the spread of HIV and to treat people who are affected. This effort has made enormous progress, but much works needs to be done.

Antiretroviral therapy (ART), though not a cure, can greatly increase the quality of life and life expectancy for people living with HIV. Yet, for years, these treatments were prohibitively expensive for most of the people living in the developing world. Recent efforts have mobilized billions of dollars to provide treatment and to prevent transmission of HIV; however, deciding how to most effectively spend these funds remains an important concern. Progress has been made in recent years getting medicine to pregnant women, dramatically decreasing the mother-to-child transmission rates. In 2013, approximately 70% of pregnant women living with HIV (970,000 women)

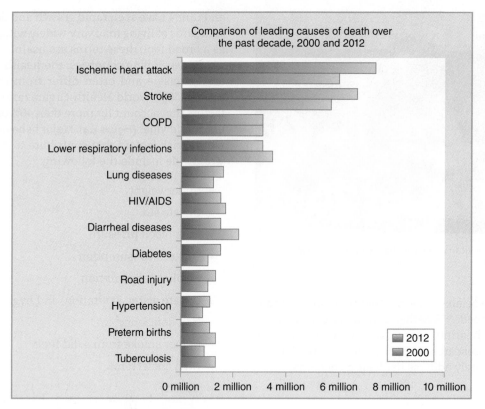

Figure 3.4   Global causes of death, comparison of 2000 and 2012.

Data from World Health Organization. (2014). Available at: http://www.who.int/mediacentre/factsheets/fs310/en/index4.html

received antiretroviral drugs, according to the WHO.[7a] Private companies are working with both **nongovernmental organizations (NGOs)** and governments to address the issue. The World Bank defines NGOs as "private organizations that pursue activities to relieve suffering, promote the interests of the poor, protect the environment, provide basic social services, or undertake community development." In wider usage, the label NGO can be applied to any nonprofit organization that is independent from government, including a large charity, community-based self-help group, research institute, church, professional association, or lobbying group.

Diseases caused or influenced by the local environment, such as cholera and tuberculosis, often occur when people do not have access to clean water or regular trash removal and lack regulations providing bacteria-free meat and food sources. People in developed countries often take for granted the infrastructures that make these systems available and reliable in their countries. In contrast, many developing countries have no system in place for sanitation and often use the same polluted water sources for bathing, drinking, and washing clothes. Parasitic infections from contaminated water and food sources are major causes of death and injury in countries throughout the world. Increasing access to preventive care, vaccinations, safe drinking water, and proper sanitation has been a primary focus of global health initiatives. Making this challenge even more difficult is the

fact that the developing world faces a chronic shortage of trained healthcare providers, particularly physicians.

Despite the very real differences between the developed world and developing countries, many health risks are the same around the world. Risk factors for mortality such as high blood pressure, tobacco use, physical inactivity, and overweight/obesity were once considered "diseases of excess," or problems that were only of concern in wealthy, developed countries. Over the past 40 years, however, these same risk factors have become the leading risks for death around the world.

Additionally, women are the primary caregivers for children and elderly family members globally. Although family composition varies from culture to culture, women consistently shoulder the burden of reproduction and feeding, clothing, and caring for children and elderly relatives. The health risks associated with motherhood in developing countries are many times higher than those experienced by women in more developed countries. Iron deficiency, one of the most prevalent nutrient deficiencies in the world, most severely affects young children and their mothers because of the high iron demands of infant growth and pregnancy. Sources of iron, such as meat, fish, and beans, are not always regularly available to families living in developing countries. Indoor smoke from solid fuels also primarily affects women because they are inside cooking for their families and working in the home far more often than men. In developing countries, about

700 million people—mainly women and children in poor rural areas—inhale harmful smoke from burning wood and other fuels. These and other factors put women at high risk for developing acute respiratory infections, especially pneumonia.[8] According to WHO:

> In some communities, inequality of girl children and women is the transcending risk factor that explains the prevalence not only of maternal mortality and morbidity, but also of higher vulnerability of girls to childhood mortality. Risk factors like malnutrition of girl children resulting in anemia, and early marriage resulting in premature pregnancy, can be traced to the fact that women do not enjoy the status and significance in their communities that men enjoy.

Barriers to improving women's health are often rooted in social, economic, cultural, legal, and related conditions that transcend health considerations. Social factors, such as lack of literacy and of educational or employment opportunities, deny young women alternatives to early marriage and early childbearing, and economic and other means of access to contraception. Women's vulnerability to sexual and other abuses, in and out of marriage, increases risks of unsafe pregnancy and motherhood.[9]

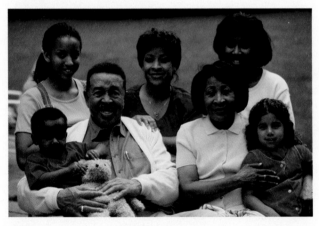

Health risks and concerns change as a woman develops from a child to an adolescent, from a young adult to an older adult.
© Photodisc

STAGES OF LIFE

Health risks and concerns change as a woman ages. Reaching women with effective health promotion, or even taking care of oneself as one ages, requires some knowledge of these differences. Accidents, for example, are the leading cause of death for women aged 10 to 34 but drop to the ninth leading cause of death by age 65. As women age, the risks for diseases also change, as do their consequences. Many factors related to age have indirect effects on health: Women in their twenties face very different social pressures, challenges, and opportunities than women in their fifties.

However, some factors remain constant at any age. Good nutrition, regular physical activity, and adequate sleep are essential for health at all stages of life. Healthy

living also encompasses avoidance of harmful substances, such as tobacco, drugs, and excessive alcohol. Mental health is equally as important as physical health. Maximizing mental health requires recognizing signs and symptoms of mental health threats, such as depression, drug or alcohol abuse, and physical or mental abuse. In addition, healthy sexuality and responsible sexual behavior are important for a woman's overall health. Healthy sexuality is expressed throughout life by exploring one's sexuality in adolescence, establishing long-term intimate relations in adulthood, and maintaining sexual pleasure in the senior years.

Health risks and concerns change as a woman develops from a child to an adolescent, and then from a young adult to an older adult. The risk of disease often varies throughout life, and, therefore, the methods of prevention differ depending on one's age as well as multiple other factors. **Table 3.2** highlights the major primary preventive measures that should be taken throughout one's life span.

Adolescence

The transition from childhood to adolescence is a time of major change. Adolescence begins with the onset of puberty and continues until the approximate age of 17, when adult physical development is generally realized. During adolescence, a girl becomes a woman and begins to form her identity and sense of independence. Parents should provide guidance and support during this time and help their children make appropriate decisions but should also encourage adolescents to learn on their own and begin to understand how to take responsibility for themselves and their actions.

Table 3.2   Primary Preventive Measures Throughout the Life Span
Avoid tobacco and other drugs.
Moderate alcohol intake to one drink per day or less. Avoid alcohol completely if you are pregnant.
Consume a healthful, balanced diet.
Participate in regular physical activity.
Learn appropriate and effective weight-management techniques.
Practice safe behaviors, such as using seat belts, wearing motorcycle and bicycle helmets, not driving under the influence of alcohol, and not riding with someone under the influence of alcohol.
Learn nonviolent measures to achieve conflict resolution.
If engaging in sexual activity, use condoms to reduce the risk of STIs, HIV/AIDS, and pregnancy.
Maintain an overall sense of well-being through stress reduction techniques, relaxation methods, socializing with friends and family, and seeking counseling if needed.
Balance work, school, family, friends, and time for yourself.

Puberty encompasses changes in nearly every aspect of development, from physical to intellectual maturation. During this period in life, girls begin to differ in appearance from boys. Secondary sexual characteristics appear, such as widening hips, breast development, height and weight gain, and body hair growth. Perspiration and body odor increase, and vaginal discharge creates a new awareness of sexuality for girls. Menstruation, the onset of a woman's reproductive capability, also begins. As these changes occur, adolescents begin to separate from their parents and assume greater independence. Teens may display rebelliousness, with friends often influencing decision making. Peer pressure also affects self-esteem and self-perception. Adolescent girls often focus on and define themselves through their relationships with both friends and romantic interests. Their concerns often revolve around popularity, attractiveness, and body weight. They face many challenges as they adjust to their sexual maturation and their increased independence.[10]

Table 3.3	Leading Causes of Death for U.S. Females Aged 10–24		
Rank	**10–14**	**15–19**	**20–24**
1	Unintentional injuries 26.2%	Unintentional injuries 42.1%	Unintentional injuries 39.9%
2	Cancer 15.6%	Suicide 12.4%	Suicide 10.3%
3	Birth defects 7.6%	Cancer 8.4%	Cancer 8.3%
4	Suicide 7.4%	Homicide 7.9%	Homicide 7.9%
5	Heart disease 4.7%	Heart disease 3.2%	Heart disease 4.6%
6	Homicide 4.4%	Birth defects 2.6%	Pregnancy complications 2.9%
7	Chronic lower respiratory diseases 2.5%	Pregnancy complications 1.2%	Birth defects 1.7%
8	Influenza & pneumonia 2.1%	Stroke 1.0%	Influenza & pneumonia 1.5%
9	Stroke 1.7%	Benign neoplasms (9) 0.9%	Stroke 1.1%
10	Diabetes 1.3%	Influenza & pneumonia (9) 0.9%	Septicemia (10) 1.0% Diabetes (10) 1.0%

Note: Numbers in parentheses indicate tied rankings.

Source: Centers for Disease Control and Prevention. http://www.cdc.gov/Women/lcod/.

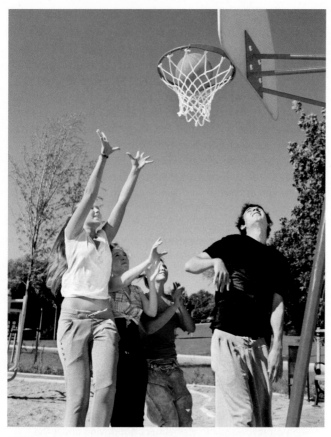

Adolescence is a time when friends become an important influence in a girl's life.
© Anatoliy Samara/Shutterstock

Specific Health Concerns for Adolescents

Adolescence is generally a healthy time of life, especially for young women. In the United States, the top four causes of death for females ages 15 to 19 are accidents (unintentional injuries), cancer, assault, and suicide (see **Table 3.3**). Mortality rates for boys in the same age group are more than twice as high as for girls.[11] Behaviors such as not using seat belts, not wearing motorcycle and bicycle helmets, riding with a driver who has been drinking alcohol, and driving after drinking alcohol are responsible for many of the injuries that result in death. Homicide is the third leading cause of death for adolescents ages 15 to 19 years and the sixth leading cause of death for adolescents ages 10 to 14 years.[10] On average, guns kill 10 to 12 children (ages 0–19) in the United States every day. About 25% of these children and teenagers take their own lives, while the other deaths are homicides or unintentional injuries. In contrast, in the developing world, major health issues for young people typically involve infections, diarrheal diseases, and other communicable diseases like tuberculosis.

It's Your Health

Challenges of Adolescence

Increased independence from parents

Adjustment to sexual maturation

Establishment of new and changing relationships with peers

Decisions regarding educational and career goals

Developing a sense of self-identity

Coping with stress

Threats During Adolescence

Smoking and substance abuse

Sexually transmitted diseases, including HIV/AIDS

Pregnancy and decisions regarding keeping the baby or having an abortion

Unhealthy eating behaviors and poor body image leading to eating disorders

Unhealthy quest for thinness

Mental health, anxiety, depression, and suicide

Source: Crockett, L. J., & Crouter, A. C., eds. (2014). *Pathways through adolescence: Individual development in relation to social contexts.* Philadelphia: Psychology Press.

Although many adolescents display moody behavior and signs of rebelliousness (normal behaviors during the teenage years), this should not be confused with depression, a significant concern during adolescence. As girls reach adolescence, there is a noted increase in the rate of depression and the rate of suicide attempts. At any given time, between 10 and 15% of children and adolescents have some symptoms of depression, with approximately 11% having a depressive disorder by age 18.[10a] After age 15, depression is twice as common in girls and women as in boys and men.[11] Suicide is the second leading cause of death for adolescents girls ages 15–19 years and the third leading cause of death for younger adolescents.[10] A national survey found that 14% of high school students have seriously considered attempting suicide and 7% of students had attempted suicide. Of the students surveyed, girls were more likely than boys to have considered attempting suicide (17% versus 10%) and more likely to actually attempt suicide (8% versus 5%).[12]

Trying new behaviors during adolescence is essential for healthy development; however, risky behaviors, such as sexual experimentation or drug and alcohol abuse, may have dangerous, life-altering consequences. Sexual relations often occur before adolescents have experience and skills in self-protection and in setting and expressing the kinds of behaviors they feel comfortable with, before they have acquired adequate information about sexually transmitted infections (STIs), and before they have access to health services and supplies (such as condoms). Almost one-half (47%) of U.S. high school students have had sex at least once, and more than one-third (34%) are currently

sexually active.[12a] Of these, 41% did not use a condom the last time they had sex, while 15% had had sex with four or more people during their life.

Of the female high school students who were currently sexually active and not using condoms, they are at high risk for various STIs, including HIV infection.[12] Approximately 3 million cases of STIs occur annually among teenagers.[13] HIV infection is the seventh leading cause of death among persons ages 20 to 24 years in the United States.[10] Chlamydia infection during adolescence is more likely to result in pelvic inflammatory disease and, potentially, lead to infertility. Some sexually transmitted infections caught by teenagers are carried throughout their life, like herpes virus, while others can be cleared with antibiotic treatment.

In addition to the risk of sexually transmitted diseases, teenage girls who are sexually active are at risk for getting pregnant. Although teen pregnancy rates dropped for much of the 1990s and into the 2000s, each year approximately 1 million U.S. teenagers become pregnant.[14] Increased condom use, the adoption of the effective injectable and implantable contraceptives, and the leveling of teen sexual activity are some of the factors believed to be driving this downturn in teen pregnancies. Young girls in developing countries also face risks associated with early sexual exposure, either recreationally or via early marriages. Practicing safe sex can be more challenging in developing countries, where girls typically have less access to health care and information. Globally, young people ages 15 to 24 account for approximately 40% of new HIV infections, and young women have HIV infection rates twice as high as in young men. They account for 22% of all new HIV infections and 31% of new infections in sub-Saharan Africa.[14a] In one study in Zambia, more than 12% of the 15- and 16-year-olds seen at antenatal clinics were already infected with HIV. Girls appear to be especially vulnerable to infection.

Adolescents may also engage in substance use, another risky behavior. Alcohol and drug use are detrimental activities on their own, but they also lead to other situations that may compromise one's health. The Youth Risk Behavior Survey, an annual national survey of high school students, found that 35% of high school students currently drank alcohol, and 21% had drunk five or more alcoholic drinks in a row in the past month. Almost one-quarter (22%) of sexually active students had had at least one drink the last time they had intercourse. Just over 10% of students had driven a car or other vehicle while drinking, while almost 3 in 10 (28%) had been in a car while the driver had been drinking.[12] In addition to direct effects on health, alcohol and drug use increase the likelihood that a person will choose casual, high-risk sexual activities.

Cigarette smoking, the cause of one in every five deaths in the United States every year, typically begins during adolescence, before it is legal to smoke and before the mind is fully capable of making rational decisions.

It's Your Health

Tattoos

The following advice has been prepared by professional tattooists working with local, state, and national health authorities.

1. Always insist that you see your tattooist remove a new needle and tube setup from a sealed envelope immediately prior to your tattoo.

2. Be certain that you see your tattooist pour a new ink supply into a new disposable container.

3. Make sure your artist puts on a new pair of disposable gloves before setting up tubes, needles, and ink supplies.

4. Satisfy yourself that the shop furnishings and tattooist are clean and orderly in appearance—much like a *medical facility.*

5. Feel free to question the tattooist about any of his or her sterile procedures and isolation techniques. Take time to observe the tattooist at work and do not hesitate to inquire about his or her *experience* and *qualifications* in the tattoo field.

6. If the tattooist is a qualified professional, he or she will have no problem complying with standards above and beyond these simple guidelines.

7. If the artist or studio does not appear up to these standards or if the person becomes evasive when questioned, seek out a different professional tattooist.

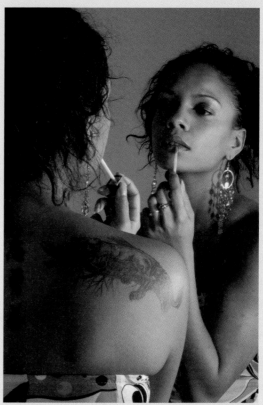

© Patricia Malina/Shutterstock

Source: Alliance of Professional Tattooists, www.safe-tattoos.com. Reprinted with permission.

Nearly one-half (46%) of surveyed high school students admitted to trying cigarettes and 20% had smoked in the past month. More than one-half (51%) of these students had tried to quit at least once in the past year.[12]

Overweight and obesity have steadily grown to epidemic proportions among adolescents over the past 40 years (**Figure 3.5**; **Table 3.4**). Increased consumption of high-fat, high-sugar foods, as well as reduced physical activity, appear to be the primary culprits behind this increase. However, this does not mean that American children and adolescents today are inherently lazier or less disciplined than they were in previous generations. Instead, epidemiologists believe the environment in which Americans grow up has made it more difficult to eat a healthful diet and to engage in regular physical activity. The CDC has identified many environmental factors contributing to child and adolescent obesity and overweight, including:

- Sugary drinks and unhealthful foods on school campuses
- Reduced access to healthful, affordable foods
- Fewer safe, appealing places to play and be active

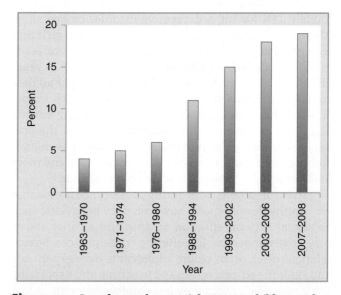

Figure 3.5 **Prevalence of overweight among children and adolescents aged 6–19 years.**

Data from Ogden, C., Carroll, M., Kit, B., et al. (2012). *Prevalence of Obesity in the United States, 2009–2010.* NCHS Data Brief 82. Hyattsville, MD: National Center for Health Statistics.

Table 3.4	Percentage of Obese and Overweight U.S. High School Students by Sex and Race/Ethnicity			
	Obese		Overweight	
	Female	Male	Female	Male
White	9.7%	16.5%	14.3%	16.9%
Black	16.7%	14.8%	22.8%	15.2%
Latino	11.4%	19.0%	19.2%	17.4%
Total	10.9%	16.6%	16.6%	16.5%

Source: U.S. Centers for Disease Control and Prevention. (2014). Youth risk behavior surveillance—United States, 2013. *Morbidity and Mortality Weekly Report* 63(SS04): 1–168.

- Growing numbers of high-calorie foods and sugary drinks
- Less daily, high-quality physical activity in public schools
- Increased portion sizes in restaurants, grocery stores, and vending machines
- Increased advertising of high-calorie, high-fat foods
- Lack of breastfeeding support
- Increased presence and use of television, video games, and electronic media

Obese children are at risk for type 2 diabetes, low self-esteem, and many other adverse health outcomes. In 2013, 13.7% of high school students were obese, and 16.6% were overweight. Nearly half (44%) of high school students were attempting to lose weight. Although male students are more likely than female students to be overweight, female students are twice as likely to attempt to lose weight. Female students are also more likely than male students to try to lose weight using dangerous, unhealthy methods (going more than a day without food; vomiting or taking laxatives; or taking diet pills, powders, or liquids).[12]

Tattoos and piercings have also become popular with adolescents and young adults. These activities hold inherent risks of infection and have been associated with serious complications. Increasingly, people are choosing to have body parts such as the lips, eyebrows, septum, or genitalia pierced, in addition to the more standard ear piercing. These piercings increase risks of infections, scarring, and nerve damage. Individuals can minimize the risks associated with these behaviors by choosing experienced professionals who uphold high safety and cleanliness standards. Some primary care physicians have ear-piercing kits and can perform the service in the safety of a clinical setting. Anyone getting either a piercing or a tattoo should be fully sober, both for safety reasons and to ensure this permanent decision is made with a clear mind.

Preventive Behaviors

Behavioral decisions are by far the greatest influence on adolescent health. Harmful behaviors include smoking, alcohol and drug use, unhealthy dietary behaviors, inadequate physical activity, and risky sexual behaviors. Many of them are contributing factors to major killers among other age groups, such as heart disease, cancer, and injuries.

Regular physical activity and good nutrition are two especially important aspects of health promotion for adolescents. However, comparatively few young Americans are engaging in these behaviors, despite their numerous, well-documented benefits. Just over one-third (37%) of U.S. high school students met the recommended levels of physical activity (were active for a total of 60 minutes or more for at least 5 days in the past week). A roughly equal percentage of high school students watch 3 or more hours of television a day. Nationwide, 23% of high school students do not exercise for 1 hour or more on any given day in the past week.[12] Female students are significantly less likely than male students to be physically active. Only 22% of high school students eat five servings of fruits and vegetables per day. Almost one-third (30%) of students drink at least one can of soft drinks per day.[12]

Although all of the essential nutrients are important for good health, calcium is especially important for adolescent girls. Girls need to consume enough calcium to develop good bone health and protect themselves from osteoporosis in their later years. Unfortunately, many adolescent girls become concerned about their widening hips and weight gain and consequently follow diets that lack sufficient nutrients. The average calcium intake of adolescent girls is about 800 mg per day, just two-thirds of the Recommended Dietary Allowance for adolescents of 1200 mg per day.[16] Millions of teenage girls face even greater long-term consequences when they develop eating disorders as a result of poor body image, unhealthy eating habits, and dangerous purging behaviors.

Heavy sun exposure during early life has been strongly correlated with an increased lifetime incidence of both **melanoma** and **nonmelanoma** skin cancers. Tanned skin remains fashionable, however, and many teenagers and young adults regularly visit beaches or tanning salons. A major study of more than 10,000 young people found that sunscreen use was low (about 35%) but was likely to be higher among girls than boys. Eighty-three percent of survey respondents reported a recent sunburn, and 36% of respondents reported three or more sunburns. About one-tenth of teenagers indicated use of tanning beds. This use was mostly among girls and increased as the girls approached age 18.[17]

Generally, adolescence is a period of good health; however, millions of teens experience the health concerns mentioned here. In addition, behaviors started during adolescence can become habits that continue throughout life. Therefore, adolescence is an excellent time for

It's Your Health

Safe Piercing

Here are 10 things to look for that will help you choose a safe piercer or piercing studio.

1. Cleanliness: A good studio should have a separate counter, waiting room, piercing room, bathroom, and an enclosed sterilizing room. All of these, as well as studio staff, should be neat and clean.

2. An autoclave and spore tests: Studios should have an autoclave (a steam sterilizer) and a spore test to check whether the autoclave is working correctly. Chemical soaks or "dry heat" systems do not provide adequate sterilization.

3. Single-use needles: Needles should be opened while you are present, as well as individually packaged, sterile, and single-use. Used needles should go into an approved sharps container.

4. Good piercing room practices: Ideally, watch the piercer prepare for the piercing. Beforehand, the piercer should wash his or her hands and then wear latex gloves, changing gloves if he or she touches anything nonsterile.

5. No ear-piercing guns: In many cases, ear-piercing guns cannot be adequately sterilized.

6. Knowledgeable staff: Ask the staff questions. Do they seem knowledgeable and friendly? How long has the piercer been doing his or her job? Does he or she seem well informed?

7. An after-care sheet: Studios should have a sheet that explains how to best take care of your new piercing. Make sure this sheet is up to industry standards.

8. Listen to your instincts (and friends): Have your friends had experience with a given studio or piercer? What did they think, and how does their piercing look? Do you feel comfortable with the studio/piercer? If not, go somewhere else.

9. A license: States and cities have different requirements for a studio or piercer, usually requiring regular inspections. Call your local health department to find the standards in your area.

10. APP recognition: Studios or piercers that have joined the Association of Professional Piercers have agreed to standards of cleanliness and jewelry quality set forth by the organization. APP members should have a membership certificate displayed on the premises; make sure this certificate is up to date.

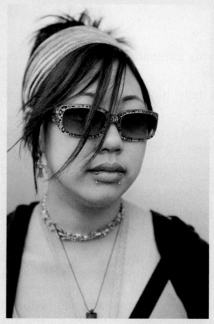

© IS Stock/Valueline/Thinkstock

young men and women, with guidance from their parents and healthcare providers, to make healthful and sensible choices about their own lives and behaviors (**Table 3.5**).

Young Adulthood

As adolescents become adults, they generally become independent of their parents and gain rights that were not afforded to them as children. Yet, the age of adulthood is often confusing considering that one can vote and can enlist in the military service at the age of 18, yet cannot legally drink alcohol until age 21. In addition, postsecondary school and the high financial burdens associated with advanced education keep many people at least partially dependent on their parents well into their twenties. Nevertheless, as a woman ages, her increased independence and age bring new health challenges and risks.

For some women, the first stage of young adulthood occurs in college. College can be an extension of

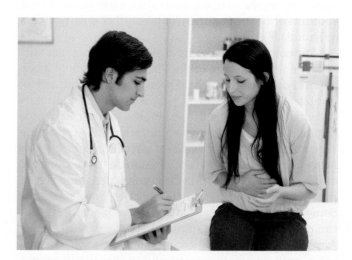

Many young women avoid routine health examinations.
© wavebreakmedia ltd/Shutterstock

Table 3.5	**Secondary Preventive Measures for Adolescents**

Pap test 3 years after onset of sexual activity or by age 21.

Annual STI screening for sexually active adolescents.

HIV screening for high-risk adolescents with their consent.

Annual preventive services visit to screen for depression, risk of suicide, abuse (emotional, physical, and sexual), eating disorders, learning or school problems, and drug use.

Physical exam recommended at least once between ages 11 and 14, once between 15 and 17, and once between 18 and 21.

Annual screening for high blood pressure, cholesterol (if risk factors are present), and tuberculin test (PPD) if risk factors are present.

Annual screening for anemia if any of the following risk factors are present: heavy menstruation, chronic weight loss, nutritional deficit, or excessive athletic activity.

adolescence in the sense that many women continue to experiment with new behaviors and explore their sense of self. Some use the freedom of being away from home to engage in behaviors that were not permitted in high school. Young women experience many of the same health threats that affect them as adolescents, including drug and alcohol use, smoking, violence (such as date rape), risky sexual behaviors, poor nutrition, and lack of exercise. Different health challenges face women who graduate from high school and then directly enter the workforce or begin parenting, as well as women after graduation from college.

SPECIFIC HEALTH CONCERNS FOR YOUNG ADULTS

For women between the ages of 15 and 24, accidents, assault, and suicide are the top three causes of death, followed by heart disease and cancer. Many accidents can be avoided. (See **It's Your Health** on texting and driving.) As women reach

It's Your Health

Texting and Driving

A major cause of injury and death in adolescence is motor vehicle crashes. In recent years, texting while driving has become a common and dangerous habit among many teens.

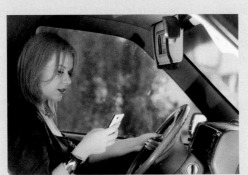

© Voyagerix/Shutterstock

According to a recent article, "About 80% of US teens aged 16 to 17 years own a cell phone. More than half of US teens have talked on the phone while driving and about one-third report texting and driving. Texting and driving is dangerous because it distracts drivers and takes their eyes away from the road. It is estimated that the minimal amount of time a driver's attention is taken away from the road when texting is 5 seconds, which, at a speed of 55 mph, equals driving about the length of a football field without looking at the road. It is estimated that teens who text while driving spend approximately 10% of driving time outside of their lane. The first year of having a driver's license is a high-risk time for crashes and texting while driving is estimated to increase the risk of a crash by 23 times."

There are several strategies to reduce texting and driving:

- Turn the sound off while driving, without alerts teen drivers are less likely to be tempted to text.
- Many states have laws against use of handheld phones while driving, or prohibit texting directly. (A state-by-state list is available at www.textinganddrivingsafety.com/texting-laws/.)
- There are also several anti–texting and driving mobile apps that aim to reduce texting and driving behavior. A few examples include Live2Txt, an Android app that blocks incoming texts and calls while driving and sends a message to senders that the driver cannot respond right now, as well as TXT Shield and AT&T DriveMode, two apps that use a global positioning system to monitor the speed of the car and shut down the phone's ability to text when the car is going faster than a certain speed, usually between 10 and 25 mph.
- Other groups are dedicated to texting and driving awareness, including Facebook, Twitter (@DistractionGov, @NHTSAgov, and @DriveSafely), and the following blogs: "From Reid's Dad," www.fromreidsdad.org/; Rookie Driver, http://rookiedriver.wordpress.com/; and End DD, http://enddd.org/.

Adults and teens can work together to cut down on this dangerous habit. Some families sign a text-free driving pledge, encouraging both teens and parents to put the phone where it cannot be reached when driving. Modeling safe behavior is important for all adults driving with teens.

Source: Megan A. Moreno, MD, MSEd, MPH. (2014). Texting and driving. *JAMA Pediatrics* 168(12): 1172. doi:10.1001/jamapediatrics.2013.3385

their mid-twenties, deaths from heart disease, cancer, and other chronic diseases increase. **Chronic diseases** (as opposed to **acute diseases**) are diseases or conditions that are permanent or semipermanent. They include heart disease and cancer, as well as diabetes, HIV/AIDS, and **autoimmune diseases**. Although chronic diseases are generally thought of as afflictions of the elderly, they are significant causes of death for all age groups; additionally, healthful behavior choices and prevention strategies begun early in life can often prevent these diseases from developing later in life or reduce the harm that these diseases cause.

Causes of death for young adult women vary dramatically by race and ethnicity. These variations are especially pronounced during the young adult years. HIV-related diseases are the leading cause of death for Black women ages 25 to 34, but only the seventh leading cause for Hispanic women, and the tenth leading cause for White and Asian American women in that same age group (see **Table 3.6**).[10] White women ages 25 to 34, meanwhile, are more likely to die from suicide or accidents than other women their same age. Black women are more likely than any other racial or ethnic group to die during these years, followed respectively by White, Hispanic, and Asian women.[10] Cultural, economic, social, and individual factors all contribute to these differences.

In developing countries, young adult women are at high risk from reproductive health–related disease and infectious disease. The top causes of death for young adult women in developing countries in this age group are six infectious diseases:

- Pneumonia
- Tuberculosis
- Diarrheal diseases
- Malaria
- Measles
- HIV/AIDS

Young adulthood can be rewarding as well as stressful. During this time, many women seek or develop long-term intimate relationships. They may start a family and have children. Women may be defining their career path, advancing within their career, or still searching for the right career. Many women face obstacles along the way, such as a lack of adequate child care and the juggling of family and work responsibilities. As women with disabilities enter the workforce, they may encounter new challenges, including discrimination from employers and employees, difficulty moving throughout the workplace, and adjustment to new tasks. Some women find it difficult to cope as their friends transition into different stages of life while they feel as if they are standing still. Managing stress and maintaining emotional well-being are important for achieving a healthy perspective.

Although women and men report similar levels of stress, causes of stress and coping mechanisms often differ between women and men. A study of 1600 Americans found that women are more apt to attribute stress to family and health issues than are men. Most women surveyed (52%) were personally concerned about the effect of stress on their health and 30% (versus 24% of men) said that they found it "very challenging" to manage the stress and tension they confront. Men were more likely than women to report watching more television (42% versus 36%) and drinking alcohol (29% versus 18%) as a way of dealing with the stress in their lives. Women report either increased eating of "comfort foods" or decreased contact with the stressor as common strategies of coping.[18]

Table 3.6   Leading Causes of Death for U.S. Females Aged 25–44

Ages 25–34		Ages 35–44	
Cause	Percentage of Total Deaths	Cause	Percentage of Total Deaths
1. Accidents	27.3	1. Malignant neoplasms (cancer)	25.7
2. Malignant neoplasms (cancer)	14.8	2. Accidents	16.5
3. Heart disease	7.9	3. Heart disease	12.0
4. Suicide	7.3	4. Suicide	4.9
5. Assault	5.8	5. HIV/AIDS	3.8
6. HIV/AIDS	3.5	6. Cerebrovascular disease (stroke)	3.4
7. Pregnancy and childbirth	2.5	7. Liver disease and cirrhosis	2.9
8. Diabetes	2.3	8. Diabetes	2.6
9. Cerebrovascular disease (stroke)	1.9	9. Assault	2.4
10. Congenital and chromosomal abnormalities	1.4	10. Chronic respiratory disease	1.4

Source: Centers for Disease Control and Prevention. (2010.) *Leading causes of death in females.* Available at: http://www.cdc.gov/women/lcod/. Accessed on: 1/20/15.

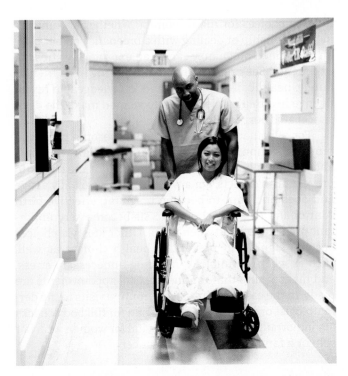

Women with disabilities often face condescending attitudes or discrimination when visiting healthcare providers.
© Photos.com

Alcohol and drug abuse affect the lives of many young women, including women who have children. An estimated 6 million children younger than 18 years of age have a parent who has used illicit drugs in the past month. Marijuana is the drug parents are most likely to use. Heavy drinking, defined as consumption of five or more drinks at one time on at least three occasions in the past 30 days, was reported by 5.2 million parents (3% of mothers and 14% of fathers).[19]

Young women deal with health-related issues associated with dating and sexual relationships, including sexual violence, STIs, and pregnancy. Consider these statistics:

- Almost 18% of the women in the United States have been the victim of rape or attempted rape at some point during their lives. Victims and assailants know each other in 80–90% of cases.

- In college, one in four female students is a rape survivor; experts estimate about 60% of the victims in reported rapes know their assailant.

- One-third of the 333 million global cases of STIs that occur every year occur among young people under 25 years of age.

- According to Planned Parenthood International, nearly 4 in 10 pregnancies are unplanned.

- The WHO estimates that between 8 and 30 million unplanned pregnancies result from inconsistent or incorrect use of contraceptive methods or from method-related failure.

Women who desire children may face fertility problems or other complications regarding pregnancy or childbearing. Infertility can lead to physical and emotional stress, financial burdens, and the anxiety and discomfort that often accompany fertility tests and treatment. Lesbians and women with disabilities may face disapproval from healthcare providers as well as friends and family members who feel they should not have children. Lesbians who want to have children may run into opposition or prejudice while they explore options for sperm donors or adoption agencies.

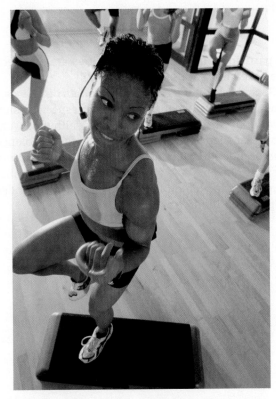

Physical activity is important for both physical and mental well-being.
© image100/age fotostock

Preventive Behaviors

Because many chronic diseases can be prevented or controlled by behavioral changes, a young woman should continue following a healthful diet, participating in regular physical activity, avoiding smoking and drug abuse, and moderating her alcohol intake. Secondary preventive measures, such as screenings for cancer, Pap and human papillomavirus (HPV) tests, and blood pressure screenings, are essential during this time as well (see **It's Your Health**).

As in all stages of life, positive mental well-being is essential for a young woman's overall health. Finding ways to cope with stress and addressing any mental health issues will help to establish a more balanced sense of well-being. Physical activity, healthy relationships with an intimate partner as well as close friends,

It's Your Health

Contributors to Improved Life Expectancy for Women

Identification, treatment, eradication, and control of some infectious and parasitic diseases

Better prenatal and antenatal care

More efficient, effective methods for assisting childbirth

Greater awareness, identification, and control of threats to health and ways to promote and maximize health

Improved protection from environmental and workplace toxins and hazards

and participation in enjoyable activities are all effective ways of reducing stress.

Sexual assault is a concern for women of all ages, but women in their late teens and twenties especially should be aware of this possibility. It is not healthy for women to consider themselves victims or targets for violence at all times, but education about how to avoid compromising situations and how to fight off an attack if it should occur can help women to maintain their independence and peace of mind.

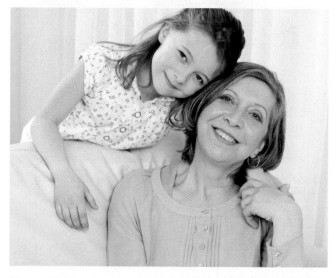

Many women no longer choose to begin their families in their twenties.
© CandyBox Images/Shutterstock

During this period of life, some women have multiple sexual partners or may be sexually involved with someone who has multiple partners. These women are at high risk for contracting STIs if they do not protect themselves by using latex condoms or other barrier contraception methods. Most sexually transmitted infections can exist with or without symptoms and, if untreated, cause infertility or other health problems.

Many women experience pregnancy for the first time in their twenties and thirties. Roughly one-half of all pregnancies are unplanned, causing anxiety and

difficult choices for many women. Whether a woman is in a relationship or dealing with a pregnancy on her own, an unplanned pregnancy can be an enormously stressful experience. Seeking advice and counseling from friends, family, healthcare providers, and knowledgeable reproductive health agencies can help women make the decision that is best for them.

For a woman who is planning to become pregnant, proper nutrition and consumption of essential minerals and vitamins like folic acid are important measures to prevent birth defects. For a woman who is sexually active and does not want to become pregnant, effective birth control and risk reduction for STIs become very important preventive health behaviors. Other lifestyle choices become significant preventive health choices as well, such as wearing sunblock, reducing unnecessary stress, and making sure that routine medical appointments are made. In the case of skin cancers, routine visits to the dermatologist or primary care physician for full body checks are important for all women, but vital for women with fair skin or a family history of skin cancer.

Midlife

Many women in their forties have completed their families and either remain at home or continue working outside of the home. Some have established productive careers, whereas others struggle to find and maintain a job with decent wages, advancement opportunities, and a satisfactory work environment. Women in this stage of life are often busy raising children, caring for elderly parents, and working to keep their relationships healthy. As they reach their fifties and sixties, many must deal with the mortality of their parents as well as their own aging. Some may be fearful of getting older, while others are looking forward to retirement. Some grandparents, often women in their fifties and sixties, are raising their grandchildren. The parents of these children, for various reasons, have left the responsibility of childrearing with the grandparent, creating a different dimension of aging for these women.

The recent economic recession, along with continuing high unemployment, has increased the number of students living at home while attending college and the number of adult children who return home after a divorce or loss of job. These "boomerang" children change the dynamics of life for many women in their middle years who assumed their children would grow up, leave home, and live as independent, self-supporting adults. Instead, many women must deal with a child at home again precisely at the time when their caregiver roles increase for their own parents.

Thanks to increasing physical fitness and greater access to effective medical treatment, many women discover midlife to be an ideal time to focus on themselves. They realize some of the benefits of the healthier lifestyles they have adopted over the past 20 years and consequently find their retirement years to be filled with physical activity, travel, healthy sexuality, and relaxation.

Specific Health Concerns for Women During Midlife

Between the ages of 45 and 64, the top five causes of death for women are chronic diseases. Cancer, heart disease, cerebrovascular disease (stroke), chronic obstructive pulmonary disease, and diabetes all benefit from behavioral changes (**Table 3.7**). In developing countries, the leading causes of death for women in this age group are a mix of infectious diseases, diseases of the reproductive system, and chronic diseases. Chronic diseases such as cancer and heart disease are increasingly dominant causes of death for women in this age group in developing countries as well.

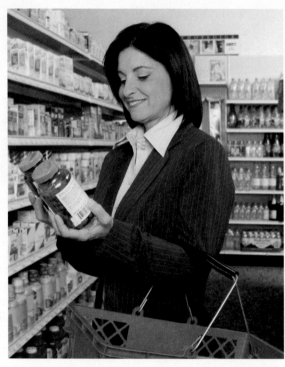

Significant controversy and confusion remain over the use of hormone replacement therapy and dietary supplements for perimenopause and menopause.
© Thinkstock Images/Cornstock/Thinkstock

Menopause, the cessation of the menstrual cycle, is a significant transition for women during their midlife years. For some women, menopause is a welcome change, eliminating their menstrual cycle and the need for contraception. Other women experience bothersome symptoms or more serious health concerns associated with menopause and have difficulty finding an effective therapy. Women entering menopause today are encountering more confusion than in the past due to recent controversy surrounding hormone replacement therapy (HRT). The controversy has limited the medical options for dealing with the distressing side effects of menopause. Women in perimenopause, the period just before menopause, may find themselves experiencing discomfort during sex or lack of libido.

Table 3.7	Leading Causes of Death for U.S. Females Aged 45 and Older

Ages 45–54

Cause	Percentage of Total Deaths
1. Malignant neoplasms (cancer)	35.8
2. Heart disease	15.3
3. Accidents	8.4
4. Cerebrovascular disease (stroke)	4.1
5. Liver disease and cirrhosis	3.1
6. Diabetes	3.1
7. Chronic respiratory disease	2.8
8. Suicide	2.6
9. HIV/AIDS	1.6
10. Septicemia (blood infections)	1.5

Ages 55–64

Cause	Percentage of Total Deaths
1. Malignant neoplasms (cancer)	41.0
2. Heart disease	18.1
3. Chronic respiratory disease	5.3
4. Diabetes	4.2
5. Cerebrovascular disease (stroke)	4.1
6. Accidents	3.2
7. Liver disease and cirrhosis	1.9
8. Kidney disease	1.7
9. Septicemia (blood infections)	1.7
10. Influenza and pneumonia	1.1

Ages 65 and older

Cause	Percentage of Total Deaths
1. Heart disease	28.7
2. Malignant neoplasm (cancer)	19.3
3. Cerebrovascular disease (stroke)	7.6
4. Chronic respiratory disease	5.8
5. Alzheimer's disease	5.2
6. Diabetes	2.9
7. Influenza and pneumonia	2.9
8. Kidney disease	2.0
9. Accidents	1.9
10. Septicemia (blood infections)	1.5

Data from Heron, M. (2010). Deaths: Leading causes for 2006. *National Vital Statistics Reports* 58(14). Hyattsville, MD: National Center for Health Statistics. Available at: http://www.cdc.gov/nchs/data/nvsr/nvsr58/nvsr58_14.pdf

Preventive Behaviors

As a woman ages, secondary preventive measures, such as mammograms and colonoscopies, become extremely important to ensure early detection of disease and, consequently, timely treatment. **Table 3.8** lists secondary preventive behaviors for middle-aged women.

As in other stages of life, maintaining mental wellness is a critical part of maintaining health. Women who are caregivers for children, elderly relatives, or both often find themselves suffering from severe stress, depression, and anxiety. Many of these women may see the effects spill over from their home life into their work life. Finding support groups, seeking professional help, and establishing time to take care of oneself are effective means for improving the mental health of many women.

Discussing options with a healthcare provider can help improve sexual functioning and desire, if necessary. Many women may still require contraception for preventing pregnancy or STIs if they are not in a mutually monogamous relationship.

The Senior Years

Over the past 110 years, the average life expectancy in the United States has increased by more than 30 years, from 48 in 1900 to 78 in 2010.[10] Public health initiatives are responsible for 25 of those years; all the medical advances over the past century have only increased the average life expectancy by about 5 years.[1]

On average, women live several years longer than men. The life expectancy for women in 2010 was 81 years, while the life expectancy for men was 76. Cardiovascular disease typically appears later in women than in men, accounting for part of this difference. In addition, women are less likely to engage in dangerous behaviors such as drinking to excess or not wearing seat belts or motorcycle helmets.

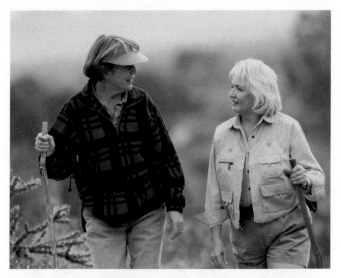

Living a healthy life from childhood on may lead to fulfilling and enjoyable senior years.
© Photodisc

Life expectancy also varies by race (**Figure 3.6**). In 2010, life expectancy was 81 years for non-Hispanic White women, 78 for Black women, and 84 for Hispanic women.[10] Social factors, rather than any biological differences between these groups, appear to be responsible for these differences. These differences shrink as women age. By age 65, the difference in life expectancy between

Table 3.8	Secondary Preventive Measures for Women During Midlife

Annual screening for high blood pressure.

Periodic height and weight measurement to monitor for overweight and obesity.

Clinical breast examinations yearly.

Periodic screening for high cholesterol levels, at least once every 5 years.

Behavioral assessment to detect depression and other problems.

Annual fecal occult blood test plus sigmoidoscopy every 5 years or colonoscopy every 10 years or barium enema every 5 to 10 years; a digital rectal examination should also be performed at the time of screening—for adults age 40 years or older with a family history of colorectal cancer and all adults age 50 years or older.

Annual mammography for women at high risk beginning at age 35 and for all women after age 50. Some authorities recommend screening mammograms every 1 to 2 years for women 40 to 49 years of age.

Annual Pap test or HPV test; after three or more consecutive normal exams, the Pap test may be performed less frequently in low-risk women at the discretion of the patient and clinician.

Counseling about the benefits and risks of postmenopausal hormone replacement therapy.

Bone density measurements for women at risk of osteoporosis.

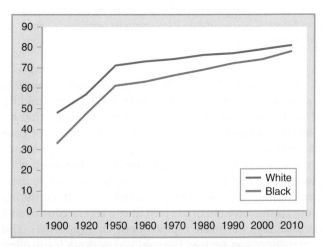

Figure 3.6 Life expectancy for Black women and White women, 1900–2010.

Data from Murphy, S., Xu, J., & Kochanek, K. (2012). Deaths: Preliminary data for 2010. *National Vital Statistics Reports* 60(4). Hyattsville, MD: National Center for Health Statistics.

non-Hispanic White and Black women shrinks from more than 3 years to 1.6, and by age 85, life expectancy for the two groups is nearly equal.

Increasing life expectancies have led to a "graying" of the U.S. population. Today, nearly one out of seven people in the United States is 65 or older. By 2030, one in four American women will be older than 65.[20] Furthermore, the fastest growing section of the population is people over age 85. In 2050, an estimated 18 million people over the age of 85 will live in the United States; in this year people in this age group will make up 4.6% of the U.S. population.[20] Because of their longer life expectancies, women constitute a majority of both these populations. The aging of the population presents a unique challenge to society, individuals, and healthcare providers, along with opportunities to allow this growing population to live healthier, more satisfying lives.

Health Concerns During the Senior Years

Women 65 or older face a spectrum of health issues. Some women remain healthy into their eighties and beyond, while other women struggle with continual health issues as they age. From the age of 65 on, chronic diseases are the leading cause of death for women in the United States (Table 3.7).[3] For women ages 65–74, the five leading causes of death are cancer, heart disease, chronic lower respiratory diseases, stroke, and diabetes. For women 75 and older, heart disease becomes the leading cause of death. As women's bodies grow more frail with age, Alzheimer's disease, influenza, and pneumonia become increasingly common killers.

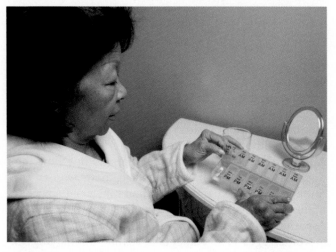

A major health concern related to aging is the side effects of taking multiple drugs.
© michellegibson/iStockphoto.com

Debilitating conditions such as osteoporosis and arthritis often make it harder for women over 65 to maintain their independence. Fall-related fractures are a major concern for anyone, but they can be extremely detrimental to a woman whose bone health is suffering. Arthritis can impede a woman's ability to perform daily activities, such as opening jars, lifting objects, bending to pick up an item that has fallen, or lifting herself from the toilet seat. A woman also may begin having problems with vision or hearing, creating new challenges in performing everyday tasks and maintaining independent living.

Women over the age of 65 often take multiple medications on a regular basis. The combination of these drugs may produce serious side effects. The risk of side effects is especially high for women who have multiple conditions or who take a medication that requires other medications to treat side effects it causes. Healthcare providers are not always aware of harmful drug interactions. Harmful effects of drug interaction may include abnormal heart rate and/or rhythm, depression, dizziness and impaired balance, constipation, increased blood pressure, and confusion.

Healthcare providers and other caregivers can also harm elderly people by treating them with a lack of respect. This lack of respect is not necessarily deliberate. It can include a nurse withholding medical information from an elderly woman on the assumption that a woman "won't understand" the information, or a physician who calls her elderly patients names like "dear" or "sweetie" in an effort to be friendly. Research has found that these kinds of habits reduce elderly patients' self-esteem and perceptions of themselves; these reduced perceptions in turn actually lower patients' life expectancies.[21]

The loss of a spouse and close friends may affect a woman's well-being as she ages. The number of women who are widowed doubles after the age of 65. Learning to cope with grief and loss is essential for physical and mental well-being. Maintaining independence and fostering social relationships may help women deal with feelings of grief, sadness, and loneliness. Diagnosable depression, however, is not the same as sadness, grief, or the emotional effects of loss. Depression is a significant health concern for aging women and may result from medication interactions, chronic disease, pain, or loneliness; it should not be viewed as a normal part of aging. The CDC estimates that 7% of Americans age 65 or older suffer from diagnosable depression in any given year.[11]

Women typically bear the responsibility of caring for their parents or loved ones when they need help. Women account for more than 80% of the family caregivers for chronically ill elders, and 73% of these women caregivers are 65 or older.[22] The value of services caregivers provide is estimated to be more than $350 billion per year. Some women may experience cognitive decline and depression as a result of being the primary caregiver for a partner, relative, or friend.[23] Healthcare providers also need to be aware of the possibility of abuse by a relative or caregiver and help provide protection when a woman is unable or is afraid to protect herself.

As women age, their skin becomes thinner, loses some of its elastic quality, suffers injury more easily, and heals more slowly. Women who have spent a lot of time in the sun during their lives may develop skin cancers at this stage of their lives. Most skin cancers can be removed

GENDER DIMENSIONS: Health Differences Between Men and Women

On average, a woman born in the United States can expect to live almost 7 years longer than a man born under the same conditions. Two major contributors to this discrepancy are women's lower rates of death from accidents and suicide. Accidents cause about 6.5% of total deaths for males, but only 3.5% of deaths for females, roughly half that amount. More than 2% of men, but only 0.6% of women, die from suicide.[11] Suicide and accidents dramatically reduce life expectancy because they typically happen while men are relatively young.

A man who dies at age 25 from a work-related accident reduces the average life expectancy for males far more than a woman who dies from a heart attack at age 70.

Compared to men, women are significantly more likely than men to die of stroke (6.7% of women's deaths versus 4.5% of men's deaths) and Alzheimer's disease (4.2% of women's deaths versus 1.8% of men's deaths), in large part because women are likely to reach the ages at which these diseases typically strike.[11]

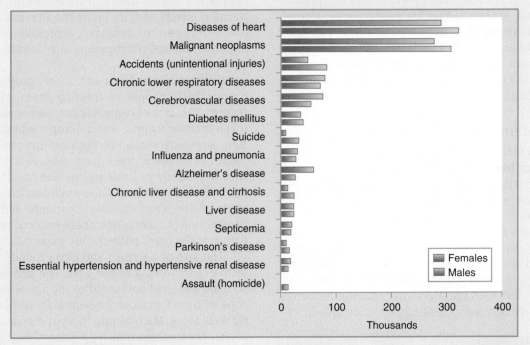

Data from CDC/NCHS, *National Vital Statistics System, Mortality 2013*. Available at: http://www.cdc.gov/nchs/data/dvs/LCWK2_2013.pdf. Accessed on: 1/20/15.

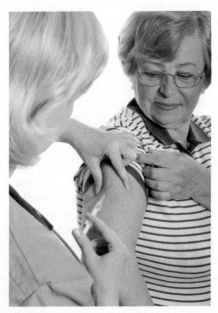

Flu immunizations significantly reduce the chance of an older woman getting influenza or pneumonia.
© Alexander Raths/Shutterstock

safely and easily with a simple procedure if they are found early. If left untreated, however, skin cancers can pose a serious health risk. Proper attention to skin care throughout life can prevent serious consequences as women age.

Sexuality also remains an issue for older women. Although many healthcare providers do not view their patients as sexual beings at this age, many women continue to desire sexual relations and may need advice for maintaining healthy sexuality as they age. An American Association of Retired People (AARP) study found that 61% of women ages 45 and older believe that "a satisfying sexual relationship" is important to their quality of life.[24]

Preventive Behaviors

The senior years can be a time of relaxation and fulfillment for women who are fortunate enough to have achieved financial stability, who have maintained their physical and mental health, and who are surrounded by loving family and friends. Other women may be less fortunate and experience considerable concerns regarding their future. Planning for one's future and maintaining

Table 3.9   *Secondary Preventive Measures for Seniors*

Annual screening for high blood pressure.

Cholesterol screening every 3 to 5 years or as recommended by the healthcare provider.

Periodic height and weight measurement to monitor for overweight and obesity.

Clinical breast examinations yearly or as recommended by one's healthcare provider.

Initial assessment of cognitive function and monitoring of changes as part of a routine preventive visit.

Behavioral assessment to detect depression and other problems.

Annual fecal occult blood test plus sigmoidoscopy every 5 years or colonoscopy every 10 years or barium enema every 5 to 10 years; a digital rectal examination should also be performed at the time of screening.

Routine mammography screening as recommended by the healthcare provider.

Periodic evaluation for hearing loss and visual acuity.

Thyroid-stimulating hormone test every 3 to 5 years.

Bone mineral density test as recommended by the healthcare provider; counseling on fall prevention.

Annual influenza and pneumococcal pneumonia vaccines.

one's health from childhood on may help women to have an easier time in their later years.

As throughout life, good nutrition, exercise, and avoidance of harmful substances can prevent harmful diseases and reduce their consequences in old age. Regular healthcare screening and preventive checkups are essential, as is continual monitoring for drug interactions and signs or symptoms that may signal a health concern. Additionally, women living in their senior years may wish to consider lifestyle changes, such as making safety arrangements to reduce the danger of falling, thus reducing their risks of accidents while maintaining their independence. Getting a flu vaccination and paying close attention to colds and minor illnesses can help keep a woman safe from pneumonia and influenza (**Table 3.9**).

Women should also take special care of their skin as they age, using proper moisturizers and barriers to protect against skin breakdown. In addition, women should get bone density screenings to make sure they are not at risk for developing osteoporosis.

INFORMED DECISION MAKING

To take personal responsibility for their own health and wellness, all women should educate themselves about their health status. Integrating primary prevention methods into one's daily life can improve both present and future health (see **Self-Assessment 3.1**). By understanding their own secondary prevention needs, such as the

appropriate screening methods for women at certain ages, women can better inform their healthcare providers about their health status and demand the healthcare services that they require and deserve.

The Internet has evolved into a valuable resource for health information. Yet the quality of health information on websites and shared through social networks like Facebook is extremely variable and difficult to assess. Evaluating the information can be a significant challenge, even for experienced users. Being able to identify the validity of the material in a given website is crucial, because it could potentially affect health outcomes for millions of people. Most online material is posted without any form of approval or review for accuracy and reliability, or it is posted by a company having a financial stake in the information being communicated (for example, pharmaceutical firms or physicians offering specific surgical procedures). Individuals must often rely on their own common sense and judgment. Keeping a critical eye and relying on trustworthy sources can help women find reliable information online. In addition, women should understand that open communication with their physicians is their right. Better communication between physicians and patients can improve both the quality of the care women receive and their health promotion knowledge base.

Self-Assessment 3.1
Rate Your Preventive Practices

Answer the following questions:

1. Do you eat a healthful diet consisting of the appropriate servings of fruits and vegetables, grains, protein, vitamins, and minerals?

2. Do you participate in moderate-intensity physical activity at least 4 days a week?

3. Do you get enough sleep so that you do not feel tired throughout the day?

4. Do you avoid using tobacco products and drugs?

5. If you consume alcohol, do you do so in moderation?

6. If you are sexually active, do you use condoms or other barrier contraceptives to protect against STIs?

7. Do you employ methods to reduce stress, find time to socialize with friends and relax, and maintain an overall sense of mental wellness?

8. Do you practice safe behaviors, such as using seat belts, wearing motorcycle and bicycle helmets, not driving under the influence of alcohol, and not riding with someone under the influence of alcohol?

9. Do you use nonviolent methods of conflict resolution?

10. Do you receive routine preventive care from a healthcare provider?

The more questions to which you answered "yes," the better off you are! If you answered "no" to any questions, try to change that behavior to achieve a better state of overall health.

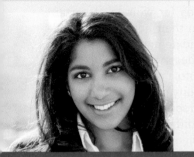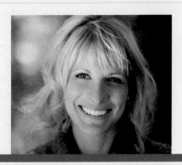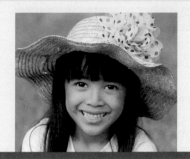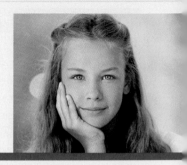

CASE STUDY

One of the most successful tobacco cessation programs ever created is a called The Truth Campaign. It leverages media to share messages about the dangers of smoking, the impact it can have on an individual's health, and the role of Big Tobacco in targeting youth. The campaign's goal, funded with millions of dollars from the Tobacco Settlement, is to prevent young people from taking up smoking and to help those who have started prioritize stopping. The campaign has been credited with lowering the rates of smoking among teenagers across America by leveraging innovating marketing, producing great ads, partnering with music venues and concert tours, and using social media to spread the word.

Meghan just started a job working for The Truth Campaign after finishing up college and working at the Department of Public Health for 3 years. Her new boss came in to her office a few days ago and explained that the most recent research showed that although smoking rates had dropped among teenagers aged 12 to 18, smoking rates were beginning to rise among young adults aged 18 to 24. Rates were especially high among young women. She asked Meghan to think up three strategies to target women in this age range.

Questions

1. What should Meghan think about as she considers how to target 18- to 24-year-old young women with an antismoking campaign?

2. What messages do you think would resonate? What are good ways to get those messages out?

3. Who would be good spokespeople for the campaign and why?

4. Why do you think smoking rates are rising in this age group? How would you go about answering the question of why?

■ Summary

Health promotion is the act of encouraging people to improve their health and maintain a healthy lifestyle. Health promotion may consist of an individual effort, such as a young woman learning how to protect her health, or it may consist of a large public health effort, such as a study to prevent deaths from lung cancer by educating teenagers about the dangers of smoking.

Health prevention may occur at the primary, secondary, or tertiary level. Primary prevention consists of avoiding a disease or injury, secondary prevention consists of early detection and prompt treatment, and tertiary prevention consists of managing a disease once it has advanced.

Global inequities in access to proper health care, including preventive services, medical treatments, family planning, or proper maternal and child health, threaten and reduce women's quality of life. These services are essential to women who seek to lead active, healthy, and happy lives at all stages of life.

Many factors, including race, age, and sexual orientation, influence women's health needs. Certain preventive measures, such as a balanced, healthful diet; regular physical activity; positive, healthy relationships; and avoidance of drugs, tobacco, and alcohol, are important for any stage of life. Other preventive measures, such as cancer screening tests, are recommended for women at specific ages. All women should take responsibility for their own health and wellness by educating themselves about their health status and risks.

Profiles of Remarkable Women

Margaret Chan (1947–)

Margaret Chan is the director-general of the World Health Organization (WHO), the United Nations organization that directs global health efforts.

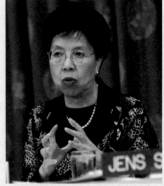

Chan was born in Hong Kong in 1947 and obtained her medical degree from the University of Western Ontario in Canada. She started working in public health in 1978, when she joined the Hong Kong Department of Health.

Chan became director of Hong Kong's public health system in 1994. There, Chan introduced initiatives to improve recording of and response to disease outbreaks, train public health professionals, and improve relationships between Hong Kong's public health department and local and international groups. She effectively managed outbreaks of avian influenza (bird flu) and of severe acute respiratory syndrome (SARS).

Chan's position leading public health efforts in Hong Kong required making difficult decisions on a daily basis. To avoid a possible outbreak of influenza among humans, Chan ordered the slaughter of 1.5 million chickens in Hong Kong.[25] Chan had no way of knowing at the time how many chickens were infected or whether the outbreak would occur. The decision to destroy Hong Kong's poultry population

© Rick Gershon/iStockphoto.com

also brought considerable economic consequences. But the consequences of a new influenza outbreak, both for Hong Kong and the world, would have been catastrophic. Today, many public health experts believe that Chan's actions may have prevented a global disease outbreak.

In a 2007 interview, Chan said, "In public health, especially when you're dealing with new and emerging infections, science is always lagging behind time and in the absence of solid evidence. But based on the best available information and evidence, one has to make difficult and often times unpopular decisions. Of course the recommendation … was a very difficult decision we took, but all in all, that was the right decision."[26]

Chan joined WHO in 2003 and was nominated as director-general in November 2006. Her first term ran through 2012; her second term will run through 2017.

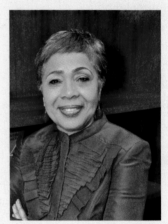

Profiles of Remarkable Women

Eleanor Hinton Hoytt

Eleanor Hinton Hoytt has served as president and CEO of the Black Women's Health Imperative since 2006. The Imperative is the only organization devoted solely to advancing the health and wellness of America's 19.5 million Black women and girls through advocacy, education, and leadership development. Before she joined the Imperative, Hinton Hoytt spent 10 years as the president of Hinton Hoytt & Associates. The firm provided strategic counsel to nonprofit organizations, foundations, and government agencies on effective organizational infrastructure, programs, and strategies for working with women of color. Before establishing this consulting firm, Hinton Hoytt was a director at the National Council of Negro Women, where she expanded their national presence as an active voice in women's health, including reproductive health and HIV/AIDS. She is a member of the Alliance for Nonprofit Management, has served as chair of the board of directors of the Avery Institute for Social Change, and is the founding chair of the board of directors of the Imperative (formerly known as the National Black Women's Health Project). Hinton Hoytt also produced the groundbreaking book *Tomorrow Begins Today: African American Women as We Age* for the National Council of Negro Women. She has received the NAACP's Thurgood Marshall Legacy Award and the Keystone Award for Women's Research Advocacy from the NIH Office on Women's Research. Most recently, she is the co-author of *Health First! The Black Woman's Wellness Guide*. The guide explores Black women's most critical

Courtesy of Eleanor Hinton Hoytt

health challenges today and features discussions with experts and the uncensored voices of real women—from adolescence through elderhood. The focus is on prevention and awareness, across generations and circumstances—from candid conversations about reproductive health and HIV/AIDS to frank explorations of Black women's top 10 health risks, including cancer, obesity, and violence.

■ Topics for Discussion

1. How can parents, healthcare providers, and health educators encourage adolescents to follow healthy behaviors? How can they convince adolescents that their present behaviors will affect their future health?

2. What are ways that smart phones are making us healthier and what ways are they making us unhealthier?

3. What are some ways in which you can improve your health? Are there preventive practices from which your parents can benefit that they are not practicing?

4. How do the health needs of women in developing countries differ from those of women in the United States? How are they similar?

5. What are some barriers to health care experienced by lesbians? What are some barriers experienced by physically challenged women?

6. Some health behaviors are detrimental to well-being. Should policies such as restricting smoking or mandating bicycle helmets be mandatory or voluntary? How should these decisions be made?

■ Key Terms

Acute disease

Autoimmune disease

Chronic disease

Incidence

Melanoma

Morbidity rate

Mortality rate

Nongovernmental organization (NGO)

Nonmelanoma

Prevalence

Primary prevention

Puberty

Secondary prevention

Tertiary prevention

Underweight

■ References

1. Steen, J. (2007). *The primacy of public health.* American Public Health Association: Community Health Planning and Policy Development. Available at: http://www.apha.org/membergroups/newsletters/sectionnewsletters/comm/spring07/primacyph.htm

1a. World Health Organization (WHO). (n.d.). Global health observatory data repository. Available at: http://apps.who.int/gho/data/?theme=country&vid=20800; Accessed on: 1/19/2015.

2. Finkelstein, E., Trogdon, J., Cohen, J., et al. (2009). Annual medical spending attributable to obesity: Payer- and service-specific estimates. *Health Affairs* 28(5): w822–w831.

3. Barrington, L., & Rosen, B. (2008). *Weights and measures: What employers should know about obesity.* New York, NY: The Conference Board.

3a. Goodarz, D., Ding, E. L., Mozaffarian, D., et al. (2009). The preventable causes of death in the United States: Comparative risk assessment of dietary, lifestyle, and metabolic risk factors. *PLoS Medicine* 6(4).

4. U.S. Census Bureau. (2014). *National population projections.* Available at: http://www.census.gov/population/projections/data/national/2014.html

5. Buchmueller, T., & Carpenter, C. S. (2010). Disparities in health insurance coverage, access, and outcomes for individuals in same-sex versus different-sex relationships, 2000–2007. *American Journal of Public Health* 100(3): 489.

6. Smeltzer, S. C. (2007). Perspectives of women with disabilities on reaching those who are hard to reach. *Journal of Neuroscience Nursing* 39(3): 163–171.

7. WHO. Available at: http://www.who.int/features/factfiles/hiv/facts/en/index8.html; Accessed on: 01/19/15.

7a. WHO. Available at: http://www.who.int/features/factfiles/hiv/facts/en/index8.html; Accessed on: 01/19/15.

8. Murphy, S., Xu, J., & Kochanek, K. (2012). Deaths: Preliminary data for 2010. *National Vital Statistics Reports* 60(4). Hyattsville, MD: National Center for Health Statistics.

9. Freedman, L. P. (2007). Practical lessons from global safe motherhood initiatives: Time for a new focus on implementation. *The Lancet* 370(9595): 1383–1391.

10. Benderly, B. L., for the Institute of Medicine. (1997). *In her own right: The Institute of Medicine's guide to women's health issues.* Washington, DC: National Academy Press.

10a. National Institute of Mental Health. (n.d.). Depression in children overview. Available at: http://www.wasd.k12.pa.us/common/pages/DisplayFile.aspx?itemId=631149; Accessed on: 2/22/16.

11. Centers for Disease Control and Prevention (CDC). (2010). Current depression among adults—United States, 2006 and 2008. *Morbidity and Mortality Weekly Report* 59(38): 1229–1235.

12. CDC (2014). Youth risk behavior surveillance 2013. *Morbidity and Mortality Weekly Report* 63(4). Available at: http://www.cdc.gov/mmwr/pdf/ss/ss6304.pdf; Accessed on: 1/20/15.

12a. CDC. (2012). Youth risk behavior surveillance—United States, 2011. *Morbidity and Mortality Weekly Report* 61(SS-4).

13. Lautenschlager, S. (2013). Sexually transmitted infections: Update 2013. *Praxis* 102(5): 273–278.

14. Santelli, J. S., & Melnikas, A. J. (2010). Teen fertility in transition: Recent and historic trends in the United States. *Annual Review of Public Health* 31: 371–383.

14a. UNAIDS. (February 2012). UNAIDS World AIDS Day report 2011. Available at: http://search.unaids.org/search.asp?lg=en&search=adolescent%20girls.

15. WHO. (2011). *Global HIV/AIDS response: Epidemic update and health sector progress towards universal access: Progress report 2011.* Geneva: World Health Organization.

16. CDC. (2011). School health guidelines to promote healthy eating and physical activity. *Morbidity and Mortality Weekly Report* 60(RR-5): 1.

17. Balk, S. J. (2011). Ultraviolet radiation: A hazard to children and adolescents. *Pediatrics* 127(3): e791–e817.

18. Adam, T. C., & Epel, E. S. (2007). Stress, eating and the reward system. *Physiology & Behavior* 91(4): 449–458.

19. Ward, B. W., et al. (2013). *Early release of selected estimates based on data from the January–March 2014 National Health Interview Survey.* National Center for Health Statistics.

20. National Center for Health Statistics. (August 21, 2007). Expectation of life at birth, 1960–2004, and projections, 2010 and 2015. *National Vital Statistics Reports* 55(19): 246–254.

21. Leland, J. (October 6, 2008). In "sweetie" and "dear," a hurt for the elderly. *New York Times.* Available at: http://www.nytimes.com/2008/10/07/us/07aging.html

22. Hooyman, N. R., & Kiyak, H. A. (1996). *Social gerontology* (4th ed.). Boston: Allyn and Bacon.

23. Gross, J. (October 14, 2008). Who cares for the caregivers? *New York Times.* Available at: http://newoldage.blogs.nytimes.com/2008/10/14/who-cares-for-the-caregivers/

24. American Association of Retired People. (2010). *Sex, romance, and relationships: AARP survey of midlife and older adults.* Washington, DC: AARP.

25. Associated Press. (November 8, 2006). Margaret Chan rose to prominence in Hong Kong's battle with bird flu. *International Herald-Tribune.* Available at: http://www.iht.com/articles/ap/2006/11/08/news/UN_GEN_UN_WHO_Chan_Profile.php

26. CNN. (April 16, 2007). Interview with Dr. Margaret Chan. Available at: http://www.cnn.com/2007/WORLD/asiapcf/04/13/talkasia.chan.script/index.html

PART TWO

Sexual and Reproductive Dimensions of Women's Health

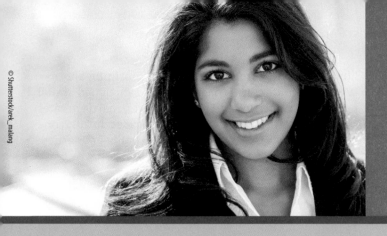

CHAPTER 4

Sexual Health

Learning Objectives

On completion of this chapter, the student should be able to discuss:

1. The ways that cultural values, stereotypes, and socialization define or influence sexual behavior.

2. The economic, legal, and political dimensions of sexual health.

3. The difference between sex, gender, and gender identity and the concept of gender roles.

4. Homosexual, heterosexual, and bisexual orientation and issues surrounding homophobia.

5. The location and function of the major external and internal female genital structures.

6. The three phases of the menstrual cycle.

7. The well-woman examination and the procedures involved.

8. The four basic phases of the female sexual response cycle.

9. Several examples of sexual expression.

10. Expression of sexuality throughout a person's life span.

11. Sexual dysfunction in women and its treatment.

12. The importance of research on sexual behavior and major contributors to this body of research.

13. Sexual violence as a public health problem.

14. The significance of communication in intimate relationships and with a woman's healthcare provider.

INTRODUCTION

Sexual health refers to the physical, psychological, social, cultural, and emotional facets of sexual human interactions. The World Health Organization (WHO) defines sexual health as:

> A state of physical, emotional, mental and social well-being related to sexuality; it is not merely the absence of disease, dysfunction or infirmity. Sexual health requires a positive and respectful approach to sexuality and sexual relationships, as well as the possibility of having pleasurable and safe sexual experiences, free of coercion, discrimination, and violence. For sexual health to be attained and maintained, the sexual rights of all persons must be respected, protected, and fulfilled.[1]

Both scientific and psychological perspectives are needed to understand sexual health. Sexual health entails the need for responsible sexual behavior to avoid sexually transmitted infections (STIs); unintended pregnancy; and sexual abuse, coercion, or violence. Positive sexuality requires thoughtful and respectful discussion of issues that may be difficult or awkward for some people to talk about. Learning about the physical and emotional aspects of sexuality and respecting the variations in sexual preferences and expression can improve sexual health and responsible sexual behavior.

CULTURAL AND RELIGIOUS PERSPECTIVES ON SEXUALITY

Cultural values often influence sexual behavior and how men and women interact sexually. The structure of various societies affects sexuality in many ways by creating normative sex roles, accepted types of sexual activity, preferences for sexual arousal, and sanctions and prohibitions on sexual behavior. One consistent theme exists,

however, that of "marriage" in some form or another. Within all cultures, marriage provides sanctioned sexual privileges. In the United States, however, marriage rates have been declining over the past 4 decades. In 2012, one in five adults ages 25 and older had never been married, compared with one in 10 adults in 1960.[2]

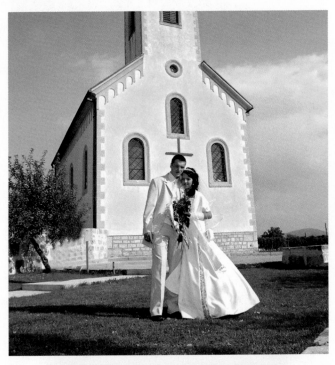

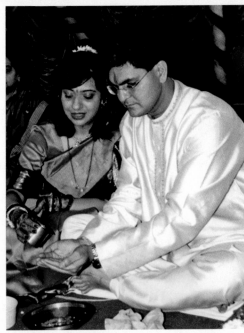

Marriage is a central social underpinning of most societies.
(top) © PhotoCreate/Shutterstock; (bottom) Courtesy of Therese Connell

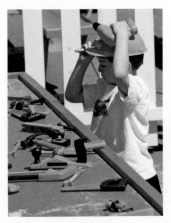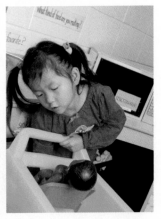

Society influences how boys and girls think, act, and express themselves as they grow up.
(left) © jcamilobernal/iStockphoto.com; (right) © ktaylorg/iStockphoto.com

Some cultures have strong values warning against premarital sex. People, especially women, who participate in sexual activity before marriage bring shame to themselves and their families, and they may be ostracized from their communities. Other cultures insist on modesty and sexual restraint for females but have a greater acceptance for male sexual behavior. Many cultures stigmatize the open display of certain behaviors, such as relationships with same-sex partners, while offering greater acceptance for those behaviors as long as they occur behind closed doors. Other cultural influences extend into contraceptive decision making. Some cultures consider it acceptable for a woman to decide what form of birth control to use, as well as to purchase condoms and ask her partner to use them. In other cultures, men take charge of this decision and consider it disrespectful for a woman to mention the use of contraception to her partner. The tremendous cultural diversity in the United States results in a spectrum of perspectives, values, and messages to women about sexual practices.

Economic Dimensions

Historically, marriage was not simply the union of two people but a formal arrangement made for financial, political, or social reasons between two families or within society as a whole. Whereas many marriages are now a celebration of the romantic bond between two people, other unions continue to be for reasons other than love. In some cultures, lengthy financial transactions taking the form of a bride-price or dowry are still common.

Throughout history, and even today in some parts of the world, the value of a bride often depends on her virginity. A girl who has lost her virginity before marriage, either willingly or unwillingly, can be seen as less valuable to both her family and the groom's family she is entering. In the United States and other Western countries, it has become extremely common for young women to have sex before marriage, though rates for U.S. teens ever having sexual intercourse have decreased over the past 20 years. In 1991, 54% of U.S. high school students surveyed had ever had sexual intercourse, while in 2013,

46% of students had ever had sexual intercourse. Rates for teens ever having sexual intercourse have not changed much since 2001[3] (**Figure 4.1**).

Sexuality can be viewed within a frame of power and economic dynamics. The less power a woman has, based on either cultural or individual factors, the less able she is to control a given sexual encounter. Significant power imbalances, like those seen between rich and poor, educated and uneducated, and young and old, have been strongly associated with sexual violence and abuse. For example, within the commercial sex industry in Thailand, the highest incidence of sexual violence is documented between Western adult males and native girl sex workers under the age of 12. Social and economic factors that give men power over women can undermine women's abilities to say "no" to unwanted sexual advances or aggression. Educating men and women about healthful, mature relationships and about how women can empower themselves in relationships has helped reduce sexual violence and has given women greater power in contraceptive decision making.

One direct relationship between sexuality and economics occurs between a commercial sex worker, or prostitute, and a sex consumer. In this relationship, sexual acts, with prices attached to them, are delineated between sex workers and their clients. Some intellectuals have argued that prostitution creates the ultimate power inversion, whereby women take control of sexuality and reap the financial rewards of performing sexual acts. The reality for most sex workers is quite different. The vast majority of sex workers are working under some level of indentured servitude, with a male pimp typically taking a portion of their earnings in exchange for protection and limiting competition. Pimps are individuals who act as brokers and supposed protectors for sex workers. They often require their sex workers to perform sexual acts on them for free, and they use physical abuse and threats to maintain power in the relationship.

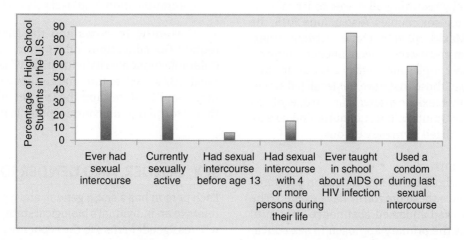

Figure 4.1   **Sexual behaviors among U.S. youth, 2013.**

Data from Centers for Disease Control and Prevention. (2014). Youth risk behavior surveillance—United States 2013. Surveillance summaries, June 13, 2014. *Morbidity and Mortality Weekly Report* 63(SS-4).

Legal Dimensions

Laws criminalizing sexual intimacy once existed in all 50 states. These laws were enacted to impose norms on the lives of the nation's citizens and, sometimes, to prevent sexual activity not intended for procreation. Cohabitation, or unmarried sexual partners sharing a living space, and fornication, defined as sexual intercourse between unmarried partners, were illegal in most states. Although these laws still exist in a handful of states, they are rarely enforced. Cohabitation is common today. By age 20, 26% of U.S. women have cohabited; by age 25, 55% have cohabited; and by age 30, 74% have cohabitated.[4] Sodomy laws, laws that define certain sexual acts as sex crimes, no longer exist in the United States. In 2003, the Supreme Court struck down state laws that ban sodomy, calling them an unconstitutional violation of privacy. Many sodomy laws had explicit rules, but courts typically interpreted the term to include any sexual act that does not lead to procreation, such as oral sex, anal sex, and bestiality; in practice, such laws were rarely enforced against heterosexual couples.

Same-sex partners face discrimination when it comes to legalizing their partnership. Marriages between same-sex couples are currently legal in only some countries around the world. The Netherlands was the first country to legalize marriage for same-sex couples in 2001. Other countries that have since legalized marriage for same-sex couples include Belgium, Canada, Spain, South Africa, Norway, Sweden, Iceland, Portugal, Argentina, Denmark, Uruguay, New Zealand, France, Brazil, England/Wales, Scotland, Luxembourg, Finland, Greenland, Ireland, and the United States. In the United States, Massachusetts became the first state to legalize marriage for same-sex couples. As of early 2015, 36 states and the District of Columbia had passed similar laws, meaning more than 70% of Americans lived in jurisdictions that permit unions for same-sex couples. On June 26, 2015, the United States became the 21st country to legalize same-sex marriage. The Supreme Court ruled that states cannot ban same-sex marriage, thereby requiring all states to issue marriage licenses to same-sex couples. Also in June 2015, the Supreme Court in Mexico ruled that laws restricting marriage between a man and a woman were unconstitutional. This means that gay couples may marry by court injunction in any state, even those that have not legalized same-sex unions. The only Mexican states that have legalized same-sex unions are Quintana Roo, Coahuila, and Jalisco; Mexico City also legalized same-sex unions.

Political Dimensions

Controversy about school-based sex education programs has been intense since these programs have existed. The federal government had endorsed abstinence-only until marriage (AOUM) as the primary approach to sex education starting with President Bill Clinton and continuing with President George W. Bush. Federally funded AOUM programs promote abstinence from sexual activity until marriage and limit discussion of condoms and contraception. In 2007, a congressionally mandated study found no statistically significant impact from Title V funded programs on the sexual behavior of young people.[5] One study of African American middle school students found for the first time that abstinence-only could be effective in delaying sexual initiation for some populations. However, the curriculum used in the study differed from the federally supported abstinence programs. Students in the study were provided with medically accurate information, given ways to resist the pressure of having sex, and educated on HIV; in addition, the curriculum did not negatively portray sex or advocate abstinence until marriage.[6] Proponents of AOUM programs have argued that comprehensive sex education might lead to an increase in teens having sex; however, research shows that comprehensive sexual education programs either delay or have no effect on initiation of sexual activity. Studies have also shown that teaching about contraception was not associated with increased risk of adolescent sexual activity or STIs; in fact, adolescents who received comprehensive sex education had a lower risk of pregnancy than adolescents who received abstinence-only or no sex education.[7] In addition, one large survey showed that parents support comprehensive sex education programs in public schools.[8]

In 2010, two provisions were included in the Patient Protection and Affordable Care Act (ACA):

- Congress renewed the Title V abstinence-only program run by the Administration on Children, Youth, and Families. The program provides grants to states for abstinence-only until marriage programs. States who agree to participate in the program must match 75% of the funds with state dollars.

- Congress created a 5-year Personal Responsibility Education Program to educate adolescents on both abstinence and contraception. The program also teaches about healthy relationships, parent–child communication, and decision making.

Currently, 22 states and the District of Columbia require sex education and 33 states and the District of Columbia mandate HIV education. When sex education is taught, 37 states require that sex education include abstinence and 18 states and the District of Columbia require that information on contraception is included.[9]

SEX, GENDER, AND GENDER IDENTITY

Each person has a sex, a gender, and a gender identity. Sex refers to an individual's biological status as male or female, whereas gender refers to the economic, social, and cultural attributes and opportunities associated with being masculine or feminine or a person's social and legal status as man or woman. **Gender identity** refers to an individual's personal, subjective sense of being male or female. Biological sex, along with many other variables, clearly influences gender identity; however, a person's gender identity is not necessarily consistent with his or her biological sex. Issues surrounding sex and gender differences in health have been evolving for the past several decades.

Biological Sex

The genetic material in a fertilized egg is organized within structures known as chromosomes. Chromosomes give rise to the process of sexual differentiation, whereby an individual develops distinct physical male or female characteristics. The physical femaleness or maleness is not just a result of this chromosome mix, however, but rather the result of processes that occur at various levels of sexual differentiation. In early prenatal development, male and female external genitalia are undifferentiated and will remain so unless a specific gene on the Y chromosome involved in sex determination is present and is activated. This gene is necessary for the development of the testes, and therefore is involved in initiating the male sexing process. Through a series of complex interactions involving gonadal sex hormones, both the internal and the external sex structures differentiate into male or female genitalia. Because the external genitals, gonads, and some of the internal structures of males and females originate from the same embryonic tissues, it is not surprising that they have homologous, or corresponding, parts (**Figure 4.2**).

Scientists have found important structural and functional differences in the brains of males and females. Sex differentiation in human brains occurs largely during prenatal development but takes place at a much later stage in development than sexual differentiation of the genitals. Sex differences in the brain and sex hormones contribute to differences in processes such as thinking, remembering, language use, and ability to perceive spatial relationships. Other gender differences such as sensory perception and emotional responses may also affect sexual behavior. Clearly, environmental factors and psychosocial factors can also affect these differences. It is premature to suggest which factors play the most important role in determining these female–male differences.

Intersex refers to a person who is born with sex chromosomes, external genitalia, or internal reproductive organs that are not considered "standard" as male or female. This condition can be manifested as a girl without ovaries, a boy without testes, or a child with genitalia that may appear as neither a vagina nor a penis. For intersex individuals, recent activism has drawn attention

> *I used to feel confused about what was feminine or what was masculine. I finally decided that it didn't matter. How I talk and dress, and what I do in the bedroom, are my business. That really does not make me less of a woman.*
>
> **—18-year-old student**

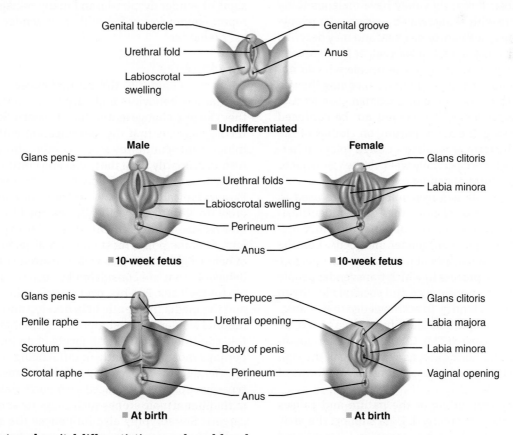

Figure 4.2   External genital differentiation—male and female.

to medically unnecessary childhood surgeries performed to "assign" a sex to an infant.

Gender and Gender Expression

Gender is often thought of in two terms: masculine and feminine. Gender expression refers to the "way in which a person acts to communicate gender within a given culture; for example, in terms of clothing, communications patterns, and interests."[10] **Androgyny** refers to having characteristics of both sexes but appearing gender neutral (or not specifically male or female). Androgyny has physiological, behavioral, and psychological aspects. Physiological androgyny describes an individual whose appearance suggests gender ambiguity; behavioral androgyny refers to the manner in which people present themselves, such as a male who displays traditionally feminine behaviors; and psychological androgyny describes an individual whose gender identity may differ from his or her sex. Androgynous individuals of both sexes are more likely to engage in behavior typically ascribed to the other sex than are gender-typed individuals.

Gender Identity and Transgender

Gender identity represents how people identify themselves. The traditional gender binary offers two identities: man or woman. Transgender is an umbrella term for anyone whose biological sex is not aligned with the person's sense of self or gender identity. People who identify as transgender often feel as if they've been born into the wrong biological sex; they may have male anatomy yet identify more with being female. Transgender people can be straight, gay, lesbian, or bisexual and may describe themselves as transgender, transsexual, or genderqueer. The term *genderqueer* refers to those people who do not fit within the traditional gender binary, meaning they do not identify with being a man or a woman. (See **It's Your Health**.) A transgender person should not be confused with cross-dressing, the act of putting on clothes of the opposite sex. The term cross-dresser often refers to heterosexual men who occasionally wear clothes associated with women as a form of gender expression.

Gender dysphoria is a psychological term used to describe a strong and persistent cross-gender identification. This term replaces the use of gender identity disorder when referring to transgender and focuses on the fact that distress is not inherent in a transgender person. **Transitioning** is the process in which transgender people work to change their appearance and societal identity to match their gender identity. To acknowledge their transition, transgender people self-identify as male to female (MTF) or female to male (FTM). Changes are often medical, via surgery and hormones, as well as legal, through name and sex changes on legal documents and forms of identification.

No clear understanding of the nature and causes of transgender has yet emerged. Data support the view that structures in the brain are sexually differentiated

It's Your Health

In early 2015, the University of Vermont recognized a third gender—neutral. The system allows students to select their own identity—male, female, or neutral—and choose a new first name if desired along with chosen pronouns. This enables professors to access this information in the university's information system and then use the correct terminology with each student. Activists on numerous college campuses are working toward raising consciousness of the existing social structures and associated language issues surrounding gender identity, resulting in gender-awareness campaigns around the country. Along with finding the correct language for one's identity and for the associated pronouns to use with that identity, transgender people face other issues such as which bathrooms to use, how to explain why their student ID or driver's license says a different gender, and receiving appropriate health care from providers who may not be aware of how to treat someone whose biological sex and gender identity do not conform. Many researchers have argued that gender identity should not be viewed as a male–female binary but as a continuum. The addition of gender-neutral options to the University of Vermont's information system represents a chance for students who identify as neither male nor female to finally be recognized and validated.

in a manner opposite to a transgender person's genetic and genital sex.[11] Children as young as age 3 can show signs of gender dysphoria, and many transgender people report feeling discomfort with their gender in their earliest memories.

Gender Roles

Gender roles refer to the cultural expectations of male and female behaviors and vary from society to society; they can also change as a culture develops. Social-learning theory suggests that the identification with either feminine or masculine roles or a combination (androgyny) results primarily from the social and cultural models and influences to which the individual is exposed from birth. Parents typically dress boys and girls differently. Children grow up with toys specifically designed for their gender and receive reinforcement for gender-expected behaviors. At some point, most children develop a firm sense of being a girl or a boy, as well as a strong desire to adopt behaviors that are considered by society to be appropriate for their sex. Parents, peer groups, schools, textbooks, and the media frequently help develop and reinforce traditional gender-role assumptions and behaviors. Gender-role conditioning affects all facets of an individual's life, perhaps most importantly in influencing sexuality.

Gender-role expectations and their resulting stereotypes have clearly influenced a woman's ability to succeed in traditional male arenas such as sports and professional careers. Stereotyping also influences the sexual health and behavior of women, who naturally find conflict with expectations that they be passive, submissive, dependent, emotional, and subordinate. Stereotypical expectations of men and women clearly influence gender-role expectations. These expectations hinder both men and women in becoming mature individuals and in establishing fulfilling relationships. Despite the constraints associated with rigid, stereotypical gender roles, many men and women behave in a manner that is remarkably consistent with the norms that these roles establish (see **It's Your Health**).

It's Your Health

Sexual Stereotypes of Women and Men

Women are undersexed, and men are oversexed.

Women are inexperienced, and men are experts.

Women are recipients, and men are initiators.

Women are controllers, and men are movers.

Women are nurturing and supportive, and men are strong and unemotional.

Women are sensitive, and men are insensitive.

Women are dependent, and men are independent.

Women are passive, and men are aggressive.

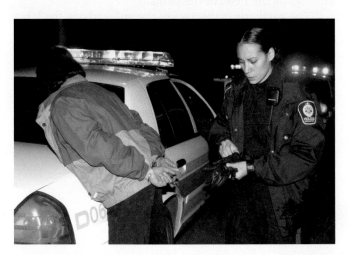

Cultural expectations of gender roles and behaviors evolve over time.
© Jack Dagley Photography/Shutterstock

SEXUAL ORIENTATION

Sexual orientation refers to a person's sexual and romantic attraction to other people, whether the attraction is to members of the opposite sex, the same sex, or both sexes. People attracted to same-sex partners refer to themselves as gay, lesbian (for women who are gay), or **homosexual**. People attracted to members of the opposite sex refer to themselves as straight or **heterosexual**. A **bisexual** person is attracted to both sexes. Although these concepts imply a clear distinction between the terms, the actual delineation is not always so precise. In Alfred Kinsey's landmark

studies in the 1940s and 1950s, he described a seven-point continuum that ranged from exclusive contact with and attraction to the other sex to varying degrees of heterosexual and homosexual orientation.[12,13] Although Kinsey's methodology and conclusions have been criticized, the continuum of orientation provides a model for understanding differences in sexual orientation. The presumption that most people are heterosexual and the idea that heterosexuality and homosexuality represent sharply distinct behaviors are inconsistent with the complex, often unpredictable arena of human behavior.

> *I am a lesbian. I am still "in the closet." I would like to be more open about my identity, but I am afraid. I still hear jokes and comments about lesbians from friends and family, like how someone "acts like a lesbian," or how shoes or an outfit looks "like something a lesbian would wear." I know they would say they don't mean any harm, but it scares me—and pisses me off.*
>
> **—27-year-old woman**

There is no profile that fits all lesbian women. They may be of any ethnicity, single, married, divorced, rich, poor, teenage, middle-age, or senior. The extent to which a lesbian decides to be secretive or open about her sexual orientation has a significant effect on her lifestyle. There are various degrees of being "in the closet" and several steps in the process of "coming out." These steps are usually incremental and include self-acknowledgment, self-acceptance, and disclosure. These steps are particularly difficult because of **homophobia**, an irrational fear or hatred of homosexuality.

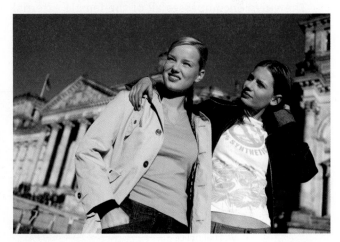

There is no profile of a lesbian woman. Women of all ages, classes, races, and body types are lesbians.
© bilderlounge/Yashoda/Alamy Images

Healthcare Needs of the Lesbian, Gay, Bisexual, and Transgender Community

Although people who are lesbian, gay, bisexual, and transgender (LGBT) are diverse, a common need exists for culturally competent health care and sensitivity from healthcare professionals. Misconceptions, stigma, and discrimination toward the LGBT community can result in missed disease, insensitive care from healthcare providers, and unfair treatment. For example, many healthcare providers, as well as women who self-identify as lesbians, believe that lesbians are not at risk for sexually transmitted infections, gynecological infections, or cancers, and therefore do not require contraception education, regular cervical cancer screening, or pelvic exams. Some healthcare providers do not address the issue of sexual orientation and assume that any sexually active woman of reproductive age should practice methods of birth control to prevent pregnancy. After encountering physicians who either ignore the facts or respond negatively, many lesbians hesitate to disclose their sexual orientation or even to visit a healthcare provider regularly. Recent focus on understanding the specific needs within the LGBT community has helped healthcare providers as well as patients begin to eliminate these disparities.

BIOLOGICAL BASIS OF SEXUAL HEALTH

Female Sexual Anatomy and Physiology

External Structures

Unfortunately, many females not only harbor misconceptions about their bodies but also are unfamiliar with their own genitalia. Gaining knowledge and understanding of how her body functions and performs is an important aspect of sexual health and well-being. One way to begin understanding female sexual anatomy is to examine the vaginal area with a mirror.

The **vulva** encompasses all of the female external genital structures, including the pubic hair, folds of skin, and urinary and vaginal openings. The **mons veneris**, or "mound of Venus," is the area covering the pubic bone. It consists of pads of fatty tissue between the bone and the skin. Nerve endings in this area are responsible for the pleasure sensations from touch and pressure. At puberty, the mons becomes covered with pubic hair that varies in color, texture, and thickness.

The **labia majora** consist of outer lips that extend downward from the mons and extend toward each side of the vulva. The color of the labia majora is usually darker than the color of the thighs. The nerve endings and underlying fatty tissue are similar to those in the mons. The **labia minora**, or inner lips, are located within the outer lips and often protrude between them. There are individual variances in terms of color, shape, and texture of the external genital structures (**Figure 4.3**).

The **clitoris** consists of an external shaft and glans and parts known as internal crura; its function is sexual arousal. The shaft and glans of the clitoris are located just below the mons area, where the inner lips converge. They are covered by the clitoral hood, or prepuce. Initially, it may be easier for a woman to locate her clitoris by touch rather than by sight or location because of its sensitive nerve endings and small size. The external part of the clitoris, although tiny, has about the same number of nerve endings as the head of the penis.

The vestibule is the area of the vulva inside the labia minora. It is rich in blood vessels and nerve endings. Its tissues are also sensitive to touch. Both the urinary and the vaginal openings are located within the vestibule.

The urinary opening is also called the urethral opening. Urine passes from the bladder through the body via this opening. The **urethra** is the short tube connecting the bladder to the urinary opening, located between the clitoris and the vaginal opening.

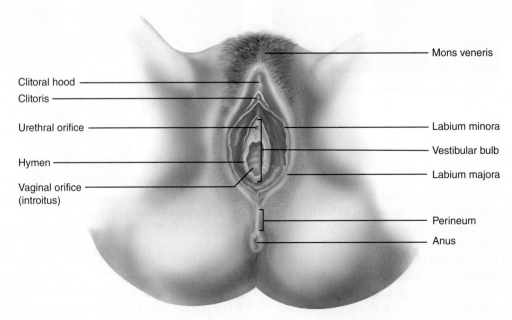

Clitoral hood

Clitoris

Urethral orifice

Hymen

Vaginal orifice
(introitus)

Mons veneris

Labium minora

Vestibular bulb

Labium majora

Perineum

Anus

Figure 4.3   **External female sexual anatomy.**

GENDER DIMENSIONS: Health Differences Between Men and Women

Role Conflict

Researchers continue to study role-conflict issues and challenges for women. Over the past 30 years, many women have assumed traditional male roles in the workplace, often becoming the primary breadwinners for their families; others have proven their abilities to succeed in areas historically associated with males, such as athletics. The migration of women into these traditional male environments has been largely studied from the perspectives, needs, issues, and challenges of working women. Researchers are appreciating now that women's entry into these domains has created significant disruption and confusion for many men.

Men with deeply entrenched expectations of gender roles for themselves are most affected. Traditional career men have more conservative gender-role attitudes for themselves and for women. They are more likely than other men to believe in traditional masculine ideology; as a result, they are more likely to experience gender-role conflict with their female colleagues, friends, and sometimes their partners. Adherence to traditional gender roles and the societal pressure to conform can lead to high levels of internal conflict and conflict with others.

A "traditional male ideology" typically includes three core beliefs. First, a man's work is the measure of his masculinity. Second, male power, control, and competition are the way to success and respect. Third, intimacy should be avoided. The more that men embrace these concepts, the greater their potential for gender-role conflict, and resultant stress and negative feelings, when females enter the workplace or assume positions of power.

Further research into the understanding of gender-role attitudes and beliefs will be essential to successfully integrate men and women into the work environment.

The vaginal opening is located between the urinary opening and the anus. The **hymen**, a thin piece of tissue, partially covers the opening. It is typically present at birth and usually remains intact until first penetration, although the vaginal opening is partially open and flexible enough to insert tampons before the hymen has been broken. Although the hymen may protect the vaginal tissues early in life, it has no other known function. Nevertheless, many cultures have traditionally placed great significance on its presence or absence. A common misconception is that a woman's virginity can be proved or disproved by the pain or bleeding that may occur with initial coitus. Although discomfort and spotting sometimes occur with first coitus, the hymen can be partial, flexible, or thin enough that there is neither discomfort nor bleeding. This very sensitive tissue also may stretch or break while performing activities such as bike riding, horseback riding, and gymnastics.

The **perineum** refers to the area of smooth skin between the vaginal opening and the anus. This tissue is rich with nerve endings and is sensitive to touch.

Internal Structures

Several structures lie along the vaginal opening. The vestibule refers to the area of the vulva inside the labia minora. The vaginal walls are lined with a vast network of bulbs and vessels that engorge with blood during sexual arousal, causing the vagina to increase in length and the vulvar area to become swollen. These bulbs are similar in structure and function to the tissue in the penis that engorges with blood during male sexual arousal and causes penile erection.

The **Bartholin's glands** are located on each side of the vaginal opening. They secrete a liquid that lubricates the tissues at the vaginal opening. The glands are usually not noticeable. Occasionally, the duct from the gland becomes blocked and enlargement results. Medical intervention may be indicated if the condition does not subside within a few days.

In addition to the glands, a complex musculature underlies the genital area. The pelvic floor muscles have a multidirectional design (**Figure 4.4**) that permits the vaginal opening to expand during childbirth and contract after delivery. These muscles can lose muscle tone during childbirth or over time. A series of exercises known as **Kegel exercises** can help restore the muscular tone, reduce involuntary urinary incontinence, and enhance sexual sensations (see **It's Your Health**).

Internal female sexual anatomy consists of the vagina, cervix, uterus, fallopian tubes, and ovaries (**Figure 4.5**). The **vagina** opens between the labia minora and extends upward into the body, angling toward the lower back. The vagina is approximately 3 to 5 inches in length when not aroused. The folded walls of the vagina, known as rugae, form a flat tube. These walls are warm, soft, and moist, and they produce secretions that help maintain the chemical balance of the vagina.

The vagina consists of three layers of tissue—mucosal layer, muscular layer, and fibrous tissue—all of which are richly endowed with blood vessels. The mucosa is a layer of moist membrane inside the vagina. During sexual arousal, lubricating fluid exudes through the mucosa. The muscular tissue is concentrated around the vaginal opening. Fibrous tissue surrounds the muscular layer. This layer aids in vaginal contraction and expansion and also serves as connective tissue to other structures in the pelvic cavity.

The **cervix**, located at the back of the vagina, is the mouth of the uterus and looks like a small, pink, glazed doughnut. Glands line the cervical canal and produce a constant downward flow of mucus to protect the uterine

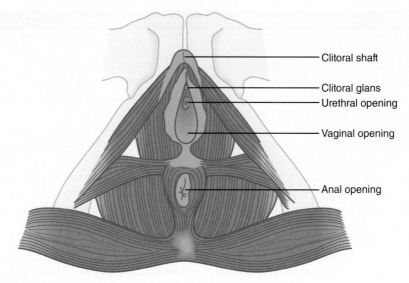

- Clitoral shaft
- Clitoral glans
- Urethral opening
- Vaginal opening
- Anal opening

Figure 4.4 **Pelvic floor muscles.**

cavity from bacterial invasion. The cervix is composed of fibrous tissue that is capable of dramatic stretching. During childbirth, the cervical canal is 50 or more times its normal width.

The **uterus**, also known as the womb, is a thick, pear-shaped organ. It is approximately 3 inches long and 2 inches wide, about the size of an orange, in a woman who has never had a child; after a pregnancy, it is somewhat larger. The uterus is suspended within the pelvic cavity by a series of six ligaments. The alignment of these ligaments permits some movement of the uterus within the

cavity. The uterine wall consists of three layers: the endometrium, the myometrium, and the perimetrium. The endometrium is the lining of the uterus. In preparation for fertilization, the endometrium thickens in response to hormone changes during the monthly menstrual cycle. The endometrium is also a source of hormone production. The myometrium, the middle layer, consists of the longitudinal and circular muscle fibers of the uterus. These muscle fibers are interwoven and enable the uterus to expand during pregnancy and contract during labor and childbirth. A thin membrane known as the perimetrium

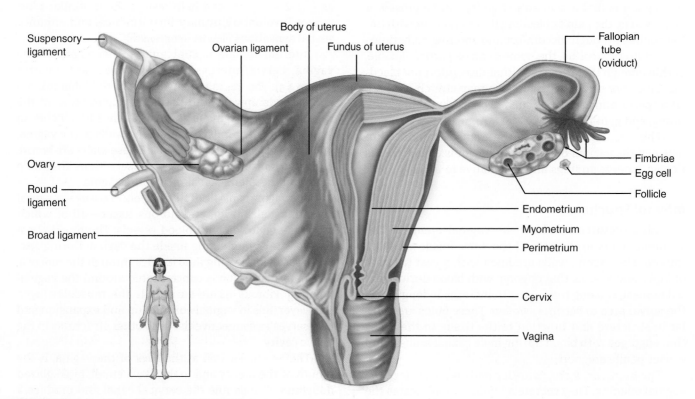

- Suspensory ligament
- Body of uterus
- Ovarian ligament
- Fundus of uterus
- Fallopian tube (oviduct)
- Ovary
- Round ligament
- Broad ligament
- Fimbriae
- Egg cell
- Follicle
- Endometrium
- Myometrium
- Perimetrium
- Cervix
- Vagina

Figure 4.5 **Internal female sexual anatomy.**

covers the myometrium. The perimetrium functions as the external surface of the uterus.

The **fallopian tubes**, which are thin, pale, pink filaments, connect the uterus with the ovaries. The outside end of each tube is like a funnel, with fingerlike projections called fimbriae that draw the egg from the ovary into the tube. The **ovaries** are located at the end of the fallopian tubes and are about the size of a small walnut in premenopausal women. The ovaries are endocrine glands that produce two classes of sex hormones: estrogens and progesterones. The estrogens influence the development of female physical sex characteristics and help regulate the menstrual cycle, while the progesterones help regulate the menstrual cycle and stimulate development of the uterine lining in preparation for pregnancy. During puberty, these hormones play a critical role in the maturation of the reproductive organs and the development of secondary sex characteristics, such as pubic hair and breasts.

The Menstrual Cycle

Women usually begin to menstruate in their early teens. During the **menstrual cycle**, the body prepares the uterine lining for implantation of a fertilized egg. If **conception** does not occur, the lining sloughs off and is discharged as menstrual flow. This menstrual discharge consists of blood, mucus, and endometrial membranes that sometimes present as small clots. The amount of menstrual flow varies but is usually 6 to 8 ounces in volume per cycle (about half a can of soda). The cycle is often 28 days in length but can vary from 21 to 40 days.

A complex series of interactions among the hypothalamus and the pituitary gland in the brain, the adrenal glands on top of the kidneys, the ovaries, and the uterus regulates the menstrual cycle. The hypothalamus produces and secretes hormones and releasing factors that act directly on the pituitary gland. One such releasing factor, gonadotropin-releasing hormone (GnRH), is responsible for reproductive hormone control. GnRH varies in amount and frequency during each menstrual cycle. In addition, this hormone plays a role in the timing of puberty. Alterations in the GnRH pulse release may be the mechanism by which stressors such as athletic training or dieting influence menstrual cycles.

The menstrual cycle is a self-regulating and dynamic process in which the level of a particular hormone impedes or increases the production of the same and other hormones.

Problems with Menstruation

For most women, menstruation creates no medical problems, but some women experience certain physical and emotional difficulties. **Dysmenorrhea**, meaning "painful menstrual flow," is a term for what most women call "cramps." Dysmenorrhea may be caused by the normal production of prostaglandins that produce strong contractions of the uterus (primary dysmenorrhea) or by problems in the uterus, fallopian tubes, or ovaries (secondary dysmenorrhea). Women with primary dysmenorrhea experience pain in the lower abdomen and back, while those with secondary dysmenorrhea often feel pain during urination and bowel movements. Relief from primary dysmenorrhea may be found through regular aerobic exercise; stress reduction techniques; adequate sleep; and decreased fat, caffeine, and sodium in the diet. Some women with primary or secondary dysmenorrhea may need anti-inflammatory medications or oral contraceptives to relieve the pain. Secondary dysmenorrhea is treated based on the underlying condition.

Premenstrual syndrome (PMS) is a group of symptoms linked to the menstrual cycle. PMS symptoms occur 1 or 2 weeks before the menstrual period, and they usually dissipate after menstruation starts. PMS can affect menstruating women of any age. It is also different for each woman. Most women of reproductive age have some physical discomfort, but about 5–8% of women suffer from severe premenstrual syndrome, where symptoms interfere with daily activities.[14] Although the root causes of PMS are not known, PMS is clearly linked to changing hormones during the menstrual cycle. Stress and emotional problems do not seem to cause PMS, but they may make it worse.

It's Your Health

Kegel Exercises

To identify the pelvic floor muscles:

1. Try stopping a flow of urine in midstream while urinating. The muscles that are tightened in this effort are the muscles of the pelvic floor.

2. Tighten the ring of muscles around the rectum, as if trying to stop a bowel movement. The muscles that are tightened in this effort are also muscles of the pelvic floor.

3. While lying down, place a hand over the abdomen. Tighten all of the muscles of the abdomen and pelvis. Notice that the hand will move. These are not muscles of the pelvic floor, and they should be relaxed during Kegel exercises. During the first few practice sessions, it is helpful to check with a hand to make sure that the abdominal muscles are relaxed.

To practice Kegel exercises:

1. Take deep breaths—do not forget to breathe.

2. Tighten the anal muscle, pulling inward and outward.

3. Tighten the vaginal muscle, pulling inward and outward.

4. Hold these muscles tight, counting slowly to 10, and then relax.

    Do Kegel exercises in sets of 5 to 10 at a time, several times a day. Build up to being able to hold the contraction for 20 seconds at a time.

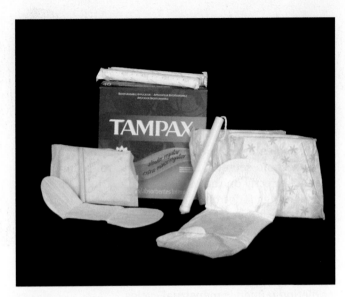

A wide variety of products are available for use during menstruation, including many different styles, sizes, and absorbencies of sanitary napkins or pads, tampons, and menstrual cups.

Diagnosis of PMS is usually based on a woman's specific symptoms, when they occur, and how much they affect her life. Symptoms include acne, breast swelling and tenderness, feeling tired, having trouble sleeping, upset stomach, bloating, constipation or diarrhea, headache or backache, appetite changes or food cravings, joint or muscle pain, trouble concentrating or remembering, tension, irritability, mood swings, crying spells, anxiety, and depression. Tracking the severity of these premenstrual problems daily on a calendar can assist clinicians with diagnosing PMS.[15]

PMS is more likely to present in women who are between their late twenties and early forties, have at least one child, and have a family history of depression or a personal history of either postpartum depression or a mood disorder. Research also suggests that cigarette smoking, especially in adolescence and young adulthood, may increase the risk of moderate to severe PMS.[16]

A single universal treatment is not yet available for PMS. Experts recommend basic health measures such as a nutritious diet, adequate sleep, daily exercise, a daily multivitamin that includes 400 micrograms of folic acid, a calcium supplement with vitamin D, and cessation of cigarette smoking to reduce PMS symptoms. (All of these measures are also excellent steps for improving general health.) Over-the-counter pain relievers such as ibuprofen, aspirin, or naproxen may ease cramps, headaches, backaches, and breast tenderness. In more severe cases of PMS, prescription medicines can ease symptoms. One approach has been to use hormonal oral contraceptives. Women using oral contraceptives report fewer PMS symptoms, such as cramps and headaches, as well as lighter periods. Further research is needed to ascertain the efficacy of this approach.[17]

Premenstrual dysphoric disorder (PMDD) is a severe form of PMS. The condition can be disabling with emotional symptoms, such as intense sadness, despair, tension, anxiety, mood swings, irritability, anger, and physical symptoms consistent with PMS. There is evidence that a brain chemical called serotonin plays a role in PMDD. Studies have found continuous dosing regimens of selective serotonin reuptake inhibitors (SSRIs) to be effective in treating these symptoms.[18] Studies also suggest that cognitive behavioral therapy in the forms of individual counseling, group counseling, and stress management may also help relieve symptoms.[19]

Amenorrhea is the lack of menstrual flow. Primary amenorrhea occurs in women who have not yet begun menstruation and may result from hormone-related problems or extremely low body fat. Secondary amenorrhea is the lack of blood flow for 3 or more consecutive months, outside of pregnancy, breastfeeding, and perimenopause; it may result from conditions such as anorexia nervosa, ovarian cysts or tumors, substance abuse, stress, or use of oral contraceptives. Healthcare providers will want to work with a woman to first establish the cause of her amenorrhea and then consider options for treatment.

Physical Health and the Well-Woman Examination

A woman's annual visit to her gynecologist typically begins with a medical history and a general physical examination, including a clinical breast examination and a pelvic examination. The pelvic exam should be timed to avoid the menstrual period. It is also advisable to avoid douching at least 24 hours before an examination; some clinicians recommend avoiding vaginal intercourse for at least 48 hours before the examination as well. These precautions ensure a more accurate visualization of the cervix and greater likelihood of diagnosing an infection if it is present. The American College of Obstetricians and Gynecologists (ACOG) recommends pelvic exams for women 21 year of age or older. For the pelvic exam, the woman lies on her back with her bottom at the very end of the examining table and her legs supported in foot stirrups. The pelvic examination consists of three phases:

- The first phase is the external examination, in which the clinician inspects the vulva and perineum visually for any evidence of infection or injury.

- The use of a speculum, a device that holds the vaginal walls apart to permit visual inspection of the cervix, is the second phase. The provider inserts the speculum with the blade closed. Once inside the vagina, the provider opens the blades and locks them into place at the correct width. With the speculum open, the clinician inspects the vaginal walls and cervix for redness, irritation, unusual discharge, or lesions. The provider collects specimens for laboratory tests while the speculum is in place and then removes the speculum.

■ The third phase of the examination is the bimanual examination, which involves the insertion of two gloved fingers of one hand into the vagina while the other hand presses downward on the abdomen. The purpose of this activity is to locate and feel the size, consistency, and shape of the uterus and ovaries and to check for any abdominal masses or tender areas.

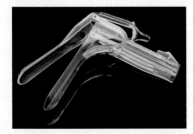

The speculum permits visual examination of the vagina and cervix during a gynecological visit.
© Elizabeth Dover/Shutterstock

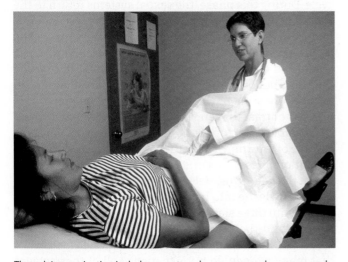

The pelvic examination includes an external exam, a speculum exam, and a bimanual exam.
© Michael Newman/PhotoEdit

A healthcare provider may also perform a rectal examination to evaluate the muscular wall separating the rectum and vagina, the position of the uterus, and any possible masses or tenderness in the area.

In 2014, the American College of Physicians published new evidence-based clinical practice guidelines recommending against performing routine pelvic exams, which includes the speculum and the bimanual exams, in women who are not pregnant and have no symptoms.[20] This recommendation does not apply to women who are due for cervical cancer screening or women with any symptoms that need to be evaluated (see **It's Your Health**). The guidelines were based on an analysis of numerous studies showing that the harms may outweigh the benefits of pelvic examinations. The analysis showed that pelvic exams in asymptomatic women do not reduce morbidity or mortality rates, based on the lack of diagnostic accuracy of the pelvic exam for detecting ovarian cancer or bacterial vaginosis; the exam also rarely detects noncervical or other treatable conditions and was not

It's Your Health

Aside from the annual well-woman visit, a woman should plan to visit a clinician for the following sexual health concerns:

If menarche has not occurred by age 16

At age 20 or earlier for first coitus

Heavy menstrual flow

Menstrual period lasting longer than 10 days

If risk for sexually transmitted diseases is present or if there is a history of abnormal Pap smears or positive HPV test

Any time there is vaginal itching, redness, sores, swelling, unusual odor, or unusual discharge

Painful intercourse

Missed menstrual period if there is a chance of pregnancy

Three missed menstrual periods if there is no chance of pregnancy

Burning or frequency of urination

Sexual partner has a genital infection or sore

Rape

Vaginal or rectal injury

associated with improved health outcomes. Harms associated with the pelvic exam include unnecessary follow-up procedures, fear, anxiety, embarrassment, pain, and discomfort. ACOG reviewed these guidelines and released a statement that they will continue to recommend annual pelvic examinations for their patients.[21]

SEXUAL AROUSAL AND SEXUAL RESPONSE

Sexual arousal and response are physical, emotional, and mental processes that individuals experience very differently. The female sexual response is not a geographically isolated phenomenon of the vaginal area. Instead, the brain, senses, and hormones all play an integrated role in the response cycle.

The brain mediates thoughts, emotions, and fantasies that provide the psychological "stage" for the sexual experience. Hearing, touch, smell, sight, and taste influence the level of sexual arousal. In addition to performing their primary role of regulating the menstrual cycle, hormones also affect sexual arousal. The function of certain hormones in the sexual response cycle—specifically, estrogens and androgens—has been studied extensively for many years. Estrogens promote cell growth and replication in the vaginal cells, increase blood flow in the vagina and urethra, and maintain vaginal lubrication in postmenopausal women. Androgens, also known as male sex hormones, affect the brain by influencing sexual behavior and libido. Evidence supports the role of androgens, specifically testosterone, for improving libido in postmenopausal women.[22] Additional studies are needed to determine the specific roles of estrogen and androgen and the effects of estrogen–androgen therapy on a woman's health. Currently, no testosterone product is approved in the U.S. for use in women.

The sexual response cycle has been described in several ways, most notably by Masters and Johnson in the 1960s.[23] Masters and Johnson were primarily interested in studying the biology of sexuality. They focused their sexual response cycle on the physiological reactions occurring during sexual activity. They developed a linear four-phase model of sexual response: excitement, plateau, orgasm, and resolution. Masters and Johnson reported three variations among women in the sexual response cycle (**Figure 4.6**): Pattern #1 demonstrates that some women are able to have one or more orgasms without dropping below the plateau level of sexual arousal; pattern #2, a variation of this response, includes an extended plateau with no orgasm; and pattern #3, which most closely resembles the typical male cycle, describes a rapid rise to orgasm with no definitive plateau and a quick resolution.

In the excitement phase of the female sexual response cycle, the clitoris swells with blood engorgement. This change ranges from slight to very distinct. The clitoral glans is highly sensitive. Some women find that the entire sexual response cycle can be set into motion and maintained to orgasm by light stimulation of the glans alone. In addition to clitoral swelling, the labia majora fatten and separate during the excitement phase. The labia minora increase in size, and lubrication begins.

Lubrication is a unique feature of the vagina and an important aspect of sexual arousal. It is often the first physiological sign of sexual arousal in women. Vaginal lubrication serves two primary functions. First, it enhances the possibility of conception by helping to alkalinize the normally acidic vaginal chemical balance; sperm are able to move faster and survive longer in an alkaline environment. Second, vaginal lubrication helps to increase sexual pleasure.

Many women cannot reach orgasm by penis insertion alone and therefore prefer other forms of stimulation in addition to coital stimulation. The "G" spot, or Grafenberg spot, is a sensitive area that can lead to orgasm when stimulated. Orgasm is the shortest phase of the sexual response cycle, though female orgasms often last slightly longer than male orgasms. Orgasmic experiences vary widely in intensity, frequency, and duration among both men and women. The female physiological responses in the orgasmic phase include an elevated blood pressure, heart rate, and breathing pattern. These physiological responses are consistent whether they originate from direct clitoral stimulation or from coital stimulation, although women report wide differences in subjective feelings and preferences.[24,25]

Resolution is the final phase of the sexual response cycle. During this phase, the sexual systems return to the nonexcited state. A significant male–female response difference occurs in the resolution period. After orgasm, the male typically enters a refractory period—a time when no amount of additional stimulation will result in orgasm. This time period has considerable variability among men and depends on physiological and psychological factors. In contrast to men, women generally experience no comparable refractory period, so they are physiologically capable of returning to another orgasmic peak during the resolution phase.

In the late 1970s, Helen Singer Kaplan introduced the concept of desire into her response cycle, which she condensed into three stages: sexual desire, followed by sexual arousal, and then orgasm. Both Masters and Johnson's model and Kaplan's model have been criticized for the fact that many women do not experience all of these stages or move through the phases sequentially.[26] Later models looked to encompass not only the biological processes

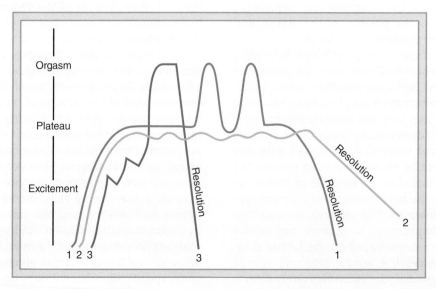

Figure 4.6 **Masters and Johnson's model lists three variations among women in the sexual response cycle.**

but also the psychosocial and emotional elements as well. In the 1990s, Whipple and Brash-McGreer proposed a circular model, overlaying the phases of desire, excitement, plateau, orgasm, and resolution with the stages of seduction (creating the desire), sensations (which include excitement and plateau), surrender (orgasm), and time for reflection (during resolution).[27] The circular aspect of the model demonstrates the reinforcing effect that satisfaction and pleasure have on leading to another sexual experience. Upon reflection, a woman may or may not circle back to the seduction stage based on whether or not she has the desire to repeat the experience.

Another framework, proposed by Basson, is an intimacy-based cyclical model and incorporates the interaction between the mind and the body.[28] A woman may enter the sexual response cycle at various points; for example, she may not feel desire, but after being aroused through sexual stimulation, she may become desirous. The model acknowledges the importance of psychosocial issues, such as relationship satisfaction, need for emotional intimacy, and previous sexual experiences. Basson's model recognizes that intimacy needs may drive a woman's sexual response more than the need for physical sexual arousal. It also acknowledges that the goal of sexual activity may be physical satisfaction (orgasm) or a combination of physical and emotional satisfaction (connectivity with a partner).

The female sexual response cycles described here are simply frameworks for understanding the physiological events of sexual response. Sexual response cycles of individual women can vary considerably from these models. Also, as women age, physiological changes in the female sexual response cycle occur, such as diminished lubrication and decreased blood flow and thus decreased swelling of the clitoris and labia. In addition to a reduction in estrogen that may be the cause of these changes, increased use of medications as well as incidence of medical conditions may interfere with a woman's overall libido. Despite these issues, however, many women report being satisfied with their overall sexual relationship well into old age.

Forms of Sexual Expression

Society has traditionally restricted the "appropriate" forms of sexual expression. Missionary (vaginal intercourse with the male on top of the female) heterosexual sex is only one of many sexual expression options. Women may elect many different forms of sexual expression depending on their experience, life situation, and personal preferences.

Masturbation refers to erotic self-stimulation, usually to the point of orgasm. Historical records indicate that both genders have engaged in masturbation since ancient times. Masturbation practices begin early in life with infants exploring their genitals and receiving pleasure from touching them. Often self-stimulation continues throughout life, whether or not the individual is in an intimate relationship. Studies vary greatly regarding

masturbation statistics, although all studies show that this practice is more common in males than in females.

Even though masturbation is widespread, many women feel ashamed or embarrassed about the practice. Folklore has often labeled masturbation as sinful, evil, and even physically or mentally harmful. Such ideas are entirely false. Many therapists and sex experts believe that masturbation can be helpful as a sexual outlet and a means to become comfortable with one's own body.

Petting is the erotic stimulation of a person by a sexual partner, without actual sexual intercourse. Petting can include kisses, genital caresses, and oral–genital contact. Petting may culminate in orgasm. During adolescence, petting is often a way to experience intense sexual excitement without actually engaging in intercourse. Petting is carried over into adult sexual experiences as foreplay or for sexual variety.

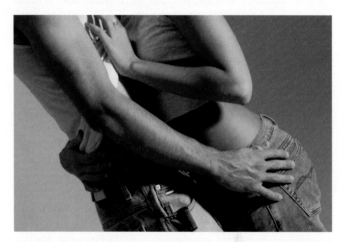

During adolescence, petting is a way to experience intense sexual excitement.
© LiquidLibrary

Oral–genital stimulation, also known as oral sex, takes two basic forms. **Cunnilingus** is the act of sucking or licking the vulva, particularly the clitoris. **Fellatio** is the act of sucking or licking the penis and scrotum. A common sexual practice among both heterosexual and homosexual couples, oral sex is often believed to be a "safe" sexual activity. However, sexually transmitted infections such as genital herpes, human papillomavirus, and gonorrhea all can be transmitted through oral–genital sex.[29]

Anal intercourse is another form of sexual expression. Because the anal opening is richly endowed with nerves, this area can be very sensitive and sexually arousing. A couple needs to be careful, however, in performing anal intercourse for many reasons. The anal sphincter tends to be tight and when stimulated can tighten even more, resulting in pain upon penetration. In addition, the anal region has no natural lubrication of its own, which increases the possibility of pain and injury. Usually anal intercourse can be accomplished without discomfort if precautions are taken. A water-based lubricant (not petroleum-based products, which weaken condoms) should be used. Unprotected anal intercourse has a high risk of transmitting many STIs, including HIV. Anyone engaging in anal intercourse should use a latex condom. In addition, care should be taken to avoid contamination of the vaginal area once anal penetration has occurred. After anal penetration, the genitals should be washed thoroughly before resuming vaginal or oral sex.

SEXUALITY THROUGH THE LIFE SPAN

In many Western societies, childhood has traditionally been considered as a time of unexpressed sexuality and behavior, and adolescence has been viewed as a time to restrain immature sexual drives. However, current evidence suggests that sexuality and sexual capacity are not "awakenings" that suddenly appear at a definitive time in development but rather that both male and female infants are born with the capacity for sexual pleasure and response.

Childhood

Individuals experience considerable variation in sexual development during childhood and adolescence. The pleasures of genital stimulation are generally discovered in the first few years of life. Besides self-stimulation, prepubescent children may engage in play that has sexual elements. The activities range from exhibition and inspection to simulating intercourse by rubbing genital regions together. Both natural childhood curiosity and curiosity about what is forbidden probably play a role in these behaviors. As children get older, they become more keenly aware of and interested in body changes, particularly those involving the genitals and secondary sex characteristics.

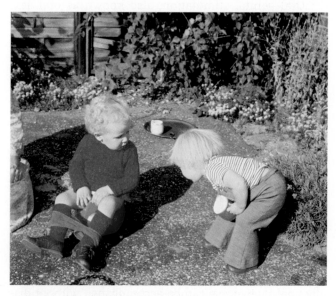

Children are innately interested in their bodies.
© David Noble Photography/Alamy Images

Adolescence

Adolescence, the period from about 12 to 19 years of age, is the most dramatic stage for physiological changes and social-role development. The first few years of adolescence are known as puberty, and this is a time of dramatic physiological change, including breast development, the growth of public hair, and the first menstrual period. Over the past 30 years, the average age of puberty has decreased. One study determined that the number of girls entering puberty at ages 7 and 8 years increased markedly between 1997 and 2010. The onset of puberty generally occurs 2 years earlier in girls than in boys. Secondary sex characteristics appear at this time in response to higher levels of hormones. In females, estrogen levels result in pubic hair growth and breast budding. The study found that 10% of White girls, 23% of Black girls, 15% of Hispanic girls, and 2% of Asian girls had started breast development by age 7.[30] Early breast development, however, has not been accompanied by earlier ages of first menarche, which has remained nearly constant since the 1970s. A number of environmental factors may contribute to the earlier age of puberty, including higher rates of childhood obesity; increased intake of animal protein and meat; high dairy and soft drink consumption; and exposure to endocrine-disrupting chemicals found in plastics, pesticides, and other chemicals.

Hormone stimulation during adolescence causes additional internal changes. Vaginal walls gradually become thicker, and the uterus becomes larger and more muscular. The vaginal pH changes from alkaline to acidic as vaginal and cervical secretions increase in response to the changing hormone status. Eventually, menstruation begins. The first menstrual period is known as menarche. Initial menstrual cycles may be irregular and occur without ovulation. Most girls menstruate at about the age of 12 or 13, but considerable variation exists in this timing. Most of the time, a girl will get her first period about 2 years after breasts first start to develop and by the age of 15.[31]

The difficulties of adjusting to new physical characteristics pale in comparison to the psychological adjustments of adolescence. This period is characterized by evolving responsibilities and assimilation of societal expectations. In Western cultures, these expectations include inherent double standards for women. Sexual overtones are impossible to escape in society, appearing on everything from ads for jeans to magazine photos to television shows. However, society also communicates the message that young women should maintain their virginity and not be sexually adventurous. In contrast, society tends to be more tolerant of experimentation and overt sexual behavior in young men.

Young to Middle Adulthood

Both personal and cultural factors influence sexual behavior in adults. Several factors have contributed to a

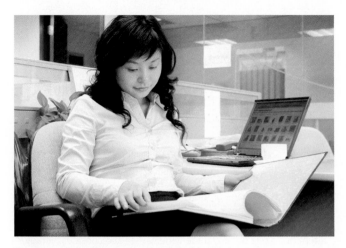

Many women are placing career goals before marriage.
© zhu difeng/ShutterStock, Inc.

dramatic increase in single, sexually active adults over the past 50 years:

- The trend toward marriage at a later age
- An increase in the number of women who never marry
- More women placing career goals before marriage
- An increase in the number of cohabiting couples
- A rise in divorce rates
- A greater emphasis on advanced education
- A greater number of women who no longer must depend on marriage to ensure their economic stability

Sexual relationships in adulthood can occur among single adults, within a marriage, or among married people having interactions with people other than their own

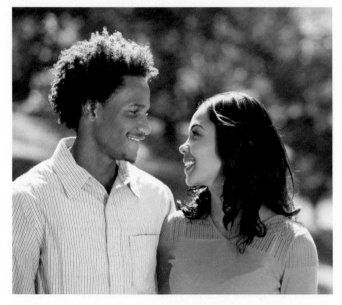

Communication contributes greatly to the satisfaction of an intimate relationship.
© Ron Chapple Studios/Dreamstime.com

spouses. However, in the absence of definitive data, it is difficult to draw conclusions about how these arrangements affect and are affected by satisfaction, sexual behaviors, and other factors.

Older Adulthood

The term **climacteric** refers to the physiological changes that occur during the transition period from female fertility to infertility. At about age 40, the ovaries begin to slow the production of estrogen and androgens. **Menopause**, one of the climacteric events, refers to the cessation of menstruation and generally occurs at about 45 to 55 years of age. The hormonal changes of menopause affect the sexual response of most women. In general, all phases of the response cycle continue at a decreased intensity. The depletion of hormones associated with menopause can result in several vaginal changes, including dryness, thinning of the walls, and delayed or absent lubrication during sexual excitement. Hormone therapy may help some women cope with symptoms; however, hormone therapy may have side effects or health risks for some women. In some cases, prescription estrogen creams applied directly to the vagina may help prevent dryness and thinning. Water-soluble lubricants and vaginal moisturizers can help solve problems related to dryness, and Kegel exercises can help make sex more pleasurable by toning the pelvic floor muscles that support the bladder and uterus, which tend to relax as estrogen declines.

In later years, a decline in frequency and intensity of sexual activity often occurs. However, the opportunities for sexual expression in a relationship often increase in later years, as pressures from work, children, and fulfilling life's goals may be reduced and more time becomes available for sharing with a partner. Couples may increasingly emphasize quality rather than quantity of sexual expression, and intimacy may find new and deeper dimensions in later years.

The perception that old age and sex are incompatible is erroneous. All too often, women dismiss sexual problems as a consequence of aging. In truth, most people can enjoy an active sex life no matter their age. Misconceptions about aging may have evolved for a number of reasons. Culturally, the United States still often equates sexuality with procreation. For older people who are neither capable of nor interested in the reproductive facets of life, this viewpoint offers little sensitivity or insight into their personal needs. Society also sends the message via the media that love, sex, and romance are only for the young and "sexy." The implicit message is that this scenario excludes older individuals.

Studies have found that sexual expression in older adults can provide relaxation, reassurance, and companionship and can reduce depression and social isolation.[32] A comprehensive national survey of seniors found that most people between the ages of 57 and 85 think of sexuality as an important part of their lives. The study also found that many older adults are sexually active, with sexual activity closely related to overall health.[33] Societal expectations can complicate sexual communication with older adults. Elders who are single may meet with disapproval from their family and friends when dating or engaging in sexual relations, and people in long-term care facilities may feel deprived of their right to privately engage in sexual behavior.

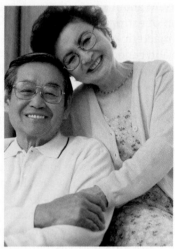

Sexuality is an important dimension of aging.
© Photodisc

SEXUAL DYSFUNCTION

Sexual dysfunction is the inability of an individual to function adequately in terms of sexual arousal, orgasm, or in coital situations. The medical and scientific community once classified women's sexual problems under the general label of "frigidity." These problems were severely misunderstood and thought to be symptomatic of a neurosis or some other psychological disorder that required long-term psychiatric therapy. This traditional approach persisted despite the absence of a demonstrated relationship between the psychiatric treatment and the alleviation of the sexual problem. More recently, however, the pharmaceutical industry has gained interest in understanding and treating female sexual problems with the hopes of uncovering a new market as lucrative as that for male-targeted medications such as Viagra.

Today, four major areas of sexual dysfunction are recognized among women: sexual desire disorders, sexual arousal disorders, orgasmic disorders, and sexual pain disorders. One large study found that 44% of women reported sexual problems. Low desire was the most common sexual problem (38.7%); less common problems were low arousal (26.1%) and orgasm difficulties (20.5%). Older women experienced the highest prevalence of sexual dysfunction (80.1% compared with 44.6% for middle-aged women and 27.2% for women 18 to 44), but the lowest level of associated distress (12.6% compared with 25.5% for middle-aged women and 24.4% for younger women).[34] Treatments for each of these conditions require understanding the complex relationships between physiological

and psychological considerations. Any form of sexual dysfunction or discomfort with intercourse or sexual stimulation should be evaluated to rule out underlying pathology (see **Self-Assessment 4.1**). In addition, the evaluation should include efforts such as counseling or therapy, if needed, to seek resolution of the condition.

Sex Therapy

Professional help may be indicated in cases where individual efforts, couple efforts, or both do not produce the desired effects. Sex therapy has evolved as a legitimate method for understanding sexual problems and increasing sexual satisfaction. Communication about sexual issues and finding ways to solve problems are critical but often difficult steps toward achieving a satisfying sex life; sex therapy can make such communication easier. Strategies with a therapist may range from expanding self-knowledge to sharing more effectively with a partner.

Therapy can also benefit individuals or couples by providing them with information. By providing specific, accurate, and reassuring information, a therapist is often able to address thoughts and feelings interfering with the person's ability to enjoy or respond to sexual activity. A therapist is also able to provide specific activities or homework "assignments" that enable the client to reduce anxiety, enhance communication, and learn new sexually enhancing behavioral techniques. Intensive therapy may be indicated in some situations in which personal emotional difficulties or significant relationship problems interfere with sexual expression.

I used to fake orgasms. I am not sure why, but somehow I felt it was necessary. My current partner figured it out, and we have spent a lot of time talking about this. I am seeing a therapist. With a few sessions, I was able to climax with masturbation, and I know that I am much more comfortable with my sexuality. I know that "faking it" was not fair to my partner or me.

—35-year-old woman

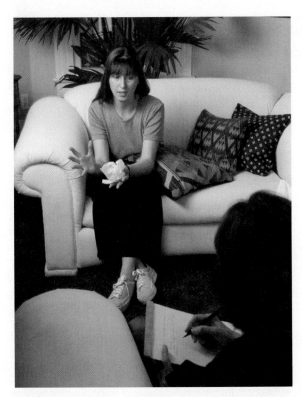

A trained counselor or clinician can often provide valuable assistance for a woman who is experiencing sexual dysfunction.
© David Buffington/Photodisc/Getty Images

SEX RESEARCH

Despite its importance, there has been less systematic, scientific research on the sexual behavior of Americans than on most other health and social topics of importance. The AIDS epidemic has improved the accuracy and increased the availability of information on sexual behavior, but the collection of scientific information on sexual matters continues to face strong political opposition.

Researchers attempting to understand sexual behavior face many of the same problems that handicap all research on human social behavior. Human subjects cannot be placed in a laboratory setting where variables that influence outcome measures can be controlled. Human behavior is complex, and studies, particularly on human behavior, are prone to contamination and bias. As a personal, private behavior, sex is more limited than other areas of behavioral research. Clearly, many problematic issues arise with any attempt to understand the prevalence and nature of contemporary sexual behavior.

Even with these limitations, there are ways to measure or analyze sexual activity and study sexual behavior, such as case studies, direct observation, experimental laboratory research, and surveys. Studies can address sexual research directly, for example, by determining the prevalence of sexual activities such as oral sex or same-sex couplings. Indirect assessments, such as adolescent pregnancy rates or sexually transmitted disease rates, provide insight into the consequences of sexual behavior.

Definitions create another technical difficulty in research. For years, researchers used the term "premarital sex" to describe penile–vaginal intercourse that takes place before a couple is married. However, as a measure of sexual activity outside of marriage, this definition is misleading because it excludes many noncoital sexual activities. Heavy petting can include extensive types of sexual contact, often resulting in orgasm. The traditional definition of "virginity" as not having had sexual intercourse, therefore, may not reflect a lack of sexual activity. The term "premarital" has connotations that may be inappropriate to some individuals, especially to couples in same-sex relationships or relationships in cultures that offer commitments equal to marriage. Not all couples that engage in sexual activity have intentions toward long-term commitment with that partner. Any review of sex studies must consider the inherent limitations of such research.

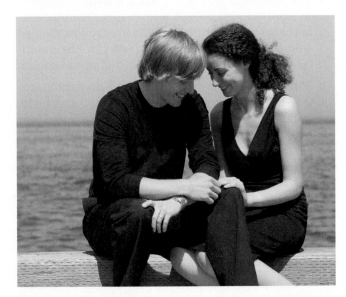

Definitions of "virginity" are subjective and may include (or exclude) a number of sexual behaviors.
© AbleStock

Well-Known Studies

Several important studies on sexual behavior have provided valuable information and insight into sexual practices, behaviors, and attitudes.

- In 1948 and 1953, Alfred Kinsey conducted the most comprehensive taxonomic surveys of human sexual behavior to date.[12,13] The 1948 study researched sexual behavior in men, and the 1953 study researched sexual behavior in women. Both studies attempted to present objective data on sexual behavior. The researchers interviewed thousands of people of various socioeconomic statuses, educational levels, marital statuses, and sex education experiences. The results showed how factors such as age, religious adherence, and gender influenced the incidence, frequency, and patterns of sexual behavior.

- In 1966, through direct observation techniques, Masters and Johnson observed and recorded more than 10,000 completed sexual response cycles.[23] Before their work, no significant empirical data had been gathered about male and female sexual arousal. Masters and Johnson are considered pioneers in sexual research for determining the four phases of the sexual response cycle: excitement, plateau, orgasm, and resolution.

- In 1976, the Hite Report, a questionnaire survey on female sexuality, also provided extensive narrative answers to several important questions about the sexual practices of American women.[35] The report, which brought to light the fact that the majority of women can reach orgasm through self-stimulation but not during sexual intercourse, helped fuel the sexual revolution of the 1970s.

- The *Redbook* Survey (1977) was a questionnaire sent to more than 100,000 U.S. women that examined sexual behavior and attitudes.[36] This survey documented women's sexual fulfillment in respect to their marital status, age at sexual initiation, and sexual fidelity.

- Blumstein and Schwartz (1983) elicited excellent information about sexual and nonsexual components of relationships from a large national sample. Their book, *American Couples: Money, Work, Sex*, explored couples as cohabitating, married, or same-sex, comparing the dynamics of decision making between partners on the major issues faced by couples.[37]

- In 1992, the National Health and Social Life Survey interviewed more than 3400 adults. The survey asked about sexual behavior over the lifetime, including childhood and adolescence, as well as sexually transmitted infections, sexual dysfunctions, and sexual attitudes and opinions. This landmark survey had significant implications for public health and provided further insight into the sexual behavior of American adults.[38]

- In 2001, the Surgeon General released the *Call to Action to Promote Sexual Health and Responsible Sexual Behavior*. The Call to Action contained strategies and information for promoting sexual health and responsible sexual behavior.[39] The Call to Action was the first time that the promotion of responsible sexual behavior and the improvement of sexual health were addressed as significant public health challenges (see **It's Your Health**).

- In 2003, Bancroft and colleagues conducted The National Survey of Women in Heterosexual Relationships.[40] Nearly 1000 women ages 20 to 65 were surveyed, assessing the prevalence and predictors of sexual distress among women; it found that the best predictors of sexual distress were a woman's emotional well-being and her emotional relationship with her sexual partner, as opposed to physical aspects of the sexual response cycle.

It's Your Health

Call to Action to Promote Sexual Health and Responsible Sexual Behavior

Individual responsibility includes the following duties:

- Understanding and awareness of one's sexuality and sexual development
- Respect for oneself and one's partner
- Avoidance of physical and emotional harm to oneself or one's partner
- Ensuring that pregnancy occurs only when welcomed
- Recognition and tolerance of the diversity of sexual values within any community

Community responsibility includes assurance that its members have the following characteristics:

- Access to developmentally and culturally appropriate sexuality education as well as sexual and reproductive health care and counseling
- The latitude to make appropriate sexual and reproductive choices
- Respect for diversity
- Freedom from stigmatization and violence on the basis of gender, race, ethnicity, religion, or sexual orientation

Source: *The Surgeon General's Call to Action to Promote Sexual Health and Responsible Sexual Behavior*. (2001). U.S. Department of Health and Human Services.

- In a 2004 *ABC News Primetime Live* poll, more than 1500 adults were randomly queried in a telephone survey about sexual activities, fantasies, and attitudes. The vast majority of respondents said they were monogamous and that they were happy about it.[41]

- The 2010 National Survey of Sexual Health and Behavior (NSSHB) is one of the most comprehensive and nationally representative studies on sexual and sexual-health behaviors. It includes the sexual experiences and condom-use behaviors of more than 5800 adolescents and adults ages 14 to 94.[42]

Although some of the above studies have been criticized for overrepresenting or underrepresenting certain population segments, these studies have provided valuable information and insight into sexual behavior and attitudes. With any study of sexual behavior, however, it is important to consider the quality of the study method and the sampling techniques employed.

SEXUAL VIOLENCE AS A PUBLIC HEALTH PROBLEM

Sexual violence violates a person's fundamental human rights and freedoms. Sexual violence can occur against men or women of any age. The perpetrator is often someone the person knows and can be a family member or friend, a respected member of the community, a colleague at work, or someone in a health facility or educational institution. Sexual violence can also occur in the highly organized and lucrative form of forced prostitution or trafficking.

Sexual Assault and Rape

Sexual assault and rape are crimes of aggression. **Sexual assault** often refers to forced sexual contact, while **rape** is usually defined as an event occurring without consent, involving the use of force or the threat of force to sexually penetrate the victim's vagina, mouth, or rectum. Rape may occur among strangers or intimates; it can also happen in a marriage, during a legal separation, or after a divorce. In addition, rape can occur between people of the same sex. About three out of every four victims of sexual violence knows their offender; between 2005 and 2010, about 34% of all rape or sexual assaults were committed by an intimate partner, 6% were committed by a relative or family member, and 38% were committed by a friend or acquaintance.[43] Women are disproportionately affected by such sexual violence. In 2010, women experienced 270,000 rape or sexual assaults, adding up to about two victimizations per 1000 women ages 12 or older.[43]

Rape and sexual assault crimes occur throughout the world. Many women who are raped or assaulted blame themselves for the attacks. In some cultures, especially in countries where women have a low place in society, families blame the girl or woman who is raped. Every year, as many as 5000 women and girls around the world are murdered by members of their own families in honor killings, for the "dishonor" that the rape has brought to the family.[44] Chapter 14 provides more information on sexual violence, abuse, and harassment.

Female Genital Mutilation

Female genital mutilation (FGM) is also known as female circumcision or female genital cutting. These procedures involve partial or total removal of the external female genitalia or other injury to the female genital organs for nonmedical reasons. The practice is usually performed on women by traditional circumcisers, who often play other central roles in communities, such as attending childbirths. Increasingly, however, medically trained personnel perform FGM. FGM is nearly always carried out on girls between infancy and age 15 without their consent or under coercion.[45]

These practices, which destroy or cripple a woman's ability to feel sexual pleasure, are usually performed for cultural or religious reasons. Girls or infants suffer short-term and long-term consequences, including infections and other conditions ranging from lasting psychological harm to death. More than 125 million girls and women alive today have suffered FGM in the 29 countries in Africa and the Middle East where the practice is most prevalent.[46] UNICEF estimates that more than 130 million women are living with the consequences of FGM. FGM is now illegal in the United States, but in 2013, nearly 507,000 U.S. women and girls either had undergone FGM or were at risk of the procedure.[47]

Over the last several decades, many governments, nongovernmental organizations, local communities, and religious and civil society groups have been working to address FGM and helping populations across countries to abandon the practice. In 2012, the United Nations General Assembly adopted the resolution *Intensifying global efforts for the elimination of female genital mutilation*, demonstrating the political will of a unified international community to eliminate FGM. Some form of legislation prohibiting FGM is in place in 26 countries in Africa and the Middle East, as well as 33 countries on other continents.[48]

Forced Sterilization

Forced sterilization, performed throughout the world for population control and eugenics (the Darwinian notion of producing a "perfect" race of humans), is a violent crime against the reproductive rights of women and men. People have been targeted for surgeries for being poor and/or illiterate; or for suffering from alcoholism, chronic disease, or mental and physical challenges. In countries with high rates of poverty, forced sterilization has been used to control population growth. Women have been bribed with payments of food, clothing, or money. Women have also been unknowingly sterilized during childbirth or other medical procedures. Over the past 100 years, forced sterilizations have occurred all over the world, including Germany, Sweden, Japan, Peru, China, and the United States.

INFORMED DECISION MAKING

Sexual well-being encompasses more than sexual arousal and response. It includes effective decision making across the spectrum of issues affecting sexual health. A health checkup with a gynecologist is a good place to start for guidance in reproductive and sexual health matters, as well as preventive health screening. A woman can maximize the benefits of a well-woman visit by selecting a clinician who is sensitive to her needs. Often that means changing clinicians until the "right" one is found. Even so, it is better to "shop" while feeling well than to wait until a pressing medical problem requires immediate attention.

Understanding personal feelings, thoughts, and symptoms and articulating concerns and questions are essential for effective personal communication and preventive health. Communication is critical for promoting sexual health and responsible sexual behavior. Being able to talk about needs, feelings, concerns, and fears is an essential component of a healthy relationship. Sexual communication can contribute greatly to the satisfaction of an intimate relationship. Unfortunately, American language lacks a comfortable sexual vocabulary. Available language seems to be either "clinical" or "medical" in nature, which may be perceived as too cold and unfeeling, or "street language," which may be perceived as too crass or juvenile. Beyond the handicaps imposed by socialization and language limitations, difficulties in sexual communication may be rooted in fears of too much self-exposure. Any sexual communication involves a degree of risk and vulnerability to judgment, criticism, or rejection. The willingness to take risks may be related to the amount of trust that exists within a relationship.

Responsible sexual behavior is also essential for promoting positive sexual health. Children look to their parents as a first resource; a healthy, loving, committed relationship can serve as a blueprint for children. Although communication between parents and children can be helpful, many parents find it difficult to discuss sexual health issues. Some parents are unsure of their own knowledge about sexual health and therefore they fear that they may not benefit the child by sharing their own experiences and information.

As girls grow up, they begin picking up information from television, movies, books, magazines, and friends. Although this is a natural behavior, parents should maintain an open dialogue with their children to ensure that they continue to learn accurate information and have the maturity and emotional control to make good decisions. Although television and radio often suggest sexual behavior, the media typically depict sexual behavior in short-lived romances without the use of contraception.

According to the Institute of Medicine, "The Code of Silence has resulted in missed opportunities to use the mass media to encourage healthy sexual behavior."[49] It is important to realize that sexual relationships should include negotiation and communication skills, safe sex practices, and healthy and positive relationships.

Healthcare providers also can be a good source of information for adolescent girls and women. Women should articulate the reason for their visits (such as fears about STIs) and address their specific questions or concerns. Clinicians will not necessarily ask a standard set of questions or ascertain by examination the nature of a sexual concern or automatically detect an underlying fear or anxiety. Insisting that all questions be answered and persisting when answers are not clear are equally important avenues for a satisfactory visit. Women are often eager to please their healthcare providers and will nod as if understanding when they actually do not. This behavior results in more confusion and an increased likelihood of problems. Many women find it helpful to write down their questions and concerns and deal with them one by one with the clinician in the office before clothes are removed and the examination begins. Unfortunately, many healthcare providers do not address important topics regarding sexual health and appear uncomfortable when questions are asked of them. Healthcare providers need to find ways to broach the subject in a respectful, and culturally sensitive manner.

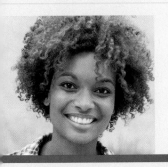
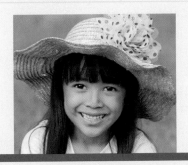
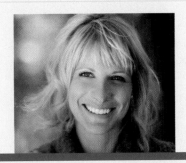
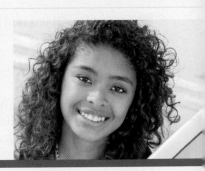

CASE STUDY

Michelle is a 47-year-old woman who has not been to see any healthcare provider since the birth of her third child 6 years ago. She is considering making an appointment to discuss medical options for female sexual dysfunction. Based on this information, answer the following questions.

Questions

1. What are some questions her healthcare provider may ask her when she goes for an appointment?

2. Is there anything her healthcare provider could learn about her sexual dysfunction from a physical exam?

3. What are other factors (e.g. non-physical) that could lead to a lack of vaginal lubrication?

4. Could Michelle's age be a factor? If so, why?

■ Summary

Sexuality pervades every aspect of a person's life. It evolves throughout the life span, from the beginnings of sexual urges in girlhood to maintaining a fulfilling sexual life into old age. Understanding the biological, psychological, power, and sociological dimensions of sexual health enhances total wellness. Women must understand the unique facets of their own sexuality, from their physiology to their desires. Both positive and negative sexual experiences can affect a woman's overall well-being. Communication and awareness of sexuality are key factors to resolving these experiences in a healthful way. Incorporating open communication and awareness of sexuality into personal relationships, informed decision making, and preventive health care can enhance a woman's sexual health throughout her life span.

Profiles of Remarkable Women

Eve Ensler (1953–)

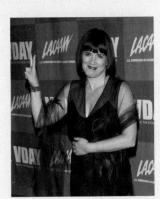
© Featureflash/Shutterstock

Eve Ensler is a playwright, performer, and activist whose work grows out of her own personal experiences with violence. Ensler's Obie-Award-winning play, *The Vagina Monologues,* is based on her interviews with more than 200 women about their intimate anatomy. The piece celebrates women's sexuality and strength and exposes the violations that women endure throughout the world. The play has been translated into more than 48 languages and has been performed in more than 140 countries. Ensler's performance in *The Vagina Monologues* can be seen in the 2002 HBO original documentary.

Ensler is also the founder of V-Day, which grew from her conversations with women who approached her after performances of *The Vagina Monologues* to tell her of their own experiences of violence. Today, V-Day is a global movement that helps antiviolence organizations continue and expand their core work on the ground, while drawing public attention to the larger fight to stop worldwide violence (including rape, battery, incest, FGM, and sexual slavery) against women and girls. V-Day has raised more than $100 million and funded more than 13,000 community-based antiviolence programs and safe houses in Democratic Republic of Congo, Haiti, Kenya, Egypt, and Iraq.

In 2010, V-Day and UNICEF opened the City of Joy, a facility for the survivors of sexual violence in Democratic Republic of the Congo (DRC). Conceived, created, and developed by the women on the ground, the City of Joy supports women survivors of sexual violence to heal and provides them with opportunities to develop their leadership through innovative programming of educational training and political activism. The women experience extensive literacy and communications courses as well as civics and politics training that teach them about human rights, women's rights, and psychotherapy to help them recover from their trauma.

In November 2009, Ensler was named one of *US News & World Report*'s "Best Leaders" in association with the Center for Public Leadership (CPL) at Harvard Kennedy School, and in 2010 she was named one of "125 Women Who Changed Our World" by *Good Housekeeping Magazine.*

■ Topics for Discussion

1. How have sexual norms affected you as an individual? Have there been positive as well as negative influences?

2. Should sex education be taught in the nation's public schools, and, if so, what kind of education should be provided? Which topics do you think are appropriate for school-based sex education courses?

3. How can schools and public institutions better address gender identity concerns? Do you believe that we as a society should start moving away from a binary system and raising awareness toward a gender identity continuum?

4. Gender-neutral parenting is a form of raising a child without letting others around the child know his or her sex. Proponents of gender-neutral parenting point out that a child can choose clothes, toys, and behaviors freely, without the constraints imposed by society. Opponents of this type of rearing are concerned with isolation, bullying, or other social concerns among peers, as well as confusion for the child in other organized settings. Is gender-neutral parenting beneficial or detrimental to a child and why?

5. It is a paradox that women appear to have a greater capacity for orgasm and can experience orgasm from a wider range of stimulation, yet seem to have more difficulty experiencing orgasm than men. Is this true? If so, which factors may contribute to this paradox?

6. How is homophobia displayed in modern society?

7. Many researchers have proposed nonlinear models of sexual response patterns. Identify two of these models.

8. What are ways to maintain healthy relationships while being aware of risks of sexually transmitted disease, pregnancy, and rape?

■ Key Terms

Amenorrhea

Androgyny

Bartholin's glands

Bisexual

Cervix

Climacteric

Clitoris

Conception

Cunnilingus

Dysmenorrhea

Fallopian tube

Fellatio

Gender dysphoria

Gender identity

Gender role

Heterosexual

Homophobia

Homosexual

Hymen

Intersexuality

Kegel exercises

Labia majora

Labia minora

Masturbation

Menopause

Menstrual cycle

Mons veneris

Ovaries

Perineum

Premenstrual dysphoric disorder (PMDD)

Premenstrual syndrome (PMS)

Rape

Sexual assault

Sexual dysfunction

Sexual health

Sexual orientation

Transitioning

Urethra

Uterus

Vagina

Vulva

■ References

1. World Health Organization (WHO). (2006). *Defining Sexual Health. Report of a technical consultation on sexual health 28–31 January 2002.* Geneva, Switzerland: WHO. Available at: http://www.who.int/reproductivehealth/publications/en/

2. Pew Research Center. (n.d.). Analysis of the 1960–2000 decennial census and 2010–2012 American Community Survey, Integrated Public Use Microdata Series (IPUMS). Available at: http://www.pewsocialtrends.org/2014/09/24/record-share-of-americans-have-never-married/#fn-19804-1

3. Centers for Disease Control and Prevention (CDC). (2014). Youth risk behavior surveillance—United States, 2013. Surveillance Summaries. *Morbidity and Mortality Weekly Report* 63(SS-4): 1–168.

4. Copen, C. E., Danils, K., & Mosher, W. D. (2013). *First premarital cohabitation in the United States: 2006–2010 National Survey of Family Growth.* National Health Statistics Reports, No. 64. Hyattsville, MD: National Center for Health Statistics.

5. Mathematica Policy Research, Inc. (2007). *Impacts of four title V, section 510 abstinence education programs: Final report.* Available at: http://www.mathematica-mpr.com/~/media/publications/PDFs/impactabstinence.pdf

6. Jemmott, J. B., Jemmott, L. S., & Fong, G. T. (2010). Efficacy of a theory-based abstinence-only intervention over 24 months.

Archives of Pediatric and Adolescent Medicine 164(2): 152–159. Available at: http://archpedi.jamanetwork.com/article.aspx?articleid=382798#ArticleInformation

7. Kohler, P. K., Manhart, L. E., & Lafferty, W. E. (2008). Abstinence-only and comprehensive sex education and the initiation of sexual activity and teen pregnancy. *Journal of Adolescent Health* 42(4): 344–351.

8. Eisenberg, M. E., Bernat, D. H., Bearinger, L. H., et al. (2008). Support for comprehensive sexuality education: Perspectives from parents of school-age youth. *Journal of Adolescent Health* 42(4): 352–359.

9. Guttmacher Institute. (2015). *State policies in brief: Sex and HIV education.* Available at: http://www.guttmacher.org/statecenter/spibs/spib_SE.pdf; Accessed on: 1/10/2015.

10. American Psychological Association. (2012). Guidelines for psychological practice with lesbian, gay, and bisexual clients. *American Psychologist* 67(1): 10–42.

11. Johnson, C. V., Mimiaga, M. J., & Bradford, J. (2008). Health care issues among lesbian, gay, bisexual, trans-gender and intersex (LGBTI) populations in the United States: Introduction. *Journal of Homosexuality* 54(3): 213–224.

12. Kinsey, A., Pomeroy, W., & Martin, C. (1948). *Sexual behavior in the human male.* Philadelphia, PA: W. B. Saunders.

13. Kinsey, A., Pomeroy, W., Martin, C., et al. (1953). *Sexual behavior in the human female.* Philadelphia, PA: W. B. Saunders.

14. Yonkers, K. A., O'Brien, P. M., & Eriksson, E. (2008). Premenstrual syndrome. *Lancet* 371(9619): 1200–1210.

15. Borenstein, J. E., Dean, B. B., Yonkers, K. A., et al. (2007). Using the daily record of severity of symptoms as a screening instrument for premenstrual syndrome. *Obstetrics and Gynecology* 109: 1068–1075.

16. Bertone-Johnson, E. R., Hankinson, S. E., Johnson, S. R., et al. (2008). Cigarette smoking and the development of premenstrual syndrome. *American Journal of Epidemiology* 168(8): 938–945.

17. Lopez, L. M., Kaptein, A., & Helmerhorst, F. M. (2008). Oral contraceptives containing drospirenone for premenstrual syndrome. *Cochrane Database System Review* 23(1): CD006586.

18. Shah, N. R., Jones, J. B., Aperi, J., et al. (2008). Selective serotonin reuptake inhibitors for premenstrual and premenstrual dysphoric disorder. *Obstetrics and Gynecology* 111: 1175–1182.

19. Busse, J. W., Montori, V. M., Krasnik, C., et al. (2008). Psychological intervention for premenstrual syndrome: A meta-analysis of randomized controlled trials. *Psychotherapy and Psychosomatics* 78(1): 6–15.

20. Qaseem, A., Humphrey, L. L., Harris, R., et al. (2014). Screening pelvic examination in adult women: A clinical practice guideline from the American College of Physicians. *Annals of Internal Medicine* 161(1): 67–72.

21. American College of Obstetricians and Gynecologists (ACOG). (2014). *ACOG Practice Advisory on annual pelvic examination recommendations.* Available at: http://www.acog.org/About-ACOG/News-Room/Statements-and-Advisories/2014/ACOG-Practice-Advisory-on-Annual-Pelvic-Examination-Recommendations

22. Garefalakis, M., & Hickey, M. (2008). Role of androgens, progestins and tibolone in the treatment of menopausal symptoms: A review of the clinical evidence. *Clinical Interventions of Aging* 3(1): 1–8.

23. Masters, W., & Johnson, V. (1966). *Human sexual response.* Boston, MA: Little, Brown.

24. Tavris, C., & Sadd, S. (1977). *The Redbook report on female sexuality.* New York, NY: Delacorte Press.

25. Blumstein, P., & Schwartz, P. (1983). *American couples: Money, work and sex.* New York, NY: William Morrow.

26. Kaplan, H. S (1979). *Disorders of sexual desire and other new concepts and techniques in sex therapy.* New York, NY: Brunner/Hazel Publications.

27. Whipple, B., & Brash-McGreer, K. (1997). Management of female sexual dysfunction. In M. L. Sipski & C. Alexander (Eds.), *Maintaining sexuality with disability and chronic illness: A practitioner's guide* (pp. 509–534). Frederick, MD: Aspen Publishers.

28. Basson, R. (2001). The new model of female sexual response. *Sex Dysfunction in Medicine* 2: 72–77.

29. ACOG. (2008). Addressing health risks of noncoital sexual activity. *Obstetrics and Gynecology* 112: 735–737.

30. Biro, F. M. (2010). Pubertal assessment method and baseline characteristics in a mixed longitudinal study of girls. *Pediatrics* 126(3): e583–e590.

31. Office of Women's Health, Department of Health and Human Services. (2014). *Menstruation and the menstrual cycle fact sheet.* Available at: http://www.womenshealth.gov/publications/our-publications/fact-sheet/menstruation.html#f

32. Laumann, E. O., Anirudda, D., & Waite, L. J. (2008). Sexual dysfunction among older adults: Prevalence and risk factors from a nationally representative U.S. probability sample of men and women 57–85 years of age. *Journal of Sexual Medicine* 5(10): 2300–2311.

33. Lindau, S. T., Schumm, L. P., Laumann, E. O., et al. (2007). A study of sexuality and health among older adults in the United States. *New England Journal of Medicine* 357(8): 762–874.

34. Shifren, J. L., Monz, B. U., Russo, P. A., et al. (2008). Sexual problems and distress in United States women. *Obstetrics and Gynecology* 112: 970–978.

35. Hite, S. (1976). *The Hite Report: A nationwide study of female sexuality.* New York, NY: Dell Books.

36. Tavris, C., & Sadd, S. (1977). *The Redbook report on female sexuality.* New York, NY: Delacorte Press.

37. Blumstein, P., & Schwartz, P (1983). *American couples: Money, work and sex.* New York, NY: William Morrow.

38. Laumann, E. O., Gagnon, J. H., Michael, R. T., et al. (1992). *National Health and Social Life Survey, 1992: [United States].* Ann Arbor, MI: Inter-university Consortium for Political and Social Research.

39. U.S. Department of Health and Human Services. (2001). *The Surgeon General's Call to Action to promote sexual health and responsible sexual behavior.* Hyattsville, MD: Department of Health and Human Services.

40. Bancroft, J., Loftus, J., & Long, J. S. (2003). Distress about sex: A national survey of women in heterosexual relationships. *Archives of Sexual Behavior* 32(3): 193–208.

41. ABC News. (2004). *Primetime live poll: The American sex survey.* Available at: http://abcnews.go.com/images/Politics/959a1AmericanSexSurvey.pdf

42. Herbenick, D., Reece, M., Schick, V., et al. (2010). Sexual behavior in the United States: Results from a national probability sample of men and women ages 14–94. *Journal of Sexual Medicine* 7: 255–265.

43. Berzofsky, M., Krebs, C., Langton, L., et al. (2013). Female victims of sexual violence, 1994–2010. Bureau of Justice Statistics. Available at: http://www.bjs.gov/content/pub/press/fvsv9410pr.cfm

44. United Nations Population Fund. (2000). *The state of world population 2000 report. Lives together, worlds apart: Men and women in a time of change.* Available at: http://www.unfpa.org/swp/2000/english/index.html

45. WHO. (2014). *Female genital mutilation.* Factsheet #241. Available at: http://www.who.int/mediacentre/factsheets/fs241/en/

46. UNICEF. (2013). *Female genital mutilation/cutting: A statistical overview and exploration of the dynamics of change.* Available at: http://www.unicef.org/publications/index_69875.html

47. Mather, M., & Feldman-Jacobs, C. (2015). *Women and girls at risk of female genital mutilation/cutting in the United States.* Population Reference Bureau. http://www.prb.org/Publications/Articles/2015/us-fgmc.aspx

48. UNICEF. (2013). *Female genital mutilation/cutting: A statistical overview and exploration of the dynamics of change.* Available at: http://www.unicef.org/publications/index_69875.html

49. Institute of Medicine. (2001). *No time to lose: Getting more from HIV prevention.* Washington, DC: National Academies of Science.

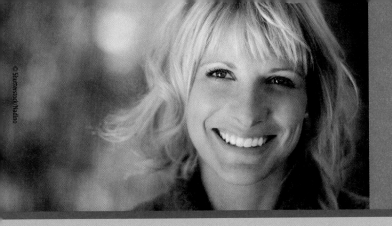

CHAPTER 5

Reproductive Health

Learning Objectives

On completion of this chapter, the student should be able to discuss:

1. The four primary mechanisms for achieving birth control.

2. The prevalence of contraceptive use among American women today and sociodemographic differences among women.

3. Contraceptive efforts from historical and legal perspectives.

4. How sociocultural and religious considerations influence contraceptive use.

5. Economic perspectives associated with contraception.

6. The importance of family planning services to demographic segments of American women, including adolescents.

7. The concept of fertility awareness for contraception.

8. The mechanisms, risks, benefits, side effects, and contraindications of hormonal, barrier, permanent, and other methods of contraception.

9. Emergency contraception options.

10. The concept of contraceptive efficacy.

11. The options available for an unplanned pregnancy.

12. The difference between induced and spontaneous abortion.

13. Abortion from a historical perspective.

14. Abortion from legal and political perspectives.

15. The pro-life, pro-choice, and middle ground positions on abortion.

16. Abortion from an epidemiological perspective.

17. The major types of abortion procedures.

18. Reasons why the assessment of risks, benefits, and contraindications is an integral component of contraceptive decision making.

19. The strategies in effective contraceptive decision making.

20. The importance of careful decision making regarding abortion.

INTRODUCTION

From a personal perspective, the ability to control the body's reproductive function is a necessary part of a woman's health, career, and family management. Contraception is also important from a public health perspective. The Centers for Disease Control and Prevention (CDC) recognize contraception as one of the 10 great public health achievements in the 20th century.[1] Family planning allows today's women to have fewer children than in centuries past and to space births more widely, resulting in healthier infants, women, and children. Family planning has also helped women advance in society by enabling them to more easily integrate their educational, career, and maternal roles.

Although the terms "birth control," "family planning," and "contraception" are often used interchangeably, each term has a distinct meaning. **Contraception** is a specific term for any procedure used to prevent fertilization of an ovum. **Family planning** is a term generally used to include the timing and spacing of children. **Birth control** is a broad term that refers to procedures that prevent the birth of a baby, so it would include all available contraceptive measures as well as sterilization, the **intrauterine device (IUD)**, and abortion procedures. With the exception of condoms, none of these methods provides protection against sexually transmitted infections (STIs).

PERSPECTIVES ON BIRTH CONTROL

There are four primary mechanisms by which birth control can be accomplished:

1. Preventing sperm from entering the female reproductive tract. Strategies that use this mechanism include abstinence, withdrawal (pull-out method), male and female condoms, and male sterilization.

2. Preventing sperm from fertilizing an ovum once they have entered the female reproductive tract. Strategies that use this mechanism include the diaphragm, cervical cap, contraceptive sponge, and spermicides.

3. Preventing ovulation and/or preventing the sperm from reaching the ovum. Strategies that use this mechanism include oral contraceptives, hormone implants, hormone injectables, hormone patch, vaginal ring, some types of IUDs, some types of emergency contraceptives, and female sterilization.

4. Preventing progression or implantation of a fertilized ovum. Strategies that use this mechanism include the copper IUD, some forms of oral contraceptives, and abortion. Some studies have shown that emergency contraceptives containing both estrogen and progestin work by preventing implantation of a fertilized egg. However, other studies have found no changes or impact to the endometrium. Once implantation has occurred, emergency contraceptive pills do not interrupt the pregnancy.[2]

Some women use timing to prevent pregnancy by avoiding vaginal intercourse on fertile days. The fertility awareness method (FAM) is based on keeping sperm out of the vagina during the days near ovulation. Similarly, women who have just given birth may use continuous

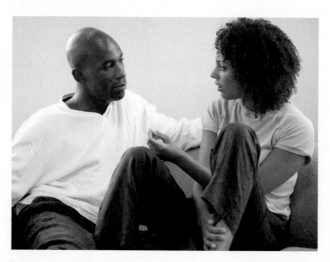

Choosing the right contraception is a decision that couples should make together.
© Creatas

breastfeeding to prevent pregnancy, because a woman will not likely ovulate while she is continuously breastfeeding in the first 6 months after pregnancy.

Some couples may elect to practice **oral sex**, outercourse, or other forms of sexual intimacy rather than engage in vaginal sex. Oral sex, or oral–genital contact, cannot result in pregnancy but can result in the transmission of sexually transmitted infections. **Outercourse** is the sharing of sexual intimacy through behaviors such as kissing, petting, and mutual masturbation without penile–vaginal penetration. These behaviors allow a couple to share pleasure and physical closeness without the risk of pregnancy; however, these activities can result in STI transmission if fluids are exchanged or if genital skin comes in contact with another person's genitals, mouth, or anus. Couples who practice outercourse require strong and motivated discipline to stay within limits: Ejaculation on, next to, or inside the vaginal opening has real risk for pregnancy and requires contraception if pregnancy is not desired.

Ultimately, decisions regarding birth control and family planning are a shared responsibility, so the best method for one woman and her partner can be different from that of another woman and her partner. The risk of STIs should also influence a couple's decision about what type or types of contraception to use.

Contraceptive Use

Contraception is an integral dimension of a woman's life. The "typical" American woman will spend about 3 years of her adult life being pregnant, postpartum, or trying to become pregnant and 3 decades of her reproductive life trying to avoid being pregnant.[3] National survey data reveal that nearly all sexually experienced women have used some method of contraception and approximately 62% of reproductive-age women in the United States are currently using some form of birth control.[4] The two most popular forms of birth control are female sterilization and the birth control pill. The 38% of women of reproductive age who are not currently using contraception includes women who are currently pregnant or postpartum; trying to become pregnant; have never had intercourse or no intercourse in the last 3 months; and are sterile for reasons other than contraceptive choice (**Figure 5.1**).

Contraceptive use among women varies by age. Nearly 31% of women in the 15- to 19-year-old range are currently using contraception, with the proportion of users rising in each successive age group through 44 years. As shown in **Figure 5.2**, a higher proportion of women under 30 use the pill compared to other methods. Female sterilization is the leading contraceptive method among women aged 30 to 44.[4] Compared to earlier generations of women, young women today are more likely to use contraceptives when they begin intercourse; this probability increases with greater maternal education and higher socioeconomic status.[5] Data indicate that 56% of women whose first intercourse occurred before 1985 used a method of contraception. That proportion increased to 76% in 2000–2004 and reached 84% in 2005–2008.

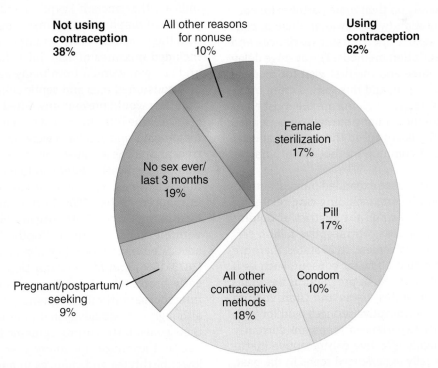

Figure 5.1   Percentage distribution of women aged 15 to 44 years, by whether they are using contraception and by reasons for nonuse and methods used: United States, 2006–2010.

Data from Jones, J., Mosher, W., & Daniels, K. (2012). *Current contraceptive use in the United States, 2006–2010, and changes in patterns of use since 1995.* National Health Statistics Reports, no 60. Hyattsville, MD: National Center for Health Statistics. Available at: http://www.cdc.gov/nchs/data/nhsr/nhsr060.pdf

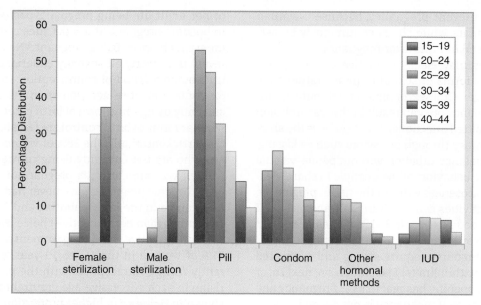

Figure 5.2   **Percentage distribution of method used by age and marital status: United States, 2006–2010.**

Data from Jones, J., Mosher, W., & Daniels, K. (2012). *Current contraceptive use in the United States, 2006–2010, and changes in patterns of use since 1995.* National Health Statistics Reports, no 60. Hyattsville, MD: National Center for Health Statistics. Available at: http://www.cdc.gov/nchs/data/nhsr/nhsr060.pdf

Special Population: Adolescents

A sexually active female teen who does not use a contraceptive has a 90% chance of becoming pregnant within a year.[6] Teens and young adults often harbor many myths and misconceptions about contraception (see **Table 5.1**). Teenage girls tend to rely on their male partners for contraceptive implementation (withdrawal and use of condoms) during early sexual intercourse experiences and only later adopt prescription methods. The average delay between first intercourse and the first visit for medical consultation is about 1 year, and this visit is often motivated by a pregnancy scare. Condoms are the most common contraceptive method among sexually experienced teen females, with 95% having used the condom at least once; the second most common method is withdrawal, followed by the pill.[7]

In recent years, states have expanded minors' authority to consent for health care, including care related to sexual activity. In 21 states and the District of Columbia, minors are able to access contraceptive health services without parental involvement. In 25 states, there are various circumstances that allow for consent, such as if the minor is a parent, married, or pregnant or has graduated high school. Two states, Texas and Utah, require parental consent for contraceptive services paid for with state funds.[8] Sexually experienced teens are currently more likely to use highly effective contraceptive methods compared to sexually experienced teens in the past; the increased use of these contraceptives may be a contributing factor to the national decline in teen birth rates.[9]

Historical and Legal Perspectives

Throughout history and across global cultures, women have attempted to control their **fertility** by using many different methods. The biblical book of Genesis contains a reference to *coitus interruptus* (withdrawal), while records indicate that ancient Egyptian and Greek women made primitive diaphragms by inserting paste-like mixtures into their vaginas. Early attempts at spermicidal agents included mixtures of acid, juice, honey, alcohol, opium, and vinegar. Women from many ages and cultures have also consumed teas and septic solutions with the hopes that they would prevent unwanted pregnancy.

Until the introduction of the birth control pill in 1960, diaphragms and condoms were the primary forms of contraception. The earliest condoms were probably made from linen sheaths; later condoms were made from animal intestines. The cervical cap and diaphragm were introduced in the 1800s. In the mid-19th century, feminists in the United States began a birth control campaign with the slogan "Voluntary Motherhood." This campaign advocated birth control by abstinence. Margaret Sanger (1879–1966) and Mary Coffin Dennett (1872–1947) were early promoters of contraceptive birth control (sexual intercourse without pregnancy) in the United States, although the two advocated different means to achieve their goals. Birth control remained within the scope of national attention for many years. In the early 1900s, lower birthrates and changes in family structure among upper-class White Americans caused some to feel anxiety about "race suicide," in which the race's death rate

Table 5.1 Myths and Misconceptions About Contraceptives

There are perhaps as many myths and misconceptions about contraceptives as there are facts. A few of the more common ones are summarized below:

Myth: Birth control pills make a woman fat.

Some women may gain a few pounds while taking the pill; some women may lose weight.

Myth: A woman cannot get pregnant the first time.

A woman can become pregnant as soon as she begins to ovulate.

Myth: A woman needs to take a break from the pill every year.

There is no medical reason to have a break from the pill; it can be taken for many years without a break.

Myth: IUDs make sex uncomfortable for men.

IUDs are rarely felt by the male partner.

Myth: Wearing two condoms will provide twice as much protection.

Using more than one condom actually increases the risk of tearing due to friction.

Myth: Condoms detract from sexual pleasure.

Some condoms are designed to increase sensitivity. Not using a condom increases the risk of sexually transmitted infections.

Myth: Male withdrawal before ejaculation prevents pregnancy.

Pre-ejaculate fluid can contain sperm and timing of withdrawal is very difficult.

Myth: Plastic wrap can be a substitute for a condom.

Plastic wrap, balloons, and plastic bags do not work as protection during sexual intercourse. They do not fit and can be easily torn or displaced during sex.

Myth: A woman can't get pregnant while she is breastfeeding.

Breastfeeding will delay ovulation and will reduce the chance of getting pregnant, but it is not a guarantee. Nursing mothers who are sure they do not want to become pregnant should use an additional form of birth control.

Myth: Douching, showering, or urinating after sex will prevent pregnancy.

Douching is not effective, and there is some evidence that it may increase the risk for pregnancy by propelling the semen toward the cervix. Showering or urinating will not stop the sperm that have already entered the uterus through the cervix.

Myth: A woman can't get pregnant during her period.

A woman is usually not ovulating during her period. But sperm can live a long time inside a woman's body and women with irregular cycles often do not know when they are ovulating.

would exceed its birth rate, and more fertile immigrants and poor people would replace the current population. Proponents of this elitist theory encouraged Anglo-Saxon women especially to have large families as a duty to their race and nation.

Today, many women take information on birth control and the availability of contraceptive devices for granted. However, for most of American history, contraceptives, as well as information about contraceptives, were illegal in parts or all of the country. Just 50 years ago, birth control pills were illegal in some states.

- In 1965, the Supreme Court's landmark decision, *Griswold v. Connecticut*, struck down a statute that banned the use of birth control and criminalized spreading information about its use. Justice William Orville Douglas based the decision on the fact that the case involved "the intimate relationship of husband and wife" and contraceptives were a logical extension of the marital relationship.

- In 1972, with *Eisenstadt v. Baird*, the Supreme Court established the right of unmarried people to possess contraception and invalidated a Massachusetts law that had made it a felony to give contraceptives to anyone other than a married person.

- In 1977, with *Carey v. Population Services International*, the court legalized the sale of nonprescription contraceptives by people other than licensed pharmacists and the sale, distribution, and advertisement of contraceptives to adults and minors under 16.

Recent legal victories in the contraceptive movement have mandated increased women's access to more contraceptive options through their health insurers. The debate about insurance coverage, and particularly contraceptive options, continues to be a major political issue with the Patient Protection and Affordable Care Act of 2010 (PPACA, or more commonly known as ACA). The ACA includes a birth control requirement, which states that all new health insurance plans must cover all FDA-approved methods of birth control, sterilization, and related education and counseling without **cost sharing**. A number of businesses have challenged this requirement under the federal Religious Freedom Restoration Act and the Free Exercise Clause of the First Amendment. One case that received much national attention in 2014 involved Hobby Lobby, a national arts and crafts chain that employs over 13,000 people. The owners of Hobby Lobby claimed that the birth control coverage requirement violated their religious beliefs and thereby the company's religious beliefs. The ruling was in favor of Hobby Lobby, stating that for-profit companies can exercise religious beliefs and providing their female employees with no-cost access to contraception violated the Religious Freedom Restoration Act.[10]

Federal restrictions on contraceptive development have resulted in the United States having fewer contraceptive options than other developed nations. Since 2000, however, several new methods of birth control have become available in the United States, including new levonorgestrel-releasing IUDs, the hormonal contraceptive patch, the hormonal contraceptive ring, the hormonal implant, an improved female condom, new emergency contraceptive pills, and a new method of transcervical female sterilization.[11] U.S. women have a responsibility to stay informed as contraceptive technology evolves and to stay aware of the political and economic forces that might affect the availability of various devices or drugs.

Sociocultural Considerations

Birth control attitudes and practices and contraceptive availability vary widely among social classes and racial and ethnic groups. In some cultures, motherhood is the ultimate status a woman can reach and is considered a personal achievement. In male-dominated relationships and marriages, a woman may have considerable difficulty in expressing and asserting her concerns and need for contraception.

Religious beliefs often influence a woman's attitudes and practices about contraception. Many Protestant denominations endorse birth control as a marital option, although a growing number of ultraconservative Protestant denominations espouse limiting its use. Teachings of Conservative and Reform Judaism emphasize the individual choice of the married couple, with couples able to limit their family size for either health or social reasons. Orthodox Jews may practice contraception under special health circumstances by consulting with medical and rabbinical authorities. The Roman Catholic Church traditionally and still officially accepts only rhythm methods, involving periodic abstinence, for contraception. According to its teachings, the primary purpose of sexual intercourse is procreation, and any interference with procreation is considered to be a violation of natural law. However, a national study shows that 98% of sexually experienced women of childbearing age who identify as Catholic have used a contraceptive method other than natural family planning at some point in their lives.[12] This practice in violation of church teachings creates emotional difficulties for some Catholic women. The Muslim faith also generally forbids contraception, teaching that reproduction is both a sacred duty and a gift. Although Muslims, on average, have the highest birth rates in the world, many Muslim couples use contraception, and some Islamic scholars approve of its use.[13]

> Birth control is a high priority for me. My family expects me to be a virgin when I marry. But we aren't ready to get married yet and I am not a virgin. I am afraid that my family will not understand this problem.
>
> **—20-year-old Hispanic American woman**

As shown in **Figure 5.3**, Hispanic, White, Black, and Asian women differ in their use of the pill and male and female sterilization. White women are more likely to use the pill compared to Hispanic, Black, and Asian women (21% for White women; 12% for Hispanic women; 10% for Black women; and 12% for Asian women). Black and Hispanic women are the most likely to undergo female sterilization (20% and 19%, respectively) compared with White and Asian women (15% and 7%, respectively). There also are significant differences in the sterilization rates of the male partners, with male sterilization rates of nearly 9% in the partners of White women but only 4% of the partners of Asian women, 3% of the partners of Hispanic women, and 1% of the partners of Black women.[4]

Economic Perspectives

Contraception and contraceptive use have three important economic considerations: (1) contraceptive costs for the couple, (2) contraceptive issues with healthcare plans, and (3) the costs and benefits that contraception provides society compared to unintended outcomes, including pregnancies and STIs.

Contraceptive costs vary significantly, depending both on the method's initial expense and how often (if at all) the method needs to be repurchased. Birth control pills and diaphragms, for example, both have required office visit costs; however, pills may cost about $15–50 per month, while a diaphragm, which should last for about 2 years, has a one-time cost of about $100. Additional costs are associated with some methods. For example, contraceptive jelly or cream should be used each time with a diaphragm for greatest effectiveness, and insertion and removal fees should be considered with an IUD. Couples may be able to save on contraceptive costs by using a publicly funded facility.

Although most contraceptives are prescriptive, not all insurance plans that provide coverage for prescription drugs include prescription contraceptive drugs and devices. Legal victories in the contraceptive movement have mandated increased women's access to contraception through their health insurers. Federal employees achieved mandated coverage for contraception via an act of Congress in 1998. In 2011, the U.S. Department of Health and Human Services (DHHS) adopted recommendations for women's preventive health care issued from the National Academies of Science and the Institute of Medicine. The ACA, based on these recommendations, requires new private health plans to cover contraceptive counseling and services and all FDA-approved methods of contraception without out-of-pocket costs to patients.

Twenty-eight states require insurance policies that cover other prescription drugs to cover all FDA-approved contraceptive drugs and devices, as well as related medical services. Twenty states allow certain employers and insurers to refuse to cover contraceptives on religious or moral grounds.[14]

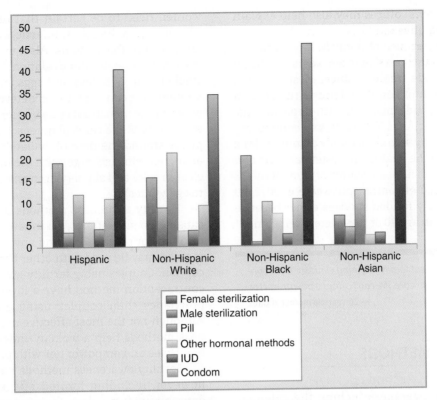

Figure 5.3 Current contraceptive status and specific method of women aged 15–44 years, according to race: United States, 2006–2010.

Data from Jones, J., Mosher, W., & Daniels, K. (2012). *Current contraceptive use in the United States, 2006–2010, and changes in patterns of use since 1995.* National Health Statistics Reports, no 60. Hyattsville, MD: National Center for Health Statistics. Available at: http://www.cdc.gov/nchs/data/nhsr/nhsr060.pdf

---

We are happily married, and someday we wish to have children, but right now our goal is to establish our careers. It would be really difficult for me to establish myself professionally if I become pregnant during the next 3 years.

—26-year-old attorney

The overall cost analysis of contraception should also include the societal costs of unintended pregnancies. Nearly one-half of all pregnancies in United States are unintended.[15] Two national studies have concluded that unintended pregnancies cost U.S. taxpayers about $11 billion per year.[16] Because these estimates are limited to public insurance costs for pregnancy, they are likely to be conservative and underestimate the true cost of unintended pregnancies. Subsidized family planning programs, such as those funded by Title X, could provide additional savings, but estimates of these savings vary widely. Existing family planning services clearly save money by preventing costs associated with unplanned pregnancies. The Guttmacher Institute estimates that without publicly funded family planning services, the number of unintended pregnancies and abortions occurring in the United States would be nearly two-thirds higher among women overall and the number of unintended pregnancies would nearly double among teens

and poor women.[17] In terms of public expenditures, for every $1 spent on publicly funded contraceptive services, an estimated $5.68 is saved.[18]

Additional cost considerations of unintended pregnancy include possible emergency contraception that may have associated prescription and office costs. The risks and costs of screening and treatment for STIs also contribute to the costs of some types of contraceptive failure. For individual women and men, contraceptive failure also has personal and emotional costs.

Contraceptive Services

Contraceptive services remain an unmet need for many women. More than one-half of the reproductive-aged women in the United States are in need of contraceptive services and supplies. These women are sexually active and able to become pregnant, but do not wish to become pregnant. Studies have found use of family planning services varies with demographic factors. Women with lower levels of education and income, uninsured women, Latino women, and non-Hispanic Black women are less likely to have access to family planning services.[19] Inequalities in use of reproductive health services are especially pronounced among young and socially disadvantaged women.[20] The underlying reasons for these differences are complex, and the geographical distribution of clinics and private practitioners' offices may also help explain disparities in contraceptive use.

In the United States, use of publicly funded family planning services has increased in recent years.[21] Publicly funded services provide free or reduced-cost services, including the provision of contraceptives to the general public. Such sites include public health departments, Planned Parenthood facilities, hospitals, and community health centers. For many women, a family planning clinic is the entry point into the healthcare system and the one that they consider for their usual source of care. Of the 38 million women in need of contraceptive care in 2012, 20 million needed publicly funded services either because they were younger than age 20 or they were low income.[21]

> *I am dependent on our local family planning clinic for birth control and my personal health care. We can't afford a private doctor.*
> **—26-year-old mother of three**

CONTRACEPTIVE METHODS

Fertility Awareness Methods

Methods of fertility awareness include the calendar method, basal body temperature, "natural family planning," and the cervical mucus or ovulation method. These methods are based on avoiding sexual intercourse during a woman's most fertile time of the month, which includes the days previous to, during, and immediately following ovulation. Understanding the female menstrual cycle is an essential foundation for using fertility awareness methods. Couples using fertility awareness tend to have more accidental pregnancies than do couples using most other contraceptive methods.

All fertility awareness methods require identifying the fertile days in a woman's menstrual cycle. On fertile days, the couple abstains from intercourse or uses a barrier method of contraception. The calendar method requires determining when ovulation occurs by calculating the average length of consecutive menstrual cycles and then predicting when ovulation is most likely to occur. This is a difficult method to use effectively, especially for women with irregular menstrual cycles. One of the most important changes during the menstrual cycle is the variation of hormones from the anterior pituitary and the ovaries. These hormonal variations cause biological alterations throughout the cycle, which lead to fluctuations in basal temperature patterns and variations in the type of cervical mucus produced. Many women are able to observe these changes during their fertility cycles and use methods of fertility awareness as birth control or a signal to use barrier methods of contraception. Measuring the body's daily temperature (basal body temperature) can help to determine that ovulation has occurred. When progesterone is released immediately after ovulation, the body's temperature increases a small amount; however,

women need to be certain that other factors, such as sexual activity, illness, or infection, are not causing these temperature fluctuations. Also, women can conceive a few days before or after ovulation, because sperm can be viable for up to 5 days and eggs are viable for 24 hours. Women also can sometimes determine the most fertile phase of the menstrual cycle by monitoring the change in the quality of the cervical mucus. During the most fertile phase around the time of ovulation, women experience an increase in discharge, with the mucus becoming more clear in color and slippery in consistency (often compared to egg whites).

Fertility awareness methods have the advantage of causing no side effects, no inherent risks, no contraindications or precautions, and anyone can use them. This method may be used with other barrier forms of contraception. Couples using fertility awareness with another contraception method have a lower risk of unintended pregnancy than couples using either method alone. Although not the most effective method, fertility awareness methods help a woman understand her body and her cycles and empower her with practical knowledge.

Fertility awareness methods have many drawbacks, however, including limited effectiveness, challenges determining fertile days, the need to abstain from sexual intercourse during many days of the month, and the lack of protection against sexually transmitted infections. For a woman who absolutely does not wish to become pregnant, fertility awareness methods for contraception have inherent liabilities: Fertility awareness methods depend on partner compliance, careful observations and calculations, personal discipline, and good luck.

Hormonal Methods

Hormonal Contraception

Combined hormonal contraception refers to contraceptive methods that include both an estrogen and progestin component. These methods include pills, patches, and

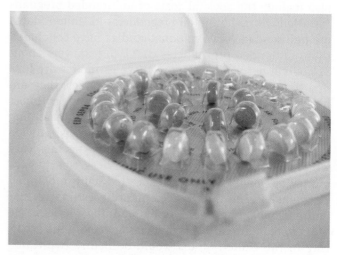

One type of birth control pills.
© Christy Thompson/Shutterstock

vaginal rings. Single hormone contraception includes progestin pills, implants, and injectables.

Combined Oral Contraception Pills

The oral contraceptive pill has changed considerably since its initial launch into the marketplace in 1962. Today, more than 30 formulations are available to American women. Although the specific hormones are the same or similar, the dosages and formulations have undergone tremendous change. Oral contraceptives are now available in packets of 21, 28, or 91 pills to be taken once a day, preferably at the same time each day—it is important to take the pills as prescribed. There are many brands, which can have different hormone levels. Different women find that they prefer different formulations of pills. Talking with a healthcare provider about symptoms and concerns may help a woman find the pill that best suits her individual needs. Pills are usually started on the first or fifth day of a menstrual cycle, or the first Sunday after a woman has started menstruating. Sometimes women need to use a backup contraceptive for the first few days after starting the pill. Backup contraception should also be used when a pill user has extended vomiting or diarrhea or is taking certain medications, including some types of antibiotics.

Birth control pills suppress a woman's natural reproductive hormone cycle, and the synthetic estrogen and progestin of the pill produce an artificial cycle to replace it. Without the natural signals, the egg follicle in the ovary cannot mature, and ovulation cannot occur. Another way the pill prevents pregnancy is by inducing development of thick cervical mucus, in contrast to the profuse, slippery mucus associated with ovulation. The thick cervical mucus impedes sperm movement through the cervical canal and inhibits chemical changes in sperm cells that would permit them to penetrate the outer layer of the egg. The pill also acts as a contraceptive by preventing the uterine lining from thickening as it normally does in the menstrual cycle. Thus, even if ovulation and conception did manage to occur, successful implantation would be unlikely.

Overall, birth control pills are highly effective in preventing pregnancy: Effectiveness rates of 99% can be expected when they are taken properly.

Side Effects   Side effects, both positive and negative, have been associated with birth control pills, including:

1. Shorter, lighter, and more regular menstrual periods. The reduced amount of uterine lining results in reduced blood loss.

2. Reduction or elimination of menstrual cramps. Cramping is often associated with ovulation; because ovulation does not occur with use of birth control pills, cramping is reduced or eliminated. Steady progestin exposure from birth control pills tends to reduce or eliminate cramps and menstrual discomfort.

3. Mood changes. Women may experience diverse reactions to birth control pills, such as irritability, depression, or mood swings. Some women, particularly those with a history of depression or premenstrual syndrome (PMS), may find these mood-related changes intolerable and choose to discontinue the pill.

4. Reduction or elimination of premenstrual symptoms. In many women, PMS tends to be significantly less severe or disappear with birth control pills.

5. Decreased libido. For some women, birth control pills may increase sex drive by reducing anxiety about pregnancy and alleviating discomfort or distaste at having to "get ready" for sex. From a biochemical perspective, however, some women may experience adverse reactions to birth control pills and experience a decrease in sex drive.

6. Spotting or bleeding between periods. The estrogen level maintained in the body by the pill is often lower than the natural level produced by the ovaries. This lower level may trigger slight uterine bleeding, generally referred to as "breakthrough bleeding." Such bleeding is more likely to occur when a pill is taken late or forgotten.

7. Weight changes. Some birth control pill users gain weight with the pill; others lose weight with its use.

8. Acne improvement. Most women who have acne notice significant improvement when they take birth control pills. In fact, some brands of pills are used to treat acne in some patients. However, birth control pills may cause chloasma, the darkening of skin pigment on the upper lip, under the eyes, and on the forehead. These pigmentation effects are not common and disappear when use of the birth control pills is discontinued.

Other effects associated with birth control pills include nausea, tender or larger breasts, headaches, and fluid retention.

Risks and Complications   Risks and complications are a major concern for oral contraceptive users, although many of these fears are unfounded. Safety issues concerning oral contraceptives are mainly based on the use of the original pills that contained high levels of hormones (although the original formulation of Enovid contained 150 mcg, current brands contain less than 50 mcg of estrogen) and the risks associated with smoking combined with use of oral contraceptives.

One concern about oral contraceptives has been that they may increase the risk of venous thromboembolism, the formation of abnormal blood clots within veins; these clots can sometimes break apart and cause blockages in a blood vessel. Venous thromboembolism, although rare, remains one of the serious possible adverse consequences of hormonal contraception. It has been estimated that venous thromboembolism rates in nonusers of reproductive age approximate 4–5/10,000 women per year, while rates in oral contraceptive users are in the range of 9–10/10,000 women per year. For comparative purposes, venous thromboembolism rates in pregnancy approach 29/10,000 overall and may reach 300–400/10,000 in the immediate postpartum period.[22] Thus, the absolute risk of this side effect is very small, and there is less danger of it occurring while on the pill than if a woman were to become pregnant and deliver.

An increased risk of high blood pressure, especially for older women and obese women, also has been associated with use of birth control pills. Other concerns identified by earlier studies of high-dose oral contraceptives include an increased risk of stroke and heart attack, though more recent studies show that there is no increased risk for either condition in women without preexisting risk factors, regardless of age. There is, however, an increased risk if the woman smokes or has hypertension. For women with cardiovascular risk factors or for women who smoke, nonhormonal methods of birth control may be the best option.[23]

Concerns have been raised about a possible connection between the pill and cancer in women. Since the pills were introduced 5 decades ago, sufficient time has elapsed to permit long-term studies on the possible association between the pill and cancer. Because some cancers depend on naturally occurring sex hormones, researchers have asked whether the hormones in oral contraceptives affect cancer risk. To date, hundreds of studies have been conducted; the results have not always been consistent. Studies have revealed that taking oral contraceptives *reduces* a woman's chances of getting endometrial and ovarian cancers but slightly *increases* her chances of getting breast cancer, cervical cancer, and benign liver tumors. Because all cervical cancers are caused by high-risk HPV, a sexually transmitted virus, the association between oral contraceptive use and cervical cancer is likely to be indirect.[24]

Some evidence has shown that long-term use of birth control pills is associated with changes in the surface of the cervix. These changes may make pill users more vulnerable to cervical cancer and sexually transmitted infections of the cervix, particularly chlamydia. Confounding factors, however, make it very difficult to draw conclusions based on this evidence. Contradictory studies have shown no significant alterations of the cervix that would lead to associated risks. Women who have more than one sexual partner or who are at risk of transmission of sexually transmitted infections should consider using condoms in combination with birth control pills.

Several drugs can reduce the contraceptive effectiveness of the pill and increase the risk of bleeding between periods. These drugs include barbiturates, some anticonvulsants, antifungal medications, phenytoin (Dilantin), and certain antibiotics such as isoniazid, rifampin, and possibly tetracycline. It is probably wise for any woman using birth control pills to employ a backup form of contraception while taking any of these medications. Oral contraceptives also may prolong the effects of caffeine, theophylline, and benzodiazepines (e.g., Librium, Valium, and Xanax).

Advantages

In addition to offering the maximum protection possible against unwanted pregnancy with a temporary contraceptive method, oral contraceptives provide additional advantages over other methods. They are woman-controlled and discreet. They do not require any additional supplies or equipment, and they do not interfere with the spontaneity of lovemaking. Also, they provide regular menstrual cycle certainty, freedom from heavy cramps and excessive menstrual bleeding, and often relief of premenstrual symptoms. Menstrual periods become regular and predictable. The hormones in birth control pills provide some long-term health benefits as well as pregnancy prevention:

- Women who take birth control pills have a lower prevalence of ovarian and endometrial cancers[24] and benign breast disease.[25]

- Ovarian cysts are also less common in women who take birth control pills; although oral contraceptives have often been prescribed for treatment of cysts, a recent review concluded that the pills are of no benefit and cysts will often go away on their own in 2 to 3 months.[26]

- Oral contraceptives may also be prescribed to help treat iron-deficiency anemia because they lighten heavy menstrual flow.[27]

For many years, scientists believed that oral contraceptives provided protection against osteoporosis because population data showed that long-term premenopausal use allowed women to enter menopause with higher bone densities than non-pill users.[28] Now, some evidence suggests that oral contraceptive use in young women may have an adverse effect on peak bone mineral density and osteoporosis.[29] More research on the relationship between pill use and osteoporosis is needed.

Contraindications

A contraindication is a medical condition that renders a treatment or procedure inadvisable or unsafe. Women who are contemplating use of birth control pills should carefully review and evaluate the contraindications before deciding to proceed. Absolute contraindications—meaning that combined hormonal contraceptives absolutely should not be taken—include:[30]

- A known cardiovascular disorder, now or in the past, such as thrombophlebitis, stroke, heart attack, coronary artery disease, or angina pectoris

- Impaired liver function
- Known or suspected cancer of the breast, uterus, cervix, or vagina
- Known or suspected estrogen-dependent neoplasia (abnormal tissue growth)
- Current or suspected pregnancy
- Abnormal vaginal bleeding
- Jaundice during previous pill use or pregnancy
- Malignant melanoma, now or in the past
- Smoking in women older than 35 years of age
- Diabetes with complications
- Headaches with neurological symptoms

Oral contraceptive use when breastfeeding has generated concern for infant safety. Although there is no current evidence of harm, the question cannot yet be definitively answered. Experts believe that the risks of combined hormone contraceptive products usually outweigh the benefits before 4 weeks postpartum. Between 4 weeks and 6 months postpartum, the advantages of using the combined contraceptive method appear to outweigh the risks, although data are lacking for definitive conclusions.[31] The National Institutes of Health (NIH) advise that progestin-only oral contraceptives are safe for use by breastfeeding mothers. A mother who is fully breastfeeding (not giving her baby any supplemental food or formula) may begin taking this medication 6 weeks after delivery; if the mother is partially breastfeeding (giving the baby some food or formula), she should begin taking this medication by 3 weeks after delivery to prevent another pregnancy.[32]

Types of Birth Control Pills

Pill packaging options are available in monophasic (each cycle provides 21 identical hormone-containing pills), biphasic (each cycle contains two levels of hormones), and triphasic (each cycle contains three levels of hormones) formulations. Triphasic pills, the most recently introduced combination pills, contain three different progestin doses for different parts of each pill cycle. The primary advantage of triphasic pills is that the overall amount of progestin in a cycle is lower than it is with regular, identical-dose pills.

Traditionally, oral contraceptives have been prescribed in 21-day cycles of active hormone pills followed by a 7-day placebo or pill-free interval that produces predictable withdrawal bleeding in most users. Some women who follow this regimen, however, experience nuisance breakthrough bleeding, spotting, or amenorrhea. New formulations of continuous oral contraceptive therapy provide continuous hormonal dosing without monthly periods of menstrual flow. Clinicians agree there is no biological basis for the original pill cycle regime, because

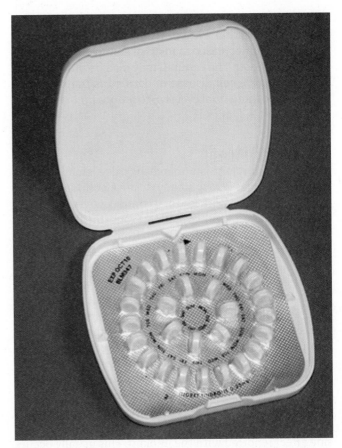

The minipill can be an effective form of birth control, but it must be taken every day, preferably at a consistent time.

monthly bleeding is not necessary either for contraceptive efficacy or patient safety reasons.[33] The most commonly prescribed regimen for extended therapy is 84 days of active pill use followed by a 7-day hormone-free interval. Patient satisfaction studies indicate that many women prefer continuous therapy, as it provides fewer and lighter bleeding days and less bloating and menstrual pain.[34]

Estrogen dose is generally considered to be the most important factor in selecting a pill. Side effects and complications are reduced with lower estrogen doses. Minipills are estrogen-free (also called progestin-only) birth control pills that provide a continuous, low dose of progestin. These pills may be a better option for women who have certain health problems, such as blood clots, and cannot take pills with estrogen. They are slightly less effective than the phasic pills and have a higher likelihood of breakthrough bleeding in the early months of use. Minipills do not totally suppress hormone production, so the natural estrogen and progesterone production usually remains sufficient to trigger menstrual periods. There is less margin of error with these oral contraceptives, however—the likelihood of pregnancy increases substantially with just one or two missed tablets. The minipill must be taken at the same time every day, and it may be less effective when taken with some drugs. Although menstrual periods tend to be less predictable with the minipills, women who use them generally experience fewer premenstrual symptoms, lighter or absent menstrual periods, decreased menstrual cramps, and less pain during ovulation. The minipill may also be prescribed to help treat sickle cell disease or dermatitis that seems to be related to menstrual cycles or to reduce iron-deficiency anemia.[35,36]

Hormonal Implants

A hormonal implant is a matchstick-like, small, flexible rod that releases a low, steady dose of hormones under the skin. Implants work like oral contraceptives, providing progestin that prevents ovulation. **Progestin** also thickens cervical mucus, preventing sperm from traveling through the cervix to the uterus. The implant is usually inserted under the skin of the upper arm, and it provides contraceptive protection for up to 3 years or until it is removed. The insertion procedure usually lasts about 5 minutes. A local anesthetic is used, and the procedure is normally painless. Hormonal implants are more than 99% effective in preventing pregnancy, but like other hormonal birth control products, they do not provide any protection against STIs. Hormonal implants are not as widely available as other forms of hormonal contraception because of the training that is needed for insertion and removal.

Irregular menstrual bleeding is the most common side effect reported with the implant. This usually occurs in the first few months of use. After 1 year on the implant, most women report that they have fewer and lighter menstrual periods, and some women stop having periods entirely, though some women will report longer and heavier periods. Another possible side effect is difficulty in removing the implants, but this is minimized with an experienced practitioner. Fertility is not affected after the implant is removed. Benefits, cautions, and contraindications for implants are similar to those for the minipill.

The hormonal implant is highly convenient. Candidates for a hormonal implant include those women who do not desire children for at least 3 to 5 years and who are seeking a highly effective and convenient form of birth control. Women for whom other methods may be contraindicated or for whom daily, regular pill-taking or monthly refills would be an issue may find the implant appealing. Women who are pregnant, or who have unexplained vaginal bleeding, serious liver disease, or a history of breast cancer should not use a hormonal implant. Although the initial cost of the implant can be several hundred dollars, this cost provides pregnancy protection for 3 years, making it a cost-effective solution in the long run. Many insurers will cover the cost of the hormonal implant.

Hormonal Delivery Methods: Injectables, Patches, and Vaginal Rings

Other hormonal forms of contraception besides the pill and the implant include injectables, patches, and vaginal rings. They all provide steady and predictable doses of contraceptive hormones that prevent ovulation and thicken the cervical mucus.

The hormonal injectable or "shot," also known as Depo-Provera, is an injection of progestin given intramuscularly. The shot lasts 3 months and has both a theoretical and actual-use effectiveness of almost 100%. Depo-Provera offers women a highly effective contraceptive that affords privacy and only requires four doses per year. Irregular bleeding for the first 6 to 12 months of use is the most common side effect; however, about half of women using the shot will stop having periods completely. Some women experience a delayed return to fertility after discontinuing the injections. Women who cannot take estrogen or who are breastfeeding are not good candidates for the injectable. As with other hormonal methods of contraception, the injection does not protect against sexually transmitted infections, and women with multiple risk factors for cardiovascular disease should consider other contraceptive options. Many women and teenagers have shown a decrease in bone density while using hormonal injections, but bone density appears to return to levels that are normal for the woman's age when the injections are stopped.[37]

The contraceptive patch is an adhesive patch that delivers hormones to the body. An advantage to the patch is that it does not require daily application: It is

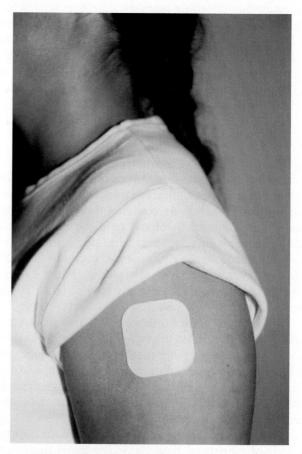

The contraceptive patch is worn on the skin for 1 week and replaced on the same day of the week for 3 consecutive weeks.

worn on the skin for 1 week and then is replaced on the same day of the week for 3 consecutive weeks. The fourth week is patch-free, and then the patch-use cycle resumes. The patch is durable and does not break away from the skin during warm weather, bathing, or vigorous exercise. Contraceptive patch users are exposed to higher doses of estrogen than pill users. Side effects to the patch are similar to oral contraceptives, although patch users report increased transient breast tenderness. Data from some studies show an increased risk of venous thromboembolism (VTE) among patch users compared to some combined oral contraceptive users.[38] The patch also was shown to be less effective in women weighing 198 pounds (90 kilograms) or more.[39] In 2014, the Ortho Evra patch was discontinued; however, a generic patch (Xulane) is still available for use.

A vaginal ring (brand name: NuvaRing) is a flexible, plastic ring that a woman inserts into the upper vagina. A provider is not needed for insertion or removal of the ring but a clinician must prescribe it. The ring is inserted in the vagina for 3 weeks and then removed for a week of menstruation, with a new ring inserted after the menstrual week. If a woman wishes to have continual protection without a menstrual week, she can insert a new ring every 3 weeks as a continuous form of birth control. The ring releases a gradual and steady dose of hormones. Women must learn to correctly insert the ring and most women do not feel the ring when it is properly inserted. Side effects to the ring are similar to those of the combination pill with additional possible effects of vaginal irritation or swelling and vaginal discharge.

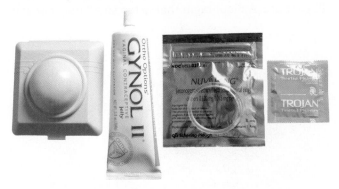

Barrier methods of birth control have virtually no associated health risks but must be used every time a couple has sex.
© michellegibson/iStockphoto.com

Barrier Methods

Barrier methods of contraception were the primary forms of contraception before the pill and IUD. After the introduction of more recent, "high-tech" birth control measures, barrier methods were seen as messy, unromantic, and less sophisticated. Barrier methods, however, do offer several advantages over other contraceptives. The condom has reemerged, particularly as a result of the AIDS epidemic, as a major form of protection against HIV infection as well as other sexually transmitted infections, such as herpes and gonorrhea. In addition, the diligent, consistent, and proper use of condoms with a spermicide has demonstrated pregnancy protection rates fairly comparable to those seen with the pill and IUD.[40] Another compelling reason for the return to barrier methods is that they have virtually no associated health risks, with the exception of rare allergic responses or localized irritation.

Barrier methods, as the name implies, provide a physical or chemical barrier that prevents sperm from fertilizing eggs. All barrier methods (except the female condom) are ideally used with **spermicide**, a chemical that breaks down the cell membranes of sperm for pregnancy prevention. Most barrier methods are used inside the vagina to cover the cervix and prevent sperm from entering the uterus. Male condoms are protective sheaths that enclose the penis during intercourse and ejaculation, while female condoms line the inside of the vagina and prevent semen from coming in contact with the vagina.

Barrier methods are very safe for the user, and problems and risks tend to be rare. One rare but important risk from barrier methods is toxic shock syndrome (TSS), which may be associated with the diaphragm, cap, and sponge. Although the TSS risk is small, the diaphragm, sponge, or cervical cap should not be used during a menstrual period or when any type of vaginal bleeding occurs. Further recommendations include delaying using these devices for 4 to 6 weeks after having a baby or until all postpartum bleeding completely stops. TSS risk also can be minimized by not leaving the devices in place in the vagina for longer than the recommended time period.

Vaginal birth control devices are also associated with some other complications. If left in place for too long, a diaphragm, sponge, or cervical cap may cause a vaginal bacterial infection. A foul-smelling discharge indicates such an infection and should be evaluated by a clinician. The diaphragm and cervical cap also may increase the risk of urinary tract infections, indicated by painful and frequent urination.

Although the diaphragm and cervical cap require fitting by a clinician, women (and men) may purchase other barrier methods in pharmacies. With the exception of abstinence, condoms are the only contraceptive method that can reliably reduce the risk of transmission of STIs. Barrier methods are seen as noninvasive contraceptive measures by those women who do not want to have an IUD and who do not want to manipulate their hormonal system. They may also be used as backup contraceptive measures for a woman who has forgotten a pill or who questions an IUD's effectiveness. Some couples have intercourse sporadically or infrequently and find barrier methods appealing because they are effective and can be used only when necessary. Barrier methods are typically more effective among older women and careful users, compared to younger women, women who have frequent intercourse, and those who are not careful users.

> *Well, I am proof that you need to follow directions. I thought that using a diaphragm was enough. I don't like that spermicidal stuff, and I thought a diaphragm alone was good protection. So I am pregnant. I can't believe that this is because I didn't follow directions.*
>
> **—21-year-old pregnant woman**

Spermicides

Spermicidal agents are available as creams, foams, films, suppositories, or gels that are inserted into the vagina. Foams, creams, and jellies are thick liquids inserted via an applicator (**Figure 5.4**), while suppositories are soft capsules that melt into a thick spermicidal liquid after being inserted by hand. Contraceptive film contains spermicide in a small, thin sheet of soluble film that is placed over the cervix, which melts in response to body temperature, and the spermicide in the film is released into the vagina. Spermicides are available without a prescription in drugstores or from online retailers. Spermicides provide some protection as mechanical barriers, by spreading over the surface of the cervix and blocking access to the cervical opening. More importantly, though, the active ingredient in most spermicides, nonoxynol-9 (N-9), inactivates sperm by breaking down the surface of the sperm cells on contact. To be effective, spermicides must be inserted deep into the vagina.

Spermicidal agents have the advantage of being effective immediately upon use, and they may provide some protection against STIs. They do have time limits, however, and their effectiveness varies. For spermicidal agents to be effective, a woman must carefully read and comply with the specific instructions for the agent she is using. An additional application of spermicide is needed for each round of sexual intercourse, and women should leave the product in place with no douching for at least 6 hours after each round. Women may use spermicidal agents alone or with diaphragms, cervical caps, or condoms. The agents are more effective when used with a barrier method. Spermicides are safe to use for extended periods of time. However, there are possible side effects with N-9, such as irritation, itching, or the sensation of burning of the sex organs (either partner); in women, urinary tract infections, yeast infections, and bacterial vaginosis are possible. In addition, spermicides containing N-9 do not protect against HIV and have even been shown to increase the risk of HIV.

Diaphragm

A **diaphragm** is a dome-shaped latex cup rimmed with a firm, flexible band or spring (**Figure 5.5**). It should be filled with a spermicidal agent before being inserted into the vagina prior to intercourse. The spermicidal agent creates a tighter seal around the cervix and inactivates sperm on contact. The pubic bone anchors the diaphragm in place. Because the diaphragm must fit the cervix it is to cover, this contraceptive method requires clinician examination, fitting, and prescription. During the fitting, women should evaluate the comfort of the diaphragm as well as practice its insertion and removal. Refitting of the diaphragm is necessary after a pregnancy, abortion, or significant weight change. A diaphragm should be replaced every 2 years.

Diaphragm effectiveness depends on proper fit and diligent use. A diaphragm that is too small may not stay

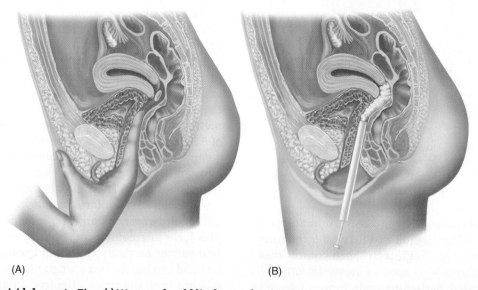

(A)   (B)

Figure 5.4   Spermicidal agents. Tips: (1) Woman should lie down after insertion; spermicide will leak out and have reduced effectiveness if she is in a vertical position. (2) No douching for 6 hours. (3) Keep extra supplies available—it is not possible to measure residual amounts of foam in containers. (4) Repeat intercourse requires repeat application of spermicide. (5) Wash reusable applicators with soap and water after use. Follow directions carefully for amounts and frequency of use.

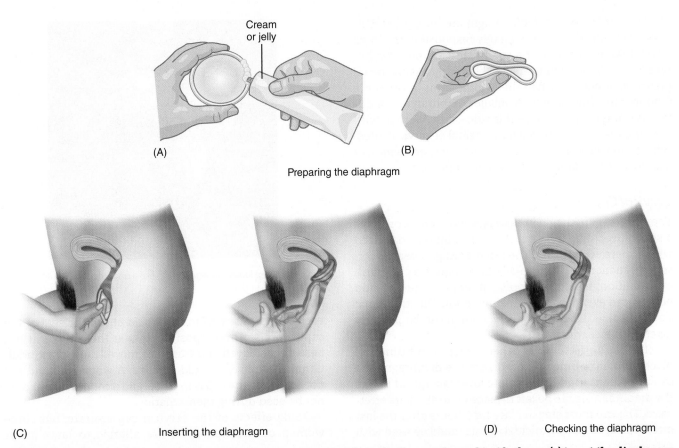

Cream
or jelly

(A)   (B)

Preparing the diaphragm

(C)   Inserting the diaphragm   (D)   Checking the diaphragm

Figure 5.5   Diaphragm. Tips: (1) Apply 1 to 2 teaspoons of spermicide to diaphragm rim and inside dome. (2) Insert the diaphragm by holding it in one hand, squeezing rim together in center. With other hand, spread labia and insert diaphragm. (3) Diaphragm is inserted deep into vagina with the anterior rim tucked into place last. (4) Check for proper placement of the diaphragm. Cervix is felt through dome–feels like tip of the nose. (5) To remove the diaphragm, assume the squatting position and break the suction by placing index finger between diaphragm and pubic bone. Hook finger behind anterior rim, bear down, and remove.

in place and slip off the cervix; one that is too large may press on the urethra and cause a urinary tract infection. Application of the spermicidal cream or gel and insertion of the diaphragm can occur up to 6 hours before intercourse. If intercourse occurs more than once, women should use an additional application of spermicide for each event, regardless of how short a time the diaphragm has been in place. The diaphragm should not be removed or dislodged to add the cream or gel for a follow-up round of lovemaking; spermicide can be inserted directly into the vagina.

A woman may insert a diaphragm up to 6 hours before intercourse; the diaphragm need not interrupt or interfere with lovemaking. It should be left in place for a minimum of 6 hours after intercourse to allow the spermicide to inactivate all of the sperm. Douching should not occur during that time. A diaphragm is not recommended during menstruation.

The diaphragm should not remain in place longer than 24 hours. After removing the diaphragm, a woman should wash it with warm water and soap, rinse it, and dry it with a towel. Women should not use petroleum jelly or oil-based lubricants with a diaphragm for lubrication

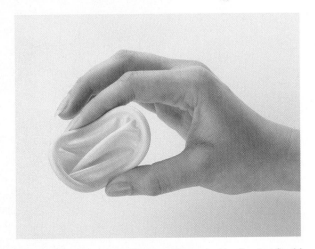

A diaphragm is a dome-shaped latex cup rimmed with a firm but flexible band or spring.
© Dorling Kindersley/Getty Images

because these products will weaken the latex of the diaphragm. Women who desire additional lubrication may use a water-soluble lubricant, such as K-Y Jelly or Astroglide.

Side effects with the diaphragm are infrequent. Urinary tract infections or an allergic response to the latex of the diaphragm or to the spermicide are possible but rare. Some diaphragm users feel bladder pressure, rectal pressure, or cramps when the diaphragm is left in place 6 hours after intercourse. A smaller diaphragm or a different rim type may relieve this side effect. Women with poor muscle tone of the vagina, a vaginal or cervical infection, vaginal bleeding, allergies to latex or spermicides, or a history of TSS should not use a diaphragm.

Cervical Cap

The **cervical cap**, shown in **Figure 5.6**, looks and works like a small, deep diaphragm. It is made of latex and is used with a spermicidal agent. The cap fits snugly over the cervix and suction holds it in place. Caps require a clinician's examination, fitting, and prescription, and they should be replaced every year for best protection. Due to normal anatomical variances, not every woman can be properly fitted with a cervical cap.

The cap's effectiveness depends on proper fitting and placement each time it is used. Like the diaphragm, the cap may be inserted hours before lovemaking, but unlike the diaphragm, it can be left in place up to 48 hours afterward. The cap must stay in place for 6 hours after the last intercourse. Fresh spermicidal agent should be used with

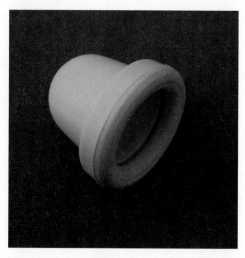

The cervical cap looks and works much like a small, deep diaphragm.

each round of sex. Women should check the seal of the cap before sex and reposition it over the cervix if it has become dislodged. If the cap has moved during sex, additional spermicide should be used. A woman should not douche while the cap is in place, and a cervical cap should not be used during menstruation.

Side effects of the cervical cap are rare, but some women or their partners are allergic to latex. After

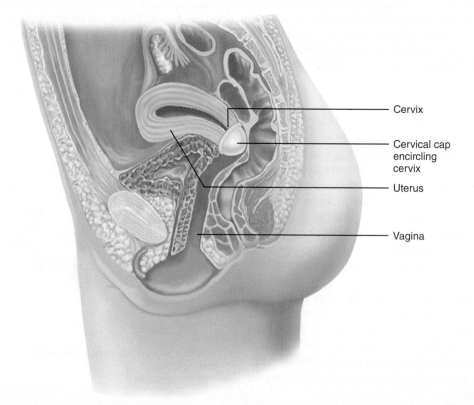

Cervix

Cervical cap encircling cervix

Uterus

Vagina

Figure 5.6   Cervical cap. Tips: (1) Fill cap approximately two-thirds full of spermicide. (2) Insert the cap by holding it in one hand, squeezing rim together in center. With other hand, spread labia and insert cap. (3) Cap is inserted deep into vagina. Use the index finger to press cap around the cervix until dome covers the cervix. (4) To avoid odor and reduce the risk of complications, remove within recommended time. (5) To remove the cap, break the suction by placing index finger between cap and pubic bone. Grasp dome and pull down and out.

childbirth, weight loss or gain of 10 pounds or more, pelvic surgery, a miscarriage, or an abortion, women should have their cervical caps refitted to ensure proper sizing. The cap is not recommended for women who have a history of TSS or a history of reproductive tract infections. Unlike the diaphragm, women with poor vaginal muscle tone or a history of urinary tract infections can use a cervical cap.

Condom

Condoms (**Figure 5.7**) are popular barrier contraceptives. The male condom is a thin sheath, usually made of latex, but sometimes made of a natural animal membrane, or a synthetic material, that fits over an erect penis. Condoms are available with lubricants and spermicides and come in a variety of colors and textures. Condoms are portable, disposable, and easy to purchase. They may be discreetly carried and are, therefore, easily available when necessary. Women do not experience any post-intercourse vaginal leaking when condoms are used, and condoms permit the male partner to take an active role in birth control. Condoms made from latex or polyurethane are also the only methods that effectively prevent STIs. For couples wishing to be especially diligent in their birth control efforts, condom use can supplement other forms of contraception.

Condoms should be stored in a cool, dry place. Condoms stored in a heated area (such as a glove compartment) can deteriorate and be less effective. Because oil-based lubricants (such as Vaseline) weaken latex, water-soluble lubricants (such as K-Y Jelly or Astroglide) should be used with latex condoms if extra lubrication is desired. Prelubricated condoms may also help to reduce

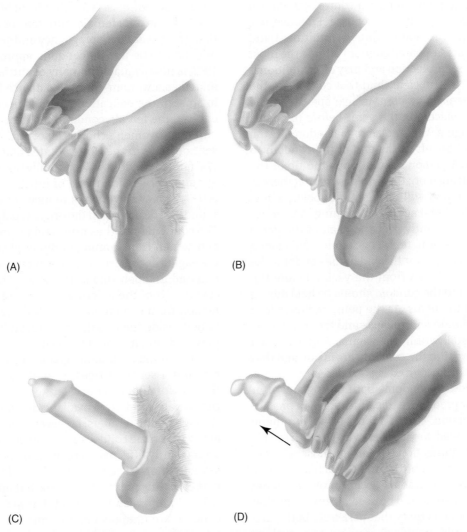

(A)   (B)

(C)   (D)

Figure 5.7   Condom use. Tips: (1) Avoid prolonged heat or pressure—condoms should not be stored in glove compartments or wallets. (2) Use only once and throw away. (3) If condom should break, use an extra dose of spermicide. (4) Put condom on an erect penis before it comes into contact with the vagina, pinching the tip of the condom to prevent air from becoming trapped. (5) Hold on to the rim of the condom as the penis is withdrawn from the vagina. (6) Do not use petroleum-based lubricants with condoms. (7) Latex condoms are better protection against HIV, although some individuals are sensitive or allergic to latex.

friction during intercourse and reduce the risk of vaginal or penile irritation.

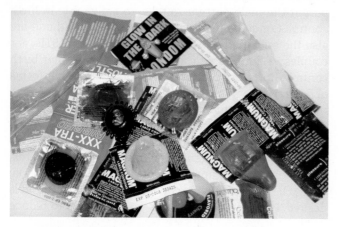

Condoms can be latex, polyurethane, or lambskin.

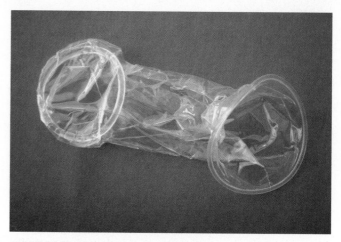

The female condom works by lining the entire vagina.

Couples using condoms for birth control should use them for every act of sexual intercourse. Effective use of this contraceptive method requires commitment and discipline. A spermicide-coated condom affords the most effective birth control protection and may offer additional protection from STIs. The clear fluid that collects on the end of an erect penis may contain live sperm, so the condom should be placed on the penis before the penis comes near the vagina. When placing a condom on the penis, room should be left at the end of the condom to collect the semen. A person should pinch the tip of the condom before putting it on; this will ensure that there is room for the semen and will prevent air bubbles, which increase the risk for breakage, from forming. A condom that is stretched very tightly over the head of the penis is more likely to break or to force the seminal fluid along the shaft of the penis and out the end of the condom. The penis should be withdrawn from the vagina before the erection subsides, and the condom should be held during this withdrawal of the penis. As the penis begins to lose its erection, the condom will collapse and the contents of the condom may spill within the vagina. A quick visual inspection to ensure that the contents are inside and that no spill or leakage has occurred is a good idea.

Couples should use condoms both during and after treatment for any reproductive tract infection as a precaution against reinfection. Use of a latex or polyurethane condom is encouraged for women who are at risk for sexually transmitted infections—even for those who are using an effective form of birth control, such as the pill. Lambskin and novelty condoms do not protect against diseases. Condoms also should be used on any items that are used during sexual activity that penetrate both partners—examples would include shared sex toys, such as vibrators and dildos. In such cases, condoms should be changed between insertions if penetrating both vaginal and anal regions. Couples should not use more than one condom at a time, and never reuse a condom.

Female Condom

The **female condom** is another form of barrier contraception. It is the only female-initiated contraceptive method that can prevent both pregnancy and sexually transmitted infections. The female condom, approved by the FDA in 1993, is now available in many countries and is often promoted as a woman-controlled device for HIV protection. In spite of the educational details necessary for individual use, the female condom has enormous potential for improving women's choices for contraception and STI prevention, both in the United States and around the world. The female condom was originally made of polyurethane, but a newer version made of nitrile became available in 2007. The newer versions reduce some of the crinkling sounds associated with the original polyurethane version. The condom lines the entire vagina, preventing the penis and semen from coming in direct physical contact with the vagina. It consists of a sheath with a closed ring at one end and an open ring at the other. The female condom covers part of the external genitals, providing extra protection from semen leakage. Although lubricant is contained inside the female condom, additional lubricant is provided, and it should be used.

The female condom gives the woman more control and a sense of freedom with her personal protection. A woman does not need to see a clinician because the female condom is available in some drugstores and through online retailers; however, it is not as widely available as the male condom and costs more. The female condom is fairly effective in preventing both pregnancy and sexually transmitted infections. The female condom can make rustling noises during sex, but additional lubricant will help diminish this effect. The size and shape of the condom are unappealing to some women. Proper insertion of the penis into the condom is essential for the condom's effectiveness. Because the female condom is not made of latex, it may appeal more to individuals who have latex allergies. Also, because both polyurethane and nitrile transmit heat well, some couples find increased pleasure with the female condom. The female condom can be inserted up to 8 hours before sex.

Use of the female condom requires paying attention to details, as well as patience and practice (see **Figure 5.8**). Before insertion, rub the sides of the female condom together to evenly distribute the lubrication inside the pouch. The female condom should be stored in a cool, dry place and it should be used only once. It should not be used with a male condom, diaphragm, cervical cap, or sponge. The only side effect to the female condom is possible allergy to the lubricant.

Contraceptive Sponge

The **contraceptive sponge** is a one-time-use barrier method that acts as both a cervical barrier and a source of spermicide; it also absorbs semen. The sponge is a soft, disk-shaped device made from polyurethane foam. One side of the sponge has a dimple that fits up against the cervix, and the other side has a nylon loop that facilitates removal. The sponge is relatively inexpensive, does not require a fitting or a prescription, and is available in drugstores and from online retailers. The sponge is portable, disposable, and can be inserted a few hours before having sex. It does not interrupt lovemaking. The sponge is designed for 24 hours of use, and it should remain in place for 6 hours after the last round of sex. It does not require repeat applications of spermicide for additional sex. The

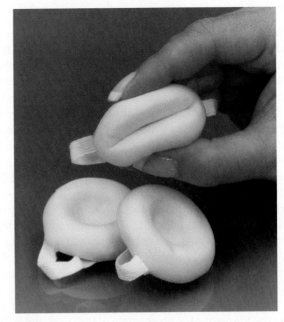

The contraceptive sponge acts as both a cervical barrier and a source of spermicide. It absorbs ejaculated semen.
Courtesy of Allendale Pharmaceuticals (http://www.allendalepharm.com)

effectiveness of sponge birth control, like all methods, varies depending on how it is used. The sponge is more effective in women who have never given birth than in women who have. Individual sponges cannot be reused.

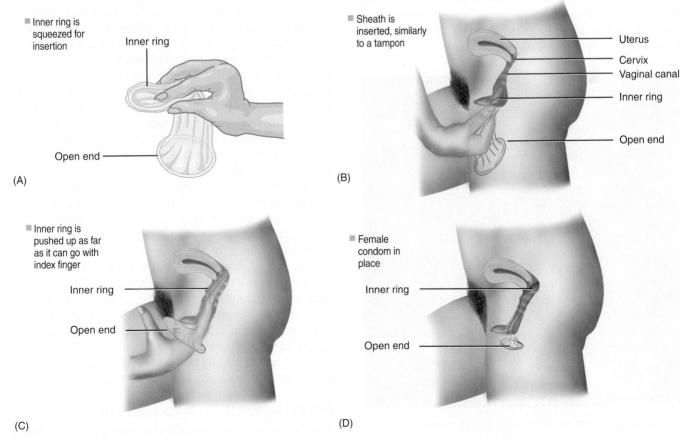

Figure 5.8   **The female condom.**

Intrauterine Devices

An intrauterine device (IUD) is a small object that a clinician inserts into a woman's uterus. Today, the IUD is the most widely used contraceptive in the world. Even though the effectiveness of the IUD is superior to that of contraceptive pills, patch, or ring,[41] the device has not been as popular in the United States as it is in the rest of the world. Its use, however, has been increasing. From 2006 to 2010, only 3.8% of U.S. contraceptive users reported using an IUD in the month they were asked; from 2011 to 2013, 7.2% of U.S. women said they used an IUD.[42] Modern forms of the IUD provide very effective, private, and reversible long-term protection from unwanted pregnancy without increasing the risk of reproductive tract infections. Although initial costs for an IUD may be higher than other forms of contraception, their long-term effectiveness is an important consideration, and IUDs yield a very low cost over time.

Because it is extremely challenging to study the exact mechanism of contraceptive action with the IUD in humans, there is not yet scientific consensus about how IUDs prevent pregnancy. Their different designs present different theories for their effectiveness. The horizontal arms of some designs gradually release small amounts of copper into the uterine cavity, preventing sperm from successfully reaching eggs from a woman's ovaries. Other types slowly release a progestin hormone, causing a thickening of the cervical mucus, preventing sperm migration to the egg. All IUDs establish a chronic sterile inflammatory reaction in the uterus that interferes with sperm function so that fertilization is less likely to occur; they may also interfere with implantation.

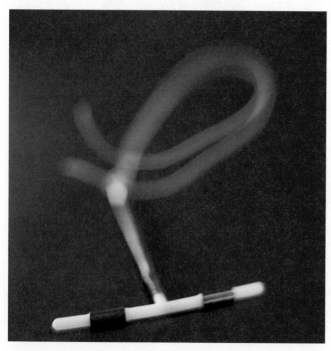

An IUD is a small object placed in the uterus through the cervix by a clinician.
© Spike Mafford/Photodisc/Thinkstock

Two highly effective forms of IUDs are available in the United States. One form is the Copper T-IUD, also know as Paragard, which is effective for 12 years. This long-term effectiveness presents a good alternative to a younger woman who might be contemplating sterilization. It can also be used as emergency birth control if inserted within 5 days after unprotected intercourse. The other type of IUD is a hormonal device, of which two brands are available, Mirena and Skyla. The Mirena IUD is effective for 5 years and Skyla is effective for 3 years. Hormonal IUDs offer the benefits of reduced period cramps and lighter periods for many women. Hormonal IUDs are sometimes used to treat endometriosis or as alternatives to hysterectomy for menorrhagia, a condition characterized by abnormally heavy and prolonged menstrual periods at regular intervals. Both IUD forms rival surgical sterilization in their effectiveness in preventing pregnancy. Fewer than 1% of users will experience an accidental pregnancy in the first year.[43] Provider education and training issues may prevent some healthcare providers from offering young women IUDs as often as hormonal contraceptives.

Permanent Methods

Healthy men and women usually have many years of fertility left after they have completed their childbearing. Surgical **sterilization** offers permanent birth control for individuals who are certain that they do not wish to have any more children. Female sterilization is second only to oral contraceptives in overall popularity as a method of birth control (see Figures 5.1 and 5.2). Advantages of sterilization for men and women include a very high rate of effectiveness and relatively quick, simple procedures that have minimal complications and side effects. Sterilization procedures do not disrupt either partner's hormones. An important disadvantage of sterilization as a form of birth control is that although it can sometimes be surgically reversed (a much more complicated procedure than sterilization), it should be considered a lifetime permanent choice to end childbearing. Also, sterilization provides no protection against STIs.

Perhaps the most important decision for a couple is which partner will undergo permanent sterilization. Women have the option of having a tubal ligation (tubes "tied"), and men have the option of vasectomy. The most common choice is for a tubal ligation. This may be due to several factors. Many couples don't realize that a vasectomy poses far less risk to men than the risks associated with tubal ligation for women. Men may also be reluctant to have this procedure that surgically disrupts the passageway of sperm into the semen; as a result, semen no longer contains sperm, so conception cannot take place. A vasectomy is usually performed in a physician's office and a ligation requires a hospital setting.

Female Sterilization (Tubal Ligation)

Trends among older, reproductive-age U.S. women using contraception show a dramatic increase in sterilization rates. Sterilization of women has been made much easier in recent years by the development of new instruments and new techniques that have replaced laparotomy, which involves surgically opening the abdomen and tying off the fallopian tubes. The procedure requires hospitalization and may take several weeks of recovery. Because unintended pregnancies occasionally occurred after this procedure, newer techniques now often destroy or remove part of the fallopian tube.

> We have three children and that is our family. The decision for sterilization was not difficult once we realized that we did not wish to become pregnant again. Our sex lives have improved—there is no need to worry about birth control anymore.
>
> **—35-year-old woman**

Laparoscopic sterilization, also known as "band-aid" surgery, is one of these techniques. A laparoscope, a tube equipped with light and magnification lenses (see **Figure 5.9**), is inserted into the abdomen to provide a view of the uterus and tubes. The doctor uses a cauterizing instrument, rings, or clips to seal the fallopian tubes. The procedure requires anesthesia and can be performed in outpatient surgical clinics.

Minilaparotomy is often performed after childbirth. It requires a small abdominal incision and is usually performed under local anesthesia. A doctor lifts the fallopian tubes out of the incision, and then cuts, seals, and replaces them. The entire procedure takes a few minutes;

the woman is able to go home after a few hours of recovery and observation.

A less invasive procedure for female sterilization, called Essure, is performed in an ambulatory clinic setting. The procedure requires the insertion of a small plug through a hysteroscope into each of the fallopian tubes. The plugs cause a local inflammatory process that results in tubal occlusion within 3 months of insertion. A backup form of birth control is needed for this period; a radiologic confirmation test can then confirm if the tubes are completely blocked. The method offers high sterilization efficacy without incisions, general anesthesia, or a prolonged recovery period for the woman.

Male Sterilization (Vasectomy)

A **vasectomy** is a procedure performed by a healthcare provider to close or block the vas deferens, preventing sperm from entering the seminal fluid and permanently sterilizing a man. Vasectomy can be performed in two ways, an incision method and a no-incision method. The incision method is a 30-minute surgical procedure usually performed under local anesthesia in a physician's office. In most cases, one or two small incisions are made just through the skin of the scrotum. The vas deferens is lifted through the incision and the two ends are tied or cauterized to seal them so that new sperm cannot enter the semen. With the no-incision method, a tiny puncture is made to reach the vas deferens. No stitches are needed and no scarring takes place. Also, fewer cases of infection, bruising, and other complications occur with the

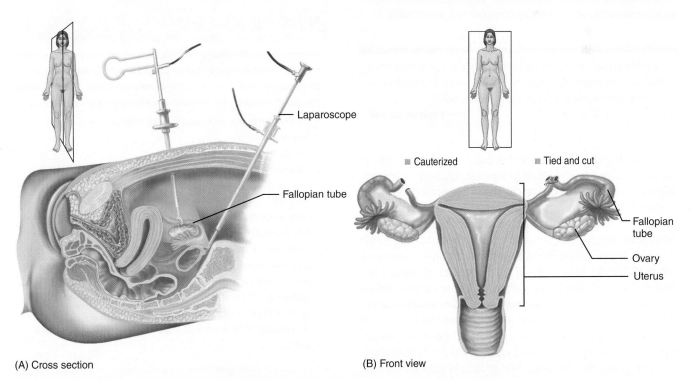

(A) Cross section

Laparoscope

Fallopian tube

■ Cauterized   ■ Tied and cut

Fallopian tube

Ovary

Uterus

(B) Front view

Figure 5.9   Female sterilization. Tips: (1) Resume normal daily activities slowly after the procedure. (2) Most sutures are dissolvable. (3) Take a mild analgesic for discomfort. (4) Resume sexual activity when comfortable. (5) Seek medical attention if temperature rises above 100°F, or if acute pain, discharge from incision, or bleeding is experienced.

no-incision method. With either procedure, most men are able to return to work and normal activities the day after surgery but are advised to avoid strenuous activities, such as straining and lifting, for the first week after surgery. Vasectomy does not provide immediate contraceptive protection. Live sperm may remain in semen temporarily because mature sperm are stored in the vas deferens above the surgical site. As a consequence, men often are advised to use backup contraception for approximately 15 to 20 ejaculations.

Vasectomy offers several advantages. It is extremely effective as a permanent form of birth control and has a very low risk of complications compared to temporary forms of birth control or tubal ligation for women. Vasectomy does not cause any change in hormone levels or in the appearance or volume of semen. It also permits the male partner to take an active role in contraceptive responsibility.

Other Forms of Contraception

Not all contraceptive methods are appropriate for general use. Some methods are valid approaches to birth control, yet are associated with fairly high failure rates. **Abstinence** refers to no penis-in-vagina intercourse and depends on a couple's sustained willpower. In theory, abstinence is 100% effective for both preventing pregnancy and protecting against STIs; unfortunately, this method requires considerable personal sacrifice and has a high rate of failure in real life. Some couples consider oral sex or mutual masturbation, which do not result in pregnancy, a form of abstinence. However, oral sex can still transmit many sexually transmitted infections.

> *He told me that he knew what he was doing. It was the first time that I had sex. He pulled out but I still got pregnant. I was so foolish to think that I would not or could not get pregnant.*
>
> **—16-year-old student**

Withdrawal, also known as *coitus interruptus*, refers to interrupting lovemaking before ejaculation of semen. Although it may seem logical that conception requires semen and therefore requires ejaculation, withdrawal often fails as a form of birth control when the man is unable to remove his penis in time or because the penis releases some sperm before ejaculation. The failure rate for withdrawal as a form of birth control is fairly high because it is difficult for a man to know exactly when ejaculation will occur. The pregnancy failure rate in withdrawal has historically been attributed to the belief that preejaculatory fluid contained sperm. While some studies have shown no sperm in preejaculatory fluid,[44] other studies contradict this finding.[45] So, a couple should assume that there is some potential for preejaculate sperm to be present. It also is mentally sand physically difficult to suddenly stop in the midst of lovemaking. Withdrawal

does not protect either partner from sexually transmitted infections.

Lactational Amenorrhea Method (LAM)

Lactational (means breastfeeding) amenorrhea (means no monthly period) is a temporary family planning option for nursing women. Breastfeeding women may use this method, alone or with other forms of contraception, for the first 6 months postpartum. For LAM to be effective, the woman must be breastfeeding exclusively (no infant supplementation) on demand, be amenorrheic (no vaginal bleeding after 8 weeks postpartum), and have an infant younger than 6 months. This method works by preventing the release of eggs from the ovary. The failure rate of this contraceptive method is reported to be less than 2% if these criteria are met.[46] If pregnancy is not desired, another method of contraception must be used as soon as menstruation resumes, breastfeeding is decreased, or the baby reaches 6 months of age.

Emergency Birth Control

Emergency contraception (EC) is known by several other names, including emergency birth control (EBC), the morning-after pill, and postcoital contraception. These terms all relate to a therapy or procedure used to prevent pregnancy after an unprotected or inadequately protected act of sexual intercourse. Emergency contraception is a critical clinical resource for sexual assault survivors. In addition, contraceptive accidents can occur with any method or any couple. As seen in **Table 5.2**, a number of

Table 5.2   Emergency Contraception
Emergency contraception is indicated when a woman does not wish to become pregnant after she has had sex without using birth control or if the birth control method failed. The following examples warrant consideration of emergency contraception:
▪ Birth control was not used during intercourse
▪ Sex was forced
▪ Condom broke or came off
▪ Diaphragm or cervical cap tore or slipped out of place
▪ Two or three consecutive active birth control pills were missed
▪ Two week or longer delay in getting hormonal injection
▪ Contraceptive patch or vaginal ring is placed too late or removed too soon
▪ Spermicide tablet did not have time to melt before sex
▪ IUD comes out
▪ Failure to abstain from sex during fertile days when using natural family planning
▪ Any reason to believe that regular birth control may have failed

Data from U.S. Department of Health and Human Services, Office on Women's Health. (2011). *Frequently asked questions: Emergency contraception (emergency birth control)*. Available at: http://womenshealth.gov/publications /our-publications/fact-sheet/emergency-contraception.cfm

conditions warrant the consideration of EC. Women, their partners, and clinicians have often had a need for measures that can provide immediate additional backup pregnancy prevention.

It is important to understand how emergency contraception works. Emergency contraception is not intended for routine use, but as a backup in the event of unprotected sex or a contraceptive failure. It provides no protection against STIs or HIV. Emergency contraception should not be confused with medical abortion. A medical abortion is used to terminate an existing pregnancy; EC is effective only *before* a pregnancy is established. Although EC is *not a medical abortion drug,* the topic has been a source of debate over abortion and contraception. Some have argued that EC is equivalent to abortion because it works by preventing implantation of a fertilized egg into the lining of the uterus. Recent analysis of scientific data shows that EC works by stalling an egg's release from the ovary until sperm can no longer fertilize it or by thickening cervical mucus, hampering the upward motility of the sperm.[47] Emergency contraception is ineffective after implantation occurs.

Plan B, which is levonorgestrel (progestin) pills, was the first product approved for use in the United States as EC by the FDA. Although the FDA approved Plan B in 1999, it was not available for over-the-counter (OTC) sale until 2006. In 2013, the FDA approved OTC sales with no age restrictions. Age restrictions on sales of generic pills similar to Plan B, such as Take Action, Next Choice, and My Way, were removed in 2014. Plan B is the most widely used form of EC in the United States. Plan B reduces the likelihood of pregnancy by 81–90% when taken within 72 hours of intercourse. It continues to reduce the risk of pregnancy up to 120 hours after intercourse, but effectiveness rates are reduced after 72 hours.[49] Additionally, Plan B may not work as well for overweight women. In 2010, the FDA approved a newer form of EC, known as ella, which is slightly less effective than Plan B but remains highly effective for 5 days. The EC ella is only available by prescription. A copper IUD also can be used as EC up to 5 days after intercourse. If a woman can estimate her time of ovulation, she can place it up to 5 days after ovulation, even if that time is more than 5 days after intercourse.

In addition to these two hormonal options and the IUD, regular birth control pills may be used for EC. A woman can take birth control pills in two doses in a 12-hour interval. The same brand must be used for both doses and the active pills, not the placebo pills, should be used from the packets. However, the number of birth control pills required to effectively work as emergency

> *I did not know that my regular birth control pills could be used for emergency contraception. I had missed a couple of them because I forgot to take them with me on a weekend trip. My pharmacist was very helpful in explaining my EC options.*
>
> **—20-year-old college student**

contraception varies from brand to brand, and not all brands can be used for EC. Additional information on birth control pills that can be used for EC is available on the Emergency Contraception website (www.not-2-late.com).

In the United States, the availability of emergency contraception has been a political story as much as a medical one. Conservative groups have organized heavy resistance to the availability and use of the product. In 2010, the federal Emergency Contraception Education Act was introduced by Congresswoman Louise Slaughter (D-NY) (see **Profiles of Remarkable Women** in this chapter) to fund national campaigns to educate women and healthcare providers about EC, but the bill was not passed. The bill would have addressed the reality that many women and their healthcare providers do not understand available options for EC. A recent survey shows that 86% of women ages 15 to 44 had heard of EC, but awareness was lower among teens than older women.[49] Some groups believe that EC availability would lead to increased sexual behavior risk taking; others have argued that EC would lead to fewer unintended pregnancies. Studies have found that women with a supply of EC are not more likely than women without a prescription or supply to have unprotected sex or to use EC repeatedly.[50]

CONTRACEPTIVE EFFICACY

Consistency and correct use are the two most important factors that determine contraceptive efficacy—how well a particular method is likely to work. However, even if used consistently and correctly, some methods are more likely to work than others, and contraceptive failure rates should have an important role in the selection of a birth control method. Failure rates are determined by following large groups of couples who use specific methods of birth control for a specified time and then counting the number of pregnancies that occur with couples using a given method. The larger the number of study participants, the more reliable the study results. A failure rate of 2% means there were 2 pregnancies per 100 women per year studied.

Two types of failure rates exist:

- The lowest observed failure rate represents a method's absolute top performance, the highest efficacy ever achieved in a reputable clinical trial. This rate is often referred to as the failure rate with perfect use.

- The failure rate for typical users is an average rate based on an analysis of a range of reputable studies. The failure rate for typical users is usually higher than the best-observed failure rates (**Table 5.3**).

Avoiding contraceptive failure is a goal of the Healthy People 2020 national health objectives. Baseline data from 2002 show that 12.4% of females experience a pregnancy despite using a reversible contraceptive method; the 2020 goal is to reduce this rate to 9.9%.[51] The effectiveness of a

Table 5.3 Contraceptive Failure Rates	
Method	**Number of Pregnancies Expected per 100 Women per Year**
Sterilization—female	< 1
Sterilization—male	< 1
Implant	< 1
IUD	< 1
Injection	< 1
Oral contraceptives	5
Skin patch	5
Vaginal ring	5
Male condom	11–16
Diaphragm with spermicide	15
Sponge with spermicide	16–32
Cervical cap with spermicide	17–23
Female condom	20
Natural family planning	25
Spermicide alone	30
Emergency contraception	1

Data from U.S. Department of Health and Human Services, Office on Women's Health. (2011). *Frequently asked questions: Birth control methods.* Available at: http://www.womenshealth.gov/publications/our-publications/fact-sheet/birth-control-methods.cfm

birth control method depends in large part on how carefully and consistently it is used. A diaphragm does not work when it is left in a drawer, pills do not work if a woman forgets to take them, and condoms may break or leak, especially if improperly stored or worn. Couples often face a choice between highly effective contraceptive methods that have side effects and other methods that have few side effects but may detract from sexual enjoyment and may have a higher failure rate.

HANDLING AN UNPLANNED PREGNANCY

Women who experience an unplanned pregnancy must face a difficult decision. They may decide to terminate the pregnancy, to carry the baby to term and keep the child, or to carry the baby to term and have the child adopted. A woman must consider the implications of each decision to feel comfortable with her choice. Having a baby brings major changes to a woman's life, and it may cause many difficulties for women who are young and single. Plans for future education, careers, or relationships may have to be sacrificed to raise a child. All of these issues must be considered so that a woman does not resent her child based on a decision she has made. A woman may be concerned about financial and emotional support during the pregnancy, especially if she does not have support from the baby's father or from family and friends. Many family planning clinics, crisis pregnancy centers, and health departments have programs to meet the needs of these women.

Unplanned pregnancies are not always unwanted pregnancies. Often, a couple is not planning to have a

GENDER DIMENSIONS: Health Differences Between Men and Women

Contraception

Historically, contraceptive options have been largely for women. This may be due in part to the reality that women, not men, get pregnant, or the fact that family planning research and contraceptive services have focused disproportionately on women. The female reproductive system has been extensively studied for centuries. Studies on male contraceptives have been seriously limited. Today, options for the male range from mildly effective (withdrawal) to highly effective (vasectomy). It could be argued that the remarkable effectiveness of modern hormonal contraceptives for women has given women high levels of protection, but that it has absolved men from participating in contraceptive protection and decision making. Men are often silent partners in preventing pregnancies.

Several factors contribute to the dominant role women play in contraceptive decision making and the availability of services for them. Modern medical care services provide ready access to contraceptive information and options for women. Women are taught and encouraged to see a gynecologist regularly in their teens; there is not a parallel system of routine health care for men. Society educates girls

and young women early that the penalty of unprotected sex will be an unwanted pregnancy, personal and family shame, and economic hardships. The educational message to boys and young men is not the same, although legal issues surrounding paternity and child support in recent years have introduced the penalty concept to an unwanted pregnancy.

Multicultural surveys demonstrate that men are willing to participate in contraception, and their female partners trust them to do so.[52] Male contraceptive research includes hormonal and nonhormonal methods. Today the most significant barriers for expanded use include limited delivery methods and perceived regulatory obstacles. Promising options include products that target sperm motility, decrease or eliminate semen emission, or interrupt sperm maturation. These products vary in delivery method and include pills, gels, ultrasound technology, and injection. Although considerable progress has been made in clinical research on male contraception, no new product is currently available.

child at the time that they become pregnant, but they want a child and happily decide to proceed with the pregnancy.

If a woman decides that she would like to carry the baby to term but not raise the child, she should look into adoption. Adoption can be "open," where the birth mother has some role in the child's future, or "closed," where the whole process remains confidential. Both public and private adoption services are available. Public adoption services are usually less costly but may be very competitive and require long waits for the adoptive parents. Parents often have to be more flexible about the age, gender, or race of the child they are willing to adopt. Private adoptions usually involve a financial arrangement negotiated by an agency or lawyer between the adoptive parents and the birth mother. Private adoptions can be faster and allow adoptive parents and birth mothers to have more options in selecting each other. Adoptions also can be domestic or international, though adoption laws vary from country to country. In all adoptions, the parties involved must consider a host of legal and ethical factors. Many adoption agencies can help match the child with an adoptive family and may be able to arrange for the adoptive parents to pay for the mother's healthcare costs during the pregnancy.

> *I am an organized and responsible person, but apparently contraceptive failure really can happen to anyone. It was impossible for me to raise a child at that time in my life. It would have destroyed everything that I had worked years for and my family could not help me. So I gave the baby up for adoption. I am not proud of it, but I am grateful that the child will have an opportunity for a decent life.*
>
> **—32-year-old woman**

Other women choose to terminate their pregnancies. In these cases, a decision should be made as early as possible to ensure a safe abortion.

PERSPECTIVES ON ABORTION

Abortion may be defined as the spontaneous or induced expulsion of an embryo or fetus before it is viable or can survive on its own. This can occur without human interference. Natural complications of fetal development, perhaps due to genetic, medical, or hormonal problems, can result in the spontaneous termination of the pregnancy. This manner of termination of pregnancy is called a miscarriage or a spontaneous abortion. In contrast to a spontaneous abortion, an induced abortion involves a decision to terminate a pregnancy by medical procedures.

Women choose to end their pregnancies for a variety of reasons. Women are most likely to choose abortion when facing an unwanted pregnancy but may also choose abortion when they learn that they have a potentially deadly ectopic pregnancy or that the fetus has a genetic disorder, neural tube defect, or some type of malformation. In a survey of more than 1000 abortion patients, 74% of women said that having a child would reduce their ability to work, finish their education, or care for existing dependents; 73% said they could not afford to have a baby at the time; and 48% said they were either having relationship problems or did not want to be a single mother. Other commonly cited reasons were that the woman had completed her childbearing (38% of women), was not ready for another child (32%), or did not want people to know she was pregnant or that she had had sex (25%).[53]

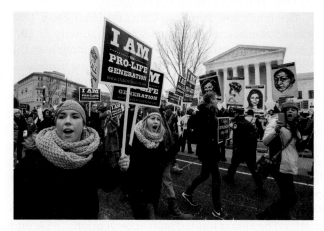

Abortion continues to be one of the greatest debates in American society.
© NICHOLAS KAMM/AFP/Getty Images

Historical Overview and Legal Perspectives

Women have ended unwanted pregnancies for thousands of years. The earliest methods used to induce an abortion were often either dangerous or used in ways to control women: Chinese legends attribute the prescription of mercury to induce abortion to emperor Shennong (c. 2737 BCE), and in the Western world, ancient Greeks and Romans generally considered abortion acceptable during the early stages of pregnancy—so long as the prospective father did not object. Saint Augustine (AD 354–386) agreed with Aristotle that abortion could be considered lawful before the fetus takes on a human-like shape and shows signs of movement, or during about the first 40 days of pregnancy. Through the 1800s, midwives and community healers in Western Europe and the United States used a variety of techniques to end pregnancies, making use of herbal abortifacients, mechanical methods (such as constriction of a girdle or introduction of foreign objects into the uterus), heat applied externally, strenuous physical activity, and starvation.[54]

Toward the end of the 19th century, physicians began leading movements to ban abortions, and by 1910, many states had passed legislation that prohibited abortion during all stages of pregnancy, with the exception of pregnancies that endangered the mother's health. Legal prohibition did not have its intended effect of reducing the incidence of abortions, however. Without a legal method of obtaining abortions, many women sought out unlicensed and unskilled abortionists or attempted to perform the procedure on themselves. Estimates of the number of illegal abortions performed annually in the 1950s and 1960s range from 200,000 to 1.2 million.[55] Illegal abortion accounted for nearly 17% of all deaths due to pregnancy and childbirth in 1965.[56] Women with greater personal financial resources were able to arrange for safer, more "legal" abortions by traveling to less rigid jurisdictions or by persuading physicians to make exceptions for "therapeutic reasons," while women with fewer financial resources were more likely to suffer from unsafe abortions and incompetent abortionists.

The landmark Supreme Court decision *Roe v. Wade* legalized abortion in the United States on January 22, 1973. This decision declared unconstitutional all state laws that prohibited or restricted abortion during the first trimester of pregnancy. The decision stated that the "right of privacy … founded on the Fourteenth Amendment's concept of personal liberty … is broad enough to encompass a woman's decision whether or not to terminate her pregnancy." That right to privacy, however, had to be balanced against a state's interest in protecting prenatal life and women's health. Arguing that the state's interest becomes stronger over the course of a pregnancy, the court sought balance by tying state regulation of abortion to pregnancy trimester. The ruling limited state interventions in second-trimester abortions and left the issue of third-trimester abortions up to each individual state. By dividing the ruling between a woman's interest and the state's interest, the Court created a heated national debate that continues today. The debate has shaped national political agendas and polarized interests into opposing camps with intense grassroots support for each perspective.

In 1976, Congress introduced and passed the Hyde Amendment. This legislation banned Medicaid funding for abortion unless a woman's life was in danger. This amendment disproportionately affected low-income women, who were (and remain) less likely than other women to be able to pay for abortion services or to receive contraception. A compromise version of the Hyde Amendment eventually added exceptions for promptly reported rape and incest cases in which two physicians would testify that the woman's health would be seriously impaired by maintaining the pregnancy.

The 1991 case of *Rust v. Sullivan* upheld the constitutionality of the "gag rule," which prohibited federally funded clinics from providing information about and referrals for abortion. In 1992, the Court's ruling in the case of *Planned Parenthood of Southeastern Pennsylvania v. Casey* reaffirmed the central holdings of *Roe v. Wade* but allowed states to restrict abortion access. This decision prompted many states to require parental consent, mandatory waiting periods, and counseling. Some state laws have also limited antiabortion demonstrators' proximity to abortion clinics. These laws attempt to ensure the safety and privacy of women seeking abortions after many attacks on women seeking abortions, abortion providers, and abortion clinics took place.

In the 2007 case of *Gonzales v. Carhart,* the Court upheld a federal ban on a rare abortion procedure known as dilatation and extraction, despite the fact that the law did not allow an exception to the ban when the procedure was necessary to protect a woman's health. **Table 5.4** provides a summary of the categories of state abortion restrictions.

The ramifications of abortion being a political issue are complex and widespread. Trained and available abortion care providers are limited, and these provider shortages may delay abortion services that are safest when provided early. A study found that 87% of U.S. counties had no abortion provider.[57] Another ramification of the intensity of the polarized views has resulted in provider murders, clinic bombings, death threats, acts of vandalism, harassment of clinic personnel, and postings of clinic patients online.

I am haunted by a story my mother told me of her friend who died years ago from a botched abortion. Her friend was desperate. It makes me realize that women will seek abortions whether they are legal or not. They should have access to safe facilities.

—27-year-old woman

Current Perspectives

Today legal abortions are very safe—markedly safer than childbirth.[58] Legal abortions are credited with decreasing

---

Table 5.4	**Categories of State Laws Restricting Access to Abortions**

- Waiting periods required between counseling and getting the procedure done
- Parental involvement required, either through notification or consent
- State-mandated counseling provided before an abortion with information that may be misleading or medically inaccurate
- Requirements for abortion to be performed by a licensed physician or in a hospital
- Prohibitions after a specified point in pregnancy with the exception to protect the woman's life or health
- Restrictions on use of state funds for abortion or coverage of abortion by private insurance plans
- Allowance for individual healthcare providers to refuse to participate in an abortion and institutions to refuse to perform abortions

Data from Guttmacher Institute. (2015). *State policies in brief: Overview of abortion laws.* Available at: http://www.guttmacher.org/statecenter/spibs/spib_OAL.pdf

It's Your Health

Reasons Women Have an Abortion

Conflict with education, work, or care for other dependents

Cannot afford to have a child

Desire not to be a single mother or relationship problems

Not ready to have a child

Data from Finer, L. B., Frohwirth, L. F., Dauphinee, L. A., et al. (2005). Reasons U.S. women have abortions: Quantitative and qualitative perspectives. *Perspectives on Sexual and Reproductive Health* 37(3): 110–118.

both maternal and infant mortality. Abortion is both one of the most common gynecological procedures women experience and ranks among the most controversial and passionately debated topics in the United States. Traditionally, people who believe that abortion should be illegal have described themselves as "pro-life," whereas people who believe that women should be able to choose abortion to end their pregnancies have described themselves as "pro-choice." Journalists, who wish to appear neutral and not imply that either group is against life or choice, use the terms "antiabortion" and "abortion rights" to describe activists on either side. Legal issues continue to evolve at the personal, state, and national levels about abortion and the challenges are likely to remain for some time.

The Antiabortion Perspective

The antiabortion (or "pro-life") position is typically based on the belief that a fertilized ovum is a human being from the moment of conception onward. From this perspective, a fetus has a right to live, and a woman does not have the ability to override that right by choosing an abortion. Antiabortion efforts to overturn abortion public policy have taken three major approaches: (1) amendments to the U.S. and state constitutions that define human life beginning at conception, (2) legislation and government action that defines human life beginning at conception, and (3) efforts to slow or restrict access to abortion services. By defining a fetus as "human," antiabortion groups hope to afford fetuses the same legal rights and protection as adults and children and ultimately outlaw (or put severe legal restrictions on) all abortions.

The Abortion-Rights Perspective

Abortion-rights (or "pro-choice") advocates favor full legalization and ready availability of abortions. Abortion-rights advocates see abortion as part of a spectrum of a woman's reproductive health care. They believe that women facing unwanted pregnancies will usually try to find a way to end them, and that legalizing abortion at least provides these women with safe services rather than putting their lives at risk. Additionally, they believe that a woman should be able to choose whether or not to end

a pregnancy because the fetus is ultimately still within and sustained by the woman's body. Abortion-rights advocates typically do not believe that a fertilized ovum qualifies as "human life."

Middle Ground

Most Americans' opinions about abortion have elements of both the antiabortion and the abortion-rights perspectives. Poll trends show that Americans tilted slightly toward "pro-choice" from the mid-1990s through 2009 when, for the first time, more people identified as "pro-life." Since then, the numbers have been evenly split, with the most recent Gallup Poll showing 47% identify as "pro-choice" and 46% identify as "pro-life."[59]

Finding a suitable compromise on such a divisive issue remains a political and personal challenge. However, research has found ways to safely prevent many abortions without increasing or decreasing women's access to safe services. The easiest of these methods may be to increase access to contraception and prevent the need for abortions of unwanted pregnancies. Allowing women and their partners to control when and if they want to have children will prevent enormous psychological and financial burdens for families as well. Increasing public assistance and access to family planning may also reduce abortion levels, because funds and aid will allow women living in poverty to better prevent unintended pregnancies as well as care for unplanned babies. In addition, allowing women access to abortion services does not necessarily increase the abortion rate; women who are determined to end their pregnancies may instead seek underground, possibly unsafe, services.

Epidemiology

Abortions are one of the most common medical procedures undergone by women of reproductive age. Each year, 1.7% of women aged 15–44 have an abortion.[60] Half of pregnancies among women in the United States are unintended, and 4 in 10 of these are terminated by abortion.[61] As **Figure 5.10** shows, the number of annual abortions has decreased since peaking in the 1980s.

Several factors appear to have affected this decline of abortion rates. Changes in U.S. demographics mean that a lower proportion of the female population is of childbearing age and at risk for having to consider abortion. The drive to educate girls about teen pregnancy and contraceptive options has also helped to reduce teen pregnancy. Other factors affecting the decline in abortions over time may include reduced access to abortion services, changing attitudes toward abortion, or more frequent decisions to continue unplanned pregnancies.

The profile of the typical abortion seeker has also changed in the last 20 years. In addition to young women who experience an unintended pregnancy, the growing number of women who get pregnant over the age of 35 has led to an increase in women who find out that their

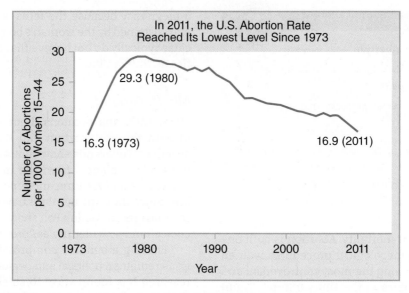

Figure 5.10 **Number of abortions per 1000 women aged 15–44: United States, 1973–2011.**

Data from Jones, R. K., & Jerman, J. (2014). Abortion incidence and service availability in the United States, 2011. *Perspectives on Sexual and Reproductive Health* 46(1). Available at: http://www.guttmacher.org/pubs/journals/psrh.46e0414.pdf

developing babies are at very high risk of birth defects or have a chromosomal abnormality like trisomy 18. Women living in poverty continue to be much more likely than wealthy women to have abortions, in large part because poor women are more likely to experience unwanted pregnancies. Additional characteristics of U.S. abortion patients include:[62]

- More than half are in their twenties, with women ages 20 to 24 having the highest abortion rate of any age group.

- Non-Hispanic Whites make up 36%, 30% are non-Hispanic Black, 25% are Hispanic, and 9% are women of other races.

- Six in 10 women already have one child and 3 in 10 have two or more children.

- Most women pay for abortions out of pocket even when they have health insurance.

ABORTION PROCEDURES

Elective abortions in the United States can be either in-clinic surgical procedures or a medical prescription that causes abortion. The type of procedure used primarily depends on how far a woman is into her pregnancy.

In-Clinic Surgical Abortions

There are two primary procedures for in-clinic abortions: vacuum curettage and dilation and evacuation (D&E). **Vacuum curettage**, sometimes called manual vacuum aspiration (MVA), is the most widely used abortion technique; nearly 80% of all legal abortions done in the United States use vacuum curettage.[63] This procedure is performed while the woman is under local anesthesia. It involves dilating the cervix and then inserting a vacuum curette, an instrument consisting of a tube with a scoop attached for scraping away tissue, through the cervix into the uterus. The other end of the tube is attached to a suction-producing apparatus, and the contents of the uterus are aspirated into a collection vessel. This procedure is usually performed during the first trimester of pregnancy, or until 13 weeks, but can be done up to 20 weeks following conception. The length of pregnancy is determined from the onset of the last menstrual flow or the last missed period. Through 13 weeks of pregnancy, this procedure can be performed in a clinical office setting with appropriate backup facilities for unexpected medical problems. The actual procedure takes about 10 to 15 minutes after the cervix is dilated.

Dilation and curettage (D&C) is a technique used for many gynecological procedures but rarely in abortions. It can be used up to 16 weeks from the last period. A sharp curette is used to scrape out the contents of the uterus. The procedure requires that the woman be under general anesthesia. Dilation and curettage is rarely used in abortions in the United States because it is more painful than the vacuum curettage method, causes more blood loss, and requires larger cervical dilation.

Dilation and evacuation is a procedure that combines the D&C and vacuum curettage approaches. It is usually done between 13 and 15 weeks' gestation but may be done through week 22. At this time, the cervix needs to be dilated to a greater extent because the products of conception are larger. This procedure is performed in the operating room of a clinic or hospital.

Oxytocin, a product produced in the posterior pituitary and also commercially manufactured, is often used to facilitate uterine contractions. It is commonly used with the D&C method and with hypertonic saline during second-trimester abortions.

As with all medical procedures, abortions carry some health risks. Abortion-related health risks are greatly reduced if the pregnancy is terminated as early as possible, the woman is healthy, and she receives care in a competent facility. The most common postabortion problems include infection, retained products of conception in the uterus, continuing pregnancy, cervical or uterine trauma, and bleeding.

Medical Abortion

A medical abortion (sometimes referred to as a medication abortion or "abortion with pills") is an abortion performed with medication instead of surgery. Medical abortion offers women the opportunity to end pregnancies safely and in a way that is less invasive than surgical abortion procedures. Two drugs called mifepristone and misoprostol, used in succession, can end an early pregnancy. The drug combo is also known as RU-486 or Mifeprex. The FDA approved mifepristone in 2000 as a safe and effective alternative to surgical abortion in the United States. Since FDA approval of mifepristone, the proportion of medical abortions has grown and the proportion of surgical procedures has declined. About 19.1% of abortions performed in the United States in 2008 were with medical abortion.[63]

Mifepristone is a hormone pill that blocks the action of progesterone, which is necessary for maintaining a pregnancy. A woman first takes mifepristone at a provider's office; this causes the uterine lining to break down. In some cases, a provider may use a medication called methotrexate instead of mifepristone. Days later, a woman takes misoprostol to induce contractions and expel the fetal tissue. Heavy bleeding and cramping ensue as a result of the misoprostol. These symptoms may last from a few hours to 2 weeks. The entire abortion is therefore considered to take anywhere from a few days to a few weeks and requires several visits to the healthcare provider's office. Possible side effects may include nausea, vomiting, diarrhea, headaches, hot flushes, and mouth sores.

Medical abortions may be performed as soon as a pregnancy is confirmed, and they must be performed within 7 weeks after a woman's last menstrual period. Medical abortions must be performed by a physician. Women who are older than 35 years of age or who smoke should not use methotrexate or mifepristone. Other conditions that may preclude a woman from having a medical abortion include history of asthma, cardiovascular disease, uncontrolled hypertension, diabetes, ovarian cysts or tumors, and severe anemia.

Currently, lawmakers in many states are moving to restrict medical abortion. At both the federal and state levels, some have proposed legislation designed to curtail the availability of mifepristone and limit the number of doctors who can prescribe it.

GLOBAL PERSPECTIVES

The World Health Organization (WHO) reports that in 2008, an estimated 21.6 million unsafe abortions took place, mostly in the developing world. Deaths due to unsafe abortion account for about one in eight (13%) of all maternal deaths. Each year, 47,000 women die from complications of unsafe abortion.[64] It has been estimated that one in three deaths related to pregnancy and childbirth could be avoided if women who wanted effective contraception had access to it.

Despite the magnitude of this problem, there are solutions: Provide women with skilled attendants (such as doctors or midwives) when they give birth, provide family planning so that women and their partners can choose when and if they want to have children, and allow women access to safe abortion services. However, poor health systems, a lack of organized political willpower, and legal restrictions and opposition have limited progress in this arena. Reductions in maternal mortality have been extremely slow over the past 20 years. Lessons can be learned from the international landscape. Countries with highly restrictive abortion laws are not associated with lower abortion rates. Abortions are generally safe in countries where abortion is permitted on broad legal grounds; in countries where abortion is prohibited or difficult to access, it is typically unsafe.[65]

INFORMED DECISION MAKING

Contraception

Many effective, yet imperfect, birth control methods are available to women today. The decision-making challenge is to determine which method or combination of methods best meets each woman's unique needs. Safety and reliability are always the first concern. Other factors, such as health status, lifestyle, financial considerations, and patterns in sexual activity, also determine which method is preferred. Many women will decide to change to a different birth control method as their preferences and

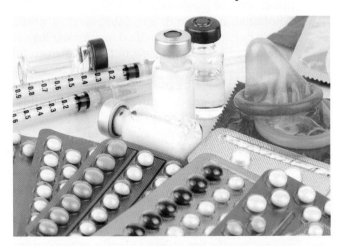

Many contraceptive choices are available today.
© areeya_ann/Shutterstock

situations change. Communication is an essential component of contraceptive decision making—couples should talk about their feelings, needs, and fears.

Determining Personal Needs

Sexual urges and sexual activity are normal, and pregnancy is a very real possible consequence of heterosexual intercourse. Both homosexual and heterosexual relationships also carry the risk of sexually transmitted infections, including HIV. For both technological and sociological reasons, women have traditionally shouldered the major responsibility for contraception. This has been unfair for women. Although most of the currently available contraceptives require primary use by women, couples can share the responsibility for contraception in many ways. Open and honest communication, sensitivity to each other's needs and feelings, and awareness of each method's strengths and weaknesses are essential components for effective decision making.

Specific strategies for informed contraceptive decision making include the following (also see **Self-Assessment 5.1**):

1. Review needs.
   - Consider when or if pregnancy is desired. Women who are sure they do not want to become pregnant now or in the future can consider sterilization. Women looking to become pregnant within the year may opt for a barrier method. And women who may want to become pregnant in a few or many years can explore hormonal options or IUDs.
   - Frequency of intercourse is another major consideration to review. If intercourse occurs frequently, barrier methods may prove to be inconvenient.
   - Number of partners should be considered. If a woman has more than one partner, or if her partner has another partner, she is at a greater risk for infection. In this case, a condom with spermicide in addition to birth control pills would provide the best protection against both sexually transmitted infections and pregnancy.
   - Emotional, behavioral, and psychological needs should be considered. A method may appear logical from a medical point of view, but if it is distasteful or undesirable, chances are that compliance with that method will be poor. The degree of partner cooperation is another important consideration, because barrier methods are more likely to succeed with partner cooperation and support.
   - Couples should be honest and realistic when deciding which kinds of contraception they will use. Couples who are unable or unwilling to use condoms every time they have sexual intercourse may wish to consider another form of contraception to supplement or replace condoms. Birth control pills will not be effective unless a woman remembers to take them every day.

Contraceptive decision making is a personal and private matter between a woman and her partner. The couple should consider several factors before deciding on what method to use. These factors include:

1. Evaluate needs:
   When/if a pregnancy will be desired
   How disruptive or difficult an unplanned pregnancy would be
   Frequency of intercourse
   Number of partners
   Risk of STIs
   Personal preferences for lovemaking
   Level of partner cooperation and interest
   Significance of spontaneity
   Comfort with touching one's own body or partner's comfort level of touching or being touched
   Manual dexterity for certain methods
   Financial considerations

2. Review medical history:
   Cardiovascular risk factors
   History of cancer
   Certain disabilities or chronic conditions
   Smoking status
   Allergies
   Circulatory disorders

3. Review reproductive health history:
   History of abortion or pregnancy scare
   Vaginal or cervical infections
   History of STIs
   Number of sexual partners or partner's number of partners
   Drug use (including alcohol)
   Past use of contraceptives

4. Put risks and benefits of methods in perspective:
   Weigh the advantages and disadvantages of each method in a personal perspective (see **Table 5.5**)

5. Reevaluate decision periodically:
   Each partner should assess level of compliance
   Each partner should assess level of satisfaction

- Perhaps one of the most important considerations is an evaluation of partner feelings and support. Ideally, the contraceptive choice will be a joint decision made by a couple following open, honest discussion of all the considerations and issues. In a less than ideal situation, a woman would be unwise to depend on her partner for contraceptive decision making or use.

Table 5.5   Comparisons: Contraceptive Options

Fertility Awareness Methods

"Perfect use" effectiveness	96%
Typical effectiveness	75%
How it works	Prevents sperm from reaching egg
Advantages	No costs; causes no health problems; no side effects or contraindications; no supplies or advance preparation; partner shares responsibility; no delay immediately before sex or extra steps during lovemaking
Disadvantages	Requires considerable discipline and partner cooperation and regular menstrual periods; does not reduce STI risk
Availability	No purchase required
Comments	Unreliable form of contraception

Withdrawal

"Perfect use" effectiveness	96%
Typical effectiveness	73%
How it works	Prevents sperm from reaching egg
Advantages	No costs; causes no health problems; no side effects or contraindications; no supplies or advance preparation; partner shares responsibility; can be used as a backup method of contraception
Disadvantages	Requires consistent discipline and partner cooperation; compromises spontaneity; may decrease pleasure; does not reduce STI risk
Availability	No purchase required
Comments	Unreliable form of contraception

Birth Control Pills

"Perfect use" effectiveness	99%
Typical effectiveness	92%
How it works	Prevents release of eggs from the ovaries; thickens cervical mucus; causes uterine lining changes
Advantages	Fairly inexpensive; lighter and less painful periods; decreased PMS symptoms; improved skin conditions; protective for some chronic diseases; does not interfere with sexual activity; no delay or interference with spontaneity; protection against ovarian and endometrial cancer; some forms may be used for emergency contraception
Disadvantages	No protection against STIs; may be contraindicated for women with cardiovascular risk problems or women who smoke; must be taken daily; inconsistent studies for breast cancer risk
Availability	Requires clinical examination and prescription
Comments	Most effective form of temporary contraception; combination pills contain both synthetic estrogen and progesterone; minipill contains only progesterone and may cause some irregular bleeding

Hormonal Implants

"Perfect use" effectiveness	99%
Typical effectiveness	99%
How it works	Prevents release of eggs from the ovaries; thickens cervical mucus; causes uterine lining changes
Advantages	Fairly inexpensive; provides protection up to 3 years or until it is removed; highly convenient—nothing to remember; protective for some chronic diseases; no delay or interference with spontaneity
Disadvantages	Must be removed by clinician; irregular menstrual bleeding may occur; no protection against STIs; may be contraindicated for women with cardiovascular risk problems or women who smoke

(continues)

Table 5.5 Comparisons: Contraceptive Options *(continued)*

Availability	Must be inserted by clinician; not all clinicians are trained for insertion and removal
Comments	Highly effective contraceptive; reversible once implant is removed

Injectable Contraceptives

"Perfect use" effectiveness	99%
Typical effectiveness	97%
How it works	Prevents release of eggs from the ovaries; thickens cervical mucus; causes uterine lining changes
Advantages	Fairly inexpensive; lasts 3 to 4 months; less bloating and mood swings than with pill; convenient—nothing to remember; protective for some chronic diseases; no delay or interference with spontaneity
Disadvantages	Must be prescribed by clinician; more weight gain and bleeding issues than with pill; no protection against STIs; may be contraindicated for women with cardiovascular risk problems or women who smoke
Availability	Clinical exam required; must be injected by clinician; not as widely available as the pill
Comments	Highly effective contraceptive; reversible once injections wear off, although there may be a waiting period; contains only progesterone, so it is an option for women who cannot take estrogen

Hormonal Patches

"Perfect use" effectiveness	99%
Typical effectiveness	92%
How it works	Prevents release of eggs from the ovaries; thickens cervical mucus; causes uterine lining changes
Advantages	Fairly inexpensive; convenient; weekly schedule is easier than daily pill; similar side effects and benefits as pill; no delay or interference with spontaneity
Disadvantages	Less effective in women weighing more than 198 lbs.; no protection against STIs; may be contraindicated for women with cardiovascular risk problems or women who smoke
Availability	Requires clinical examination and prescription
Comments	Highly effective and convenient contraceptive

Vaginal Ring

"Perfect use" effectiveness	99%
Typical effectiveness	92%
How it works	Prevents release of eggs from the ovaries; thickens cervical mucus; causes uterine lining changes
Advantages	Inexpensive; convenient; requires removal every 3 weeks; weekly schedule is easier than daily pill; similar side effects and benefits as pill; no delay or interference with spontaneity
Disadvantages	Requires clinical visit; women must learn to correctly insert and remove the ring; no protection against STIs; may be contraindicated for women with cardiovascular risk problems or women who smoke
Availability	Relatively new form of contraception; not all clinicians may be prescribing it
Comments	Highly effective and convenient contraceptive

Spermicide

"Perfect use" effectiveness	82%
Typical effectiveness	71%
How it works	Kills sperm; absorbs ejaculate; blocks sperm from entering vaginal tract
Advantages	Inexpensive; no clinical visit; able to use it only as needed; few side effects and contraindications; provides some protection against some STIs; provides additional lubrication; effective immediately
Disadvantages	Required for each sex act; messy; must be applied just before intercourse; effective for 30–60 minutes; may be awkward or disruptive to use

Table 5.5	**Comparisons: Contraceptive Options** (continued)
Availability	Easily available in drugstores and from online pharmacies in creams, foams, gels, film, or suppositories
Comments	Best contraceptive results are achieved when spermicide is used with a barrier method such as a condom or diaphragm
Diaphragm	
"Perfect use" effectiveness	94%
Typical effectiveness	84%
How it works	Blocks sperms from reaching egg; spermicide inactivates sperm
Advantages	Used only when needed; no side effects or contraindications (latex allergies are rare); can be inserted up to 6 hours ahead of time; reusable
Disadvantages	Moderately expensive one-time cost; clinical visit, fitting, and prescription required; must be used with a spermicide; may be awkward or inconvenient; may increase risk of urinary tract infections; dependent upon proper fit and diligent use
Availability	Clinical visit and fitting required
Comments	Spermicide must be used with each act of intercourse; diaphragm should be refitted when weight changes +/− 10 lbs.
Contraceptive Sponge	
"Perfect use" effectiveness	
Parous women (women who have had children)	80%
Nulliparous women (women who have not had children)	91%
Typical effectiveness	
Parous women	68%
Nulliparous women	84%
How it works	Kills sperm; absorbs ejaculate; blocks sperm from entering cervix
Advantages	Easy to use; spermicide is contained in sponge; may be inserted up to 24 hours before sex; provides continuous protection for 24 hours; relatively inexpensive; available without a fitting or prescription; less messy than other forms of spermicides; may provide some protection against STIs; disposable
Disadvantages	Less effective in women who have had children; requires some practice to insert and remove
Availability	Available in drugstores and online pharmacies
Comments	Sponges should not be reused
Cervical Cap	
"Perfect use" effectiveness	82%
Typical effectiveness	76%
How it works	Blocks sperm from reaching egg; spermicide inactivates sperm
Advantages	Easy to use once technique is mastered; may be inserted up to 48 hours before sex; some protection against STIs; few side effects (latex allergies are rare); reusable
Disadvantages	Fairly expensive one-time cost; clinical visit, fitting, and prescription required; not all women can be fitted with a cap; due to smaller size it may be more difficult to insert and remove than a diaphragm; effectiveness is dependent upon proper fitting, proper placement, and spermicide use each time
Availability	Generally available, although not all clinicians are skilled in educating women about insertion and removal
Comments	Should be replaced each year; should be refitted when weight changes +/− 10 lbs.

(continues)

Table 5.5　Comparisons: Contraceptive Options (continued)

Male Condom

"Perfect use" effectiveness	98%
Typical effectiveness	85%
How it works	Provides a physical barrier between the penis and vagina; prevents sperm and ejaculate from entering vagina
Advantages	Inexpensive; provides strong protection against most STIs; no clinical visit, fitting, or prescription required; can be used with other methods; can be used as a backup method for other contraception; no hormonal or systemic effects
Disadvantages	Can be used for only one act of intercourse; can tear or slip during use; may decrease sexual pleasure; may interrupt lovemaking; requires cooperation of male partner; latex allergies may require use of polyurethane condoms
Availability	Widely available over the counter and from online sources; available with lubricants and spermicides, in a variety of colors, textures, and flavors
Comments	More effective when used with a spermicide; can degrade with heat, light, and oxidation, so should be stored in a cool, dry place

Female Condom

"Perfect use" effectiveness	95%
Typical effectiveness	79%
How it works	Prevents sperm from entering vagina; provides best level of protection for women from STIs by covering vagina and perianal area
Advantages	Used only when needed; no hormonal or systemic effects; empowering to women; clinical visit, fitting, or prescription not needed
Disadvantages	More expensive than male condom; may feel awkward; tendency to be noisy; requires partner cooperation; can be used for only one act of intercourse; requires attention to details for woman and her partner
Availability	Widely available over the counter and from online sources
Comments	More effective when used with a spermicide

Female Sterilization

"Perfect use" effectiveness	99%
Typical effectiveness	99%
How it works	Prevents egg from traveling between ovaries and uterus
Advantages	Permanent—lifelong freedom from contraception after procedure for the woman; no interruption of lovemaking; highly effective; no need for partner compliance
Disadvantages	Expensive one-time fee; no protection from STIs; surgical risks; not reliably reversible
Availability	Widely available
Comments	Even though actual risks with female sterilization are low, vasectomies pose far less risk to men; ideal option for women who do not desire more children

Male Sterilization

"Perfect use" effectiveness	99%
Typical effectiveness	99%
How it works	Prevents sperm from being in the ejaculate
Advantages	Lifelong freedom from contraception worries for the male; no interruption of lovemaking; shared responsibility by the male

Table 5.5   Comparisons: Contraceptive Options (continued)

Disadvantages	Expensive—one-time fee; not always reversible; surgical experience; no protection from STIs
Availability	Outpatient procedure
Comments	Vasectomies pose far less risk to men than tubal ligation does for women

Lactation Amenorrhea Method (LAM)

"Perfect use" effectiveness	Uncertain
Typical effectiveness	80%
How it works	Lactation suppresses ovulation
Advantages	No clinical visit; no costs; easy for nursing mother
Disadvantages	Only effective with direct breastfeeding on demand, meeting all nutritional needs of baby; not effective when any menstrual bleeding returns or after 6 months postpartum
Availability	Only for nursing mothers
Comments	Can be used with other forms of contraception

Intrauterine Device (IUD)

"Perfect use" effectiveness	99%
Typical effectiveness	99%
How it works	Inhibits fertilization; thickens cervical mucus; inhibits sperm function; thins and suppresses the endometrium; copper ions may disrupt sperm motility
Advantages	Highly effective; does not interfere with sexual activity; no hormonal impact; long-acting; nothing to remember; decreased risk of endometrial cancer; reduced menstrual flow; reversible
Disadvantages	Clinical visit required; high insertion and removal costs; no STI protection; few days of mild cramping and light bleeding upon insertion
Availability	Dependent upon provider willingness and training for insertion; generally available
Comments	IUDs are the most widely used reversible form of contraception in the world—used by 12% of women; are much less common in the United States

No Method

"Perfect use" effectiveness	15%
Typical effectiveness	15%
How it works	Dependent upon good luck
Advantages	No clinical visit; no costs
Disadvantages	Risky for unwanted pregnancy; no protection against pregnancy or STIs
Availability	
Comments	Couples using no method of contraception should plan on a pregnancy

2. Consider medical factors. Carefully review risk factors for cardiovascular disease, smoking status, circulatory disorders, and other medical factors before deciding on birth control pills. A history of vaginal or cervical infections may rule out the use of diaphragms or cervical caps.

3. Review failure rates. The higher the failure rate is, the greater the risk of an unintended pregnancy. The difference in failure rates between "typical" and "perfect" use provides an estimate of the role human error plays for most couples. Some contraceptive methods, such as sterilization, are effective for virtually all couples; for other methods, failure rates for the average couple may be several times higher than for a consistent and diligent couple. Remember that typical failure rates are only an average, and that failure rates for couples who are less than diligent may be even higher.

4. Put the risks and benefits of the various methods in perspective. Weigh all dimensions and issues of the relationship carefully against the advantages and disadvantages of each birth control method. Carefully assess the risks and benefits of each method in terms of the individuals involved and their relationship. Some couples rank different options based on convenience, failure rates, and other factors to determine the best contraceptive that meets their unique needs.

5. Periodically reevaluate the decision. Regular gynecological checkups are opportunities to discuss contraceptive needs, options, and concerns with a clinician. At regular intervals, contracepting couples should reexamine the level of effectiveness and their individual levels of satisfaction with the selected method. A couple may want to reconsider both partners' needs, feelings, and family planning goals.

When to See a Healthcare Provider

It is necessary to see a clinician for prescription of the diaphragm, cervical cap, any hormonal methods, IUD, or sterilization. Other forms of birth control do not require a clinician's prescription, but conditions associated with these forms may warrant a clinic visit. In general, a woman should consult a clinician any time she experiences pain during intercourse or any unusual bleeding, spotting, discharge, or odor. Any burning or itching associated with spermicide use may be an indication of an allergy to the agent.

With a diaphragm, it is wise to check with a clinician any time the diaphragm does not seem to be fitting properly or there is discomfort, pain, or recurring bladder infections. After having a baby, it will be necessary to be refitted for a different-sized diaphragm because vaginal depth and muscle tone are usually altered by full-term pregnancy.

Abortion

Decisions regarding an unwanted pregnancy are private, personal, and difficult. They should not be rushed, and all options should be carefully weighed. Being able to talk through the process with a trusted person is essential. Options include terminating the pregnancy, continuing the pregnancy and raising the child, or continuing the pregnancy and choosing adoption. Many supportive services are available for each of these options.

If a woman elects to have an abortion and is confident in her decision, she can reduce her risk of medical complications from the procedure by making arrangements in a timely fashion. In selecting an abortion facility, a primary concern should be the availability of around-the-clock emergency care services. Infection, bleeding, and other complications can almost always be treated successfully if treatment begins promptly. Other ways to minimize risks from an abortion include making sure the surgeon who performs the procedure is well trained and experienced and verifying the facility provides comprehensive care, including postoperative instructions, education, and supportive services. Abortion counseling services are perhaps one of the most important features of a comprehensive facility.

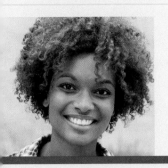
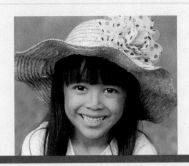
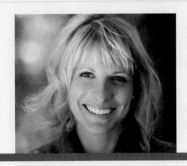
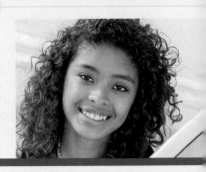

CASE STUDY

Sophie is a 16-year-old high school student who has recently become sexually active with her 17-year-old boyfriend. She comes to the family planning clinic to discuss her options for contraception. She tells the nurse that she isn't worried about sexually transmitted infections, but her mom will "freak out" if she gets pregnant. She doesn't want her parents to know that she has visited the clinic and she is worried that they will find out that she is having sex. She has heard about IUDs from a friend and wants to know if this is a good option for her.

Questions

1. What are some benefits of Sophie using an IUD as a contraceptive method?

2. What are some drawbacks to teenagers using IUDs?

3. Discuss additional barriers to prescribing an IUD to a teenager.

■ Summary

Being able to control reproductive functioning is a necessary component of women's health, career preparation, and family growth management. Many methods of contraception are available today, but no method is perfect. Table 5.5 compares the methods discussed in this chapter. The best method is one that a woman and her partner feel comfortable using and one that they will use correctly and consistently. Although ideally contraception is a shared responsibility between both partners, in today's world a woman is likely to bear the burden of an unexpected pregnancy. All women in relationships where there is the possibility of pregnancy should therefore make informed, well-thought-out decisions regarding contraception.

Abortion is something that no woman wants to face, but it is a choice that many women facing unwanted pregnancies will consider. Abortion is not just an issue for young, unmarried women; many women who have planned a pregnancy turn to abortion when they discover their developing fetus has a serious birth defect or

Profiles of Remarkable Women

Louise Slaughter (1929–)

Since 1986, Congresswoman Louise Slaughter has been serving in the U.S. House of Representatives where she holds several leadership positions. She is a former microbiologist and holds a master's degree in public health. She has been a long-time champion of science and health, particularly women's health issues.

Slaughter played a leadership role in crafting and passing the Patient Protection and Affordable Care Act, ensuring that the bill would not contribute to the national deficit. She has been a leader in addressing livestock antibiotic use and is a leading congressional expert on genetics issues. She wrote cutting-edge legislation to protect Americans from genetic discrimination, which has now become law. As one of the leading advocates in Congress for women's rights, Slaughter served as cochair of the Congressional Caucus for Women's Issues in the 108th Congress and continues to serve as cochair of the Bipartisan Congressional Pro-Choice Caucus. She was a coauthor of the historic Violence Against Women Act in 1994 and wrote legislation to make permanent the Department of Justice's Violence Against Women Office. She is leading the fight against sexual assault in the military. Slaughter has championed historic increases in funding for women's health in breast cancer research. She fought for legislation guaranteeing the inclusion of women and minorities in federal health research and for the establishment of the Office of Women's Health at the National Institutes of Health (NIH). She has introduced legislation to direct the NIH to fund up to six national centers to focus on women's health and the environment as well as a bill to increase research on the impact of hormone disrupters on women's health.

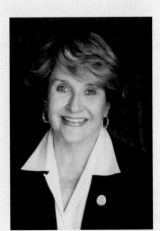

Courtesy of Congresswoman Louise M. Slaughter

chromosomal abnormality. Questions around abortion continue to be a focus for much of the women's health and women's rights movements, as well as for conservative and religious political movements.

Preventing unintended pregnancy is a primary responsibility of all sexually active heterosexual couples. In the event of an unwanted pregnancy, understanding all options and risks is a critical prerequisite for effective decision making.

■ Topics for Discussion

1. What are some of the trends in contraceptive use over the past decades since the introduction of the pill?

2. What are some explanations for the higher contraceptive failure rate among younger women compared with older women?

3. What are some of the common reasons for birth control failure?

4. What are some examples of the influence of sociocultural, sociodemographic, or socioeconomic factors on birth control choices?

5. How do politics play into the availability or options for birth control or emergency contraception?

6. What factors should be considered when calculating the cost of a contraceptive?

7. How have the trends with contraceptive use changed for first intercourse over the past decades?

8. Describe the differences between types of failure rates for contraceptives.

9. Describe some common myths and misconceptions about contraception.

10. Select one method of birth control and describe its advantages and disadvantages as a contraceptive method.

11. What health conditions are contraindicated for hormonal methods of contraception?

12. Describe the issues that surround a decision for sterilization.

13. What are the laws in your state about emergency contraception? Is EC available locally for all women?

14. Are abortion services available locally in your state? What obstacles are in place for a woman who is seeking an abortion locally?

■ Key Terms

Abortion
Abstinence
Birth control
Cervical cap
Condom
Contraception
Contraceptive sponge
Cost sharing
Diaphragm
Dilation and curettage (D&C)
Family planning
Female condom
Fertility
Intrauterine device (IUD)
Oral sex
Outercourse
Progestin
Spermicide
Sterilization
Vacuum curettage
Vasectomy

■ References

1. U.S. Department of Health and Human Services (DHHS), Centers for Disease Control and Prevention (CDC). (1999). Achievements in public health, 1990–1999. Family Planning. *Morbidity and Mortality Weekly Report* 48(50): 241–243.

2. Trussell, J., Raymond, E. G., & Cleland, K. (2015). *Emergency contraception: A last chance to prevent unintended pregnancy*. Available at: http://ec.princeton.edu/questions/EC-Review.pdf

3. Sonfield, A., Hasstedt, K., & Gold, R. B. (2014). *Guttmacher Institute—Moving forward: Family planning in the era of health reform*. Available at: http://www.guttmacher.org/pubs/family-planning-and-health-reform.pdf

4. Jones, J., Mosher, W., & Daniels, K. (2012). *Current contraceptive use in the United States, 2006–2010, and changes in patterns of use since 1995*. National Health Statistics Reports, no 60. Hyattsville, MD: National Center for Health Statistics.

5. CDC. (2010). *Use of contraception in the United States: 1982–2008*. Available at: http://www.cdc.gov/nchs/data/series/sr_23/sr23_029.pdf

6. DHHS. *Healthy People 2020. Family planning*. Available at: http://www.healthypeople.gov/2020/topicsobjectives2020/overview.aspx?topicid=13

7. Hall, K. S., Moreau, C., & Trussell, J. (2011). Determinants of and disparities in reproductive health service use among adolescent and young adult women in the United States, 2002–2008. *American Journal of Public Health* 102(2): 359–367. Available at: http://ajph.aphapublications.org/doi/abs/10.2105/AJPH.2011.300380

8. Guttmacher Institute. (2015). *State policies in brief: Minors' access to contraceptive services*. Available at: http://www.guttmacher.org/statecenter/spibs/spib_MACS.pdf

9. Guttmacher Institute. (2011). *New government data finds sharp decline in teen births: Increased contraceptive use and shifts to more effective contraceptive methods behind this encouraging trend*. Available at: http://www.guttmacher.org/media/inthenews/2011/12/01/index.html

10. National Women's Law Center. (2014). *Birth control coverage cases before the U.S. Supreme Court: An overview of the legal issues.* [Fact Sheet.] Available at: http://www.nwlc.org/sites/default/files/pdfs/bc_cases_before_us_sup_ct_overview_legal_issues_03.19.14.pdf

11. DHHS, CDC. (n.d.). *Reproductive health: Contraception.* Available at: http://www.cdc.gov/reproductivehealth/unintendedpregnancy/contraception.htm

12. Jones, R. K., & Dreweke, J. (2011). *Countering conventional wisdom: New evidence on religion and contraceptive use. Guttmacher Institute.* Available at: http://www.guttmacher.org/pubs/Religion-and-Contraceptive-Use.pdf

13. Pew Research Center. (2011). *The future of the global Muslim population.* Available at: http://features.pewforum.org/FutureGlobalMuslimPopulation-WebPDF.pdf

14. Guttmacher Institute. (2015). *Insurance coverage of contraceptives.* Available at: http://www.guttmacher.org/statecenter/spibs/spib_ICC.pdf

15. Finer, L. B., & Zolna, M. R. (2011). Unintended pregnancy in the United States: Incidence and disparities, 2006. *Contraception* 84(5): 478–485.

16. Guttmacher Institute. (2012). *Nation pays steep price for high rates of unintended pregnancy.* Available at: http://www.guttmacher.org/media/nr/2011/05/19/index.html

17. Guttmacher Institute. (2012). *Facts on publicly funded contraceptive services in the United States.* Available at: http://www.guttmacher.org/pubs/psrh/full/4309411.pdf

18. Frost, J. J., Zolna, M. R., & Frohwirth, L. (2013). *Contraceptive needs and services, 2010.* Guttmacher Institute. Available at: http://www.guttmacher.org/pubs/win/contraceptive-needs-2010.pdf

19. DHHS. *Healthy People 2020. Family planning.* Available at: http://www.healthypeople.gov/2020/topicsobjectives2020/overview.aspx?topicid=13

20. Hall, K. S., Moreau, C., & Trussell, J. (2011). Determinants of and disparities in reproductive health service use among adolescent and young adult women in the United States, 2002–2008. *American Journal of Public Health* 102(2): 359–367. Available at: http://ajph.aphapublications.org/doi/abs/10.2105/AJPH.2011.300380

21. Frost, J. J., Zolna, M. R., & Frohwirth, L. (2014). *Contraceptive needs and services: 2012 update.* Guttmacher Institute. Available at: https://www.guttmacher.org/pubs/win/contraceptive-needs-2012.pdf

22. Reid, R., Leyland, N., Wolfman, W., et al. (2010). Oral contraceptives and the risk of venous thromboembolism: An update. *SOGC Clinical Practice Guidelines* 252. Available at: http://www.sogc.org/guidelines/documents/gui252CPG1012E.pdf

23. Shufeit, C. L., & Merz, C. (2009). Contraceptive hormone use and cardiovascular disease. *Journal of the American College of Cardiology* 53: 221–231.

24. National Cancer Institute. (2012). *Oral contraceptives and cancer risk.* Available at: http://www.cancer.gov/cancertopics/causes-prevention/risk/hormones/oral-contraceptives-fact-sheet#r1

25. Vessey, M., & Yeates, D. (2007). Oral contraceptives and benign breast disease: An update of findings in a large cohort study. *Contraception* 76(6): 418–424.

26. Grimes, D. A., Jones, L. B., Lopez, L. M., et al. (2014). Oral contraceptives for functional ovarian cysts. *Cochrane Database of Systematic Reviews* 4: CD006134. doi:10.1002/14651858.CD006134.pub5

27. Mayo Clinic Patient Information. (2014). *Iron deficiency anemia: Treatment and drugs.* Available at: http://www.mayoclinic.org/diseases-conditions/iron-deficiency-anemia/basics/treatment/con-20019327

28. Corson, S. L. (1993). Oral contraceptives for the prevention of osteoporosis. *Journal of Reproductive Medicine* 38(Suppl. 12): 1015–1020.

29. Ziglar, S., & Hunter, T. S. (2012). The effect of hormonal oral contraception on acquisition of peak bone mineral density of adolescents and young women. *Journal of Pharmacological Practice* 25(3): 331–340.

30. Bonnema, R. A., McNamara, M. C., & Spencer, A. L. (2010). Contraception choices in women with underlying medical conditions. *American Family Physician* 82(6): 621–628.

31. Tepper, N. K., Curtis, K. M., Jamieson, D. J., et al. (2011). Update to CDC's U.S. medical eligibility criteria for contraceptive use, 2010: Revised recommendations for the use of contraceptive methods during the postpartum period. *Morbidity and Mortality Weekly Report* 60(26): 878–883.

32. National Institutes of Health, National Library of Medicine. (2012). *Progestin-only contraceptives.* Available at: http://www.nlm.nih.gov/medlineplus/druginfo/meds/a602008.html

33. Wright, K. P., & Johnson, J. V. (2008). Evaluation of extended and continuous use oral contraceptives. *Therapeutic Clinical Risk Management* 4(5): 905–911. Available at: http://www.ncbi.nlm.nih.gov/pmc/articles/PMC2621397/

34. Krishnan, S., & Kiley, J. (2010). The lowest-dose, extended cycle combined oral contraceptive pill with continuous ethinyl estradiol in the United States: A review of the literature on ethinyl estradiol 20 μg/levonorgestrel 100 μg + ethinyl estradiol 10 μg. *International Journal of Women's Health* 2: 235–239.

35. Mayo Clinic Patient Information. (2012). *Minipill (progestin-only birth control).* Available at: http://www.mayoclinic.org/tests-procedures/minipill/basics/why-its-done/prc-20012857

36. American College of Obstetricians and Gynecologists (ACOG). (2014). *Progestin-only hormonal birth control pill: Pill and injection.* Available at: http://www.acog.org/Patients/FAQs/Progestin-Only-Hormonal-Birth-Control-Pill-and-Injection

37. ACOG. (2014). Committee opinion number 602: Depot medroxyprogesterone acetate and bone effects. *Obstetrics & Gynecology* 123: 1398–1402.

38. U.S. Food and Drug Administration. (2012). *Ortho evra (norelgestromin/ethinyl estradiol) transdermal patch.* Available at: http://www.fda.gov/Safety/MedWatch/SafetyInformation/ucm319219.htm

39. Xu, H., Wade, J. A., Peipert, J. F., et al. (2012). Contraceptive failure rates of etonogestrel subdermal implants in overweight and obese women. *Obstetrics & Gynecology* 120(1): 21–26.

40. Planned Parenthood. (2012). *Condom information.* Available at: http://www.plannedparenthood.org/learn/birth-control/condom

41. Winner, B., Peipert, J. F., Zhao, Q., et al. (2012). Effectiveness of long-acting reversible contraception. *New England Journal of Medicine* 366: 1998–2007.

42. Daniels, K., Daugherty, J., & Jones, J. (2014). Current contraceptive status among women aged 15–44: United States, 2011–2013. *National Center for Health Statistics Data Brief*, No. 173. Available at: http://www.cdc.gov/nchs/data/databriefs/db173.htm

43. Planned Parenthood Federation of America. *IUD: How effective is the IUD?* Available at: http://www.plannedparenthood.org/learn/birth-control/iud

44. Researchers find no sperm in pre-ejaculate fluid. (1993). *Contraceptive Technology Update* 14(10): 154–156.

45. Killck, S. R., Leary, C., Trussell, J., et al. (2011). Sperm content of pre-ejaculatory fluid. *Human Fertility* 1: 48–52.

46. Planned Parenthood Federation of America. (n.d.). *Breastfeeding as birth control at a glance*. Available at: http://www.plannedparenthood.org/learn/birth-control/breastfeeding

47. Planned Parenthood Federation of America. (n.d.). *Morning-after pill (emergency contraception)*. Available at: https://www.plannedparenthood.org/learn/morning-after-pill-emergency-contraception

48. Kaiser Family Foundation. (2013). *Kaiser Women's Health Survey*. Available at: http://kff.org/womens-health-policy/fact-sheet/emergency-contraception/

49. Raine, T. R., Harper, C. C., Rocca, C. H., et al. (2005). Direct access to emergency contraception through pharmacies and effect on unintended pregnancy and STIs: A randomized controlled trial. *Journal of the American Medical Association* 293(1): 54–62.

50. DHHS, Office of Population Affairs. (2010). *Reproductive health and Healthy People 2020*. Available at: http://www.hhs.gov/opa/pdfs/reproductive-health-and-healthy-people-2020.pdf

51. Page, S. T., Amory, J. K., & Bremner, W. J. (2008). Advances in male contraception. *Endocrine Reviews* 29(4): 465–493.

52. Finer, L. B., Frohwirth, L. F., Dauphinee, L. A., et al. (2005). Reasons U.S. women have abortions: Quantitative and qualitative perspectives. *Perspectives on Sexual and Reproductive Health* 37(3): 110–118.

53. Shain, R. N. (1986). A cross-cultural history of abortion. *Clinics in Obstetrics and Gynaecology* 13(1): 1–17.

54. Cates, W., Jr. Grimes, D. A., & Schulz, K. F. (2003). The public health impact of legal abortion: 30 years later. *Perspectives on Sexual and Reproductive Health* 35(1): 25–28.

55. Gold, R. B. (1990). *Abortion and women's health: A turning point for America?* New York: Alan Guttmacher Institute.

56. National Women's Law Center. (2011). *Women in county without an abortion provider. Health Care Report Card*. Available at: http://hrc.nwlc.org/status-indicators/women-county-without-abortion-provider

57. Raymond, E. G., & Grimes, D. A. (2012). The comparative safety of legal induced abortion and childbirth in the United States. *Obstetrics & Gynecology* 119(2): 215–219.

58. Gallup. (2014). *U.S. still split on abortion: 47% pro-choice, 46% pro-life*. Available at: http://www.gallup.com/poll/170249/split-abortion-pro-choice-pro-life.aspx

59. Jones, R. K., Finer, L. B., & Singh, S. (2010). *Characteristics of U.S. abortion patients, 2008*. New York: Guttmacher Institute.

60. Finer, L. B., & Zolna, M. R. (2014). Shifts in intended and unintended pregnancies in the United States, 2001–2008. *American Journal of Public Health* 23(3): e1–e9.

61. Jones, R. K., & Kavanaugh, M. L. (2011). Changes in abortion rates between 2000 and 2008 and lifetime incidence of abortion. *Obstetrics & Gynecology* 117(6): 1358–1366.

62. CDC. (2014). Abortion surveillance—United States, 2011. *Morbidity and Mortality Weekly Report* 63(SS11): 1–41.

63. World Health Organization (WHO). (2011). *Unsafe abortion: Global and regional estimates of the incidence of unsafe abortion and associated mortality in 2008, 6th ed.* Available at: http://whqlibdoc.who.int/publications/2011/9789241501118_eng.pdf?ua=1

64. Guttmacher Institute. (2012). *Facts on induced abortion worldwide*. Available at: http://www.guttmacher.org/pubs/fb_IAW.html

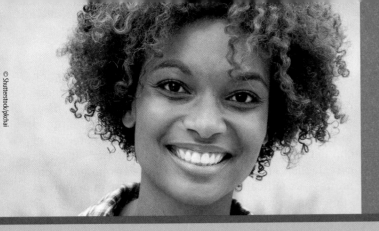

CHAPTER 6

Pregnancy and Childbirth

Learning Objectives

On completion of this chapter, the student should be able to discuss:

1. Historical dimensions of pregnancy, childbirth, and breastfeeding.

2. Conception and the process of cell division after fertilization.

3. Hormonal changes and fetal changes during pregnancy.

4. Nutritional and weight gain recommendations for pregnancy and exercise concerns with pregnancy.

5. Detrimental effects of smoking, alcohol, drugs, and various environmental risks on pregnancy.

6. Techniques for prenatal testing and complications of pregnancy.

7. The significant issues surrounding childbirth preparation, labor and delivery, cesarean section, and vaginal birth after cesarean section.

8. Physiological changes of the breast for breastfeeding.

9. Benefits and complications associated with breastfeeding.

10. The concepts of fecundity and infertility.

11. Causes and diagnoses of infertility.

12. Treatment of infertility, including assisted reproductive technologies.

13. Emotional effects of infertility.

14. Trends in birth rates, maternal mortality rates, and infant mortality rates.

15. Breastfeeding trends.

16. Prevalence of infertility, its major causes, and the types of treatments used.

INTRODUCTION

This chapter provides an overview of pregnancy, childbirth, breastfeeding, and infertility. In addition to the obvious biological aspects, social, cultural, historical, legal, and ethical dimensions influence pregnancy and childbirth.

HISTORICAL DIMENSIONS

The academic examination of childbirth as a social phenomenon did not really begin until the 1960s. Before that time, academic knowledge about childbirth came principally from the writings of medical historians who stressed the progressive history of scientific advances in obstetrics. This medical and historical account provided little insight into how the management of pregnancy or birthing affected women's experiences of birth or about women's reactions to and participation in such changes. The accounts also failed to document how the birth experience felt to the woman. Today there is considerably more focus on the social, racial, economic, and ethnic aspects of childbirth. Childbirth history is now studied in a variety of contexts—medical, demographic, cultural, social, economic, professional, and symbolic, among others. In the United States, however, the medical perspective continues to dominate. The term *childbirth* generally evokes an image of a medical environment, with physicians and nurses, surgical drapes, intravenous poles, and fetal monitors. In contrast, in the early United States, childbirth did not have an association with medical personnel or equipment except when a woman's life was threatened. Both immigrant and native populations considered childbirth to be part of a woman's domestic responsibilities.[1] Although specific cultural and ethnic variations existed in the management of the birthing process, all shared the tradition that only women attended other women. Women were the experts on birthing.[1]

> There is a realization that women's attitudes toward and behavior during birth are shaped and conditioned by the demands and expectations of family, peers, community, and often religion. What a woman expects from her childbirth experience, what she will do, what she will fear and not fear, how she will interpret what is happening to her, and what in fact will happen when she gives birth, depend in large measure upon how her society defines what birth should be and where she fits in the various hierarchies of that society.
>
> —**Janet Carlisle Bogdan (1990). Childbirth in America, 1650 to 1990. In R. D. Apple (Ed.),** *Women, health, and medicine in America.*

During the mid-18th century, the expertise of women in birthing began to be questioned. Women in France began to deliver babies in hospitals under the watchful eyes of not only traditional midwives but also physicians. Although physicians had previously witnessed or participated in abnormal deliveries, the hospitalization practices enabled them to study and understand the normal childbirth process. Through close observation, measurements, and recordings, French physicians attempted to explain what they saw as the mysterious process of childbirth.[2] During the same period, the English medical establishment became more oriented to surgical techniques—specifically, the development of instruments known as **forceps** to assist in the extraction of the fetus from the woman. The European obstetrical knowledge quickly crossed the Atlantic, and U.S. physicians began appearing at the births of middle- and upper-class urban women. At first, physicians attended along with traditional midwives, but soon physicians replaced midwives during birth. Medical schools began to certify men as birth attendants, leading to a decline in traditional midwifery. By the end of the 18th century, physicians had established roles in managing childbirth throughout urban areas, including those for poor women.

With the medical presence during childbirth came a widening array of interventions, including medications, anesthesia, and birthing instruments. Accompanying the newly introduced technologies were additional problems of birth accidents, including tears and infections. Physician attitudes had changed from observing and learning to affecting and controlling. Women continued to actively participate in determining the terms of their childbirths only as long as the home was the birthing environment. Once birthing moved to the hospital, however, women lost this power.[3] The U.S. medical management of childbirth originated in urban northeastern areas. In the South and in some religious communities, childbirth retained much of its traditional aspects during the 19th and early 20th centuries. Immigrant groups also were more likely to continue with traditional practices.

The 20th century brought additional medicalization and hospitalization to the childbirth experience, while midwives remained in the more inaccessible portions of the United States. Despite the increased technology and promises of greater safety, women were exposed to greater mystification of childbirth than they had ever known.[3] This trend was in some ways ironic because women were electing to control their fertility and have fewer children, thereby increasing the significance of the childbirth experience. At the same time, they understood less about the process and were less in control of birthing than their grandmothers had been. This trend continued until the late 1950s and 1960s, when women began to openly express dissatisfaction with "medicalized" births. Europe again was the leader in a new trend of childbirth experiences that suggested that childbirth should be anticipated with joy and knowledge, not fear and ignorance, and could be accomplished with less pain, less medication, and less of the medical and surgical control typical of U.S. births. These natural-birth relaxation techniques are the foundation of modern efforts toward "prepared childbirth."

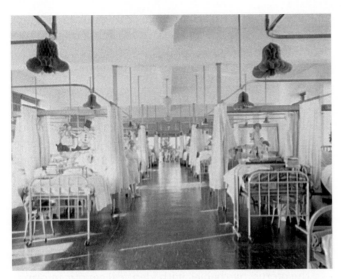

The 20th century brought medicalization and hospitalization to the child-birth experience.

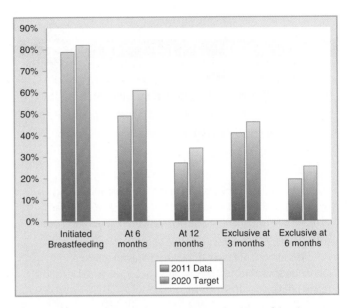

Figure 6.1 *Healthy People* 2020 Breastfeeding Objectives

Data from Centers for Disease Control and Prevention (CDC). (2014). *Breastfeeding report card—United States, 2014*. Available at: http://www.cdc.gov/breastfeeding/pdf/2014breastfeedingreportcard.pdf

Social scientists have studied many aspects of modern and traditional childbirth practices. Historically, the care pregnant women received focused on childbirth in the woman's home, and other women gave this support. But modern medical and hospital practices, while making childbirth safe in many regards, have also created situations where continuous support from physicians and nurses during labor has become routine rather than the exception. Some experts believe that childbirth has become an "over-medicalized" process as opposed to a natural process, leading to excessive health costs, extensive stays for mothers, and something to be feared and treated rather than experienced. Supportive care during labor and delivery may improve a woman's experience and possibly reduce the need for obstetric intervention. Hospital staff, such as nurses or midwives, doulas, or companions from a woman's social network, could provide this support. A review of 22 trials involving more than 15,000 women found that women who had support throughout labor were likely to have slightly shorter labors, more likely to have spontaneous vaginal births, less likely to use pain medications, and more likely to be satisfied with their childbirth experiences. The authors concluded that all women should have medical support throughout labor and birth.[4]

Other social scientists have examined the popular lay term of *natural childbirth*. Studies have found that the term natural birth, traditionally referring to childbirth without use of medications for pain relief and with minimal mechanical monitoring, also may refer to the social practices surrounding the birth. Three practices common to natural childbirth include: (1) preparation before birth, (2) activity during birth, and (3) social support.[5] A natural childbirth attempts to create a more active and supportive experience for the mother during the birth of her baby.

Breastfeeding also has seen many changes over the years. The first variation on the practice of breastfeeding was the substitution of the mother's breast with that of a wet nurse—another woman who was able and willing to breastfeed for the mother. In the 1700s, "dry nursing," the mixing of flour, bread, or cereal with broth or water, became popular, because this early form of infant formula was a cheaper option than "wet nursing." As women entered the workforce during the Industrial Revolution, substitutes for milk were produced, resulting in a decline in the practice of breastfeeding.[6] Formula substitutes remained popular for those women who could afford them, until reports surfaced on the benefits of breastfeeding in the 1970s. Since that time, breastfeeding rates have again fallen and risen as a result of various factors, ranging from a woman's place of employment to her personal finances, from her religious beliefs to her network of social support, and from her comfort with her own body to medical contraindications. Because breastfeeding has been shown to lower total healthcare costs by reducing sick care visits, prescriptions, and hospitalizations, the United States has identified breastfeeding as a major goal of the Healthy People 2020 National Health Objectives. As **Figure 6.1** shows, some progress has been made toward achieving these goals.

PREGNANCY

Pregnancy lasts an average of 266 days from the time of fertilization or 280 days from the first day of the last menstrual period (often referred to as LMP). The gestational period is divided into three phases or trimesters of approximately 3 months each. Not all women have 28-day menstrual cycles, so due dates cannot be precisely determined (see **It's Your Health**).

Conception

Conception, also known as **fertilization**, is the union of the male sperm cell and the female egg cell. The sperm cell is one of the smallest cells in the body and is produced in enormous quantities: approximately 50 million each day by a healthy male. Sperm production is a continuous, lifelong process. Sperm are produced in the testicles; they are then moved through the epididymis to the seminal vesicles, where the sperm mature into motile sperm and are stored until they are needed in the semen. Mature sperm cells swim like miniature tadpoles with an undulating movement of a threadlike tail. During the process of ejaculation, these cells are combined with secretions from the male reproductive tract to form semen. If ejaculation occurs into or around the entrance of the vagina, fertilization is possible. It has been estimated that as many as 300 million sperm are deposited with ejaculation, but fewer than 20 actually arrive anywhere near the unfertilized egg.[7]

The human egg, or ovum, is far more rare than the sperm. Each woman is born with a supply of approximately 1 million egg cells, of which only about 300,000 eggs remain by the time a girl reaches puberty. One mature egg is released from a woman's ovaries each month during ovulation, usually resulting in 300 to 500 eggs being released during a woman's lifetime.

After the sperm separates from the seminal fluid, it becomes more mobile as it travels toward the egg. If the woman is in the early or middle segment of her menstrual cycle, the cervical mucus is of a consistency that allows the sperm to pass into the uterus. If progesterone is the dominant hormone, as in the late segment of the menstrual cycle, the cervical mucus inhibits sperm penetration past the cervix. Conception usually takes place in the upper third of the fallopian tube. In a process called the acrosome reaction, the sperm releases an enzyme called hyaluronidase, which works to dissolve the outer layer of the egg cell

and allows the sperm cell to advance toward the center of the egg to join with its nucleus. Only one sperm is able to penetrate the protective coating of the egg.

Two offspring born of the same pregnancy are called twins.

- **Dizygotic twins** (also known as fraternal twins) result when two eggs are released from the ovary in one menstrual cycle and fertilized at the same time. Fraternal twins may be of the same or opposite sex and have different genetic traits and therefore different physical appearances. They are sustained through separate placentas and membranes.

- **Monozygotic twins**, also referred to as identical twins, result from a single fertilized egg splitting into equal halves. If both eggs become implanted within the uterus, two babies with identical genetic information will develop. Identical twins may share or have separate placentas and membranes.

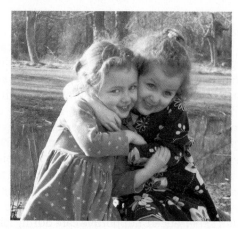

Dizygotic twins (fraternal twins) have different genetic traits and therefore different physical appearances.
Courtesy of Helaine Bader

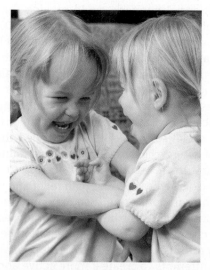

Monozygotic twins (identical twins) result from a single fertilized egg splitting into equal halves. As a result, these babies have identical genetic information.
© Photos.com

At fertilization, the 23 **chromosomes** from the sperm combine with the 23 chromosomes of the egg to form the zygote. The **zygote**, or fertilized egg, contains the full complement of 46 chromosomes. This genetic information determines the unique characteristics of the individual, including eye and hair color, height, and all the other physical characteristics that are passed from one generation to the next. One pair of chromosomes determines the sex of the individual, with the usual arrangement of males having one X and one Y chromosome and females having two X chromosomes; however, chromosomal abnormalities can occur. Among the most common chromosomal abnormalities are those that involve missing or extra sex chromosomes. Abnormalities involving the X or Y chromosome can affect sexual development and may cause infertility, growth abnormalities, and other problems (see **Table 6.1**).

Cell division of the zygote usually occurs within 36 hours of fertilization and continues as the dividing cell mass moves through the fallopian tubes toward the uterus. It generally takes 3 to 5 days to reach the uterus;

at this stage, the cell mass is known as a **blastocyst**. The blastocyst freely floats within the uterus for 1 to 2 days before implanting itself into the lining of the uterus. **Implantation** is often the marker for the beginning of a pregnancy, and the products of conception are generally referred to as the **conceptus**. For the first 8 weeks of gestation, the material is known as an **embryo**; from week 9 until birth, it is known as a **fetus**.

My niece was very short and she had some unique characteristics. It took a while for the doctors to diagnose her as having Turner syndrome. We have learned that this affects about one in every 2500 females.

—27-year-old woman

Confirming Pregnancy

The benefits of early diagnosis of pregnancy are immeasurable. When pregnancy is desired, good prenatal care can begin immediately, and efforts can be made to protect

---

Table 6.1   **Selected Sex Chromosome Abnormalities**

Sex Chromosome Abnormalities			
Female Genotype	**Syndrome**	**Male Genotype**	**Syndrome**
XX	Normal	XY	Normal
XO	Turner Syndrome	XXY	Klinefelter Syndrome
XXX	Triple X	XYY	XYY Male

Turner Syndrome

- Has only one X chromosome; also known as monosomy X or genotype XO
- Short stature and possibly certain physical features, such as webbed necks with extra folds of skin
- Lack ovarian development and infertility
- At higher risk for thyroid disease, heart or kidney abnormalities, vision and hearing problems, and diabetes
- Possible impaired intelligence

Triple X

- Increased height
- Normal fertility
- At risk for language and motor delay

Klinefelter Syndrome

- Increased height and more likely to be overweight
- Effeminate
- Decreased testicular size, normal sex function, but usually infertile
- Possible slight breast development during adolescence
- At risk for learning disabilities

XXY Male

- Increased height
- Normal sexual function, genitalia, and fertility
- Increased risk for motor delay, developmental delay, and learning disabilities

the vulnerable embryo from chemical and physical agents. When pregnancy is not desired, early detection permits early decision making; if the woman elects to have an abortion, risks of complications are reduced at this stage.

Early Signs of Pregnancy

Symptoms of pregnancy that often occur in the first 6 weeks:

Missed period(s)

Breast swelling and tenderness

Fatigue

Queasiness or nausea, vomiting

Slightly elevated body temperature

Mood swings

Need to urinate frequently

Several symptoms often occur in the first 6 weeks of pregnancy (see **It's Your Health**). Most women begin to have symptoms 2 or 3 weeks after conception. An overdue period is usually the first definitive sign of pregnancy, although it is important to note that there are many reasons for missed periods other than pregnancy. Also, some women may bleed in early pregnancy and mistake the bleeding for a normal period.

Confirming a pregnancy involves a pregnancy test and a pelvic examination. **Human chorionic gonadotropin (hCG)**, a hormone specific to pregnancy, is easily detectable in blood and urine throughout the first 3 months of pregnancy. All pregnancy tests use chemical procedures to detect its presence. Home pregnancy tests can be purchased without a prescription and are simple to use. Tests give the most reliable results when the urine

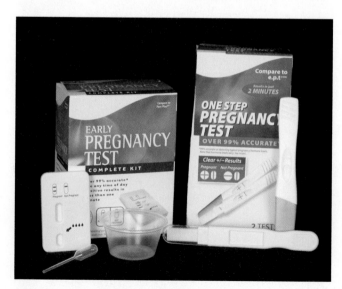

Home pregnancy tests are fairly expensive but quite simple to use.

is highly concentrated; hence, women are advised to use early morning urine as the testing sample.

Although home pregnancy tests are valuable sources of information, they are merely the beginning. If the findings are positive, it is important to set up an appointment for a pelvic examination. If the findings are negative, there is a need to determine why the menstrual period is late or missed. Urine or blood tests performed in a doctor's office are virtually 100% accurate and can be used to validate the pregnancy.

Hormonal Changes During Pregnancy

During pregnancy, a woman's hormone levels and physical characteristics change dramatically. The secretion of certain hormones involved in ovulation, such as follicle-stimulating hormone (FSH) and luteinizing hormone (LH), produced by the anterior pituitary gland, is suppressed throughout pregnancy. Shortly after implantation, specific cells in the outer portion of the developing embryo secrete hCG, a pregnancy-specific hormone. The presence of this hormone in the woman's system produces a positive pregnancy test result because, as noted earlier, hCG can be detected in the woman's blood and urine. The body produces large amounts of hCG during the first trimester to stimulate the **corpus luteum**, a structure formed on the wall of the ovary that secretes estrogen and progesterone to prepare the body for pregnancy. The corpus luteum is essential for the maintenance of early pregnancy. If it regresses, a spontaneous abortion, or miscarriage, results.

After the first 3 months of pregnancy, the corpus luteum is no longer essential to maintain the pregnancy and hCG levels drop off. This change occurs because the placenta begins producing large amounts of estrogen and progesterone. The fetus also plays a role in maintaining the pregnancy. The fetal adrenal glands produce a precursor hormone during the first 3 months of pregnancy that is converted to estrogen in the placenta. The growing fetus and placenta contribute increasing quantities of estrogen and progesterone to the maternal blood system as the pregnancy progresses; the levels of both hormones rapidly decline at birth. Estrogen helps to regulate progesterone, thereby protecting the pregnancy, and initiates one of the major processes of fetal maturation; without estrogen, fetal lungs, liver, and other organs and tissues cannot mature. Estrogen also promotes the growth of ducts in the breast to prepare for lactation. Progesterone suppresses uterine contractions during pregnancy and stimulates the alveoli of the breasts.

Another hormone unique to pregnancy is human placental lactogen (HPL), also called human chorionic somatomammotropin. The structure and function of HPL are similar to that of human growth hormone. HPL modifies the metabolic state of the mother during pregnancy to facilitate the energy supply of the fetus. It is also believed to stimulate breast growth during pregnancy and to prepare the breasts for lactation. HPL levels rise throughout pregnancy. As birth approaches, the levels decline.

Physical and Emotional Symptoms

A woman's body experiences significant changes throughout pregnancy, with each trimester bringing new physical and emotional symptoms. **Figure 6.2** shows many of the physical changes that occur during pregnancy. The first trimester is characterized by enlarged and tender breasts and, for many women, nausea and vomiting (commonly referred to as morning sickness). Women also may experience extreme fatigue, decreased interest in sex, moodiness and irritability, and skin changes such as darkening of the nipple and areola. Some women may feel no discomfort at all or may experience brief periods of nausea or fatigue while overall feeling good.

Most women find the second trimester easier than the first. During the second trimester, morning sickness usually subsides, emotions even out and both energy and sex drive usually return. The second trimester is the period in which women gain most of their weight, usually between 12 and 14 pounds. The growing fetus can lead to shortness of breath, due to pressure of the uterus and fetus on the bottom of the rib cage, and backache, caused by changes in posture to accommodate the growing fetus. Some women experience muscle and leg cramps, numbness and tingling of the hands, swollen or bleeding gums, and

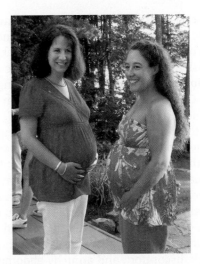

A woman's body experiences significant changes throughout pregnancy.
Photographed by Chris Bolduc

Braxton–Hicks contractions (false labor). Swelling of the feet, ankles, and hands is common and is caused by the increased weight of the uterus slowing down blood and fluid circulation. Some women experience gastrointestinal problems such as heartburn, gas, and constipation. Skin changes can also occur. Striae gravidarum (known as

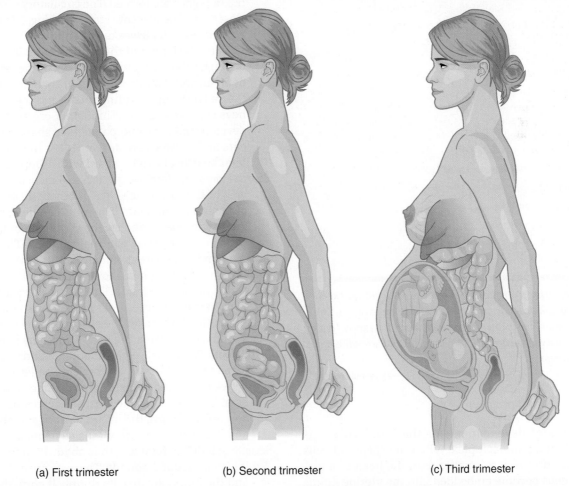

(a) First trimester   (b) Second trimester   (c) Third trimester

Figure 6.2   **Changes in a woman's body during pregnancy. Through the three trimesters, the shape of the pregnant woman's body changes dramatically.**

stretch marks) begin to appear on the abdomen, breasts, and thighs; varicose veins may appear in the legs; and chloasma (brown patches on the face or neck) and linea nigra (a dark line from the belly to the pubic area), both caused by increases in melanocyte-stimulating hormone, may occur. Changes in estrogen levels may cause redness of palms and red spots on the upper body.

In the third trimester, many of these symptoms—for example, heartburn and constipation, leg cramps, backache, breathlessness, and Braxton–Hicks contractions—continue. Each woman is different, however, and some may experience very few of these symptoms or experience them only slightly. Women may experience an increase in leukorrhea (a whitish vaginal discharge) and colostrum (pre-milk) leaking from the breasts. Hemorrhoids, pelvic and buttock discomfort, and an itchy abdomen also are common complaints. For some women, their interest in sex may decrease, while others may find themselves still interested in sex throughout the third trimester.

It's Your Health

Common Complaints During Pregnancy

- Morning sickness
- Leg cramps
- Sleep issues
- Braxton–Hicks contractions
- Bladder infections
- Backaches
- Hemorrhoids
- Skin problems
- Mouth and gum discomfort
- Dizziness and faintness
- Indigestion
- Difficulty breathing
- Headaches
- Vaginal discharge and itching

I didn't need a pregnancy test to tell me I was pregnant. I just knew it. My breasts were tender and I had some vague queasiness. Sure enough—my home pregnancy test confirmed what I knew. I realize that some women aren't as sure, but I was totally positive that I was pregnant.

—**25-year-old mother**

Fetal Development

The process of development for the fertilized egg is both fascinating and complex. When the cluster of cells reaches the uterus, it is smaller than the head of a pin. Once the cells become embedded into the uterine lining, they are collectively known as an embryo. A sac known as the **amnion** or fetal sac envelops the embryo. As water

and other small molecules cross the amniotic membrane, the embryo floats freely. The **amniotic fluid** protects the embryo from shocks and bumps and helps maintain a homeostatic, or constant, environment for the developing embryo. A primitive placenta soon forms. The **placenta** is the organ that supplies the growing fetus with oxygen and nutrients from the maternal bloodstream and serves as a conduit for the return of waste products back to the mother for disposal.

Major changes occur with the developing embryo as it evolves into a fetus (**Figure 6.3**).

First Month The embryo grows to about one-tenth to one-fourth of an inch in length and one-seventh of an ounce in weight. Foundations form for the nervous system, genitourinary system, circulatory system, digestive system, skin, bones, and lungs. The embryo has a two-lobed brain and a spinal cord. The arm and leg buds start to appear. The heartbeat appears on the 25th day. Rudiments of the eyes, ears, and nose appear. The head is disproportionately large because of the early brain development.

Second Month The embryo's length is about 1 to 2 inches, and it weighs about one-sixth of an ounce. Ears, eyelids, fingers, and toes are distinct. At 8 weeks, all the major organs are formed. The circulatory system is closed, and the placenta starts working. The neural tube closes. After 8 weeks, the embryo is called a fetus.

Third Month The length of the fetus is 2 to 3 inches and it weighs about an ounce. The sex of the fetus is defined, and it starts growing fuzzy hair, buds for future teeth, and soft fingernails and toenails. Kidneys begin to excrete urine. Other organs further develop. The nose and palate take shape, and the ears and earlobes are developed. At this time, the fetal heartbeat can be heard with a Doppler device.

Fourth Month The fetal length is 5 to 6 inches, and the weight is 2 to 5 ounces. The mother will start to discern fetal movements. The fetus can hear, move, kick, swim, sleep, and swallow. At this point, ultrasound can recognize external genitalia. The skin is pink and transparent, and eyebrows have formed.

Fifth Month Fetal length is 7 to 11 inches, and it may weigh up to 1.5 pounds. The skin is loose and wrinkled. Vernix, a white, greasy substance, and lanugo, a soft, fine hair, cover the skin for protection. Ultrasound can examine the baby's anatomy in detail.

Sixth Month The fetus weighs about 2 pounds. The skin is red and eyelids remain sealed. The fetus becomes active by kicking, punching, stretching, and turning over. It also coughs, hiccups, and responds to sudden noise. If born, the infant will cry and breathe, and it can survive with intensive neonatal care.

Seventh Month The fetal length is about 15 inches, and it weighs about 3 pounds. The eyes open and close, and the fetus can suck its thumb. If born, the infant can usually survive. Eyelids are open, and fingerprints are set.

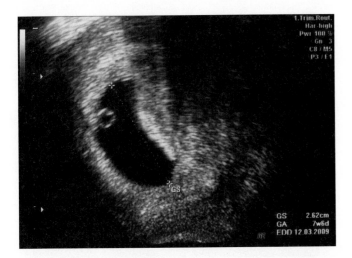

Figure 6.3A   Fetal development. Human embryo between 4 and 5 weeks of development.

© Ngo Thye Aun/Dreamstime.com

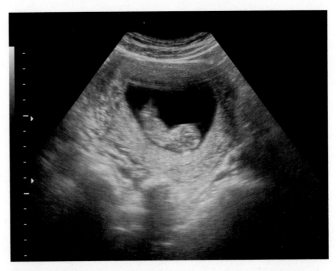

Figure 6.3B   Fetal development. Human fetus at about 11 to 12 weeks of development.

© Miroslav Ferkuniak/Dreamstime.com

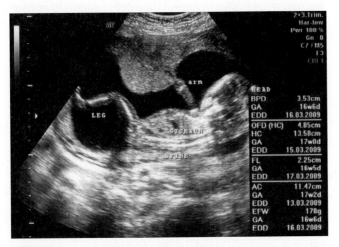

Figure 6.3C   Fetal development. Human fetus at about 5 months (20 weeks) of development.

© Ngo Thye Aun/Shutterstock

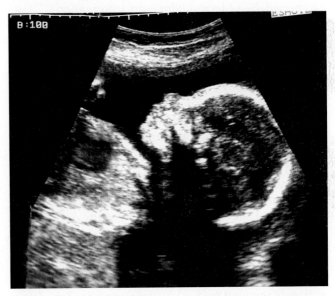

Figure 6.3D   Fetal development. Human fetus nearly full term—8 to 9 months.

© Amitai/Dreamstime.com

Eighth Month The fetus now gains about one-half pound per week and will most likely settle into position for birth. It is now about 17 inches long and weighs 4 to 5.5 pounds. The face and body have a loose and wrinkled appearance. Bones harden.

Ninth Month By the end of 37 weeks, the fetus is considered mature and ready to breathe. By 38 to 40 weeks, the fetus weighs 6 to 9 pounds and is 19–21 inches in length. In the final month, the fetus gains about an ounce per day. The skin is filled out and smooth. The skull bones have hardened, and the baby is ready for survival outside the womb. The lanugo hair and most of the vernix have disappeared.

CARE

Preconception care is the collective name for the steps a woman can take before she decides to become pregnant to ensure she is in good health when conception occurs. Many healthcare providers recommend that a woman see a clinician before getting pregnant and take a few basic steps to reduce the risk of certain problems during pregnancy. These steps include:

1. *Ensuring an adequate intake of folic acid.* The U.S. Public Health Service recommends that women of childbearing age get at least 400 mcg of folic acid daily, through food or dietary supplements. Many

healthcare providers suggest supplementing the diet with folic acid for 3 months before getting pregnant.

2. *Proper immunizations.* Women who are thinking of getting pregnant should be immunized against the communicable diseases that can harm a developing fetus, such as chicken pox and rubella, before conceiving.

3. *Healthy behaviors.* The preconception period is a good time for a woman to assess her health behaviors—smoking, alcohol use, caffeine intake, drug use, and medications. Items that should be avoided or limited during pregnancy should be minimized or eliminated in the preconception period.

4. *Nutrition.* Scientific research has shown that good nutrition is important for male and female fertility. A balanced diet including regular servings of fruits, vegetables, whole grains, lean meats, and dairy products will optimize the preconception period. Women should also get at least 1000 mg of calcium daily (three 8-ounce glasses of milk) in the preconception period. (See Chapter 9 for more information.)

PRENATAL CARE

A pregnant woman should take good care of herself to ensure proper development of her unborn child. Good prenatal care encompasses a spectrum of topics from proper nutrition to regular prenatal health care.

Nutrition

Pregnancy increases a woman's need for nutrients and calories, making a balanced diet essential for women of childbearing age (**Table 6.2**). Sensible eating during pregnancy includes the basic concepts discussed in Chapter 9. It is important not to diet during pregnancy but rather to eat sensibly. Pregnant women do not need to eat twice as much food or calories but rather consume the essential nutrients required for healthy development of the fetus.

Although it is recommended that a woman try to meet her vitamin and mineral requirements by eating a balanced diet, many healthcare providers recommend prenatal supplements to ensure adequate intake in addition to this diet. **Folate** is a B vitamin that is essential for the healthy development of the fetus; it is found naturally in green, leafy vegetables; nuts; beans; citrus fruits; and some fortified cereals. **Folic acid**, the synthetic form of the B vitamin folate, appears to help prevent **neural tube defects** such as anencephaly and spina bifida. As a result of folic acid's role in preventing neural tube defects, the Food and Drug Administration (FDA) has required enriched grain products, such as breads, pasta, and bagels, to be fortified with folic acid. This fortification has prevented many cases of neural tube defects, but the effects have not been equally seen across all racial and ethnic groups. Non-Hispanic White, non-Hispanic Black, and Hispanic births all have shown decreases in

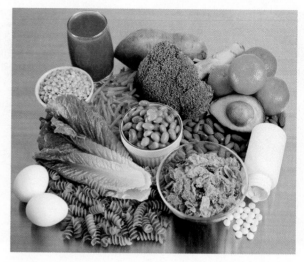

Folic acid appears to be a protective factor against neural tube defects, which develop in the first month of pregnancy. It is important for a woman to begin increasing her folic acid intake before she becomes pregnant.
© Fertnig/Getty Images

neural tube defects. Researchers emphasize that efforts to increase folic acid consumption should be continued for all racial and ethnic groups, especially among Hispanic women where rates of neural tube defects remain consistently higher than other ethnic groups.[8]

Calcium and iron are important minerals for all women, including pregnant women. Calcium is essential to the formation of bone and teeth in the fetus, and it prevents the pregnant woman from losing her own bone density while providing for the growing fetus. Iron helps carry oxygen in the blood and reduces the risk of pregnancy-induced hypertension. Women often require iron supplements, because most female iron stores are not adequate to supply both mother and fetus given the large demand for iron throughout the pregnancy. Iron supplements should be taken with vitamin C to facilitate their absorption.

Women should drink plenty of fluids throughout pregnancy. A woman's blood volume and blood fluids increase significantly during pregnancy, and drinking enough fluids will help to prevent dehydration and constipation. Pregnant women should also avoid certain foods during pregnancy, to help prevent infections that may harm the fetus (see **It's Your Health**).

Weight gain is another important prenatal nutritional issue. It is not necessary to "eat for two," but extra nutrients and calories are needed in the prenatal period. A woman should consult with her healthcare provider about how much weight to gain during her pregnancy. A woman of average weight is generally advised to gain 25 to 35 pounds during her pregnancy; an underweight woman should gain more, between 28 and 40 pounds; and overweight women may need to gain only 15 to 25 pounds. Obese women should have a total weight gain of 11 to 20 pounds. Women who are expecting multiple births will need to gain more weight than a single pregnancy. Women often average a weight gain of 4 to

It's Your Health

Foods to Avoid During Pregnancy

- Sushi and other raw fish, especially shellfish (oysters, clams).
- Hot dogs or luncheon meats (such as ham, turkey, salami, and bologna) unless they are reheated until steaming hot.
- Unpasteurized milk, unpasteurized fruit and vegetable juices, or foods made from unpasteurized milk, including soft cheese (feta, brie, Camembert, Roquefort, queso blanco, queso fresco). Soft cheeses may be eaten if they are made with pasteurized milk.
- Refrigerated pates, meat spreads, or smoked seafood. Canned versions of these products are safe to eat.
- Raw vegetable sprouts (alfalfa, clover, and radish), which can carry *Salmonella* or *E. coli*.
- Raw or undercooked meat, poultry, and eggs, as well as products made with raw or partially cooked eggs (such as eggnog, hollandaise sauce, and some Caesar salad dressings).
- Some herbal supplements and teas.
- Swordfish, shark, king mackerel, and tilefish, which have high levels of mercury.
    - According to the FDA/Environmental Protection Agency (EPA), women who are pregnant can eat up to 12 ounces (two average-sized fish meals) per week of fish or shellfish that are lower in mercury, such as shrimp, salmon, catfish, and canned light tuna. White (albacore) tuna contains more mercury than canned light tuna, so women should limit their consumption of canned white tuna and tuna steaks to no more than 6 ounces per week.
    - Women should check for local advisories about any fish caught in waters by family and friends. If no advice is available, women should limit their consumption to less than 6 ounces per week of this type of fish and not eat any other fish during the week.

Table 6.2   Healthy Food Choices for a Pregnant Woman

The foods below are the best sources of nutrients needed by pregnant and breastfeeding women.

Vegetable Group (choose fresh, frozen, canned, or dried)

- Carrots
- Sweet potatoes
- Pumpkins
- Spinach
- Cooked greens (such as kale, collards, turnip greens, and beet greens)
- Winter squashes
- Tomatoes and tomato sauces
- Red sweet peppers

These vegetables all have both vitamin A and potassium. When choosing canned vegetables, look for "low-sodium" or "no-salt-added" on the label.

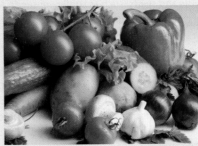

© Denis Vrublevski/Shutterstock

Fruit Group (choose fresh, frozen, canned, or dried)

- Cantaloupes
- Honeydew melons
- Mangoes
- Prunes or prune juice
- Bananas
- Apricots
- Oranges and orange juice
- Red or pink grapefruit

These fruits all provide potassium, and many also provide vitamin A. When choosing canned fruit, look for fruit canned in 100% fruit juice or water instead of syrup.

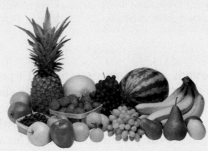

© Photodisc

(continues)

Table 6.2 Healthy Food Choices for a Pregnant Woman (continued)

Dairy Group

- Fat-free or low-fat yogurt
- Fat-free milk (skim milk)
- Low-fat milk (1% milk)
- Calcium-fortified soymilk (soy beverage)

These all provide necessary calcium and potassium. Look for choices that are fortified with vitamins A and D.

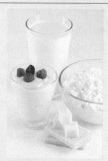

© Olga Lyubkina/Shutterstock

Grain Group

- Fortified ready-to-eat cereals
- Fortified cooked cereals

When buying ready-to-eat and cooked cereals, choose mostly those made from whole grains. Look for cereals that are fortified with iron and folic acid.

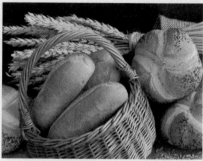

© Magdalena Kucova/Shutterstock

Protein Foods Group

- Beans and peas (such as pinto beans, soybeans, white beans, lentils, kidney beans, and chickpeas)
- Nuts and seeds (such as sunflower seeds, almonds, hazelnuts, pine nuts, peanuts, and peanut butter)
- Lean beef, lamb, poultry, and pork
- Oysters, mussels, crab
- Salmon, trout, herring, sardines, and pollock

All of these foods provide protein. In addition, beans and peas provide iron, potassium, and fiber. Meats provide heme-iron, which is the most readily absorbed type of iron. Nuts and seeds also contain vitamin E. Seafood provides omega-3 fatty acids.

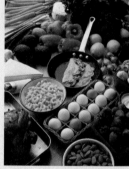

© Photodisc/Getty Images

NOTE: Do not eat shark, swordfish, king mackerel, or tilefish when you are pregnant or breastfeeding. They contain high levels of mercury. Limit white (albacore) tuna to no more than 6 ounces per week.

Source: Reproduced from U.S. Department of Agriculture. *Health and nutrition information for pregnant and breastfeeding women.* Available at: http://www.choosemyplate.gov/moms-making-healthy-food-choices

6 pounds in the first trimester and 1 pound per week in the second and third trimesters. As shown in **Table 6.3**, pregnancy weight gain is distributed throughout a woman's body. Gaining too much or too little weight during pregnancy can produce health risks for a woman and her baby. Failure to gain adequate weight is associated with higher infant morbidity, lower birth weight, and preterm delivery. Excessive weight gain can increase the likelihood of pregnancy and delivery complications, higher infant birth weight, and health-related risks in subsequent pregnancies, such as gestational diabetes.[9]

Exercise

Proper exercise during pregnancy can have many benefits. Studies show that women who exercised in the 3 months before pregnancy felt better during the first trimester than women did not exercise; similarly, women who exercised in the first and second trimesters felt better in the third trimester than those who did not exercise. Well-conditioned women often have shorter labor, less need for obstetric intervention during pregnancy and childbirth, and speedier recovery after childbirth. The American College of Obstetricians and Gynecologists

Table 6.3	Pregnancy Weight Gain Distribution
	Pounds
Baby	8
Placenta	2–3
Breasts	2–3
Amniotic fluid	2–3
Blood supply	4
Fat stores	5–9
Uterus	2–5
Total	25–35 pounds

(ACOG) recommends at least 30 minutes of daily active exercise during pregnancy to reduce backaches, constipation, bloating, and swelling. Exercise also helps prevent or treat gestational diabetes; improves energy and mood; improves posture; promotes muscle tone, strength, and endurance; and helps the pregnant woman sleep better. ACOG, however, does not recommend exercise for weight reduction while a woman is pregnant.[10]

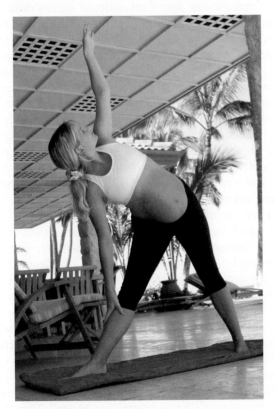

Proper exercise during pregnancy can have many benefits. Walking, swimming, and low-impact aerobics are particularly good choices for pregnant women.

The exercise program of a pregnant woman must be geared to her current level of fitness, medical history,

past pregnancies, stage of fetal development, and maternal complicating factors. Walking, swimming, and low-impact aerobics are particularly good exercise choices for pregnant women. Classes or exercise videos made specifically for pregnant women are also good options.

Activities that involve bouncing, jarring, twisting, or any activity that places the abdomen in jeopardy should be avoided during pregnancy. This includes horseback riding, scuba diving, and downhill skiing. Contact sports are too risky, as is any activity that requires rapid stops and starts or an extreme range of motion. The center of gravity for the body changes during pregnancy, increasing the risk of loss of balance. Exercises that require lying on the back, particularly after the fourth month, can be dangerous because this position can block the blood supply to the uterus and depress fetal heart rate. A resting position on the side does not compromise fetal blood supply.

Many questions regarding the safety and benefits of exercise during pregnancy remain unanswered. Although women with medical or obstetric complications should avoid rigorous physical activity, healthy women should continue exercising under their healthcare provider's supervision.

Another form of exercise, known as pelvic muscle or Kegel exercises, is important during pregnancy. Increasing the strength of the pelvic muscles decreases urine loss during late pregnancy and may speed up the rehabilitation of the pelvic floor after vaginal delivery.

Avoiding Toxic Substances

Maternal exposure to many substances during pregnancy has been shown to have detrimental effects on the developing fetus. Many of these topics are discussed in detail elsewhere in this book. Note, however, that cigarettes, alcohol, and drugs have specific detrimental effects on the fetus.

Not smoking is essential to a healthy pregnancy and birth. Smoking before and during pregnancy is one of the most preventable causes of infant morbidity and mortality. Women who smoke before pregnancy are more likely to have difficulty becoming pregnant compared to nonsmoking women. Men who smoke also are more likely to have damaged DNA in their sperm, which can reduce fertility. Smoking is also known to cause ectopic pregnancy and spontaneous abortion. Women who smoke during pregnancy are more likely to experience complications including premature rupture of membranes, early separation of the placenta from the uterus, and blockage of the cervix by the placenta.[11] In addition, babies born to women who smoke during pregnancy are more likely to be born premature and/or of low birth weight and to die of sudden infant death syndrome (SIDS). Women who smoke also are more likely to deliver babies with cleft lip or cleft palate.[12] Unfortunately, about 13% of women still smoke during pregnancy. As **Figure 6.4** shows, younger, less educated, non-Hispanic White, and American Indian women are more likely to smoke during pregnancy.

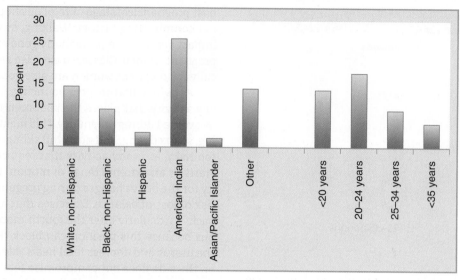

Figure 6.4   **Prevalence (%) of smoking during pregnancy by race/ethnicity and age.**

Source: Tong, V. T., Dietz, P. M., Morrow, B., et al. (2013). Trends in smoking before, during, and after pregnancy—Pregnancy Risk Assessment Monitoring System (PRAMS), United States, 40 sites, 2000–2010. *Morbidity and Mortality Weekly Report* 62(SS06);1–19.

Alcohol also is detrimental for both the mother and her developing baby. Alcohol consumption during pregnancy is known to cause alcohol-related defects among infants and **fetal alcohol syndrome (FAS)**, which is characterized by growth retardation, facial malformations, and central nervous system dysfunctions, including intellectual disabilities, speech and language delays, and poor social skills. Alcohol appears to act in concert with several other factors to promote the development of FAS in infants:

- Differences in the degree of prenatal exposure to alcohol
- Maternal drinking patterns
- Possible genetic susceptibility to FAS
- Differences in maternal metabolism of alcohol
- Time of gestation during heavy alcohol consumption
- Interactions of alcohol use with other drugs and medications
- Maternal nutritional status

The fetus is especially vulnerable to the effects of alcohol during the first trimester of pregnancy, when the development of the central nervous system occurs. Research also links maternal drinking during pregnancy with an increased risk of early stillbirth.[13] In spite of campaigns to reduce alcohol consumption during pregnancy, usage levels still remain fairly high. In a self-reported study from the Centers for Disease Control and Prevention (CDC), about 1 in 13 pregnant women in the United States reported alcohol use 30 days prior to the survey, and about 1 in 71 pregnant women reported binge drinking (having five or more drinks at one time).[14]

Consumption of other drugs also can adversely affect a developing fetus. Based on national survey data, 5.4% of pregnant women aged 15 to 44 were current illicit drug users. Drug use was highest in the first trimester (9.0%) and decreased with each trimester (4.8% and 2.4%, respectively).[15] Illicit drugs may pose various risks for pregnant women and their babies. For example, the use of cocaine is associated with fetal distress, low birth weight, and impaired fetal growth. Compared with mothers who did not smoke marijuana, smokers had smaller, sicker babies and a higher risk of stillbirths. Also, babies of marijuana smokers may be prone to excessive crying and trembling. Drug use may lead to neurochemical birth defects by disrupting normal development of the brain, and, in turn, cause long-term effects on intelligence, mental development, and learning. Some drugs also can cause a baby to have withdrawal symptoms. Women who are pregnant and using heroin should work with a physician to quit using, as abruptly stopping use of the drug can cause miscarriage.[16] Because many pregnant women who use illicit drugs also use alcohol and tobacco, which also pose risks to unborn babies, it often is difficult to determine which substance causes the adverse outcomes. Additionally, illicit drugs may be prepared with impurities that could be harmful to a pregnancy.

Many over-the-counter prescription medications can prove dangerous during pregnancy as well. The antibiotic streptomycin can cause deafness, and the antibiotic tetracycline can lead to bone abnormalities and discolored teeth. Even aspirin and acetaminophen may affect a developing fetus. Clearly, it is important for pregnant women to consult their physicians before taking any type of medication.

Environmental Risks

Although not all environmental hazards can be avoided, a pregnant woman should take some precautions to protect herself and her baby. Although data are scarce, it is believed that the rapidly developing fetus is especially vulnerable to pollutants, toxic wastes, heavy metals, pesticides, gases, and other hazardous compounds. For example, the element lead can cross the placenta and has been associated with gestational hypertension, spontaneous abortion, low birth weight, and impaired brain development.[17] Air pollution, such as secondhand smoke, can be detrimental to both a woman's health and the developing fetus. Scientists also have concluded that prenatal exposure to tobacco and environmental lead is a risk factor for attention deficit hyperactivity disorder (ADHD) in children.[18] Diagnostic X-rays should be avoided if possible throughout the pregnancy or if there is the possibility of pregnancy. X-ray exposure is associated with respiratory diseases and blood disorders in the fetus, as well as miscarriage.

Another environmental risk to consider during pregnancy is heat exposure. Women who use hot tubs and saunas or who have high fevers early in pregnancy have been found to be at greater risk of miscarriage and having children with neural tube defects such as spina bifida. Although more research is needed on this subject, it appears that the greatest risk arises early in the pregnancy when the fetal central nervous system is developing.[19]

Prenatal Testing

Prospective parents often worry whether their baby will be born normal and healthy. Most of the time, these worries are unfounded: Almost all children born in the United States are healthy. However, the CDC reports that 1 of every 33 babies is born with a birth defect.[20] A birth defect can affect almost any part of the body. The well-being of the child depends mostly on which organ or body part is involved and how much it is affected. Most birth defects occur during the first 3 months of pregnancy. Birth defects can be genetic in origin, or they can be caused by exposure to harmful agents.

Risk factors that increase the likelihood of birth defects include family or personal history of birth defects, a previous child with a birth defect, certain medications used around the time of conception, diabetes before pregnancy, and being age 35 years or older when the baby is due.

Screening tests are performed during pregnancy to assess the risk of certain birth defects. If a screening test shows an increased risk for a certain defect, further diagnostic tests can confirm whether it actually exists. Screening tests include:

- *First-trimester screening tests* combine the result of special **ultrasound** tests and maternal blood tests to detect **Down syndrome** and trisomy 18. Ultrasound is a noninvasive procedure that uses high-frequency sound waves to project an image or sonogram of the fetus. This type of ultrasound exam, called nuchal translucency screening, measures the thickness of the translucent space at the back of the fetus' neck. Babies with Down syndrome, trisomy 18, or other chromosomal problems tend to accumulate more fluid than babies without chromosomal abnormalities, causing a larger space. The exam must be performed between 11 and 14 weeks, when the base of the neck is still translucent. Increased levels of pregnancy-associated plasma protein A and hCG, found by testing the blood, also may indicate Down syndrome.

- A *second trimester screening test*, called "multiple marker screening," examines blood for abnormal levels of substances linked with certain birth defects such as Down syndrome and neural tube defects. This test, referred to as triple or quadruple screening, measures the level of three or four substances:
  - **Maternal serum alpha-fetoprotein (MSAFP)**, a substance produced by the fetal kidneys between the 13th and 20th weeks of pregnancy and found in the mother's blood.
  - Estriol, a hormone made by the liver of the fetus and the placenta.
  - Human chorionic gonadotropin, a hormone made by the placenta.
  - Inhibin-A, another hormone produced by the placenta.

Detailed ultrasound exams are usually done after 18 weeks of pregnancy and allow for a more extensive view of the fetus' organs and features.

Diagnostic tests try to detect a genetic disorder or birth defect. They are offered to women at risk of genetic disorder based on family history, advanced maternal age, or the results of screening tests. Diagnostic tests include:

- **Amniocentesis (Figure 6.5A)** is usually performed at 15 to 20 weeks of pregnancy. The doctor guides a thin needle through the abdomen and uterus and withdraws a small amount of amniotic fluid. Cells from the fluid are analyzed for chromosomal defects. Complications from the procedure are rare. One large study found that the procedure-related fetal loss rate after mid-trimester amniocentesis performed on patients in a contemporary prospective clinical trial was 0.06%. There was no significant difference in the risk of miscarriage before 24 weeks' gestation between those undergoing amniocentesis and those not undergoing amniocentesis.[21]

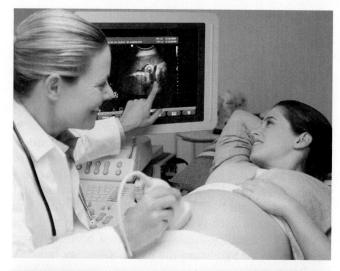

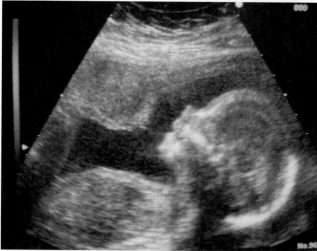

Performed at various times during pregnancy, ultrasound uses sound waves to show a picture of the fetus. Ultrasound can check the age, growth, and size of a fetus; identify multiple pregnancies; and diagnose complications or birth defects.

(top) © Simon Pederson/Shutterstock; (bottom) © Chris Ryan/OJO Images/Getty Images

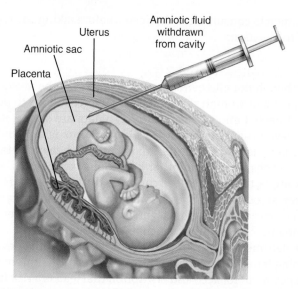

Figure 6.5A   Amniocentesis is a test for fetal abnormalities that involves withdrawing amniotic fluid and inspecting the cells contained within it.

Prenatal Testing

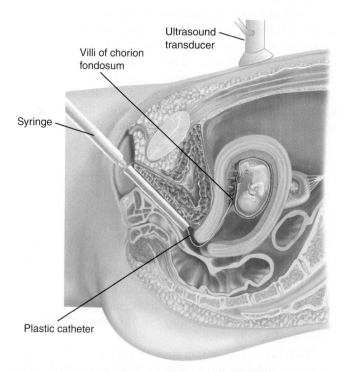

Figure 6.5B   In chorionic villus sampling, fetal cells from the chorionic villi (fingerlike projections on the developing placenta) are suctioned out through the cervix.

- Chorionic villus sampling (CVS) (**Figure 6.5B**) detects some of the same chromosomal abnormalities as amniocentesis; however, it can be performed earlier, at 10 to 12 weeks of pregnancy. The doctor guides either a small tube through the vagina and cervix or a thin needle through the abdomen and uterine wall to take a small sample of tissue from the placenta. The chorionic villi contain cells with the same genetic makeup as the fetus. The sample is studied for chromosomal or other defects. Studies show that there are no significant differences in the risk of miscarriage before 24 weeks' gestation between those undergoing CVS and those not undergoing CVS.[21]

- *Fetal blood sampling*, also known as cordocentesis, tests fetal blood for chromosomal defects and other problems. This procedure involves the insertion of a needle through the abdomen and uterine wall to take blood from a vein in the umbilical cord. Cordocentesis is usually performed when amniocentesis or CVS is not possible because results are needed quickly. There is a small chance of fetal loss after fetal blood sampling.

If the results from any of the screening or diagnostic tests are abnormal, counseling and supportive services can help the parents make decisions that best meet their needs.

Women also should be tested for **Rh incompatibility** through a simple blood test. Most people produce Rh factor, a protein located on the surface of red blood cells. A person who does not produce Rh factor has Rh-negative blood. Rh incompatibility occurs when an Rh-negative mother and an Rh-positive father conceive a baby who inherits the father's Rh-positive blood type. If the fetal Rh-positive blood cells enter the mother's bloodstream, the mother forms antibodies against the fetal blood cells in a process called maternal sensitization. This situation often occurs in a first pregnancy with an Rh-positive fetus, but because of the small amount of antibodies produced, it does not cause problems with the fetus. Future pregnancies, however, are at greater risk of antibodies crossing the placenta and causing Rh disease in the fetus. Rh-negative mothers should receive an injection of Rh immune globulin after delivery, during pregnancy, after a miscarriage, and after certain procedures such as amniocentesis. Without treatment, the most severely affected fetuses will be stillborn. In the newborn, Rh disease can result in jaundice, anemia, brain damage, heart failure, and death. Rh disease does not affect the mother's health.

COMPLICATIONS OF PREGNANCY

There are several factors that may cause complications in pregnancy. Some common pregnancy complications include Rh disease (as mentioned earlier), ectopic pregnancy, gestational diabetes, preeclampsia, and preterm labor and delivery. Various types of infections can cause complications as well. Some complications can lead to miscarriage or stillbirth. In addition, genetic disorders and congenital abnormalities can cause complications in the newborn.

> *I had some rather severe abdominal pain and some bleeding. I knew my period was late, but I was shocked to learn from my doctor that I had had a miscarriage. I didn't even know that I was pregnant.*
>
> **—24-year-old woman**

Ectopic Pregnancy

Ectopic pregnancy occurs when the fertilized egg implants outside the uterus, usually in the fallopian tube. The egg begins to grow outside the uterine cavity and presents a risk for rupture and hemorrhage. This problem occurs in about 1 to 2% of pregnancies.[22] Increased awareness and improved technologies that identify early ectopic pregnancies have greatly decreased maternal deaths;

Table 6.4 Ectopic Pregnancy Risk Factors
▪ Pelvic inflammatory disease (PID)
▪ Previous ectopic pregnancy
▪ Previous tubal or pelvic surgery
▪ Endometriosis
▪ Infertility or infertility treatments
▪ Utero or tubal abnormalities
▪ DES (a drug once prescribed to prevent miscarriage) exposure
▪ Cigarette smoking

however, ectopic pregnancy-related deaths still account for 3 to 4% of all pregnancy-related deaths.[23]

Several factors increase the risk of an ectopic pregnancy by causing disruption of fallopian tube function (see **Table 6.4**). Pelvic inflammatory disease (PID), commonly caused by gonorrhea or chlamydia, is the most common risk factor. (See Chapter 7 for more information.) Symptoms of ectopic pregnancy usually begin in the seventh or eighth week of gestation. The most common symptoms are abdominal pain and tenderness and a missed menstrual period. The abdominal pain can be subtle at first, sometimes localized on one side, and increase in severity if tearing of the fallopian tube causes internal bleeding. Abnormal vaginal bleeding or spotting occurs in most ectopic pregnancies. Blood tests and vaginal or abdominal ultrasound tests can effectively diagnose an ectopic pregnancy. In some cases, an ectopic pregnancy may degenerate and require no intervention. In most cases, however, laparoscopic surgery may be performed to remove the fertilized egg that cannot survive outside the uterus.

Gestational Diabetes

Gestational diabetes usually occurs in the second half of pregnancy. One in twenty pregnant women in the United States will be affected by gestational diabetes.[24] Most women can control their blood sugar levels with diet and exercise, but some women with gestational diabetes or women who had diabetes before pregnancy will need insulin injections to control their blood sugar levels. A woman is considered to be at high risk for gestational diabetes if she is very overweight, previously had gestational diabetes, has a strong family history of diabetes, or has glucose in her urine. The baby of a mother with gestational diabetes is at risk of being born very large and with extra fat, making delivery difficult and more dangerous, and causing an increased risk of cesarean section. The baby is also at greater risk of having breathing problems and low blood glucose after birth. For most women, glucose levels return to normal after pregnancy, but they have a 35 to 60% chance of developing type 2 diabetes in the next 10 to 20 years.[25]

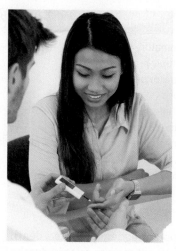

Women with diabetes are at an increased risk for complications during pregnancy.
© AndreyPopov/iStockphoto/Getty Images

Preeclampsia

Preeclampsia is pregnancy-related high blood pressure. It can also be called **toxemia**. Preeclampsia usually occurs after about 30 weeks of pregnancy. In addition to having high blood pressure, mothers with preeclampsia often experience protein in their urine, swelling of the hands and face, sudden weight gain (a pound a day or more), blurred vision, severe headaches, dizziness, and intense stomach pain. The only real cure for preeclampsia is delivery, which may not be best for the baby. Labor is usually induced if the condition is mild and the woman is near-term (37 to 40 weeks' gestation). If a woman is not ready for labor, she and her fetus will be monitored, often in a hospital setting, until her blood pressure stabilizes or the baby is born.

Preterm Labor and Delivery

Pregnancy usually lasts from 38 to 42 weeks. Labor that begins before week 37 of pregnancy is considered **premature labor**. Babies born prematurely may have problems with breathing, eating, and temperature control, and they are more likely to die within the first month of life than a full-term baby. Approximately 9.6% of babies in the United States are born preterm, a decrease of 8% since 2007.[26] Women are at higher risk of preterm birth if they have had a previous preterm birth, are pregnant with twins or more, have certain uterine or cervical abnormalities, or have certain medical conditions. Women who seek late prenatal care or no care at all, as well as women who smoke, drink alcohol, use drugs, or experience stress, are also at greater risk. Women can decrease their risk of premature birth by recognizing the warning signs of preterm labor (see **It's Your Health**).

Infections

Any infection in the mother can potentially cause harm to an unborn fetus. Sexually transmitted infections, including HIV, can be particularly dangerous during a pregnancy. (For more information, see Chapter 7.)

- Gonorrhea, chlamydia, and syphilis can cause preterm delivery and miscarriage.

- Bacterial vaginosis (BV), an infection of the vaginal area that is usually benign and asymptomatic, can lead to preterm delivery as well as low-birth-weight babies. The presence of BV also is associated with an increased risk of HIV infection.

- Perinatal transmission of HIV can occur during pregnancy, labor, and delivery, or via breastfeeding. Since medications can reduce the risk of perinatal HIV transmission, testing of pregnant women and subsequent treatment of those who are infected have dramatically reduced transmission rates. Perinatal transmission is the most common route of HIV infection in children; in 2010, 75% of children with HIV were perinatally infected.[27] The actual number of AIDS cases associated with perinatal transmission has decreased dramatically in recent years, though the disease burden remains disproportionately high for racial and ethnic minorities.

The CDC recommends that all pregnant women be tested for HIV as early in pregnancy as possible. Pregnant women should also be screened for chlamydia, gonorrhea, hepatitis B, and syphilis, as well as hepatitis C if they have a history of injection drug use or a history of blood transfusion or organ transplantation before 1992.[28]

The most common prenatal infection today is **cytomegalovirus (CMV)**, a viral infection. Cytomegalovirus causes mild flulike symptoms in adults, but in newborns, it can cause small birth size, brain damage, developmental problems, enlarged liver, hearing and vision impairment, and other malformations. Each year in the United States, about 1 in 150 children is born with CMV infection and 1 in 750 children has permanent disabilities as a result of CMV infection. About 80% of babies born with CMV never have symptoms or problems.[29]

A blood test can ascertain whether a woman already had a CMV infection. More invasive tests, such as amniocentesis, can help determine whether the fetus is infected.

Because CMV is found in body fluids, including urine, saliva, breast milk, blood, tears, semen, and vaginal fluids, a woman can become infected with CMV when she comes in contact with them. Good hygiene by pregnant women is still the best way to protect unborn babies against CMV infection.

Rubella is also linked with birth defects. A rubella infection is usually mild and often asymptomatic. The biggest danger of rubella is if a woman becomes infected during the first 20 weeks of pregnancy: She may lose the pregnancy, or the virus could cause problems to her unborn baby such as cataracts, deafness, or damage to the heart or brain. There is no treatment for rubella, but the measles-mumps-rubella (MMR) vaccine can prevent it. All women of reproductive age should be immunized against rubella if they have not had this formerly common childhood illness.

Group B streptococcus (GBS) is a bacterium that can cause illness in newborn babies and pregnant women. It is the most common cause of life-threatening infections in newborns, and it is a frequent cause of newborn pneumonia. On average, about 1000 babies less than 1 week old get early-onset group B strep disease.[30] In most cases, this disease can be prevented in newborns by administering IV antibiotics to women in labor who had a baby with group B strep disease in the past or who now have a urinary tract infection caused by group B strep. Pregnant women who carry the bacterium, as confirmed with a positive test during pregnancy, should also be given antibiotics during labor.

Miscarriage

A **miscarriage**, or spontaneous abortion, is defined as a pregnancy that ends before the 20th week of gestation. An estimated 10 to 15% of clinically recognized pregnancies end in spontaneous abortion,[31] though experts acknowledge challenges in estimating rates. Miscarriages often occur early in the pregnancy, even before women are aware that they are pregnant. Factors associated with miscarriage include advanced maternal age, chromosomal abnormalities, single gene mutations, structural uterine abnormalities, endocrine abnormalities, immunologic factors, genital infections, cigarette smoking, alcohol use, and various environmental and occupational exposures. Some of these, such as chromosomal abnormalities, are clearly related to the embryo and others, such as uterine abnormalities, are clearly related to the mother.

A miscarriage is usually characterized by bleeding and cramping. Generally, when a woman experiences bleeding or cramping early in the pregnancy, bed rest is recommended. In some cases, the symptoms subside and the pregnancy proceeds normally. In other cases, the bleeding increases, the cervix dilates, and the embryo is released from the body. If the miscarriage is complete, the bleeding stops, and the uterus returns to its normal shape and size. If the miscarriage is incomplete, any remaining tissue must be removed in a procedure known as a dilatation and curettage (D&C). The risk for miscarriage decreases after the first trimester of pregnancy.

The causes of miscarriage vary and are not always clear. This uncertainty is a source of frustration for many couples who feel the need to understand why the miscarriage happened. Grief associated with miscarriage is often underestimated, leaving many affected women with inadequate support from their partners, friends, family, and healthcare providers. The intensity of a woman's emotional distress may be related to the desirability of the pregnancy, late gestational age of the fetus, lack of social support, a lengthy period of trying to get pregnant, and use of infertility treatments. Women also may feel that they have disappointed their partners or families.

Stillbirth

Stillbirth is a common term for death of a fetus in the middle of the second trimester or later, while the fetus is still in the uterus. It is also called intrauterine fetal death or demise. There are multiple causes of stillbirth, including a mother with diabetes or high blood pressure, infection in the mother or in the fetal tissue, congenital abnormalities, and Rh disease. In addition, twin-to-twin transfusion (when twin circulations connect in a shared placenta); umbilical cord problems such as knots, tightened cord, cord wrapped around the fetal body or neck, cord prolapse (the cord falling down through the open cervix during labor); and placental problems, including poor circulation, can lead to a stillbirth.

Symptoms of a stillbirth vary, but they may include the following common signs: stopping of fetal movement and kicks, spotting or bleeding, no fetal heartbeat heard with stethoscope or Doppler, and no fetal movement or heartbeat seen on ultrasound. Treatment of the woman following a stillbirth depends on many factors such as the number of weeks of gestation, the size of the fetus, and how long since the fetal heartbeat stopped. Stillbirth is often very difficult for parents and other family members. Often, the fetus is fully formed and is delivered just as is any baby. It may be very hard emotionally for a woman to go through labor, yet not have a baby to take home. Counseling is important for all parents with a stillbirth to help them understand their feelings and begin the work of grieving.

Genetic Disorders and Congenital Abnormalities

Genetic disorders are diseases caused in whole or in part by a variation or mutation of a gene. Scientists are learning that thousands of diseases have genetic components. Genetic disorders are responsible for a significant number of miscarriages, often without being diagnosed, so calculating the total number of disorders is a complicated process. Today more than 6000 abnormalities have been identified, ranging from mild differences (as in certain hemoglobin abnormalities) to fatal or overwhelmingly disabling conditions, such as trisomy 18 (Edwards syndrome) and trisomy 13 (Patau syndrome). The risk of a single-gene disorder is estimated at 1 in 200 births.

Genetic diseases result from single-gene alterations, chromosomal abnormalities, or multifactorial errors. Single-gene disorders are caused by a mutation in a single gene. (Each chromosome contains thousands of individual genes.) The mutation may be present on one chromosome or two chromosomes where one is inherited from each parent. Sickle cell disease, cystic fibrosis, and Tay–Sachs disease are single-gene disorders. Chromosome disorders are caused by extra or missing chromosomes or chromosome parts. Down syndrome, for example, is caused by an extra copy of chromosome 21, but no individual gene on the chromosome is abnormal. Multifactorial inheritance disorders are caused by a combination of small variations in genes, often in concert with environmental factors. Heart disease and most cancers are examples of these disorders. Another multifactorial example is albinism, an inherited inability to generate the protective pigment melanin. Albinism greatly increases susceptibility to skin cancer after excessive exposure to sunlight. Behaviors are also considered to be multifactorial. Behaviors are complex traits involving multiple genes that are affected by many other factors. Researchers are learning more about the genetic contribution to behavioral disorders such as alcoholism and obesity, as well as certain mental illnesses and Alzheimer's disease.

Because early detection of these conditions is essential, states and territories mandate newborn screening of all infants born within their jurisdiction for certain disorders that may not otherwise be detected before developmental disability or death occurs. Newborns with these disorders typically appear normal at birth. The Health Resources and Services Administration issued a report that recommends screening for 32 specific conditions. Each state requires newborn screening for every infant; however, each state decides what tests to require on their screening panel.[32]

Other Considerations

Women should be aware of postpartum issues, such as depression. Many women will experience postpartum "blues," mood swings, and slight depression for several days after a baby's birth. These feelings are normal and will go away in the first few weeks. Some women experience more severe symptoms, however, which will warrant treatment. Women who are more susceptible to postpartum depression include those women who suffer from depression, have experienced postpartum depression in a previous pregnancy, have severe premenstrual syndrome (PMS) or premenstrual dysphoric disorder (PMDD), and/or are experiencing other stressors in their family, marriage, or life at the time of the birth. (See Chapter 12 on mental health.)

Women with disabilities and chronic conditions who want to become pregnant may have special considerations to discuss with their healthcare providers. Certain conditions that are common in pregnant women, such as vaginal and urinary tract infections, fluid retention, and decreased mobility, may create even more significant problems for women with preexisting conditions or disorders.

Other difficulties may also impair the mobility of women with physical disabilities. As her body changes with pregnancy, a woman with impaired mobility may experience balance problems and new pressure points if she is in a wheelchair. Each disability or condition may present with different issues, just as each pregnant woman may present with different complications and issues. Throughout the pregnancy, from preconception to postpartum, women with disabilities or chronic conditions should work with a team of healthcare providers to ensure favorable pregnancy and post-pregnancy outcomes.

> I knew that having a baby would be difficult, but I was not prepared to feel so numb, miserable, hopeless, and worried. I learned that I was one of the 10–15% of mothers who experience postpartum depression. Fortunately my doctor was really helpful. I would encourage any new mom to talk to her doctor if she is feeling really sad or "down." Sometimes it is just normal "baby blues." But sometimes it can be serious. Getting help early can make a huge difference.
>
> —30-year-old mother

CHILDBIRTH

Many women have special concerns about their childbirth experience. Experts agree that interfering with the normal physiological process of labor and birth in the absence of medical necessity increases the risk of complications for the mother and baby. Unfortunately, hospital routines and procedures have often taken priority over the needs of the laboring mother and her baby. Some experts argue that many modern medical interventions, including cesarean surgery, labor induction, electronic fetal monitoring, ultrasound examinations, episiotomies, unnatural birthing positions, pubic shaving, enemas, IV lines, drugs, and forced mother and baby separations, are too normative and often do not improve birth outcome or the labor and delivery process.[33] Six evidence-based birth practices that promote, support, and protect normal birth, making it healthier and safer for mothers and babies, have been promoted by the World Health Organization (WHO) as well as Lamaze International:[34]

- Avoiding medically unnecessary induction of labor
- Allowing freedom of movement for the laboring woman
- Providing continuous labor support
- Avoiding interventions that are not medically necessary
- Encouraging spontaneous pushing in nonsupine positions
- Keeping mothers and babies together after birth without restrictions on breastfeeding

Self-Assessment 6.1
Childbirth Considerations

Birthing issues	Very Important	Not Important	Don't Want
Hospital delivery room	_____	_____	_____
Hospital birthing room	_____	_____	_____
Birthing center	_____	_____	_____
Home	_____	_____	_____
Obstetrician	_____	_____	_____
Family practitioner	_____	_____	_____
Certified nurse–midwife	_____	_____	_____
Doula	_____	_____	_____
Partner/coach:			
Present during labor	_____	_____	_____
Present during delivery	_____	_____	_____
Present for all procedures	_____	_____	_____
Present during cesarean	_____	_____	_____
Present during recovery	_____	_____	_____
Early labor:			
Stay home as long as possible	_____	_____	_____
Arrive early and settle in	_____	_____	_____
Wear own clothes	_____	_____	_____
Perineal shave	_____	_____	_____
Enema	_____	_____	_____
Intravenous tube	_____	_____	_____
First-stage labor:			
Labor room	_____	_____	_____
Birthing room	_____	_____	_____
External fetal monitor	_____	_____	_____
Internal fetal monitor	_____	_____	_____

Birthing issues	Very Important	Not Important	Don't Want
Second-stage labor:			
Labor room	_____	_____	_____
Delivery room	_____	_____	_____
Birthing room	_____	_____	_____
Family present	_____	_____	_____
Delivery position flexibility	_____	_____	_____
Episiotomy	_____	_____	_____
After delivery:			
Prolonged holding of baby	_____	_____	_____
Warm-water bath for baby	_____	_____	_____
Breastfeeding in birthing area	_____	_____	_____
Postpartum:			
Private room	_____	_____	_____
Baby rooming in with mother	_____	_____	_____
Breastfeeding	_____	_____	_____
Bottle-feeding	_____	_____	_____
Length of stay in facility	_____	_____	_____
Sibling/family visitation	_____	_____	_____
Postpartum depression concerns	_____	_____	_____

Decisions on places of birth, birthing positions, pain relief, and breastfeeding can be made based on this checklist.

After completing the assessment, women should discuss their issues of concern with their partner and their healthcare provider.

In many areas, women can decide what type of healthcare provider they want for the birth of their baby. High-risk mothers or mothers with high-risk infants have fewer options because they may require specialists who are familiar with their particular conditions. The preferences of the mother and her partner are important considerations for making many childbirth decisions.

Self-Assessment 6.1 provides a checklist for childbirth considerations. The list can serve as a basis for further questions and decision making between a woman and her childbirth healthcare providers.

Labor and Delivery

Labor and delivery can be rewarding and satisfying when a woman anticipates the sequence of events and is prepared for the process. Long before actual labor begins, the uterus changes to prepare itself to function efficiently

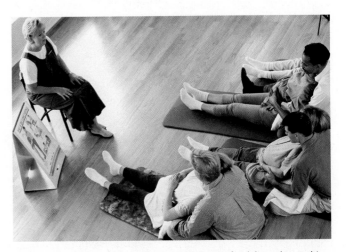

Childbirth education classes help a couple prepare for delivery by teaching relaxation and pain management techniques. The classes also provide the opportunity for the couples to discuss their concerns and excitement.
© Purestock/Getty Images

during labor and delivery. By the end of the pregnancy, the uterus measures about 10 to 14 inches. Its capacity has increased nearly 500 times during the pregnancy, and it increases in weight from 1.5 ounces to 30 ounces. The uterine muscle fibers grow to 10 times their original thickness. The uterus is one of the strongest muscles in a woman's body, and it contracts powerfully during labor. Throughout pregnancy, the uterus contracts at slightly irregular intervals. These irregular contractions, known as Braxton–Hicks contractions, differ from "real" labor contractions in that they do not gradually increase in frequency, intensity, or duration. Instead, they serve to increase the blood circulation and help the uterus to accommodate the growing baby.

Three distinctive signs indicate that labor is beginning:

■ Regular, progressive uterine contractions that occur every 5 minutes or so and last from 45 seconds to 1 minute. The contractions gradually become longer, stronger, and closer together.

■ Rupture of the membranes, or "bag of waters." This rupture may be a slow leak or a gush. The fluid is usually clear.

■ The "bloody show." It involves the passage of a small amount of bloodstained mucus, which serves as a plug in the cervix to protect the fetus from infection. As the cervix begins to dilate, this plug is released.

Other less distinctive signs of approaching labor include diarrhea, backache, and an increase in Braxton–Hicks contractions. The only confirmation that labor has begun is a pelvic examination that reveals a softening, thinned-out, and dilating cervix.

Many factors affect the progress of labor, including the position of the baby and the shape of the mother's pelvis. Although all experiences are different, each labor progresses through three distinct stages (**Figure 6.6**).

Stage I is from the onset of labor to full dilation of the cervix. The cervical canal shortens until the cervix is as thick as the uterine wall. This process, in which the cervix is "taken up" into the uterus, is known as **effacement**. Once the cervix is effaced, the force of the uterine contractions begins to dilate the cervix, although effacement and dilation may occur simultaneously. Dilation refers to the size of the round opening of the cervix. It is measured in centimeters or finger widths. Full dilation is 10 cm or 5 finger widths (**Figure 6.7**).

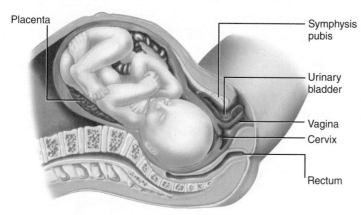

(A) Early first-stage labor

Placenta — Symphysis pubis — Urinary bladder — Vagina — Cervix — Rectum

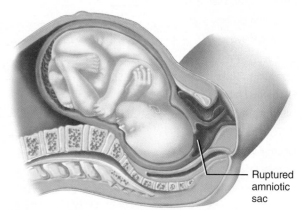

(B) Later first-stage labor: the transition

Ruptured amniotic sac

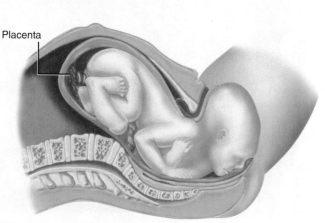

(C) Early second-stage labor

Placenta

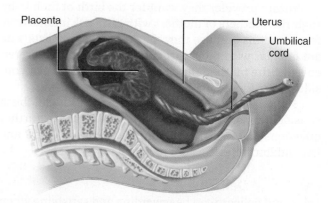

(D) Third-stage labor: delivery of afterbirth

Placenta — Uterus — Umbilical cord

Figure 6.6   Labor and delivery. Stage I: the cervix becomes fully dilated; stage II: the infant is born; stage III: the afterbirth is delivered.

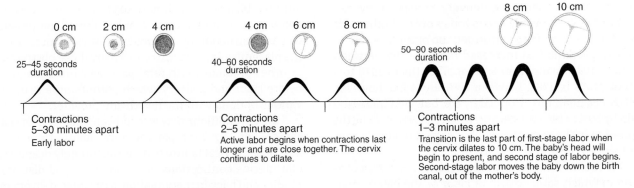

Figure 6.7   **Dilation through stages of labor.**

Stage II of labor begins when the cervix is completely dilated and ends with the birth of the baby. The presentation of the baby—the part of the body positioned to emerge first—is usually the top of the head, known as a vertex presentation. When the feet or buttocks present first, it is known as a **breech** presentation. The breech position occurs in about 3% of deliveries and usually results in a longer labor. Because a breech delivery presents greater risks to the mother and baby, a cesarean delivery is often performed.

As the baby's head appears, or crowns, an episiotomy may be performed. An episiotomy is an incision in the perineum that enlarges the vaginal opening for birth. The traditional argument for performing this procedure is that a surgical incision heals better and faster than a jagged tear. Once routine with vaginal deliveries, the practice of episiotomies has been seriously questioned as to its necessity and benefits for all pregnancies. Recent studies show that episiotomies were linked with more pain, more difficulty healing, and a longer wait for resuming sex after childbirth, with no obvious benefits for most women. Only women requiring a quick delivery for babies in distress should receive an episiotomy. Rate of episiotomies decreased from 29% of vaginal births in 1997 to 12% in 2008.[35]

Stage III lasts from the completion of delivery of the baby to completion of delivery of the **afterbirth**, or placenta. In this final stage of labor, the uterus contracts firmly after the delivery of the baby. The placenta separates from the uterine wall and is expelled. If an episiotomy has been performed, it is sutured at this time.

Pain Relief in Childbirth

Women experience different levels of pain during childbirth. The reality of childbirth is that it usually involves some physical hurt. The physical and psychological techniques promoted in childbirth preparation classes can dramatically influence the perception of pain and the confidence in dealing with labor difficulties. These pain relief measures have the inherent advantage of not producing any chemical disruption in the mother's body, which could then affect the baby or the birthing process.

Good labor support helps a woman throughout labor. Physical and emotional comfort, information, guidance, and communication with the healthcare staff are invaluable to the laboring woman and can greatly reduce her anxiety and need for pharmacological interventions. Non-drug options include:

- *Comfort measures:* These are things that a woman can do for herself, that her companion can do for her, or that can be done to the laboring environment to increase her personal comfort level.

- *Mental strategies:* Many women employ a variety of techniques, including special breathing, meditation, prayer, music, focal points, and singing to reduce anxiety and create a sense of calm during labor.

- *Medications:* A variety of pain-relieving medications are available for childbirth. Most decisions about medications are actually personal choices, not medical decisions. For this reason, it is important for the pregnant woman to learn about possible medications before she goes into labor. Tranquilizers and analgesics are often used together for general relaxation and to take the edge off contractions.

Anesthetics used during labor and delivery may be given in different forms. **Epidural anesthesia** is the most popular choice among pregnant women, and it allows the mother to be awake during the delivery. The anesthetic is injected through a catheter that is placed in a space adjacent to the spinal cord. Spinal anesthesia is injected directly into the spinal canal. Like the epidural, it prevents a woman from being able to move around in labor and often inhibits a woman from pushing. Pudendal anesthesia is injected into the area around the vagina and perineum. This method is least likely to affect the baby.

Cesarean Delivery

A **cesarean delivery** (also known as a cesarean section) is the birth of a baby through surgical incisions made in both the wall of the mother's abdomen and her uterus. Anesthesia is required for the procedure. Clearly, a cesarean birth is sometimes necessary for the safety of the mother or the baby—for example, when there are problems with the baby, problems with the woman's passage area, or problems with the delivery process. However, considerable controversy exists today over whether this type of delivery is being performed too often. The rate of cesarean sections had increased dramatically between 1970 and 1988, rising from 5.5% of all births in 1970 to a high of 24.7% in 1988. Between 1991 and 1996, however, the U.S. cesarean rate dropped by 8%, but then increased again by 50% between 1996 and 2009 to 32.9% of all births (**Figure 6.8**).[36] The cesarean rate has stayed relatively constant since 2009 and was 32.8% in 2012.[35]

One cause for cesarean section is **fetal distress**, a condition in which some aspect of labor or the baby's environment places the baby at risk. For example, the baby's oxygen supply might be cut off owing to **abruptio placentae**, in which the placenta separates prematurely from the wall of the uterus. This event threatens not only the baby but also the mother with a risk of hemorrhage. A **prolapsed cord** is another risky situation in which the umbilical cord comes through the pelvis before the baby and can disrupt the flow of oxygen to the baby due to a compressed cord.

Problems with the birth passage also influence the decision for a cesarean delivery. **Cephalopelvic disproportion**, in which the baby is too large for the pelvis, is a common reason for choosing this type of delivery. A woman in labor whose baby is in a transverse lie, a crosswise position in the uterus, will need a cesarean delivery because neither the head nor the buttocks are in the pelvis. When a baby is in a breech position, the buttocks emerge before the head. The head has a larger diameter than the buttocks, and the risk is that it will not fit well through the passage because it has not had the opportunity to mold and nestle into the pelvis throughout the labor process.

Multiple births are also more likely to require cesarean delivery. A relatively rare complication of the passageway is obstruction by a fibroid, a benign tumor, or even the placenta (**placenta previa**). Usually these obstructions or other problems with fetal passage can be diagnosed before labor and delivery, which permits time to discuss various options with the healthcare provider.

Other conditions may also indicate the need for cesarean delivery. For example, the term "failure to progress" describes cervical failure to dilate adequately despite regular uterine contractions. To avoid prolonged distress to mother and baby in this situation, a cesarean delivery may be performed. Herpes is another reason for a cesarean delivery: If a woman has active lesions in the birth canal, a cesarean delivery is indicated to avoid infecting the baby.

Vaginal Birth After Cesarean Delivery

For many years, a widely held philosophy about childbirth was "once a cesarean, always a cesarean." This philosophy may be partially responsible for the overall increase in cesarean birth rates in the United States during recent years. National data indicate a steady decline in cesarean sections through 1996, owing in part to the movement encouraging vaginal birth after cesarean delivery (VBAC). By the late 1990s, however, studies revealed that some women should not attempt VBAC for fear of uterine rupture or the need for an emergency cesarean section. Many smaller hospitals stopped offering VBAC out of medical liability concerns.[37]

The American College of Obstetricians and Gynecologists (ACOG), as well as many hospital boards, have taken a strong position on VBAC to help control the morbidity associated with major abdominal surgical procedures and to

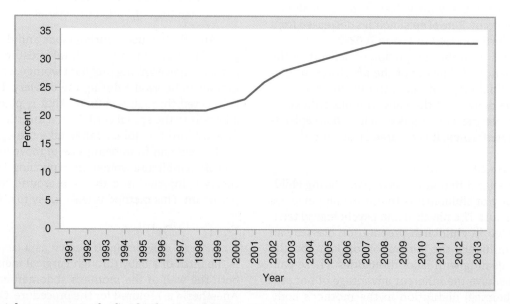

Figure 6.8 Total cesarean rates for first births: United States, 1991–2013.

Data from Menacker, F., & Hamilton, B. E. (2010). *Recent trends in cesarean delivery in the United States. National Center for Health Statistics,* no. 35. Available at: http://www.cdc.gov/nchs/data/databriefs/db35.pdf; Martin, J. A., Hamilton, B. E., Osterman, M. J. K., et al. (2015). *Births: Final data for 2013. National Vital Statistics Report,* 64(1). Available at: http://www.cdc.gov/nchs/data/nvsr/nvsr64/nvsr64_01.pdf

help reduce the spiraling costs of health care. A trial of labor is recommended for most women who underwent a previous cesarean section and have no unusual circumstances or conditions. ACOG has found that the mother usually experiences fewer complications with VBAC than with cesarean birth in terms of infection, bleeding, and anesthesia. Other advantages of VBAC include a shorter hospital stay and recovery period as well as significant cost savings. Women giving birth in hospitals that are not equipped for emergency cesarean sections and women with certain medical contraindications should not undergo VBAC.[37]

BREASTFEEDING

Physiological Changes of the Breast

During pregnancy, hormones prepare the breasts for lactation (milk production). The breasts enlarge as the cells that produce milk increase in number and the ducts that carry milk develop (**Figure 6.9**). The nipple and areola become more elastic and are protected by a natural

lubricant secreted from tiny glands under the skin. After delivery, levels of estrogen and progesterone in the body rapidly decrease, triggering the production of milk. Two hormones are released in response to a baby's suckling:

- *Prolactin*, which stimulates lactation.

- *Oxytocin*, which is responsible for the transportation of milk from the producing cells to the milk ducts to the nipple.

The composition of breast milk varies depending on the stage of lactation, the stage of feeding, and the mother's diet. Early milk, or milk produced during the pregnancy and for 3 to 5 days after birth, is called **colostrum**. Colostrum is yellowish in color, thicker than milk, and rich with protective antibodies and protein. Transitional milk leads to regular mature milk after about 10 days. During feedings, low-fat, thirst-quenching milk is released first, followed by higher-fat, more nourishing milk. The milk's vitamin content is representative of the mother's vitamin intake.

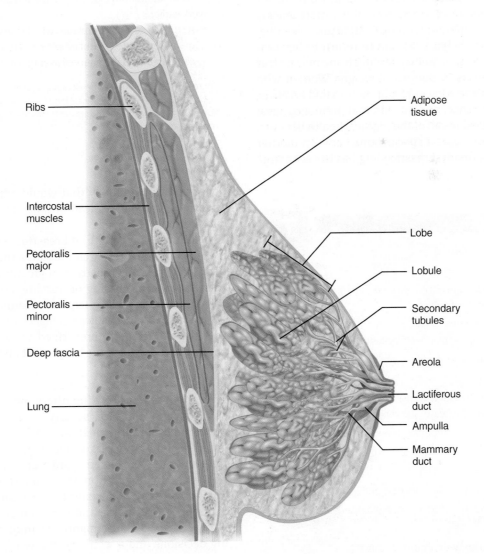

Figure 6.9   **The female breast.**

Benefits of Breastfeeding

Breastfeeding provides many benefits, including protection against many acute and chronic diseases as well as advantages for general health, growth, and development (see **It's Your Health**). Breast milk is highly nutritious, providing all of the nutrients that a growing baby needs. It is ideal as a baby's sole source of nutrients for the first 6 months of life. In addition, breast milk contains enzymes to aid the infant's digestion as well as antibodies to protect against infection. Evidence has shown that breastfed infants have fewer and less severe episodes of diarrhea; fewer cases of upper respiratory, ear, and even urinary infections; and fewer hospitalizations and doctor's visits. Studies also show the possibilities of breast milk protecting against type 1 diabetes mellitus (childhood-onset diabetes), celiac disease, SIDS, obesity, and childhood cancers (such as lymphoma and leukemia).[38] Studies have conflicting results on whether prolonged and exclusive breastfeeding improve children's cognitive development.[39,40]

New mothers may also reap benefits from breastfeeding. Due to the increased levels of oxytocin from breastfeeding, the uterus returns to its normal size more quickly and the woman experiences less postpartum bleeding. Breastfeeding also helps a woman to return to her pre-pregnancy weight more quickly, although she may be less likely to lose her last 5 pounds of weight. Women who breastfeed may have a lower risk of rheumatoid arthritis, cardiovascular disease, and ovarian and premenopausal breast cancer.[40] Besides all of the physical health benefits, breastfeeding can create a special bond between mother and infant. Additionally, breastfeeding has the economic

Table 6.5   Economic Benefits of Breastfeeding
■ One study found that the United States could save $13 million per year if 90% of mothers exclusively breastfeed their infants for 6 months.
■ Bottom line benefits noted by CIGNA Insurance Company and Mutual of Omaha, respectively, include: ○ Annual savings of $240,000 in healthcare expenses among women who breastfed their infants   ○ Savings of $2,146 per employee in healthcare costs   ○ Annual savings of $115,881 for mothers who participate in the company's lactation program
■ Companies also show lower absenteeism rates at work; 1-day absences due to illness occur twice as often among parents whose infants are not breastfed.   ○ Per year, $60,000 has been saved in lower absenteeism rates among women whose babies were breastfed, according to CIGNA Insurance Company.
■ Women who receive support for breastfeeding at work (e.g., dedicated rooms for pumping/expressing milk) are more productive and loyal to the company. They are also more likely to return from maternity leave and often come back to work earlier.   ○ A study of several companies with lactation support programs retained 92.4% of employees after maternity leave, compared with the national average of 59%.

Source: Health Resources and Services Administration's Maternal and Child Health Bureau. (2015). *The business case for breastfeeding support.* Available at: http://www.womenshealth.gov/breastfeeding/employer-solutions/business-case.html

benefit of saving money that would otherwise be spent on formula and the medical conditions that breastfeeding can prevent (**Table 6.5**).

Although any length of breastfeeding is better than no breastfeeding, research indicates that exclusive and prolonged breastfeeding have a greater protective effect than short-term nursing or nursing along with supplemental formula feeding. Experts recommend that mothers breastfeed their babies exclusively for 6 months, and that they continue to breastfeed while supplementing with solid foods until the baby's first birthday.

Optimizing Breastfeeding

Even though breastfeeding offers many advantages for children and mothers, society, and the environment, nursing mothers still must face social and cultural barriers. Education is a primary challenge, especially for first-time mothers, who benefit from prenatal and postpartum breastfeeding instruction and support. Breastfeeding is not always easy, especially for first-time mothers, but experienced guidance and care can solve problems in many cases. Worksite support also influences breastfeeding decisions and a woman's ability to continue breastfeeding upon returning to work.

It's Your Health

Benefits of Breastfeeding

Infant's Benefits

- Fewer episodes and decreased severity of diarrhea and gastrointestinal difficulties
- Decreased incidence of ear infections, urinary tract infections, and upper respiratory infections
- Fewer hospitalizations and visits to the doctor's office
- Fewer food allergies
- Possible protection against diabetes, celiac disease, SIDS, chronic digestive disease, and childhood cancers
- Possible benefits of cognitive development

Mother's Benefits

- Less postpartum bleeding
- Faster return to pre-pregnancy weight
- Possible decreased incidence of ovarian and breast cancers

Benefits for Both

- Special bond between mother and infant

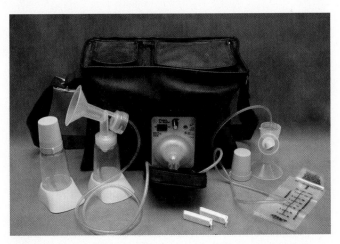

Breast pumps are useful to mothers who work or who have difficulty breastfeeding.

Complications of Breastfeeding

Breastfeeding is not always the best option for some infants. Women who are infected with HIV; have untreated active tuberculosis; are users of alcohol, tobacco, or other recreational drugs; are undergoing cancer chemotherapy or radiation treatment; or are using certain necessary medications that may not be healthy for the developing infant should not breastfeed. Infants with **galactosemia** (an inherited disease caused by a lack of enzyme for processing galactose that can lead to organ enlargement, cataracts, and mental retardation) should not be breastfed.

Women may experience difficulties with feeding, including the following problems:

- Inverted or flat nipples
- Raw or cracked nipples
- Severely swollen breasts
- Problems with the infant latching on
- Pain during latch-on

These problems often can be resolved by changing positions, massaging the breasts, or using a nipple shield to protect the breast. Other complications may require medical attention, such as **mastitis** (bacterial infection of the breast) or **thrush** (yeast infection that affects the mouth of the baby). Women should talk to their healthcare provider or a nursing lactation specialist if they experience problems with breastfeeding.

Diet, Drugs, and Alcohol During Breastfeeding

Women who choose to breastfeed should consume a healthy diet to ensure adequate intake of the necessary vitamins and minerals. Caloric intake should be increased by 500 calories per day relative to a woman's pre-pregnancy diet. Women should maintain a sufficient calcium intake (1000 mg per day) to rule out any possibility of long-term effects of breastfeeding on the mother's bone density. Note that any substance taken in by the mother can be passed to the infant through the breast milk, including harmful substances such as caffeine, alcohol, and certain drugs. For this reason, breastfeeding women should consult their healthcare providers before taking any medications.

INFERTILITY

Fecundity refers to a woman's physical ability to have a child. Women with impaired fecundity include those who find it physically difficult or medically inadvisable to conceive or deliver a child. The term *impaired fecundity* is also used to describe women who, although having sexual intercourse on a regular basis without contraception for 36 months or more, fail to become pregnant. This definition of reduced ability to bear children differs from the medical definition of infertility, which is the inability of couples who are not surgically sterile to conceive after 12 months of regular intercourse without contraception.

Causes

Fertility-related difficulties can arise at many points, including the process of ovulation in women, sperm production in men, or the maintenance of the embryo after fertilization has taken place.

- In 25 to 35% of couples, the fertility problem is in the male.
- In 25 to 35% of couples, the fertility problem is in the female.
- For the remaining couples, infertility is a result of both a male and a female factor or unknown causes.

It's Your Health

Pregnancy requires the following:

- A woman must effectively release an egg from one of her ovaries. This is known as ovulation.
- The egg must effectively travel from the ovary through the fallopian tube toward the uterus.
- A man's sperm must join with the egg—fertilization—en route to the uterus.
- The fertilized egg must effectively attach to the lining of the uterus, known as implantation. Infertility can result from problems that arise from any of these requirements.

Many factors contribute to infertility. Problems with ovulation are responsible for most cases in women. Without ovulation, eggs are not present for fertilization. Symptoms that might indicate a woman is not ovulating include irregular or absent menstrual periods. Age and other factors can affect a woman's ability to conceive. Because more women are delaying childbirth until their 30s and 40s, age is becoming a more common infertility consideration. Other possible causes of infertility or factors that increase risk of infertility include:

- Blocked or scarred fallopian tubes due to PID, endometriosis, or previous surgery for an ectopic pregnancy
- Physical or anatomical problems with a woman's uterus
- Uterine fibroids
- Poor diet
- Smoking or alcohol
- Sexually transmitted infections (STIs)
- Health problems that cause hormonal changes
- Depression and stress, which can have a direct effect on hormonal regulation and ovulation

Weight is another important factor in infertility. Women who are overweight or obese often have irregular or infrequent menstrual cycles and are at increased risk of infertility. Underweight women also have infertility issues due to low body fat levels.

Diagnosis

Various tests can often determine the cause of infertility and thus the appropriate treatment method. Tests can be used to confirm if and when a woman ovulates, as well as evaluate ovarian function and uterine receptivity to implantation. A simple method of determining whether ovulation is occurring, for example, is to monitor a woman's basal body temperature to see whether a slight increase in her temperature occurs midway through her menstrual cycle.

Tests can also examine the quality of the mucus. The ferning test involves collecting mucus near the time of ovulation to see whether, when smeared, it resembles the fronds of a fern. If so, the woman's estrogen levels are normal, and the mucus is creating a desirable environment for the sperm to travel.

A postcoital test may also be performed before ovulation. Mucus is collected within 6 hours after intercourse and is viewed under a microscope to see whether it contains multiple, active sperm.

Other tests used to diagnose infertility include the following:

- Blood tests for measuring hormone levels
- Radiograph studies, such as a hysterosalpingogram, which outlines obstructions or abnormal growths in the uterus or fallopian tubes
- Transvaginal ultrasound to check the uterus and ovaries for abnormalities
- Laparoscopic surgery to view the uterus, fallopian tubes, and ovaries

A common test used to diagnose male infertility is semen analysis. Semen is evaluated for the number of sperm present, the volume of ejaculate, the motility of the sperm, and the size and shape of the sperm. If a man has a low sperm count, blood tests may be performed to measure various hormones and proteins. A physical examination and an ultrasound of the scrotum also may be performed to detect varicose veins that may need repair.

For a couple dealing with infertility, finding the cause can be a long, complicated, and trying process. It can take months, and for couples without health insurance that covers therapy, the process can be quite expensive.

Treatment

A variety of treatment approaches can be employed depending on the cause of the infertility. The most basic form of treatment relies on a change in sexual activity.

GENDER DIMENSIONS: Health Differences Between Men and Women

Male Infertility

Problems with male fertility contribute to about one-third of cases of infertility. Many of the same factors that reduce fertility in women also affect male fertility. In most cases, producing too few sperm (oligospermia) or none at all (azoospermia) causes male infertility. Other sperm production problems include issues with sperm motility, such as abnormal structure that prevents sperm from moving correctly, or sperm's inability to fertilize the egg, oftentimes caused by abnormal sperm shape. Other factors that can play a role in infertility include:

- Paternal age
- Health problems, including sexually transmitted infections (STIs) and various medical treatments, such as chemotherapy and radiation therapy.

- Emotional factors, such as high levels of stress.
- Alcohol or drugs, smoking, and anabolic steroids. For example, studies have shown that smokers' sperm are less likely to bind tightly to an egg—a necessary step for fertilization.
- Environmental factors, such as prolonged exposure to high temperatures, radiation, or heavy electromagnetic or microwave emissions, which can decrease sperm count or affect the viability of the sperm.

By using a basal body temperature chart, for example, women can monitor their temperature changes and better determine their exact time of ovulation. About 85 to 90% of infertility cases are treated with drug therapy or surgical repair of reproductive organs. Medical approaches to infertility may involve hormones to treat cervical mucus problems or difficulties in ovulation, while ultrasound is used to monitor the response of the ovaries during treatment.

- To stimulate ovulation, a medication called clomiphene citrate (trade names Clomid and Serophene) is often prescribed. It stimulates the release of luteinizing hormone and causes an increase in estradiol, thereby triggering ovulation.

- Gonadotropin-releasing hormone (GnRH) may be administered to improve a woman's response to ovulation stimulants.

- Follicle-stimulating hormone (FSH) stimulates egg follicles in the ovaries.

- Human chorionic gonadotropin (hCG) works with clomiphene citrate to help stimulate the follicle to release its egg.

Microsurgery is a useful technique for male and female problems that require surgical intervention. Using a laparoscope, doctors can open blockages in a woman's fallopian tubes or correct structural abnormalities of the uterus or ovary. Surgery may also be used in males to open blocked sperm ducts or to repair a **varicocele** (a mesh of varicose veins in and around the testicle), which is often associated with infertility.

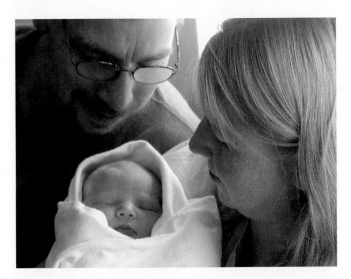

Many couples who have had trouble conceiving use assisted reproductive technologies to assist them in getting pregnant.
© Alan Heartfield/Shutterstock

Other techniques that have shown success to date include artificial insemination and **assisted reproductive technologies (ARTs)**. **Artificial insemination** is the process of implanting sperm from a donor into a woman near the time of her ovulation. Sperm donors are screened for HIV infection and various genetic disorders, as well as categorized by certain features to create as optimal a match as possible between the woman and the donor. Artificial insemination is often used when the infertility problem is based on a male factor.

Any treatment or procedure that involves the handling of human eggs and sperm for the purpose of helping a woman become pregnant qualifies as a type of ART. All ART procedures involve stimulating the ovary to produce eggs, harvesting the eggs with a microscopic needle, and then removing the eggs from the woman's body. The CDC estimates that ART accounts for slightly more than 1% of total U.S. births. More than 66,000 infants were born as a result of ART cycles performed in 2013.[41] ART methods are listed here:

- **In vitro fertilization (IVF)** involves removing the ova from a woman's ovary just before normal ovulation would occur. The woman's egg and her partner's sperm are placed in a special fertilization medium for a specific period of time and are then transferred to another medium for continued development. If the fertilized egg cell shows signs of development, it is returned to the woman's uterus within several days by means of a hollow tube placed through the vagina and cervix. The egg cell implants itself in the lining of the uterus, and the pregnancy continues as normal. IVF is the most effective and most common form of ART.

- **Gamete intrafallopian transfer (GIFT)** involves placing sperm and eggs into the fallopian tubes. This procedure is less time-consuming and less expensive than IVF. GIFT mimics nature by permitting fertilized eggs to divide in the fallopian tubes. It has a success rate similar to that seen with IVF but is more invasive than IVF.

- **Zygote intrafallopian transfer (ZIFT)** is a similar process that involves adding the fertilized egg to the fallopian tube at an earlier point than GIFT.

- **Intracytoplasmic sperm injection (ICSI)** involves injecting sperm directly into the egg with a microscopic needle. ICSI is often used for couples with male factor infertility.

- **Egg donation** is used when a woman is unable to produce eggs or she has a genetic disorder that will be passed on to the child. Egg donors must be willing to dedicate an enormous amount of time to this process because of the amount of drug treatment and monitoring that they must undergo. It is not a simple procedure for either the donor or the recipient of the egg.

- **Embryo transfer** is a procedure in which the sperm of the infertile woman's partner is placed in another woman's uterus during ovulation. Approximately

5 days later, the fertilized egg is transferred to the uterus of the infertile woman, who then carries the developing embryo.

■ **Host uterus** is a procedure in which the sperm from a man and the egg from a woman are combined in a laboratory. The fertilized egg is then implanted into the uterus of a second woman, referred to as a gestational carrier, who agrees to bear the child, which is not genetically related to her.

■ **Surrogacy** is an option for women with no eggs or unhealthy eggs. A woman, the surrogate, agrees to be artificially inseminated with the sperm of an infertile woman's partner and become pregnant using the man's sperm and her own egg. She carries the baby to term, usually for an established fee and the provision of her health care. After delivery, the baby is turned over to the couple.

Each of these procedures, while offering hope to infertile couples, can raise ethical and legal questions.

Emotional Effects of Infertility

Infertility and the procedures used to treat it are extremely stressful for most couples. In some cases, women who undergo the often arduous tests experience anger and resentment toward their partners, especially if their partners do not provide adequate support and share in their experiences. If the cause of infertility is determined, the man or woman who is experiencing the medical problem may feel guilty and blame himself or herself for failing to become pregnant. The experience of becoming pregnant and miscarrying can also lead to excitement and anticipation followed by depression and frustration. Once involved in testing, couples may become hopeful again but hesitant. The mix of emotions often leads to confusion and miscommunication between the couple.

As a couple prepares to undergo an ART procedure such as IVF, more grief may be experienced. In addition to fearing that it is the last option available, couples must shoulder the exorbitant costs of infertility treatment and face the possibility that it may be unsuccessful. Women who fail to become pregnant following any type of fertility therapy experience grief and depression before, during, and after treatment. Women may feel despair, anger, and a loss of control as their hopes of becoming pregnant fade. Effective coping behaviors and a strong network of family and friends appear to reduce a couple's emotional stress. If treatment fails, some couples accept happiness without

We had been trying to have a baby for several years. It was so frustrating because all of our friends were having babies. We felt so many things—guilt, embarrassment, fear, and anger. Finally, after a lot of testing, we tried IVF and it worked! We have a little girl. It was a long and difficult journey to have her, but we are so pleased.

—35-year-old woman

having children in their lives, whereas other couples may opt for adoption.

EPIDEMIOLOGY

Traditional epidemiological data on pregnancy and childbirth have focused on issues of maternal and child morbidity and mortality. In recent years, an expanded focus has provided insight into other important considerations of pregnancy, childbirth, breastfeeding, and infertility.

Pregnancy

In 2012, nearly 4 million births were recorded in the United States. The average age at first birth was 26 years and 40.6% of births were to unmarried women. Teenage birth rates fell to a new record low, continuing a decline that began in 1991. The rate dropped 44% from 1991 to 2010. Although rates have declined in all racial and ethnic groups, teen birth rates are still highest for Hispanic teenagers and non-Hispanic Black teenagers. **Figure 6.10** shows the decrease in birth rates for teenagers from 1960 to 2014.[26]

Pregnancy and childbirth are safe experiences for many women; however, any medical or obstetric complication is one too many. In the early 1900s, 1 in 150 women

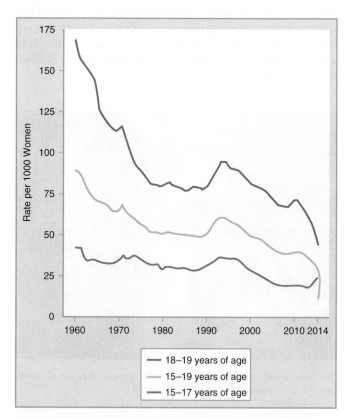

Figure 6.10 Birth rates for teenagers aged 15–19 years.

Data from Martin, J. A., Hamilton, B. E., Osterman, M. J. K., et al. (2015). Births: Final data for 2014. *National Vital Statistics Reports* 64(1). Hyattsville, MD: National Center for Health Statistics.

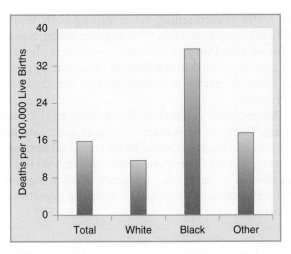

Figure 6.11 **Pregnancy-related mortality ratios, by race: United States, 2006–2009.**

Data from Centers for Disease Control and Prevention. National Center for Chronic Disease Prevention and Health Promotion, Pregnancy Mortality Surveillance System. Available at: http://mchb.hrsa.gov/chusa13/perinatal-health -status-indicators/p/pregnancy-related-mortality.html

died from causes related to pregnancy, with the death rate among women of color being nearly double that of White women.[42] These deaths were typically caused by infection, toxemia, abortion, and hemorrhage. Today, leading causes of pregnancy-related deaths include cardiovascular disease, hemorrhage, and pregnancy-related hypertension. In 1900, there were approximately 850 maternal deaths per 100,000 live births in the United States. In 2006 to 2009, there were 15.8 maternal deaths per 100,000 live births. Although this reduction in maternal mortality is

impressive, women of color are still three times more likely than White women to die of pregnancy-related causes, and the risk for Black women is the highest among all racial groups (**Figure 6.11**).[43]

The **infant mortality rate** (also called the infant death rate) is the number of children dying under a year of age divided by the number of live births that year. This rate is an important measure of the well-being of infants, children, and pregnant women because it is associated with factors such as maternal health, quality of and access to medical care, socioeconomic conditions, and public health practices. In 2010, the U.S. infant mortality rate was 6.14 infant deaths per 1000 live births.[44] As **Figure 6.12** shows, the rates range from 4.27 deaths per 1000 live births for Asian or Pacific Islander mothers to 11.46 for non-Hispanic Black mothers. Infant mortality rates for multiple births (i.e., twins, triplets, and higher-order births) were almost five times the rates for singleton births. Because of their much greater risk of death, infants born at the lowest birth weights and gestational ages have a large impact on overall U.S. infant mortality. Two-thirds of all infant

> *I cannot remember much about the birth of my first baby. I was young and scared, and I only wanted to be "knocked out." Afterwards, I realized that I had missed one of the most important events of my life. With my second baby, we went to classes and I read everything I could. I really was prepared. I felt so much more in control of what was happening to me. Birth is something too wonderful to miss.*
>
> **—30-year-old woman**

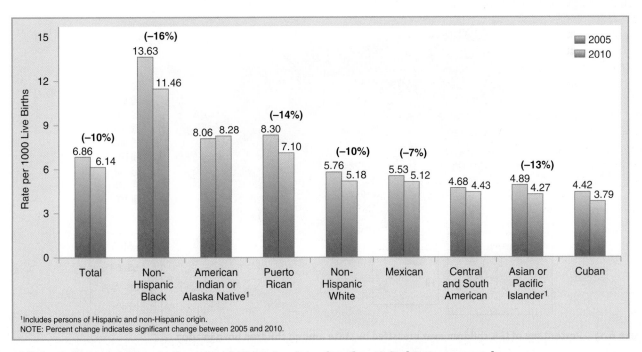

Figure 6.12 **Infant mortality rates by race and Hispanic origin of mother: United States, 2005 and 2010.**

Data from Mathews, T. J., & MacDorman, M. F. (2013). Centers for Disease Control and Prevention. Infant mortality statistics from the 2010 period linked birth/infant death data set. *National Vital Statistics Reports* 62(8).

deaths occurred in the 12% of infants who were born pre-term. Congenital malformations, low birth weight, and sudden infant death syndrome (SIDS) accounted for 46% of the infant deaths.

Breastfeeding

Breastfeeding rates in the United States have increased since 1999; however, only 17 states have achieved the Healthy People 2020 goal of 82% of new mothers initiating breastfeeding in 2011. Rates of exclusive breastfeeding at 3 and 6 months and breastfeeding at 6 and 12 months are getting closer to their 2020 targets. Among children born in 2011, 79% initiated breastfeeding, 49% were breastfeeding at 6 months (target is 61%), and 27% were breastfeeding at 12 months of age (target is 34%). Only 41% were exclusively breastfeeding at 3 months (target is 46%) and 19% were exclusively breastfeeding at 6 months (target is 25%) (see **Figure 6.13**).[45]

Worksite support for working nursing mothers is an important challenge for many women. In one national study, the availability of employer-sponsored childcare was found to increase the likelihood of breastfeeding 6 months after birth by 47%. In addition, on average, working an additional 8 hours at home per week increased the probability of breastfeeding initiation by 8% and breastfeeding 6 months after birth by 16.8%.[46]

Studies on breastfeeding in the United States have historically shown substantial racial/ethnic and socioeconomic disparities. In a national study, immigrant women in each racial/ethnic group had higher breastfeeding initiation and longer duration rates than native women of the same racial/ethnic group. Acculturation was associated with lower breastfeeding rates among both Hispanic and non-Hispanic women.[47] In another study, researchers found that immigration status was strongly associated with increased breastfeeding initiation, suggesting that cultural factors are important in the decision to breastfeed.[48]

Geographical variance is also a factor in U.S. breastfeeding. There are wide state variations in breastfeeding initiation and duration, with the western and northwestern states having the highest rates.[49] Additional research is needed to ascertain the influence of state legislation and local programs designed to promote breastfeeding practices.

Fertility

Technically, fertility simply denotes successful production of offspring. The U.S. Census Bureau collects fertility data and provides reports showing historical trends with childbearing and associated sociodemographic data. Recent fertility data indicate the following trends:[50]

- The average number of children born has dropped from more than 3 children per woman in 1976 to about two children per woman in 2012.

- There have also been recent drops in teen childbirth as well as increases in nonmarital births.

- Women 40 to 50 years old will end their childbearing years with an average of 2 children each, and 16% are childless. Hispanic women will have an average of 2.4 children each, higher than that of non-Hispanic White, Black, or Asian women.

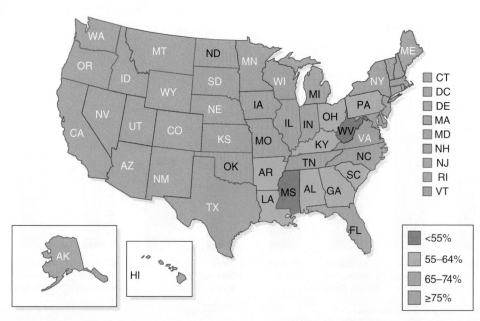

Figure 6.13 **Percentage of U.S. children ever breastfed by state among children born in 2007.**

Reproduced from Centers for Disease Control and Prevention. (2014). Breastfeeding among U.S. children born 2001–2011. *CDC National Immunization Survey.* Available at: http://www.cdc.gov/breastfeeding/data/NIS_data/index.htm

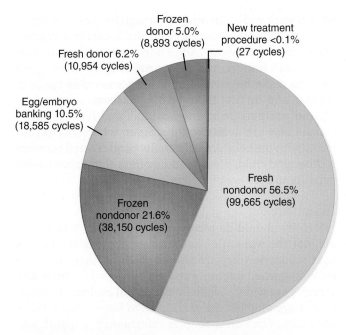

Figure 6.14   Types of ART cycles: United States, 2012.

Reproduced from Centers for Disease Control and Prevention, American Society for Reproductive Medicine, Society for Assisted Reproductive Technology. (2014). *2012 assisted reproductive technology national summary report*. Available at: http://www.cdc.gov/art/reports/index.html

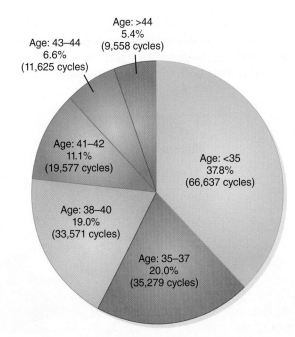

Figure 6.15   ART use by age group: United States, 2012.

Reproduced from Centers for Disease Control and Prevention, American Society for Reproductive Medicine, Society for Assisted Reproductive Technology. (2014). *2012 assisted reproductive technology national summary report*. Available at: http://www.cdc.gov/art/reports/index.html

Infertility

Infertility is usually defined as not being able to get pregnant after trying for 1 year. Among women aged 25 to 44, 17% had ever used infertility services from 2006 to 2010. Infertility services include medical tests to diagnose infertility, medical advice and treatments to help a woman become pregnant, and services other than routine prenatal care to prevent miscarriage. The most commonly used services were advice, testing, medical help to prevent miscarriage, and ovulation drugs.[51] ART is associated with a substantial risk for multiple births. **Figure 6.14** shows the types of ART cycles performed in 2012 and **Figure 6.15** shows ART use by age group.

INFORMED DECISION MAKING

Informed decision making about pregnancy should begin before conception. The newly conceived offspring depends on its mother for nutrition and well-being weeks before the mother may know that she is pregnant. If the mother is a smoker or is abusing alcohol or drugs during this critical early period of development, her child is at a decided disadvantage.

Pregnancy

A pregnant woman has to take good care of herself to provide the best care for her unborn child. Regular prenatal care that begins early in the pregnancy is essential and is associated with reduced infant morbidity and mortality. Most women see their clinician once a month during the pregnancy until week 28. In the last trimester, this frequency increases to every other week until week 36, when weekly visits until delivery are indicated. Proper nutrition; adequate and appropriate exercise; and avoidance of alcohol, tobacco, caffeine, and illegal drugs are all essential components of good prenatal care.

Childbirth

Childbirth is a personal, special, and an irreplaceable event. Preparation for birthing helps to ensure the best possible experience. Childbirth education classes provide many valuable opportunities for learning, practical preparation, and building skills for a rewarding and facilitated childbirth experience. They also provide an opportunity to share concerns and discuss plans. Local resources for childbirth options, such as birthing centers or home deliveries, can be evaluated. Classes provide motivation to learn relaxation and pain management techniques. Strategies that are taught may include breathing techniques, such as **Lamaze**; relaxation techniques; muscle-strengthening exercises; and different positions that facilitate labor, thereby promoting an uncomplicated birth. Resources in childbirth preparation vary. Some communities offer many resources; in other communities, resources are rather few and far between. To maximize the benefits from a childbirth education class, the qualifications of the instructor, class size, and class focus should be carefully evaluated.

Breastfeeding

Breastfeeding can be a very rewarding experience. Women who have difficulty beginning the process are encouraged to "stick with it" as both the mother and the infant learn

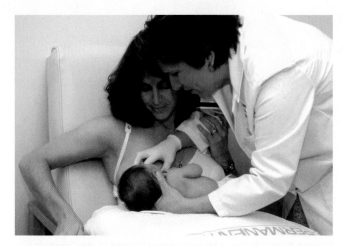

Hospitals and birthing centers often have lactation specialists on staff to help new mothers learn the ropes of breastfeeding.
© Michael Newman/PhotoEdit, Inc.

how to work with each other. Although suckling is instinctual for the infant, feeding from the breast is a learned behavior for the mother. Adjusting positions, anticipating the infant's hunger, and relaxing during the feeding are ways to make breastfeeding more pleasurable for both mother and infant. Breastfeeding assistance is usually offered postpartum at the hospital, and lactation specialists also are available for women when they return home with the baby. Aside from the bond created between mother and child, breastfeeding offers significant health benefits to both parties.

Infertility

Infertility should be recognized as a problem of a couple, not the woman or her partner. Because the factors that reduce fertility are shared, both partners must be evaluated when initiating an infertility workup. Infertility services are widely available today, and evolving technologies have enabled many couples to have a child. Infertility clinics can offer couples information, support, and procedures to address their specific needs. Identification of infertility services is often facilitated through referral from a gynecologist.

Profiles of Remarkable Women

Martha May Eliot, MD (1891–1978)

Martha May Eliot, a pioneer in maternal and child health, graduated from Radcliffe College and the medical school at Johns Hopkins University. She taught at Yale University's Department of Pediatrics until 1935, while also directing the National Children's Bureau Division of Child and Maternal Health. As bureau chief, Eliot conducted community studies, exploring issues of social medicine and ways that public health measures could prevent disease. She also drafted most of the Social Security Act's language dealing with maternal and child health in 1934. During World War II, Eliot provided care for more than 1 million servicemen's wives through the Emergency Maternity and Infant Care program. She continued her involvement with women's and children's health after the war by working with the WHO and the United Nations Children's Fund (UNICEF) in significant capacities.

After leaving her position at the National Children's Bureau, Eliot became department chair of Child and Maternal Health at Harvard University's School of Public Health. She received many honors throughout her lifetime that recognized her work as a leading pediatrician and the force behind many maternal and child health programs. She was one of the first women admitted into the American Pediatric Society, the first woman elected president of the American Public Health Association (APHA), and the first woman to receive APHA's Sedgwick Memorial Medal. APHA now awards the Martha May Eliot Award to recognize others' achievements in maternal and child health.

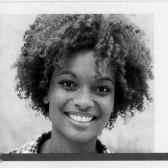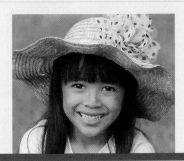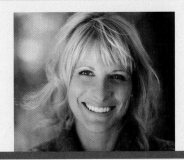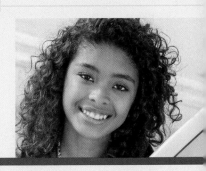

CASE STUDY

Jill, who is 32 years old, is hoping to become pregnant. She has recently stopped using birth control pills and has been having unprotected sex with her partner for the past 3 months.

Questions

1. What are some lifestyle behaviors and medical interventions that Jill may want to consider during this time?

2. What considerations should Jill be thinking about when it comes to preparing for childbirth?

■ Summary

Pregnancy, childbirth, and breastfeeding are exciting, yet complex, dimensions of women's health. Cultural, historical, legal, and ethical factors influence how women deal with pregnancy, give birth, and care for their infants. Understanding the physiological causes for the physical and emotional changes that occur in a pregnant woman can often help make the pregnancy process more manageable. Prenatal care is a vital component of a healthy pregnancy and usually includes nutritional counseling, genetic testing, ultrasounds, and ongoing monitoring of the mother and baby. Many women experience the changes of pregnancy and the birth of their child without complications. Others learn firsthand the emotional hardships of infertility, miscarriage, diagnosis of abnormalities in the fetus, premature delivery, or complications during delivery. For couples who have difficulty conceiving, a host of medical and surgical options exist to achieve a pregnancy; however, these methods are imperfect and often carry a high financial (as well as emotional) cost. As with other areas of women's health, informed decision making is critical throughout the prenatal and postnatal periods.

■ Topics for Discussion

1. What are the possible advantages and disadvantages of treating childbirth as a "medical" condition (i.e., constant medical care led by doctors and healthcare providers, hospitalization, etc.)?

2. Should pregnant women be restricted in their access to tobacco, alcohol, or drugs?

3. What should you do, if anything, if you see a young mother smoking? What if she is drinking or not wearing a seatbelt?

4. Should preparation for childbirth be required for all women?

5. Discuss the rights of pregnant teenagers as parents. What rights do a teen's parents have in regard to her pregnancy?

6. Does the father of the child have any say in pregnancy decisions if the mother and father are not married?

7. What are possible ethical and legal dilemmas associated with infertility techniques and treatments?

■ Key Terms

Abruptio placentae

Afterbirth

Amniocentesis

Amnion

Amniotic fluid

Artificial insemination

Assisted reproductive technologies (ART)

Blastocyst

Braxton–Hicks contractions

Breech

Cephalopelvic disproportion

Cesarean delivery

Chorionic villus sampling (CVS)

Chromosomes

Colostrum

Conceptus

Corpus luteum

Cytomegalovirus (CMV)

Dizygotic twins

Down syndrome

Ectopic pregnancy

Effacement

Egg donation

Embryo

Embryo transfer

Epidural anesthesia

Fecundity

Fertilization

Fetal alcohol syndrome (FAS)

Fetal distress

Fetus

Folate

Folic acid

Forceps

Galactosemia

Gamete intrafallopian transfer (GIFT)

Gestational diabetes

Group B streptococcus (GBS)

Host uterus

Human chorionic gonadatropin (hCG)

Implantation

Infertility

In vitro fertilization (IVF)

Infant mortality rate

Intracytoplasmic sperm injection (ICSI)

Lamaze

Mastitis

Maternal serum alpha-fetoprotein (MSAFP)

Miscarriage

Monozygotic twins

Neural tube defects

Placenta

Placenta previa

Preeclampsia

Premature labor

Rh incompatibility

Rubella

Stillbirth

Surrogacy

Thrush

Toxemia

Ultrasound

Varicocele

Zygote

Zygote intrafallopian transfer (ZIFT)

■ References

1. Bogda, J. C. (1990). Childbirth in America, 1650 to 1990. In R. D. Apple (Ed.), *Women, health, and medicine in America*. New York, NY: Garland Publishers.

2. Wertz, R. W., & Wertz, D. C. (1977). *Lying-in: A history of childbirth in America*. New York, NY: Free Press.

3. Leavitt, J. W. (1986). *Brought to bed: Childbirthing in America, 1750–1950*. New York, NY: Oxford University Press.

4. Hodnett, E. D., Gates, S., Hofmeyr, G., et al. (2013). Continuous support for women during childbirth. *Cochrane Database of Systematic Reviews*. Available at: http://www.cochrane.org/CD003766/PREG_continuous-support-for-women-during-childbirth

5. Mansfield, B. (2008). The social nature of natural childbirth. *Social Science Medicine* 66(5): 1084–1094.

6. Barness, L. A. (1991). Brief history of infant nutrition and view to the future. *Pediatrics* 88: 1054–1056.

7. Ansley, D. (1992). Spermtales. *Discover* 13(6): 66–69.

8. Centers for Disease Control and Prevention (CDC). (2015). Updated estimates of neural tube defects prevented by mandatory folic acid fortification—United States, 1995–2011. *Morbidity and Mortality Weekly Report* 64(1): 1–5.

9. Institute of Medicine (IOM) and National Research Council (NRC). (2009). *Weight gain during pregnancy: Reexamining the guidelines*. Washington, DC: The National Academies Press.

10. American College of Obstetricians and Gynecologists (ACOG). (2011). *Exercise during pregnancy*. Available at: http://www.acog.org/~/media/For%20Patients/faq119.pdf

11. CDC. (2007). *Preventing smoking and exposure to secondhand smoke before, during, and after pregnancy fact sheet*. Available at: http://www.cdc.gov/nccdphp/publications/factsheets/Prevention/pdf/smoking.pdf

12. CDC. (2014). *Smoking and reproduction*. Available at: http://www.cdc.gov/tobacco/data_statistics/sgr/50th-anniversary/pdfs/fs_smoking_reproduction_508.pdf

13. Bailey, B. A., & Sokol, R. J. (2011). Prenatal alcohol exposure and miscarriage, stillbirth, preterm delivery, and sudden infant death syndrome. *Alcohol Research and Health* 34(1): 86–91.

14. CDC. (2012). Alcohol use and binge drinking among women of childbearing age—United States, 2006–2010. *Morbidity and Mortality Weekly Report* 61(28): 534–538.

15. Substance Abuse and Mental Health Services Administration. (2014). *Results from the 2013 National Survey on Drug Use and Health: Summary of national findings*. Rockville, MD: Office of Applied Studies. NSDUH Series H-48, DHHS, Publication No. SMA 14-4863.

16. March of Dimes. (2013). *Street drugs and pregnancy*. Available at: http://www.marchofdimes.com/pregnancy/alcohol_illicitdrug.html

17. ACOG. (2014). *Lead screening during pregnancy and lactation*. Committee Opinion Number 533. Available at: http://www.acog.org/Resources-And-Publications/Committee-Opinions/Committee-on-Obstetric-Practice/Lead-Screening-During-Pregnancy-and-Lactation

18. Froehlich, T. E., Lanphear, B. P., Auinger, P., et al. (2009). Association of tobacco and lead exposures with attention-deficit/hyperactivity disorder. *Pediatrics* 123(60): 1054–1063.

19. Chambers, C. D. (2006). Risks of hyperthermia associated with hot tub or spa use by pregnant women. Birth Defects Research. Part A. *Clinical and Molecular Teratology* 76(8): 569–573.

20. CDC. (2008). Update on overall prevalence of major birth defects—Atlanta, Georgia, 1978–2005. *Morbidity and Mortality Weekly Report* 57:1–5.

21. Akolekar, R., Beta, J., Picciarelli, G., et al. (2015). Procedure-related risk of miscarriage following amniocentesis and chorionic villus

sampling: a systematic review and meta-analysis. *Ultrasound in Obstetrics and Gynecology* 45: 16–26.

22. CDC. (2003). Pregnancy-related mortality surveillance—United States, 1991–1999. *Morbidity and Mortality Weekly Report Surveillance Summary* 52: 1–8.

23. Berg, C. J., Callaghan, W. M., Syverson, C., et al. (2010). Pregnancy-related mortality in the United States, 1998 to 2005. *Obstetrics and Gynecology* 116: 1302–1309.

24. DeSisto, C. L., Kim, S. Y., & Sharma, A. J. (2014). Prevalence estimates of gestational diabetes mellitus in the United States, pregnancy risk assessment monitoring system (PRAMS), 2007–2010. *Preventing Chronic Disease* 11: 130415. doi:http://dx.doi.org/10.5888/pcd11.130415

25. CDC. (2011). *National diabetes fact sheet*. Available at: http://www.cdc.gov/diabetes/library/factsheets.html

26. Martin, J. A., Hamilton, B. E., Osterman, M. H. S., et al. (2015). Births: Final data for 2015. *National Vital Statistics Reports* 64(12): 1-65. 1–64.

27. CDC. (2014). HIV among pregnant women, infants and children. Available at: http://www.cdc.gov/hiv/risk/gender/pregnantwomen/facts/index.html

28. CDC. (2010). Sexually transmitted diseases: Treatment guidelines 2010. Available at: http://www.cdc.gov/std/treatment/2010/specialpops.htm

29. CDC. (2013). Congenital CMV infection trends and statistics. Available at: http://www.cdc.gov/cmv/trends-stats.html

30. CDC. (2014). Group B strep infection in newborns. Available at: http://www.cdc.gov/groupbstrep/about/newborns-pregnant.html

31. Rull, K., Nagirnaja, L., & Laan, M. (2012). Genetics of recurrent miscarriage: Challenges, current knowledge, future directions. *Frontiers in Genetics* 3: 34.

32. Advisory Committee on Heritable Disorders in Newborns and Children. (2015). *Recommended uniform screening panel*. Available at: http://www.hrsa.gov/advisorycommittees/mchbadvisory/heritabledisorders/recommendedpanel/index.html

33. Romano, A. M., & Lothian, J. A. (2008). Promoting, protecting, and supporting normal birth: A look at the evidence. *Obstetric, Gynecologic, and Neonatal Nursing* 37(1): 94–105.

34. Lothian, J. A. (2009). Safe, healthy birth: What every pregnant woman needs to know. *Journal of Perinatal Education* 18(3): 48–54.

35. ACOG. (2014). Safe prevention of the primary cesarean delivery. *Obstetric Care Consensus*. Available at: http://www.acog.org/Resources-And-Publications/Obstetric-Care-Consensus-Series/Safe-Prevention-of-the-Primary-Cesarean-Delivery

36. Podulka, J., Stranges, E., & Steiner, C. (2011). *Hospitalizations related to childbirth, 2008*. HCUP Statistical Brief #110. Available at: http://www.hcup-us.ahrq.gov/reports/statbriefs/sb110.pdf

37. ACOG. (2010). Vaginal birth after previous cesarean section. *ACOG Practice Bulletin* 115.

38. American Academy of Pediatrics. (2012). Policy statement: Breastfeeding and the use of human milk. *Pediatrics* 129(3): e827–e841.

39. Leventakou, V., Roumeliotaki, T., Koutra, K., et al. (2013). Breastfeeding duration and cognitive, language and motor development at 18 months of age: Reah mother-child cohort in Crete, Greece. *Journal of Epidemiology and Community Health* doi:10.1136/jech-2013-202500

40. Sajjad, A., Tharner, A., Kiefte-de Jong, J. C., et al. (2015). Breastfeeding duration and non-verbal IQ in children. *Journal of Epidemiology and Community Health* doi:10.1136/jech-2014-204486

41. CDC, American Society for Reproductive Medicine, Society for Assisted Reproductive Technology. (2014). *2012 assisted reproductive technology national summary report*. Available at: http://www.cdc.gov/art/reports/index.html

42. Rochat, R. W., Koonin, L. M., Atrash, H. K., et al. (1988). Maternal mortality in the United States: Report from the Maternal Mortality Collaborative. *Obstetrics and Gynecology* 72(1): 91–97.

43. U.S. Department of Health and Human Services, Health Resources and Services Administration, Maternal and Child Health Bureau. (2013). *Child Health USA 2013*. Rockville, MD:: U.S. Department of Health and Human Services.

44. Mathews, T. J., & MacDorman, M. F. (2013). Infant mortality statistics from the 2010 period linked birth/infant death data set. *National Vital Statistics Reports* 62(8): 1–27.

45. CDC. (2014). *Breastfeeding report card—United States, 2014*. Available at: http://www.cdc.gov/breastfeeding/pdf/2014breastfeedingreportcard.pdf

46. Jacknowitz, A. (2008). The role of workplace characteristics in breastfeeding practices. *Women's Health* 47(2): 87–111.

47. Singh, G. K., Kogan, M. D., & Dee, D. L. (2007). Nativity/immigration status, race/ethnicity, and sociodemographic determinants of breastfeeding initiation and duration in the United States, 2003. *Pediatrics* 119(Suppl. 1): S38–S46.

48. Celi, A. C., Rich-Edwards, J. W., Richardson, M. K., et al. (2005). Immigration, race/ethnicity, and social and economic factors as predictors of breastfeeding initiation. *Archives of Pediatrics and Adolescent Medicine* 159(3): 255–260.

49. CDC. (2010). Racial and ethnic differences in breastfeeding initiation and duration, by state—National Immunization Survey, United States, 2004–2008. *Morbidity and Mortality Weekly Report* 59(11): 327–334.

50. Monte, L. M., & Ellis, R. R. (2014). *Fertility of women in the United States: 2012*. Current Population Reports. Washington, DC: U.S. Census Bureau. Available at: http://www.census.gov/content/dam/Census/library/publications/2014/demo/p20-575.pdf

51. Chandra, A., Copen, C. D., & Stephen, E. H. (2014). *Infertility service use in the United States: Data from the national survey of family growth, 1982–2010*. National Health Statistics Reports, no. 73. Available at: http://www.cdc.gov/nchs/data/nhsr/nhsr073.pdf

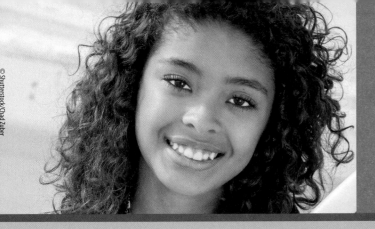

CHAPTER 7

Sexually Transmitted Infections

Learning Objectives
On completion of this chapter, the student should be able to discuss:

1. Common bacterial, viral, and parasitic sexually transmitted infections (STIs), how they are transmitted, and how they affect the body.

2. The relative frequency of major STIs, and relative infection rates among the general population, the young, and different racial and ethnic groups.

3. Biological and cultural reasons why STIs disproportionately affect and infect women and people of color.

4. How stigma associated with STIs hurts people who are infected and slows prevention and treatment efforts.

5. Routes of transmission, symptoms, and course of infection for each of the major sexually transmitted infections in the United States.

6. The links between HPV, cervical cancer, and genital warts; and the role of screening and vaccination in preventing cervical cancer.

7. How the AIDS epidemic has spread and affected the U.S. and global populations over the past three decades.

8. The course of HIV/AIDS infection and how treatment works.

9. The role of open communication, both with clinicians and with partners, in regard to STIs.

10. The importance of personal responsibility and risk reduction in making decisions about one's sexual life.

INTRODUCTION

Infections passed from one person to another through sexual intimacy are known as **sexually transmitted infections (STIs)**. STIs are a major public health problem, especially for young men and women; most people who are sexually active will be infected with an STI at some point in their lives.[1] Women are at a higher risk than men for contracting many STIs; they also suffer greater complications from these conditions. At least 20 distinct infections are transmitted through sexual contact. Sexually transmitted infections include chlamydia, gonorrhea, herpes, hepatitis B, human papillomavirus (HPV), and human immunodeficiency virus (HIV). Sexually associated infections, which may be acquired sexually or nonsexually, include trichomoniasis, yeast infections, and bacterial vaginosis.

The consequences of STIs depend on the organism causing the infection. HPV, the most common sexually transmitted infection, is the primary cause of cervical cancer, yet most cases of HPV will be transitory and harmless. Gonorrhea and chlamydia can permanently damage the reproductive system, even in the absence of symptoms, but can be cured easily with medical treatment. Herpes is an incurable disease with painful and often emotionally devastating symptoms, but it usually does not pose a long-term health risk. HIV, once a life-threatening infection, can now be held in check with daily medications, but it remains a serious, chronic condition. STIs also differ in how they attack the body: Some infections affect a single structure, such as the labia or cervix, while others can spread throughout the reproductive tract. Some bacteria and viruses may enter the bloodstream and result in systemic effects.

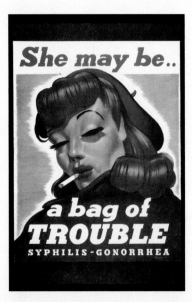

Historically, society has looked on STIs as punishment for engaging in immoral activity. In addition, women, or women's behaviors, have been viewed as the source of the disease.

Reprinted with permission of the American Social Health Association. www.ASHAstd.org

Having one STI increases a person's risk of acquiring another STI. For example, an individual with herpes or gonorrhea may be up to seven times more likely than an uninfected person to acquire HIV through sexual contact.[1] STIs also increase a person's infectiousness: An HIV-positive individual infected with another STI is more likely to transmit HIV through sexual contact and to acquire other STIs if exposed.[2]

Sexually transmitted organisms know no class, racial, ethnic, or social barriers. All individuals are vulnerable if exposed to the infectious organism. Society, however, has a tendency to look on STIs as punishment for immoral activity. In addition, women have been viewed as either the source of disease or deserving of infection. Common reactions to finding out about an STI include disbelief, hurt, guilt, embarrassment, anger, fear, shame, and a feeling of loss of control over one's sexuality and health. The emotional effects of some infections are often as serious or worse than the physical consequences.

Viral STIs, which are incurable, bring the added pressure of worry over how the lingering virus will affect not only one's own body but also present and future relationships. Knowledge and prevention are the best defenses against STIs, followed by early diagnosis and treatment to reduce or eliminate the consequences of infection.

PERSPECTIVES ON SEXUALLY TRANSMITTED INFECTIONS

Historical Overview

Although STIs are a modern epidemic, they are not modern infections. Historical references to STIs reach back thousands of years. The oldest books in the Bible describe diseases that probably were gonorrhea and syphilis. Ancient Greek and Roman physicians identified genital warts and sexually transmitted chancres in their writings; Hippocrates described the mechanism for gonorrhea transmission as "excesses of the pleasures of the Venus." Susruta, an ancient Hindu, also described gonorrhea. In ancient Rome, Tiberius issued a decree outlawing public kissing to curb an epidemic of cold sores caused by a herpes virus. Spanish explorers may have brought syphilis to Europe from the New World; between 1495 and 1500, syphilis ravaged Europe. Several characters in William Shakespeare's plays appear to have the disease.

Epidemiological Data and Trends

The United States has the highest rate of STI infection in the industrialized world. More than 110 million Americans are now living with a sexually transmitted infection.[1] Young people make up one-fourth of the sexually experienced population but have nearly 50% of the country's STIs (see **Figure 7.1**).[1] There are many reasons for this. Adolescents and young adults are more likely to be sexually active; adolescents also appear to have a greater

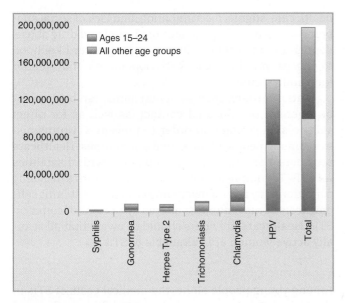

Figure 7.1   **Estimated number of new cases per year of major STIs among youth.**

Source: Satterwhite, C., Torrone, E., Meites, E., et al. (2013). Sexually transmitted infections among US women and men. *Sexually Transmitted Diseases* 40(3): 187–193.

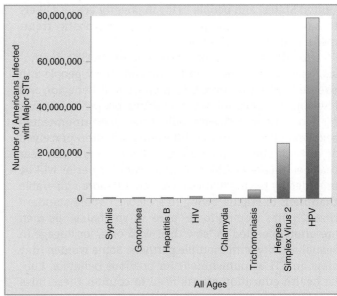

Figure 7.2   **Estimated number of American men and women currently infected with major STIs.**

Source: Satterwhite, C., Torrone, E., Meites, E., et al. (2013). Sexually transmitted infections among US women and men. *Sexually Transmitted Diseases* 40(3): 187–193.

biological risk of infection. Other factors, such as difficulty accessing appropriate health care, the increased risk of multiple short-term sexual relationships, and inconsistent use of barrier contraception, also increase their risk of exposure.[3]

Measuring the scope of the STI epidemic is a difficult task. Some STIs are reportable conditions (diseases required by federal law to be reported to prevent and control their spread), and national data on them are available. Other STIs are not reportable, and actual incidence rates can only be estimated (**Figure 7.2**). Healthcare providers are required to report cases of chlamydia, gonorrhea, and syphilis, but healthcare facilities vary widely in the manner that they report these diseases. Many STIs are asymptomatic, so many infected individuals are not diagnosed.

Sexually transmitted infection estimates that do exist provide a startling picture of the epidemic. For example, 18% of women between the ages of 15 and 19 have HPV, and 4% have chlamydia.[4] One in six Americans has genital herpes. The Centers for Disease Control and Prevention (CDC) estimate that there are almost 3 million new cases of chlamydia each year in the United States.[4]

There are significant racial disparities in rates of STI infection. Chlamydia is more than seven times more common among Black females than among White females, and 69% of the recorded cases of gonorrhea in the United States occur among Black Americans.[4] Sexually transmitted infections also affect Hispanic and Native American women at higher rates than non-Hispanic Whites.

These disparities exist for many reasons. In general, people of color have reduced access to testing and care.

They are also more likely to live in poverty, reducing their chances of receiving effective treatment and increasing the likelihood of complications and disease progression. In general, Americans are more likely to choose a partner of the same race—and for people of color, this means that a person's sexual partner is more likely to have an STI and to face similar obstacles to testing and treatment. Taken together, these factors multiply the chances of infection for people in at-risk groups. In addition to these legitimate disparities, reporting bias may also affect the data collected. Minorities are more likely than Caucasians to visit public clinics, which are often the main source of STI estimates, accounting for some increased reporting of disease among these groups.

Social Issues and Dimensions

Sexually transmitted infections are biologically sexist, presenting greater risk and causing more complications for women than for men. Women experience most of the STI burden and complications, including infertility, perinatal infections, cancers of the reproductive tract, and death. In women, STIs are often silent, presenting as asymptomatic but remaining damaging and infectious. Sexually transmitted infections in pregnant women frequently place fetuses at risk of illness, congenital anomalies, developmental disabilities, and death. Because STIs are most prevalent among women aged 15 to 24, these women experience the greatest burden of chronic pelvic pain, pelvic inflammatory disease (PID), ectopic pregnancy, and infertility.[1,4] Women constitute the majority of individuals living at or below the poverty line in the

United States, and people living in poverty are less likely to have access to comprehensive STI diagnostic, treatment, and follow-up services.

Considerable stigma accompanies an STI diagnosis, regardless of the culprit organism. Many people still equate STIs with immorality, promiscuous behavior, and low social status. All sexually active people are at risk for acquiring an STI, especially if they have unprotected sex. Sexually transmitted infections are often perceived as dirty or shameful, and an infected woman may fear that healthcare providers will not care for her or will be offended by having to do so. Women are more vulnerable than men to stigma owing to society's double standard that requires women to be "pure" or virginal, while men are often expected to "sow their wild oats," or engage in sexual activity with multiple partners. Some women may view an STI as punishment for previous behavior. Public health education efforts need to counter these false perceptions.

Cultural issues often complicate public health and education efforts. Men in cultures or regions that are intolerant of homosexuality may identify themselves as "straight" while having secret, high-risk encounters with other men, ultimately infecting their girlfriends or wives. Many women may unknowingly put themselves at risk by engaging in sexual activities with philandering or infected partners. Drug-related sexual behaviors (selling or trading sex for drugs), as well as risky sexual activity while under the influence of alcohol and other drugs, greatly increase the risk for STI transmission. Emotions often dominate logical behavior and rational thinking—for example, among sex workers who wear condoms with clients but not with boyfriends, and among partners of both genders that get "caught up in the moment" during a sexual encounter and neglect to consider how they are putting themselves at risk.

Healthcare providers may also neglect some populations of women when it comes to screening for STIs. Women who identify as lesbian, gay, bisexual, or transgender (LBGT) often encounter problems when attempting to access health care. Healthcare providers may assume that their female patients are straight, they may not know how to discuss risk reduction for female-to-female sexual encounters, or they may simply not believe that lesbians are at risk for STIs. (Although women who have exclusively female partners do have lower rates of some STIs, they are still at risk for infection and should be aware of risk reduction methods. Whereas HIV, for example, is unlikely to be transmitted from one woman to another woman, other STIs, such as herpes or HPV, can be easily spread this way.)

Transgender women—women whose self-identified gender does not conform to their physical sex—face even greater challenges. Transgender women often face stigma and ignorance within the medical community that either prevents them from receiving testing, treatment, and other medical care or causes them to avoid seeking care altogether. In addition to affecting their access to health care, stigma, discrimination, and lack of social support contribute to higher rates of alcohol and drug abuse, depression and mental illness, and a greater likelihood to engage in risky sexual behaviors among transgender men and women.

Latex barriers, such as dental dams, can be used for oral–genital or oral–anal contact, as well as for direct skin-to-skin contact, in order to prevent STI transmission among people of all sexual orientations. Healthcare providers also may not screen women with disabilities for STIs. To complicate matters, a woman with a disabling condition may have sensory impairments that limit self-diagnosis or may manifest altered symptoms of common STIs. Healthcare providers should be aware that all sexually active women are vulnerable to STIs.

Economic Dimensions

Among young people alone, the medical costs of STIs in the United States are more than $16 billion each year.[5] This estimate does not include lost wages, loss of productivity due to STI-related illness, out-of-pocket costs, or costs incurred by the transmission of STIs to infants, which can result in significant lifelong expenditures.

For bacterial STIs, complications of untreated chlamydia and gonorrhea present the greatest costs. Without medical attention, these STIs can lead to PID and future fertility problems, leading to even more costs and health concerns. Because viral STIs cannot be cured and may require treatment for years, they tend to cost more than bacterial STIs. The greatest expenses associated with viral STIs result from treatment of precancerous cervical lesions caused by HPV infection and treatment of sexually transmitted HIV infection. In addition to their economic dimensions, STIs carry a high human cost of pain, suffering, and grief. Chlamydia and gonorrhea complications can lead to chronic pain, infertility, and other complications that can affect a woman's health and well-being throughout her lifetime.

HIV/AIDS creates enormous costs at both the societal and individual levels. The rapid spread of HIV in many parts of the world, especially sub-Saharan Africa, has brought catastrophic economic consequences as the primary wage earners have fallen ill or died. In the United States, treatment regimens for HIV can cost thousands of dollars per month. In addition to coping with the physical and psychological consequences of infection, people living with HIV face the additional challenges of finding and maintaining health insurance and prescription drug coverage.

Over the past 15 years, global spending on HIV has grown dramatically, allowing more people to receive treatment, get tested, and reduce their chances of infection. From 2004 to 2013 the number of people receiving treatment for HIV in low- and middle-income countries grew by more than 10 million.[6] Increased access to treatment has helped to reduce AIDS-related deaths by 19% during the same time period. The mobilization of this money, as well as the logistical efforts to provide and distribute

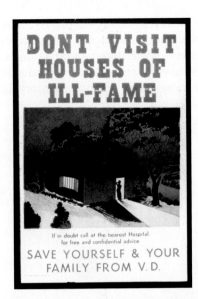

Although this public service announcement is more than 50 years old, people still equate STIs with immorality, promiscuous behavior, and low social status.
Reprinted with permission of the American Social Health Association. www.ASHAstd.org

treatment, is a major global achievement. Yet this effort is only the beginning: More than 20 million people living with HIV still need treatment, and a lasting recession in many parts of the world, as well as a sense that the crisis is now over, has eliminated or threatened many sources of funding.[6] Continuing the fight against HIV will require a renewed commitment, as well as effective use of resources where they are most needed.

Clinical Dimensions and Treatment

Considerable variation exists in the course of infection, symptoms, and optimal treatment of STIs, depending on the responsible organism. This section reviews the clinical and treatment perspectives of each major STI.

Infection Process

Sexually transmitted infections can be caused by bacteria, viruses, or parasites. Each organism requires a unique diagnostic strategy and treatment.

Bacteria, which cause gonorrhea, chlamydia, syphilis, vaginitis, and many other infections, receive nourishment from the fluid or tissue in which they reside. The infected area becomes warm, red, and swollen owing to the increased circulation and the accumulation of **pus**. Eventually, the body's **immune system** senses the presence of the foreign bacteria and mobilizes white blood cells to attack them. This may or may not be successful in eliminating infection. The local host cells may be destroyed directly from the bacteria, indirectly from the excessive swelling and waste products, or even by the body's own overzealous immune response. In many cases, bacterial waste products are toxic beyond the local area and may result in systemic conditions of aches, fever, chills, and malaise. An example of a systemic illness produced by bacterial waste products

is **toxic shock syndrome (TSS)**, which is caused by certain strains of *Staphylococcus aureus* bacteria.

Although the immune system routinely fights off invading organisms throughout the body, bacterial infections in the reproductive tract are particularly challenging. The pelvis contains ideal media for bacterial growth and proliferation, especially during menstruation and after a miscarriage or abortion. In addition, many kinds of bacteria normally live in the intestine and vaginal area, so the normal ecosystem of these areas involves a delicate balance of organisms. Harmful bacteria that upset this balance can be killed by antibiotics, but taking such drugs to kill one organism often results in the death of the normal bacteria as well. When these bacteria levels are reduced, yeast colonies may proliferate, and additional treatment may be necessary.

Viruses, which cause herpes, HPV, hepatitis, and HIV, follow unique invasion patterns. These tiny organisms are made of DNA or RNA protected by an outer coat and are hundreds to thousands of times smaller than bacteria. Their attack mechanism also differs from that of bacteria. Viruses invade normal cells and take over the metabolic functions, replicating themselves thousands or millions of times in the process. As this replication occurs, viruses often destroy their host cells. The body's immune system eventually recognizes invading viruses and responds to them. The immune response is often effective at controlling a viral invasion, but in some cases viruses can stay dormant inside human cells, where the immune system cannot reach them. Viral STIs, especially HIV, present difficult challenges to medical researchers. HIV weakens and even subverts the host immune system, allowing **opportunistic infections** that normally the body easily fights off to invade and proliferate. Because antibiotics are ineffective against viral organisms, researchers are constantly looking to develop effective antiviral drugs that do not cause harm to the human host, or vaccines, which can prevent infection.

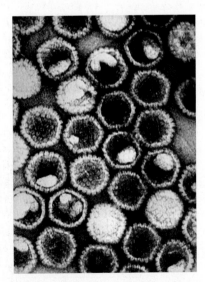

Magnified view of herpes simplex virus. About one in four young people in the United States will be affected by a viral STI.
Courtesy of CDC

Ectoparasitic infections are caused by tiny parasites that reside on the skin and survive on human blood and tissue. Although small or invisible to the naked eye, these parasites are many times larger than bacteria or viruses. Parasitic infections include scabies and pubic lice ("crabs"). Parasites cause itching and may cause bumps or a rash but are easily treated with a topical cream. Parasitic infections are not considered major STIs; although they affect many people, they are more an annoyance than a serious health threat.

BACTERIAL STIS

Chlamydia

Chlamydia is both the most common bacterial sexually transmitted infection and the most commonly reported infectious disease in the United States—about 1.2 million cases are reported every year. Young women are most likely to be infected (**Figure 7.3**). More than 1 in 35 women between 15 and 24 years of age in the United States has chlamydia.[7] Chlamydia infections are the leading cause of preventable infertility and ectopic pregnancy.

Many women with chlamydia do not experience symptoms; instead, infections are often detected at routine gynecological screenings or when a male partner develops symptoms that lead to clinical treatment. When symptoms do present in women, they may include unusual vaginal discharge or bleeding, painful urination, painful intercourse, bleeding after intercourse, pelvic pain or tenderness, or fever.

The bacteria that cause chlamydia and gonorrhea thrive in moist, warm cavities. As a consequence, infections may present in the reproductive tract, throat, eyes, and rectum. Accurate diagnosis requires a culture taken from the cervix and urethra, and from the throat and anal area if those areas may have been exposed. Either of these infections can invade the uterus, fallopian tubes, cervix, urethra, and even liver. When an infection of chlamydia or gonorrhea moves into the upper reproductive tract, the condition is known as pelvic inflammatory disease (PID).

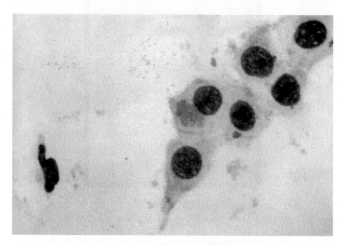

Magnified view of the bacteria that cause chlamydia. Bacterial STIs can be treated with antibiotics, but they often appear without symptoms.
Courtesy of Dr. Wiesner, Dr. Kaufman/CDC

Chlamydia screening remains one of the most important national efforts to maintain and improve fertility. Routine chlamydia screening could prevent up to 60% of new cases of PID in the United States.[8] To screen for chlamydia, a healthcare provider may obtain a culture using a cotton swab in the genital area. Newer, more accurate urine-based tests that identify the genetic makeup of the chlamydia bacteria are becoming more common; these tests also make screening easier for men. Because gonorrhea and chlamydia often coexist, culture for gonorrhea is a standard procedure when chlamydia is suspected.

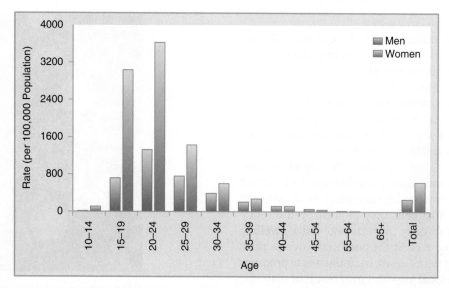

Figure 7.3   Chlamydia rates by age and sex, 2013.

Reproduced from Centers for Disease Control and Prevention. (2014). *2014 sexually transmitted diseases surveillance*. Available at: http://www.cdc.gov/std/stats14/

A woman may be treated for chlamydia, even without a confirmed diagnosis, based on symptoms and physical examination. The affected woman's partner(s) should be treated at the same time, with follow-up examinations usually performed about 4 weeks after treatment to ensure that the therapy was successful. Sexual intercourse should be avoided until after the chlamydia has been cured.

Aggressive treatment is necessary with chlamydia because uterine invasion occurs fairly rapidly, and the invasion process may be asymptomatic. Treatment delay may result in the organism reaching the fallopian tubes with resultant scarring, tubal obstruction, infertility, and ectopic pregnancy. Pregnant women infected with chlamydia may be at increased risk for spontaneous abortions, stillbirth, preterm delivery, and delivery of low-birth-weight infants. Transmission of the organism to the baby may result in eye infections and pneumonia in the infant.

Gonorrhea

Despite decades of knowledge about how **gonorrhea** is transmitted and an effective cure in the form of antibiotics, gonorrhea remains prevalent in the United States. In 2013, there were 303,000 reported cases of gonorrhea in the United States—about one-fourth of the number of reported cases of chlamydia.[4] Women, adolescents, and young adults bear the highest burden of this disease. Symptoms of gonorrhea, if present, are often similar to symptoms of chlamydia; however, like chlamydia, gonorrhea typically appears without symptoms.

There are several treatment options for gonorrhea, but treatment is complicated by the frequent coexistence of unrecognized chlamydial infection and the growth of gonorrheal antibiotic-resistant strains. Because neither gonorrhea nor chlamydia may be apparent upon physical examination, gonorrhea treatment usually includes screening for antibiotic resistance and prescribing additional antibiotics to treat infections effectively. The sequelae of gonorrhea are so severe and threatening to general health and reproductive capability that any woman exposed to a partner with gonorrhea, even in the absence of symptoms, should be treated. Symptoms may indicate gonorrhea has spread, so longer and more intensive antibiotic treatment, often including hospital admission for intravenous antibiotic therapy, may be required. About a week after antibiotic treatment for gonorrhea, reculture is necessary for a woman and her partner(s). This follow-up is especially important because gonorrhea is now often resistant to certain antibiotics, and further treatment may be necessary to eliminate the disease.

Reinfection with gonorrhea is common, so a person being treated should avoid sexual contact until cultures on both partners confirm that treatment was successful. Untreated or unsuccessful treatment of gonorrhea may result in PID or a syndrome caused by disseminated gonococcal infection, which can include septicemia (blood poisoning), joint infection, skin problems, and heart and brain infections.

Pelvic Inflammatory Disease

Pelvic inflammatory disease (PID) is a frequent, serious complication of the female reproductive tract (**Figure 7.4**). The infection process may be located in specific areas

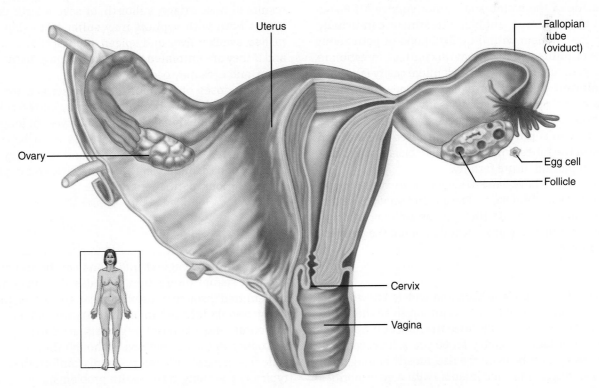

Figure 7.4   **Pelvic inflammatory disease can affect any or all of a woman's reproductive organs.**

or spread throughout the pelvic cavity. About 1 million women in the United States experience PID every year.

Chlamydia and gonorrhea are responsible for most cases of PID, which is a major cause of infertility and hospitalization in young women. Medical costs related to PID in the United States come to an estimated $4 billion a year. National efforts to screen women at risk seem to be helping to prevent PID, with documented decreases in hospitals, clinics, and doctor's offices over the past 15 years.[4]

Pelvic inflammatory disease symptoms vary considerably. Many women with PID have no symptoms at all, while some women have symptoms that can easily be overlooked or mistaken for something else, such as vaginal discharge, mild but persistent abdominal or back pain, or pain during intercourse. Other women experience sudden and severe pelvic pain, fever, shaking chills, or heavy vaginal discharge or bleeding. Chlamydial PID is more likely to present with the former, more subtle symptoms, and gonorrheal PID is more likely to present with the latter, more severe set of symptoms.

Clinical evaluation is necessary for PID diagnosis. The first step in confirming the presence of PID is eliminating the possibility of other serious conditions that may manifest themselves in a similar manner. Although uterine tenderness and discharge indicate possible infection, bacterial culture is necessary to identify the causative bacterium and determine the most appropriate treatment course.

The most serious complication of PID is infertility, which occurs in about 10 to 15% of cases.[4] Pelvic inflammatory disease from chlamydia is also a leading cause of ectopic pregnancies—pregnancies where the fetus develops outside of the womb and cannot survive.[9] If PID is limited to the uterus, antibiotic treatment can usually resolve the problem with little likelihood of permanent damage or future complications. In contrast, infection in the fallopian tubes, ovaries, or abdominal cavity is a cause for significant concern. Permanent damage from PID is especially likely if the infection has invaded the fallopian tubes, because the tubes are fragile and easily damaged by the infectious process. Infection causes swelling and scarring of the tubes, which can lead to blockage and distortion, impairing future fertility.

Women who have had PID should take extensive precautions to avoid reinfection. Present and previous sexual partners must be treated with the same antimicrobial regimen as the infected woman, whether or not the partners have symptoms.

Syphilis

Once one of the more common and widely known STIs, **syphilis** has become much less common since the 1940s, when antibiotics that easily cured the infection were discovered. After falling steadily for 60 years, however, new syphilis cases have been on the rise, mostly among men, but also among women and infants.[4] Although minorities are still more likely than their White counterparts to be infected with syphilis, these differences have shrunk over the past decade.[4]

Syphilis is caused by the bacterial organism *Treponema pallidum*. It is highly infectious and has a long, varied clinical course. If untreated, it may cause serious consequences, including cardiac and neurological damage and even death. Although the syphilis bacterium can be killed with antibiotics, the damage caused by long-term infection is permanent. There are three major stages of syphilis: primary, secondary, and tertiary.

Primary syphilis, the first disease stage, usually occurs 3 to 12 weeks after sexual contact with an infected individual. The first symptom is a painless open sore, called a chancre, at the site of sexual contact. The chancre heals within 2 to 6 weeks, whether or not the individual receives treatment. *Secondary syphilis*, which occurs from 1 week to 6 months later, includes a variety of symptoms, most notably a rash on the palms of the hands, the soles of the feet, and the external genitals; these rashes may develop into open sores. Individuals are highly infectious in this stage. Symptoms usually last 3 to 6 months but may reappear temporarily for several years. This latent phase of syphilis may be temporary or permanent. A few people progress to the most dangerous phase, *tertiary syphilis*, which can occur a decade or more after infection. These symptoms include heart disease, nerve and brain damage, spinal cord damage, blindness, and death.

Syphilis can pass from an infected woman to her developing fetus. Early screening and treatment of pregnant women are essential to prevent congenital syphilis. Untreated syphilis infection during pregnancy often results in miscarriage, stillbirth, or severe birth defects. Babies born with syphilis may suffer from skin sores, rashes, swollen liver and spleen, **jaundice**, and anemia, and if they are untreated after birth, damage to the heart, brain, and eyes may occur.

High doses of antibiotics are prescribed for early-stage syphilis; more prolonged, intensive treatment is indicated for individuals infected for a year or longer. For all stages of syphilis, sexual partners must be concurrently treated. Effective treatment and follow-up in the primary and secondary stages of the disease can prevent further serious, permanent damage.

VAGINITIS

Several kinds of vaginal infections can be transmitted through sexual interaction. Because they may also be transmitted through nonsexual means, however, they are not generally referred to as STIs. Trichomoniasis, yeast infection, and bacterial vaginosis are fairly common reproductive tract infections. Although they are responsible for physical and emotional discomfort, they do not typically pose long-term health problems.

Trichomoniasis

Trichomoniasis is caused by a one-celled protozoan and is usually transmitted via sexual contact, but the infectious organism is capable of surviving outside a human host in a wet environment, such as on a swimsuit or wet towel, and transmission between individuals can occur via these objects.

Some women do not experience any symptoms with trichomoniasis. When symptoms do occur, they typically include a frothy, thin, grayish, or greenish vaginal discharge; intense vaginal itching; an objectionable odor; pain during urination and intercourse; and urinary frequency. Diagnosis is confirmed with a wet smear of vaginal secretions.

Trichomoniasis can be effectively treated with antibiotics in either a single- or multiple-dose format. Because many women and most men infected with trichomoniasis do not experience symptoms, sexual partners should be treated at the same time, and condoms should be used until treatment is complete. Recurrent infections are common with trichomoniasis in pregnant women. This disease may result in premature rupture of membranes, preterm delivery, low birth weight, or a genital or lung infection in the newborn.

Yeast Infections

Yeast organisms (also known as *Candida albicans*, fungus infection, monilia, and candidiasis) normally exist in the microscopic ecosystem of a woman's body. A yeast infection occurs when the population of yeast organisms grows large enough to irritate the vagina and vulva. Yeast infections are very common; most women will have at least one during their lives. While yeast infections are usually temporary, the symptoms can be painful and irritating, and include a thick, white, cottage-cheese-type vaginal discharge, redness, swelling, and itching. Diagnosis is generally made by microscopic examination of a sample of the vaginal discharge or a culture. Although yeast infections affect the female reproductive tract, yeast infections are usually not sexually transmitted. **Yeast infections** are usually treated with antifungal vaginal cream (Monistat, Gyne-Lotrimin, Vagistat, Femstat). Treatment of partners is usually unnecessary. Medications for yeast infections are available in over-the-counter forms; for women with chronic and recurrent infections, this has made treatment easier, cheaper, and faster by reducing the waiting time for a prescription and the expense of a clinical visit. For women who are not sure what type or kind of vaginal infection they may have, self-treatment is not a good idea, however.

Although yeast infections do not usually affect fertility, reinfection is common. Recurrent attacks may occur shortly after treatment or be delayed for a considerable period of time. What causes yeast to grow out of control is not always known. Women taking antibiotics may experience yeast infections when the antibiotics kill off the populations of "good" or healthy vaginal bacteria, allowing small populations of yeast to overgrow. Persistent yeast problems often present during pregnancy and in women who take oral contraceptives. Women with diabetes and women who are overweight also report higher frequencies of such infections. For women with recurrent infections, prolonged or intermittent treatment is often recommended to keep yeast growth under control. Concurrent treatment for yeast whenever antibiotics are prescribed may also help women with chronic yeast infections.

Bacterial Vaginosis

Bacterial vaginosis (BV) is an overgrowth of several species of vaginal organisms, which may be transmitted by sexual activity.[10] BV is known by many terms, including nonspecific vaginitis, *Gardnerella vaginalis*, bacterial vaginitis, *Haemophilus vaginalis*, *Corynebacterium vaginalis*, and anaerobic vaginosis. While the bacteria that cause BV may be spread in a sexual manner, BV has a variety of nonsexual causes, such as douching and recent antibiotic use. Although BV does not usually cause complications on its own, it does increase a woman's risk for acquiring other sexually transmitted infections, including HIV.[11] In addition, the presence of genital herpes may increase a woman's odds of developing BV. Bacterial vaginosis is more prevalent among women with more than one sexual partner, intrauterine device (IUD) users, and women who have cervicitis.[12]

Globally, BV is very common and may be present in 10 to 40% of women worldwide.[10] It is the most common cause of abnormal vaginal discharge. Symptoms include a gray or white frothy discharge that may be thick or watery and that may have an objectionable odor. Painful urination, vaginal pain or burning during intercourse, redness, and itching may also be present.

While many women complain of vaginal odor, discharge, or irritation, as many as 50% of women with BV may be asymptomatic; thus, routine screening is recommended whenever STI testing is indicated.[3] Pregnant women with bacterial vaginosis may have an increased risk of delivering preterm, low-birth-weight infants.

Bacterial vaginosis may coexist with other STIs and has been identified as a possible factor in HIV transmission. Because BV also may be associated with PID, definitive diagnosis is important to ensure adequate treatment.

Recommended treatment regimens consist of antibiotics. Treatment of sexual partners is not standard procedure, although it may be indicated if reinfection occurs after treatment or if sexual transmission is suspected.

Regular douching can increase a woman's risk of bacterial vaginosis. Douching may harm the vaginal flora and can increase the risk for bacterial vaginosis as well as other infections.[13]

VIRAL SEXUALLY TRANSMITTED INFECTIONS

Human Papillomavirus

Human papillomavirus (HPV) is an extremely common virus spread by skin-to-skin contact. There are more than 100 strains or types of HPV. Some strains of HPV are transmitted through nonsexual means and can cause warts on the hands, feet, and other parts of the body. About 40 strains of HPV, however, are transmitted sexually and affect the genital area. It is these sexually transmitted types of HPV that will be discussed in this chapter.

There are two broad types of sexually transmitted HPV. "High-risk" HPV can cause cervical dysplasia, a form of abnormal cell growth that can lead to cervical cancer. Whereas most women who get HPV never develop cervical cancer, almost every single case of cervical cancer is linked to high-risk HPV. "Low-risk" HPV can cause warts on or around the genital area but does not increase the risk for cervical cancer.

Each year, more than 7 million people in the United States, most of them in their teens or early twenties, are infected with HPV. Both high- and low-risk HPV are present in 20 to 40% of women of almost all age groups (see **Figure 7.5**). Most people who are sexually active will acquire HPV at some point in their lives; most of these people will never know it.[1]

Cervical cancer is the second most common cancer among women around the world. Fortunately, almost all cases of cervical cancer are preventable. Cervical cancer is typically preceded by abnormal cell growth called cervical dysplasia, which can be found during a routine Pap smear; in addition, a DNA test is available to detect whether a person has a high-risk strain of HPV. A screening program that includes Pap smears and HPV DNA testing (see **It's Your Health**) can identify women at risk and almost always find cervical dysplasia before it becomes cancerous.

In addition, two vaccines, Gardasil and Cervarix, provide protection against the most common strains of HPV. The development of HPV vaccines represents a major, but incomplete, step toward eliminating cervical cancer. Both vaccines prevent infection from HPV types 16 and 18, which are responsible for 70% of cases of cervical cancer. Additionally, Gardasil prevents infection from HPV

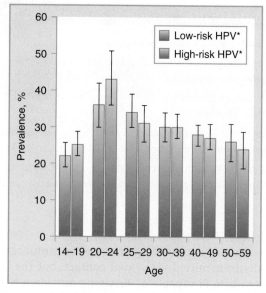

*HPV = human papillomavirus.

Note: Error bars indicate 95% confidence interval. Both high-risk and low-risk HPV types were detected in some females.

Figure 7.5 HPV—Prevalence of high-risk and low-risk types among women aged 14–59, 2003–2006.

Data from Hariri, S., Unger, E., Sternberg, M., et al. (2011). Prevalence of genital HPV among females in the United States, the National Health and Nutrition Examination Survey, 2003–2006. *Journal of Infectious Diseases* 204(4): 566–573.

types 6 and 11, which cause about 90% of cases of genital warts in men and women. The Food and Drug Administration (FDA) has approved Gardasil and Cervarix, and both vaccines have been shown to be safe and well tolerated. However, either vaccine requires a series of three injections to be effective and is most effective if given before a person becomes sexually active. In addition, neither vaccine prevents infection from the high-risk types of HPV responsible for the other 30% of cervical cancer cases. Additionally, Gardasil and Ceravix are expensive compared to other vaccines, making widespread vaccination a relatively costly option.

Current medical knowledge has the potential to eliminate cervical cancer. Vaccination, if implemented widely, could prevent most cases of HPV infection, while widespread screening involving a combination of Pap tests and HPV testing could find the remaining cases of cervical dysplasia before they develop into cancer. However, although the potential to end this disease exists, a considerable challenge remains with educating the public about cervical cancer, overcoming misplaced fears about vaccination, and expanding women's access to screening and care.

There is no cure for HPV, but symptoms of both high-risk and low-risk HPV can be treated. Additionally, the body's immune system can often rid the body of the virus, effectively "curing" an individual. HPV infections are often asymptomatic, and a person can have HPV for years without the virus causing harm to the body. Left untreated, however, cervical dysplasia caused by high-risk HPV can cause serious harm or death, so prevention and screening efforts are extremely important for women's health.

For many women, the first indication of a high-risk HPV infection is a routine Pap smear. For a woman with an inconclusive Pap test, HPV DNA testing conducted on the residual material collected from a Pap can help identify the presence of HPV to determine whether she is at risk for cervical dysplasia. The United States Preventive Services Task Force and the American Cancer Society currently recommend Pap smears every 3 years for women between the ages of 21 and 65. Women who are between the ages of 30 and 65 can reduce this frequency to every 5 years if they receive HPV DNA testing along with the Pap test. Women who are negative on both tests can be reassured that they do not have HPV and they are not at risk for developing cervical cancer in the near future. If the HPV DNA test is positive, a gynecologist may look for evidence of warts or abnormal cell growth in the cervix or vagina. While the Pap test is routinely used in gynecological exams, it can produce false positive results, indicating possible dysplasia while none is present, and it cannot identify the presence of high-risk HPV unless dysplasia is present. For this reason, a negative HPV test provides a degree and duration of reassurance not achievable by any other diagnostic method.[14] (See **Table 7.1** for a more detailed explanation of results for HPV DNA tests and Pap smears.)

While many women with cervical dysplasia will never develop cervical cancer, some women may need aggressive treatment to prevent cancer development. Colposcopic examination and biopsy of suspicious areas are indicated. Women at risk for cervical cancer should be diligent about personal care, medical follow-up, and annual Pap smears and pelvic examinations.

HPV infection with low-risk HPV is usually characterized by single or multiple lesions or warts, which may first appear as small, round elevations in the skin; later these warts may grow in size and number and blend together into a cauliflower-like growth. Genital warts vary in size, may exist in single or multiple units, and may be raised

Table 7.1	Understanding Cervical Cancer Screening: Pap and HPV Test Results and What They Mean	
Result	**What It Means**	**Recommended Course of Action**
Negative HPV test and normal Pap test	▪ Your cervical cells are normal. ▪ You do not have HPV. ▪ Your chances of getting cervical cancer in the next few years are very low.	▪ Wait 3 years before getting your next Pap smear and HPV test; ask your doctor about when to come in for your next visit.
Negative HPV test and unclear ("ASC-US") Pap test	▪ Something besides HPV (and unrelated to cervical cancer) is causing abnormal cell changes in the cervix, but you do not have HPV.	▪ Get another Pap test in a year or ask your doctor about when to receive another test.
Negative HPV test and abnormal Pap test	▪ You have abnormal cell changes in the cervix, but you do not have HPV.	▪ Have your doctor investigate the cell changes for further information and possible treatment.
Positive HPV test and normal Pap test	▪ You have HPV, but your cervical cells are currently normal. ▪ In most cases, your body will fight off the HPV infection within 2 years; however, there is a small chance for cell changes that could lead to cervical cancer.	▪ Get another Pap test and HPV test in 1 year.
Positive HPV test and unclear ("ASC-US") Pap test	▪ You have HPV, and you might have early cell changes that could lead to cervical cancer on your cervix.	▪ Schedule an appointment with your doctor, who will examine the abnormal cells further and possibly provide treatment, or watch the area over time to make sure the cells do not get worse.
Positive HPV test and abnormal Pap test	▪ You have HPV as well as abnormal cell growth that can lead to cervical cancer.	▪ The best course of action depends on the extent of cell growth (in most cases this will *not* be cancerous). ▪ Minor cell changes may simply require a follow-up visit for the doctor to look more closely. ▪ Major cell changes may require further treatment to remove the abnormal cell growth.

Source: Centers for Disease Control and Prevention. (2012). *Making sense of your Pap and HPV test results.* Available at: http://www.cdc.gov/std/hpv/pap/default .htm#sec5

GENDER DIMENSIONS: Health Differences Between Men and Women

HPV Vaccination: Who Should Get It?

Since the introduction of the HPV vaccines Gardasil and Cervarix, public health experts have debated whether males should be vaccinated for this virus. While low-risk HPV can cause genital warts in both men and women, high-risk HPV is less of a public health concern (high-risk HPV is linked to anal and penile cancers in men but these cases, while still important, are less frequent than cervical cancer). Vaccinating males for high-risk strains of HPV could protect them from acquiring the virus, reduce the risk of these rarer cancers, and prevent transmission to their female partners. However, the vaccines are relatively expensive. Parents of children who have difficulty paying for their children's vaccination may be eligible for free vaccines under the government's Vaccines for Children (VFC) program. Regardless of how the costs of vaccination are split by parents, state and federal governments, or other groups, vaccinating both men and women for HPV would cost hundreds of millions of dollars that some experts argue could be better invested in prevention or other public health efforts.

The CDC recommends that preteen girls and young women receive either vaccine and that preteen boys and young men receive the Gardasil vaccine. Gardasil appears to protect both men and women from most cases of genital warts in addition to preventing women from contracting most cases of high-risk HPV. Offering the vaccine before sexual contact has begun provides the best chance of preventing infection. The CDC also recommends vaccination for people who have not received the vaccine up to age 26 for women, and age 21 for men (up to age 26 for men with compromised immune systems). Because the vaccines only offer partial protection, however, screening procedures are still necessary to find cervical cancer caused by the high-risk strains of HPV that are unaffected by the vaccines. While the HPV vaccines are an important advance, they alone will not be the answer to eliminating cervical cancer.

It's Your Health

HPV Testing and Vaccination

Pap Tests (Pap Smears)

The Pap test is an examination that looks for signs of abnormal cell growth in the cervix. In the 5 decades they have been in use, Pap smears have prevented millions of women from dying of cervical cancer.

   Strengths: A national screening program based on Pap tests is already in place. Pap tests find most cases of abnormal cell growth before they become cancerous.

   Limitations: Pap tests sometimes produce positive results in the absence of dysplasia; because the tests look for abnormal cell growth, not the actual virus, frequent screenings are required. Because so many screenings are necessary, the Pap test is not an especially cost-effective solution. In addition, Pap tests can be painful and embarrassing for the women taking them.

HPV Testing

Instead of looking for cervical dysplasia, an early sign of disease, the HPV test looks for the DNA of the virus itself.

   Strengths: Studies consistently show that HPV tests outperform Pap testing. A combined program of HPV testing and Pap tests is nearly 100% effective at identifying women at risk.

   Limitations: The current screening infrastructure in the United States is based on Pap testing; implementing a new system will require political will and financial investment. The presence of high-risk HPV does not guarantee that cancer will develop.

HPV Vaccination

There are two vaccines, Gardasil and Cervarix, each of which prevents infection from the two types of HPV that cause most cases of cervical cancer. Gardasil also prevents infection from most cases of genital warts. Both vaccines are given as a series of three injections over a 6-month period. The CDC recommends vaccination with either vaccine for preteen girls and young women, and vaccination with Gardasil for preteen boys and young men.

   Strengths: Gardasil and Cervarix both prevent infection from the high-risk strains 16 and 18, which are responsible for 70% of current cases of cervical cancer, and the low-risk HPV strains 6 and 11, which are responsible for 90% of current cases of genital warts. Studies have shown the vaccine to be safe and effective.

   Limitations: Screening programs still need to be in place to find the other 30% of cervical cancers caused by high-risk strains of HPV not covered by the vaccine. The vaccine does not protect women who have already been infected, and it requires three doses to be effective. The vaccines are relatively expensive (about $400) to complete.

or flat. In women, these painless lesions may occur on the buttocks, anus, inner thighs, vulva, vagina, and cervix; depending on their location, symptoms can be present without a woman knowing about them.

When warts regress, HPV may still be present, just not readily apparent. Once contracted, the virus has a variable incubation period during which no symptoms are visible and the person is not yet infectious. Warts usually appear 1 to 8 months after exposure, but may take years to appear. Diagnosis of low-risk HPV is usually based on visual detection during clinical examination.

Although warts may regress spontaneously, they are frequently distressing. Treatment is often indicated to remove visible warts for psychological and aesthetic reasons, as well as to reduce the likelihood of transmission. HPV infections are sometimes persistent and can recur regardless of which treatment method is selected. Treatment is easier and less painful in earlier stages. The particular treatment depends on the extent of HPV infection and its location. Options include topical agents applied by the patient or provider, cryotherapy (freezing of warts), laser surgery, electrosurgery, and surgical removal.

HPV can present problems in pregnancy, although this is relatively rare. A pregnant woman with low-risk HPV has a small chance of passing the virus to her child during vaginal delivery. In these cases, a doctor may treat warts before childbirth to reduce these risks.

Only a small percentage of the millions of women who contract high-risk HPV every year will ever develop cervical cancer. Although no treatment can "cure" HPV, most individuals' immune systems will eventually clear the virus without treatment. At this point, a person would no longer have HPV, though he or she could be reinfected with an exposure to a new strain. The strength of the immune system appears to affect the course of infection: Conditions that alter or slow the immune response may encourage dysplasia. Men infected with high-risk strains of HPV may still transmit the virus, even if the virus never affects them or causes symptoms.

Special Precautions

Although latex condoms may reduce the likelihood of transmission, they probably do not provide reliable protection from HPV. HPV is spread by genital skin-to-skin contact, not bodily fluids—because a latex condom does not cover all of the genital skin, it cannot guarantee prevention of transmission, even if no visible symptoms are present. A female condom may provide more protection than a traditional condom that covers the penis, but there are no guarantees with either type of condom use.

Herpes Simplex Virus

Herpes simplex virus (HSV) is a common STI. Herpes can be caused by two distinct, closely related viruses: HSV-1 and HSV-2. HSV-1 is the main cause of recurring sores in the mouth, known as cold sores or fever blisters, while

HSV-2 typically causes similar symptoms that appear in the genital area and is responsible for most cases of "genital herpes." However, if HSV-1 is exposed to the genital area of an uninfected person (for example, through oral sex), HSV-1 can infect the genital area of that person; similarly, exposure to HSV-2 can infect the oral area of a person as well. Both HSV-1 and HSV-2 cause similar symptoms and have similar courses of infection, though HSV-1 tends to be milder in severity and frequency of symptoms.

More than half (53%) of the U.S. population has an infection of HSV-1, and one in six (16%) has an infection of HSV-2.[15] Most people with herpes do not know they are infected. While the number of cases of genital herpes increased rapidly from the 1960s to the turn of the century, since that time there has actually been a slight decrease in new cases (see **Figure 7.6**).[15]

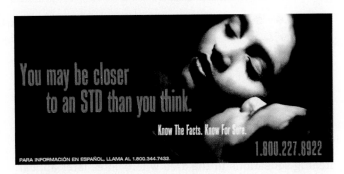

Honest communication before sexual intimacy is essential for assessing risk behaviors and avoiding transmission of disease.
Reprinted with permission of the American Social Health Association, www.ASHAstd.org

> *My husband of 22 years and I divorced recently, and so I'm new to the dating scene. I've started seeing a very sweet guy who later told me that he has herpes. I was very shocked at first, but now that I know about the disease, it's not nearly as bad as I first thought. My daughter, who's in college now, and I had a real heart-to-heart conversation about safer-sex practices afterward. She actually knew more than I did!*
>
> **—50-year-old mother of two**

Herpes is incurable, and it can be extremely painful and psychologically devastating. Yet for the vast majority of cases, herpes is not a serious medical condition. Symptoms are usually most severe just after acquiring the infection. They may appear anywhere from 1 day to 4 weeks after exposure. Lasting about 12 days, herpes generally presents as single or multiple small, painful blisters that appear in the vulva or buttocks. If sores are present on the cervix, they often go unnoticed. The blisters evolve into painful ulcers in a couple of days. These symptoms may be accompanied by vulvar swelling, fever, and enlarged and tender lymph nodes. Sores usually heal in 1 to 4 weeks with little or no scarring. The time between outbreaks is referred to as the latent or inactive phase.

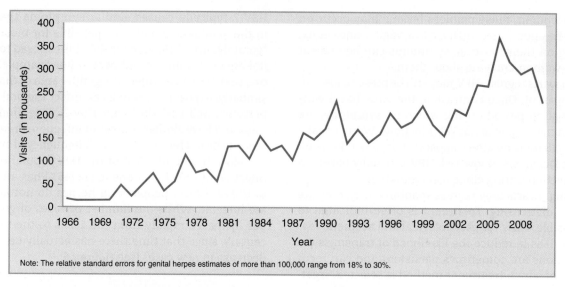

Note: The relative standard errors for genital herpes estimates of more than 100,000 range from 18% to 30%.

Figure 7.6   **Genital herpes—Initial visits to physician's offices: United States, 1966–2010.**

Data from IMS Health, Integrated Promotional Services. *IMS Health Report*, 1966–2010.

During this time, genital sores have healed but the infection remains.

A **prodrome** or warning phase often precedes a herpes outbreak. The warnings may consist of tingling or itching sensations in the area where sores later appear. It is not known what causes repeat outbreaks of herpes. Some people find that irritating stimuli to the infected area, such as tight clothing, menstrual changes, or exposure to sunlight or extreme heat or cold, can trigger an outbreak, whereas others do not notice any such effects.

The human body can never rid itself of the herpes virus. Between outbreaks, the virus evades the immune system by lying dormant within host nerve cells, where the immune system cannot reach it; however, in most cases the immune system does get better at fighting the virus. Recurrent outbreaks are usually milder and shorter than the original outbreaks, and people with herpes generally have fewer outbreaks as time goes by. Although there is no surefire way to prevent all outbreaks, maintaining a healthy lifestyle helps the immune system keep the virus in check. Any stress on the body can also stress the immune system; indeed, many people report that outbreaks begin when they are already sick with a cold or flu, have gone a long time without getting enough sleep, or are experiencing stressful times in their lives—all things that can burden the immune system. Ironically, refraining from obsessing or worrying excessively about a herpes infection, while still remaining knowledgeable about the disease, may help prevent outbreaks.

Herpes outbreaks show considerable variability from person to person. Some outbreaks last as long as 3 weeks; others are as short as a few days. Outbreaks may involve many blisters or just a few, or even a single blister. Some individuals experience outbreaks every few months; others have one or more each month. Some individuals never experience recurrent outbreak symptoms after the initial event, though this is an uncommon occurrence. Infectiousness remains an important concern, even for individuals who are unaware of their herpes symptoms.

Active herpes sores are very contagious during both the initial attack and the recurrences. Both HSV-1 and HSV-2 can be spread from sores to the eye, where serious infection is possible. An oral infection can be spread to infants and children via kissing or casual contact. People infected with herpes undergo periods of **asymptomatic viral shedding**. During these periods, active herpes virus is present on a person's infected area and may be infectious, whether or not symptoms are present. Viral shedding typically lasts for 2 to 20 days after an initial outbreak and for 2 to 5 days after recurrent outbreaks. Researchers have not been able to determine exactly how infectious an individual is when asymptomatic shedding occurs, but it is known that the risk of transmission is highest when active sores are present. Active sores contain hundreds of times more virus than viral shedding from genital secretions. Diagnosis of herpes is typically made based on the patient's history, or from a culture or examination of symptoms. Because clinical diagnosis is often inaccurate, viral culture and type-specific serology may be used as confirmation.

There is no cure for herpes. Several potential vaccines are in early development or clinical trials, but even if one or more of these vaccines prove effective, it will likely be years before they can be fully tested and mass produced. Prescribed antiviral medications may reduce or suppress symptoms, and antibiotic ointment may help prevent a secondary bacterial infection of the sores. Herpes medication may also reduce the chance of transmission between outbreaks.[16] Acyclovir, valacyclovir, and famciclovir are the current treatments of choice for herpes and can relieve symptoms and shorten healing time. All three medications inhibit the ability of the virus to use proteins, thereby interfering with its ability to replicate. Clinicians may prescribe acyclovir to women who acquire herpes during pregnancy or who have severe outbreaks around the time of delivery.[3] The FDA has approved three different treatment regimens for herpes: (1) therapy for an initial outbreak, (2) episodic therapy to speed healing and relieve discomfort during recurrences, and (3) suppressive therapy on a daily basis to attempt to prevent outbreaks. Because the effects of a herpes transmission are usually limited to symptoms and transmission, a woman with herpes should take an active role in deciding the treatment regimen, if any, that is right for her. Women with severe symptoms may wish to take suppressive therapy, whereas women who have outbreaks that are mild or not noticeable may opt for episodic therapy or seek to manage the virus without medication.

Special Precautions

Good personal hygiene is essential during a herpes outbreak. If you have herpes and are experiencing an outbreak, wash your hands after touching a herpes sore to avoid possible transmission to another mucous membrane, such as the eyes or mouth. Take care to avoid spreading the virus to others, including infants and children. If you have a cold sore on or around your mouth, avoid kissing another person. As a precautionary measure, avoid sharing personal objects such as washcloths, toothbrushes, drinking cups, and towels. Although clinical studies have not demonstrated effective indirect transmission, the virus can remain alive outside the body for several hours in a moist environment.

There are no guarantees of "safe sex" with herpes, but there are ways to reduce risk. At a minimum, sexual intercourse, including oral sex, should be avoided when active herpes sores are present. Because sores contain high populations of viruses, if you have herpes, wait until sores are completely healed before resuming sexual activity. Because it is difficult to tell when a herpes outbreak is beginning, open communication about risks and feelings is another key risk-reduction strategy. Condoms appear to provide some protection, with female condoms providing better coverage than male condoms.[17] Because herpes sores can be present in areas not covered by either condom, however, there are no guarantees against transmission. Condoms and other risk-reduction strategies are especially important in a situation in which the male partner has herpes and the female partner does not and is pregnant. An initial attack of herpes during pregnancy presents serious risks to the developing fetus, including possible pregnancy loss or preterm delivery. Women with herpes should be diligent about protecting themselves from further infection by other STIs. Such women are at increased risk for acquiring HIV and other STIs because of the open sores associated with the herpes virus.

Pregnant women with herpes should begin prenatal care early. The risk is greatest for women who contract herpes during their pregnancy. If active lesions are present in the vaginal canal at the time of birth, a cesarean delivery may be performed to avoid exposing the infant to the virus. Infant exposure to the virus may cause infections of the eyes, skin, mucous membranes, and central nervous system, and even death. However, most pregnant women with herpes deliver vaginally and give birth to healthy babies.[3]

Although no one wants to get genital herpes, in most cases the stigma of the disease vastly outweighs its physiological effects. Herpes is closely related to the viruses that cause chickenpox and mononucleosis (mono), yet because herpes is sexually transmitted, people with herpes may describe themselves as "dirty" or "tainted." Others may feel that they will never be lovable or able to enter a sexual relationship again. The truth is that many people with herpes have strong relationships and healthy sex lives. Although there is no way to guarantee prevention of sexual transmission, there are many ways to reduce risk, from avoiding sex or wearing condoms between outbreaks, to taking suppressive therapy to reduce outbreaks and asymptomatic shedding. Some people decide to enter relationships with other people who have herpes to avoid infecting another person, although other STIs would still be a potential concern. Because the symptoms of herpes infections are transient and often ultimately quite mild, some couples with one infected partner decide that the benefits of a healthy, unique, loving relationship outweigh the drawbacks of possible herpes transmission.

Comfort Measures

Keeping the genital area clean and dry minimizes discomfort during a herpes flare-up. A hair dryer on a cool setting may dry the area thoroughly without irritation or discomfort. Genital cleansing must be gentle because rubbing can cause lesions to break and bleed. Many women find **sitz baths** comforting during outbreaks of herpes. Domeboro solution or Epsom salts may be added to the sitz bath. Cold, wet compresses or cleansing pads containing glycerol and witch hazel applied to the sores may also provide temporary relief. In addition, some women find icepacks helpful during outbreaks.

> *I don't sleep around a lot. I have been with only three guys. But I have herpes. I can't tell where I got it … I mean, it's like I have slept with not only those guys, but everyone else they have had sex with. How can a person really trust someone not to have an STI these days?*
>
> **—21-year-old woman**

Hepatitis

Hepatitis, an inflammation of the liver, is caused by infection with one of several viruses—type A, B, C, D, E, F, or G. Hepatitis B and C may be spread through sexual intimacy or contact with infected blood (such as sharing needles to inject drugs).

Hepatitis B, the type of hepatitis most likely to be spread sexually, remains the one STI that can be entirely *prevented* via vaccination; a three-shot vaccine can provide lifetime immunity to both hepatitis A and hepatitis B. Since the early 1980s, infants have routinely been vaccinated for hepatitis A and B. Most individuals who have not been vaccinated as infants may safely receive the vaccines as adults.

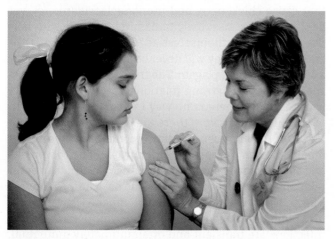

Both hepatitis A and B can be prevented with immunization.
Courtesy of James Gathany/CDC

Vaccination and other preventive efforts have dramatically reduced the number cases of hepatitis A and B. Over the past 25 years, new cases of hepatitis A have fallen by 95%, and new cases of hepatitis B have fallen by more than 85%.[18]

Progression of hepatitis B varies from person to person. For some, hepatitis B is an acute infection, lasting for 6 months or less; for others, hepatitis B can be a chronic infection, lasting for years or decades. Chronic hepatitis B can lead to chronic liver disease, permanent liver scarring, and even death.

Hepatitis C is both the most common cause of chronic liver disease and the most common bloodborne disease in the United States. It is mostly transmitted through contact with infected blood, intravenous drug use, or contaminated blood transfusion but may be spread sexually if exposure to blood occurs. Hepatitis C, like hepatitis B, can cause an acute or chronic infection, but hepatitis C is more likely to be persistent and cause complications.

HIV/AIDS

AIDS (acquired immune deficiency syndrome), a progressive disease caused by **HIV (human immunodeficiency virus)**, is characterized by the destruction of the

It's Your Health

AIDS Facts: Dispelling AIDS Myths

AIDS is not a disease of gay men.

Women are susceptible to AIDS.

AIDS may not be spread by casual contact.

AIDS cannot be transmitted to humans from insects.

There is no risk of acquiring AIDS by donating blood.

Information and education are the best weapons against AIDS.

Confidential, anonymous testing for AIDS is available.

immune system. There are no constant, specific symptoms associated with this condition, and no effective cure or vaccine is available. The best way to stop HIV is to prevent infection. Recent therapeutic advances have allowed people living with HIV to live long, full lives; however, HIV remains a serious, lifelong infection.

HIV is a **retrovirus**, a virus that incorporates its genetic material into the genome of the cell it attacks. When HIV enters the bloodstream, it attacks specific white blood cells called CD4 or T lymphocytes. The virus also replicates. The CD4 cells are no longer able to stimulate a cellular defense response, and the body's systemic immune system is compromised. The number of CD4 cells in an infected person's body decreases as the number of HIV-infected cells increases. AIDS is the final stage of HIV; it is diagnosed when the person has a positive test for antibodies to HIV and a low T-lymphocyte count. An HIV-positive person also may be diagnosed with AIDS when one of 26 known infections, called opportunistic infections, is present. Opportunistic infections present a potentially fatal risk to individuals with AIDS.

HIV is transmitted from one person to another through sexual intercourse; shared intravenous needle use; contaminated blood or blood products; or from mother to child during pregnancy, birth, or breastfeeding. HIV is not spread by casual, social, or family contact. Although HIV is a sophisticated and elusive killer within the body, the virus quickly dies when exposed to the open air; unbroken human skin provides excellent protection from HIV.

An individual with HIV may have no physical symptoms, so it is impossible to tell whether a person is infected just by looking at him or her. In fact, one out of five people living with HIV do not know they are infected.[19] HIV-infected individuals can transmit the virus, however, even in the absence of symptoms. The HIV incubation period ranges from months to years. No individual or groups of individuals are immune to HIV/AIDS.

Perspectives on AIDS

Historical Overview   AIDS was first diagnosed in the United States in 1981. By the 21st century, AIDS had gone from being an unknown disease to a national and global epidemic. Over the past 15 years, scientists, health workers, doctors, and activists have united to fight this disease. These efforts have made an enormous difference: People are now living longer, healthier lives with HIV, and the rate of new infections in the United States and around the world has fallen. The challenge of the next generation will be to sustain these advances and make further progress.

For years, the origins of HIV were unknown. It is now believed that HIV is a mutated descendant of SIV, a virus present in wild African chimpanzees. Genetic analyses of the oldest known specimens of HIV indicate that the virus probably first began spreading among humans between 1884 and 1924 in what is now the Democratic Republic of the Congo.[20] These cases went unnoticed because they spread at low levels among relatively unexamined populations, and because technology to identify the virus was nonexistent.

Men who have sex with men still constitute a disproportionate percentage of people infected with HIV. However, anyone who engages in risky sexual behavior or intravenous drug use is at risk. HIV epidemics in other countries have been spread primarily by intravenous drug users or heterosexual sex. A complicating factor is that, like many intravenous drug users, many men who have sex with men hide or deny their risky behaviors and pose as noninjecting, straight men.

Global Perspectives   In the 1980s and 1990s, HIV spread with alarming, destructive rapidity throughout the world. Developing countries—sub-Saharan Africa especially—were hit the hardest. In the year 2000 alone, 3 million people died from HIV/AIDS. Of those deaths, 80% occurred in sub-Saharan Africa, home to just 10% of the world's population. More than 12 million children in sub-Saharan Africa have lost their parents to AIDS, and sickness and deaths among the current generation of young adults will affect local economies for decades.[7] The primary manner of transmission has varied from region to region. In the United States and much of Europe, AIDS was at first most common among gay and bisexual men. However, in Russia and parts of Asia, intravenous drug use has been a major mode of transmission, and in sub-Saharan Africa and many other regions, heterosexual contact has been the primary mode of transmission.

As the epidemic has spread, governments, scientists, activists, health workers, humanitarian organizations, and others have worked to identify the areas in greatest need, improve access to treatment, provide better care, and encourage testing and prevention. This effort has curbed the growth rate of HIV. Since its peak in 1999, the number of global new cases has fallen by more than 20%; in many sub-Saharan African countries, new cases have fallen by more than 25%.[7] Access to medications has improved the life span of people living with HIV and reduced transmission rates, especially from mothers to their infants. Over the past decade, increased access to HIV medications in low- and middle-income countries has saved an estimated 4.2 million lives and prevented an estimated 800,000 child infections.[7] However, these gains are fragile and incomplete, with only one in three adults and one in four children in low- and middle-income countries receiving treatment, and millions more lacking access to latex condoms and other forms of prevention. The global fight to control this catastrophic disease is only getting started.

Today, close to 35 million people—95% of whom live in developing countries—are living with HIV (see **Figure 7.7**).[7] More than half of all people currently living with HIV are women and girls. In 2013, 2.1 million people

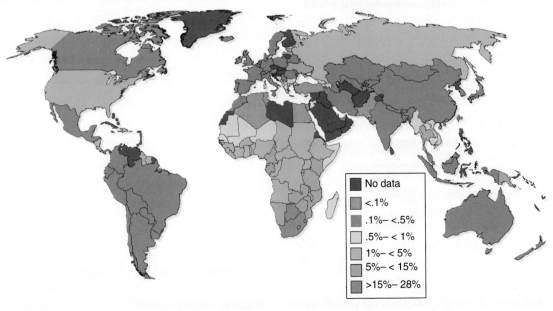

Figure 7.7   **Global prevalence of HIV.**

Source: Reproduced from UNAIDS. (2010). UNAIDS Global Report.

were newly infected, and 1.5 million people died of HIV-related causes.[7]

Epidemiological Data and Trends In the United States, almost 50,000 people are infected with HIV each year, and about 1.2 million people are living with HIV.[21] About 84% of HIV-infected women acquire the virus through heterosexual contact; almost all of the rest acquire it through injection drug use.

AIDS and HIV infection rates present different epidemiological patterns by sex. Women did not constitute a sizeable proportion of the total number of HIV cases in the United States until several years into the AIDS epidemic, but this number has grown since then. In 1992, women accounted for 13.8% of people infected with HIV; by 1998, they represented 20% of this total. Over the past decade, this proportion has stabilized at about 24%.[21] Black, and to a lesser extent Hispanic, women make up a disproportionately large percentage of people living with AIDS, as well as new infections of HIV (see **Figure 7.8**).

The number of people living with HIV and AIDS in the United States has steadily increased over the past 25 years, even as the number of new infections has plateaued (see **Figure 7.9**). This is largely due to improved treatment regimens as well as better access to treatment and care; with new infections continuing even as fewer people are dying of the disease, the total number of people with HIV/AIDS is growing.

> I've had HIV for almost 10 years now, and I'm doing pretty well. I'm staying healthy and I just got a new job. An older guy I know who's had HIV for even longer than I have says I don't know how lucky I am: medicines are better, people aren't afraid of getting AIDS from touching you, and we know a lot more about it. I don't quite feel "lucky," but I'm not letting HIV define who I am.
>
> —**24-year-old woman living with HIV**

Special Concerns for Women Women are an at-risk, HIV-susceptible population. A focus on male homosexuality as a risk factor, along with a failure to focus on women as a unique high-risk group for HIV, has created significant obstacles in diagnosis, prevention, and treatment, which can delay appropriate medical care. In the United States, women are more likely to die from AIDS than men; however, when both groups have equal access to health care, no differences in rates of survival are expected.

Women are far more likely than men to contract HIV from a man through heterosexual intercourse. This difference in part reflects a woman's exposure to a greater quantity of secretions that carry the virus (i.e., semen) and the greater mucosal surface area of the vagina and cervix in which infection can occur. In addition, women are likely to experience small tears in the vaginal lining during intercourse, increasing their susceptibility to infection by HIV-positive semen.

Women who partner with women are not free from risk, however. Many women who consider themselves lesbians, gay, bisexual, or transgender have had heterosexual intercourse and may have received HIV through that avenue without knowing it. Women who have sex with women are also at-risk populations for infections such as HPV and herpes even if they are at reduced risk for HIV.

Social Issues HIV and AIDS disproportionately affect men and women of color. Black women are more than 15 times more likely than White women to be infected with HIV, and Hispanic women are about five times more likely than White women to be infected.[22] As Figure 7.8 shows, the number of AIDS diagnoses disproportionately affects Black and Hispanic women. More than 30 years after the disease was first diagnosed, AIDS continues to be a leading cause of death for Black men and women aged 35–44.

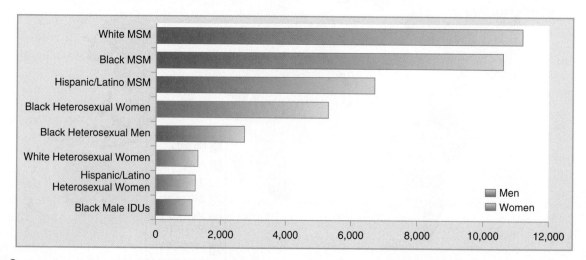

Figure 7.8 **Estimates of new HIV infections per year in the United States by subpopulation.**

Source: Centers for Disease Control and Prevention. (2012). Estimated HIV incidence among adults and adolescents in the United States, 2007–2010. *2012 HIV Surveillance Supplemental Report* 17(4).

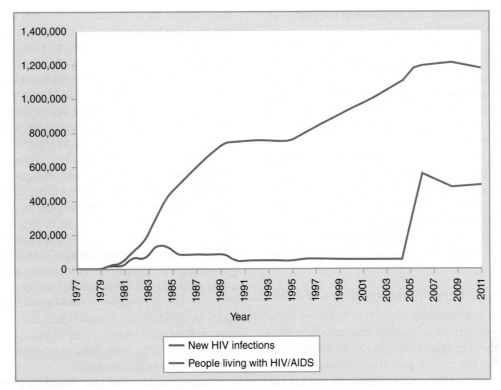

Figure 7.9 **Number of people living with HIV/AIDS and new infections of HIV: United States.**

Source: Centers for Disease Control and Prevention. (2013). Diagnoses of HIV infection in the United States and dependent areas, 2011. *HIV Surveillance Report* 23. Available at: http://www.cdc.gov/hiv/library/reports/surveillance/2011/surveillance_report_vol_23.html

There are many reasons for these disparities, many of them similar to the reasons for ethnic disparities for other STIs. As discussed earlier in the chapter, people of color are more likely to have reduced access to testing and treatment and are more likely to choose a partner of the same race, increasing the chance of exposure. In addition, many of the first AIDS-related resources and treatment centers were geared toward a White, gay male audience. Reducing these continuing racial disparities will be an important public health challenge over the next decade.

Black women with HIV face the dual stigma of being neither White nor male. Black women who have HIV are less likely to receive treatment than other ethnic groups and are more likely to die early. About one-half the people in the United States who die from AIDS are Black.[21] Class undoubtedly plays a large role in this disparity. Women who are economically deprived often have inadequate access to healthcare facilities and are more likely to be unhealthy in general. Many do not have health insurance, are chronically underinsured, or lack information on how to access and use scarce public healthcare facilities.

Early limitations of the male-based CDC diagnostic criteria for AIDS prevented many women with AIDS from being correctly diagnosed. Even with the revised criteria, few studies have provided clear diagnostic criteria for women. As a consequence, women are sometimes ineligible for benefits and services available to others diagnosed early with AIDS, and they may be excluded from clinical trials.

It's Your Health

Anonymous Versus Confidential Testing*

Anonymous testing: The person receives an identification number, provides no name or personal information, and may provide information for demographic use only. An identification number is used to receive test results.

Confidential testing: Test results are kept in confidence (not disclosed to others); however, the patient is identified and results are part of the patient's medical records. These records may be made available to certain people under certain conditions.

*Some facilities may offer both confidential and anonymous testing.

Epidemiological efforts at the beginning of the AIDS epidemic largely viewed women as vectors of AIDS transmission to their offspring and male sexual partners. Early studies were limited to perinatal assessment efforts and surveys of prostitutes. As a consequence, women were not considered as victims of transmission from their male partners. The identification of "high-risk groups" (homosexual and bisexual men, intravenous drug users, hemophiliacs, prostitutes, inmates, and people from specific geographical areas) both stigmatized the members of these groups and denied risk among nongroup members. Even if they practice high-risk behaviors women are often unaware of the risks to themselves or others because they do not consider themselves part of these high-risk groups.

Likewise, some women may not be aware of the high-risk behaviors or histories of their partners.

In 2010, the U.S. government launched the first national HIV/AIDS strategy. The priorities of this coordinated effort between federal, state, and local governments, as well as activists, the medical community, people living with HIV, and others, have been to reduce the rate of new infections, increase access to testing and care, and reduce the continuing HIV-related health disparities in the United States. Over the past 5 years, there has already been progress in some areas, such as the number of people with HIV who know their status and the number of people with HIV with access to care. Continuing this progress, however, will take a renewed, persistent effort on the part of federal, state, and local governments, as well as activists, medical organizations, and ordinary citizens.

Clinical Dimensions and Treatment Issues of AIDS

Diagnosis of HIV is extremely important both for early treatment and prevention of further transmission. Persons with HIV are contagious whether or not they have symptoms. In fact, the month just after infection is generally one of the most contagious periods in the course of infection. Tests for HIV usually attempt to detect HIV antibodies, which are found in the blood and other bodily fluids of an infected person. The **enzyme-linked immunosorbent assay (ELISA)** is an HIV screening test that determines whether a person's serum contains antibodies to one or more HIV antigens. It is used for screening large samples of blood and as a preliminary screening test for individuals because of its low cost and fast results. If an ELISA test gives positive results, a confirmatory **Western blot test** should be performed. When used together, the two tests are highly accurate. Other tests may look for presence of HIV directly, or look for both HIV antibodies and the virus; however, these tests are generally more expensive and are rarely used for screening purposes.

Because the ELISA test does not look for HIV itself, but rather for HIV antibodies, the longer a woman waits after a risk to get tested, the more confidence she can place in a negative result. It takes about 25 days for the average person with HIV to develop detectable antibodies. An early negative HIV antibody test is not a guarantee against infection. Those at risk of HIV should have a repeat test at least 3 months after the initial test to confirm their results. HIV tests are available at local blood banks, AIDS research programs, physician's offices, clinics, and health departments. The FDA has approved four different rapid antibody tests for HIV. These tests have the advantages of offering testing at a lower cost and provide a patient with results on the same visit as the test.

Home testing kits, which can be purchased at drugstores or ordered online, are available for people who are reluctant to visit a healthcare provider or have limited access to healthcare facilities. A woman can collect her own blood sample through a finger prick; the sample is then mailed to a laboratory. She can use an identification number to obtain anonymous results over the phone. After hearing her results, the caller can speak to a counselor to discuss the meaning of the test.

Once infected with HIV, symptoms vary. Some women experience a temporary flu-like illness 1 to 2 months after exposure to the virus; these symptoms typically disappear on their own without treatment. Without treatment, a person will typically begin to experience symptoms of AIDS 5 to 10 years after infection. These symptoms may include swollen lymph nodes, fatigue, recurring yeast infections, weight loss, and chronic diarrhea. Although studies suggest that gynecological symptoms are often the first signs of HIV infection in women, symptoms in women have only recently been included in the CDC criteria for diagnosis. When women seek treatment for these gynecological conditions, HIV testing may be delayed or avoided because it is not suspected. Potential indicators of HIV infection in women include gynecological infections such as candidiasis (yeast infection), PID, HPV, genital ulcers, HSV, pneumonia, and sepsis. When AIDS develops, opportunistic infections often begin to further break down the immune system.

Early treatment of HIV delays or prevents the onset of AIDS and can reduce the virus to unmeasurable levels in the blood. Approved in 1987, AZT (also known as zidovudine) was the first anti-HIV drug. Since then, combination drug therapy—multiple medications that work together—has greatly improved the quality of life for many people. New types of drugs, including nucleoside analogs and protease inhibitors, are now used together as part of an "AIDS cocktail" or HAART (highly active antiretroviral therapy). HAART therapy usually consists of three medications that attack HIV in distinct ways; this "triple attack" helps prevent HIV, which mutates rapidly, from developing resistance to any one type of medication. Newer therapies have combined these three medications into a single pill that can be taken once or a few times a day. These drugs still have significant limitations and side effects, however, and the search continues for more effective and more affordable treatment regimens.

Perinatal transmission of HIV is a special concern for women because the majority of HIV-infected women are of reproductive age. If an HIV-infected woman has a low T-cell count and becomes pregnant, she is more likely to develop HIV-associated illness during pregnancy. Without treatment, approximately one-fourth of all babies born to HIV-infected mothers will be infected with the virus.

My partner had a long-term relationship with a friend from high school, and they broke up last year. I used to worry about that relationship, but now I am more worried about the insignificant encounters he had after they broke up. He doesn't know anything about these women, and neither do I. How do I evaluate my risk?
—23-year-old woman

Prompt treatment can greatly reduce the chance of transmission; perinatal transmission of HIV has decreased over the past 20 years, but unfortunately it continues to exist. In one study of HIV-infected women, HAART therapy regimens prevented perinatal HIV transmission among all women who were compliant with their treatment regimens.[23]

INFORMED DECISION MAKING

Making clear decisions about sexual intimacy can be very difficult. There are many reasons for this. Sexual arousal, the desire to be liked, societal expectations, drugs and alcohol, individual experiences, and other factors all affect how people think and make decisions. Even on a practical level, deciding what constitutes "sexual intimacy" and what form of intimacy would be comfortable and appropriate (Kissing alone? Kissing and touching? With or without clothing? Oral sex? Vaginal intercourse? Something else?) depends on the preferences and morals of each partner and on the specific occasion (see Chapter 5 for a more in-depth discussion of sexual decision making). Adding the possibility of receiving (or transmitting) an STI adds another layer of complexity to this process.

Women who choose to become sexually active are responsible for their decision. Every woman who engages in sexual activity should understand how to communicate what she wants (and what she does not want) and know about basic STI risks, symptoms to look out for, and prevention strategies. Prevention is especially important because many STIs are either incurable or can have permanent consequences.

Apart from abstinence, the most reliable prevention strategy for STIs is long-term mutual monogamy with a single partner. The most significant risk factor for any STI is the woman's partner(s). The risk of contracting an STI increases when a woman has more than one sex partner and when her partner(s) has more than one sex partner. Sexually transmitted infections should be considered a distinct possibility whenever a woman is not in a strictly exclusive, monogamous, long-term relationship.

Safer sex practices are important for any sexual relationship where there is any doubt about a partner's or one's own monogamy or status of HIV and other STIs. Safer sex entails any form of sex in which semen, blood, or vaginal secretions are prevented from passing from one person to another. Latex or polyurethane condoms (or a polyurethane female condom) with spermicide are the key ingredient of safer sex. Condoms must be used correctly each time a person has oral, anal, or vaginal intercourse. If a condom breaks or falls off, its protective effect is lost. Data show that these condoms, when used consistently and correctly, greatly reduce the chances of transmission of HIV and many other STIs.[24] The risk of acquiring an STI increases with the number of partners a person has, but a person only needs to be exposed once to acquire an STI.

Sexually transmitted infections are transmitted by sexual intimacy. Sexual intimacy includes genital-to-genital contact, oral or anal sex, and other forms of intimate skin-to-skin and mucous membrane-to-mucous membrane contact. Sexually transmitted infections can be transmitted in encounters between men and women, men and men, or women and women. Although the notion of safe sex is misleading, safer sex practices can greatly reduce the overall risk of acquiring an STI. **Table 7.2** defines common sexual activities and compares safer, risky, and dangerous sex practices.

Latex or polyurethane condoms prevent fluid exchange and, used properly, can greatly reduce the risk of transmission of HIV. However, condoms probably provide less protection for some STIs, such as herpes and HPV, which are spread by contact with symptoms or infected genital skin. Some practices are more risky for contracting some STIs than for others. A person is extremely unlikely to get HIV from receiving oral sex even without a condom, for example, but could easily get herpes or syphilis in this way.

It's Your Health

Questions to Ask Potential Sex Partners

- What do you know about STIs, including HIV/AIDS?
- Have you ever suspected that you had an STI?
- Have any of your partners (or their partners) suspected that they were infected?
- Have you ever been tested for STIs? If so, when were you tested and what tests did you receive?
- Have you or a sex partner ever shared needles to inject drugs, even once?
- How many sex partners have you had?
- What kind of sexual activities did you engage in with previous partners?
- What do you know about the sexual history of your partner(s)?

Consistent condom use can greatly reduce risk, but there are no guarantees; viruses located at sites other than the penis, such as the scrotum, anal region, vulva, or inner thighs, are not covered by condoms, and transmission from these sites can still occur.

Frank, honest communication before sexual intimacy is essential. Although it may be difficult to have an honest discussion about infections and previous risk behaviors, the price of not communicating can be high. Honest communication is a mark of personal maturity. If a potential partner is unable or unwilling to discuss infections and intimacy concerns, it may indicate a lack of maturity that should be present in a trusted sex partner.

Table 7.2   Common Sexual Activities and Ways to Reduce Risk

Activity	Definition	Level of Risk	Ways to Reduce Risk
Abstinence	Avoiding all sexual activity with another person that would involve touching of the genital or anal areas, or the removal of clothing	None	By definition, abstaining from sexual contact eliminates the risk for STIs. However, maintaining abstinence often ends up being more difficult than many people anticipate. If you choose to be abstinent, think about how you will handle the temptations to engage in sexual contact. In addition, at least be aware of other risk reduction strategies in case you do decide in the heat of the moment to engage in sexual activity.
Mutual monogamy with an uninfected partner	Any sexual activity involving a single partner who is the only person with whom you have sexual activities (and who only has sexual actitivies with you) and who is free from infection	None	Mutual monogamy carries no risk of STIs—provided that both partners stay monogamous and that neither partner has an STI. Trust and open, honest communication are critical for this strategy to work. In addition, both partners should consider testing to confirm their status—many people have STIs without knowing about it.
Kissing	Kissing a partner on the mouth, or on unbroken skin (not on the genital area)	Almost none—some slight risk of an oral herpes or syphilis infection if symptoms are present	Realistically, the only major risk of kissing is of transmitting or receiving an oral herpes infection (a common cold sore).
Mutual masturbation	Touching another person in the genital or anal area, or having another person touch yours	Almost none—assuming no symptoms or cuts in the skin are present	Refrain from sexual activities if symptoms or cuts in the skin are present.
Genital-to-genital contact	Having another person's genital (or anal) area touch, rub against, or otherwise come in contact with yours (without penetration)	High—genital-to-genital contact can easily spread an STI, even if there is no penetration or in the absence of noticeable sexual fluids	Use a latex or polyurethane condom, a dental dam, or a female condom to reduce the chances of exchanging fluids or coming in contact with an infected area; alternatively, only have sexual contact with a tested, mutually monogamous partner.
Oral sex	Licking, sucking, kissing, or otherwise touching another person's genital/anal area with your mouth, or having another person touch yours with his or her mouth	High—most STIs can be spread through oral sex (although the risk for HIV is lower, especially for receiving oral sex)	Use a latex or polyurethane condom, a dental dam, or a female condom to reduce the chances of exchanging fluids or coming in contact with an infected area; alternatively, only have sexual contact with a tested, mutually monogamous partner.
Vaginal or anal intercourse	Sexual contact where a man inserts his penis into a partner's vagina or anus	Very high	Use a latex or polyurethane condom, a dental dam, or a female condom to reduce the chances of exchanging fluids or coming in contact with an infected area; alternatively, only have sexual contact with a tested, mutually monogamous partner.
Oral, anal, or vaginal sex with a latex condom or other safe barrier	Any of the above activities with a latex or polyurethane condom covering a partner's penis, or a dental dam or female condom covering your or a female partner's genital area, used properly and from start to finish	Low for most STIs—latex and polyurethane "male" condoms and female condoms, used properly, will almost always prevent the transmission of HIV; the risk for STIs spread through genital skin-to-skin contact, such as herpes or HPV, may be higher.	To further reduce risk, refrain from these sexual activites, or only have sexual contact with a tested, mutually monogamous partner.

Sexual closeness should be avoided if either partner has any symptoms of infection or if there are any suspicions of infection. Delaying activity for a few days and having symptoms evaluated may prevent lifelong consequences. Because many people with STIs honestly do not know they are infected, many couples now see a clinician together for examination and STI testing before initiating a sexual relationship.

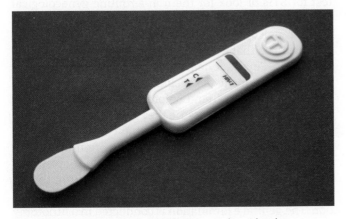

Home testing is an important option for women who wish to be anonymous.

Talking about incurable STIs such as herpes and HPV can be especially difficult. The timing of communication is important. Waiting until after sex to tell someone about a herpes infection may understandably upset a partner.

However, because of the stigma of the disease, a person with herpes may want to wait until some level of trust has been established before informing a potential sex partner. Being calm and knowledgeable about an infection also aids in communication. Many people are ignorant about the course of infection of STIs or the means by which they are spread. Open and frank discussion benefits both partners; studies have found that sharing a herpes diagnosis with a supportive spouse or lover and avoiding denial as a coping mechanism help people with herpes come to better and healthier terms with their infections.

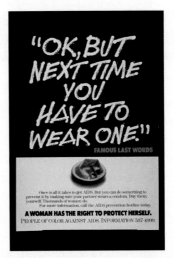

"OK, BUT NEXT TIME YOU HAVE TO WEAR ONE."

FAMOUS LAST WORDS

Once is all it takes to get AIDS. But you can do something to prevent it by making sure your partner wears a condom. Buy them yourself. Thousands of women do. For more information, call the AIDS prevention hotline today.

A WOMAN HAS THE RIGHT TO PROTECT HERSELF.

PEOPLE OF COLOR AGAINST AIDS. INFORMATION 587-4900.

Latex condoms, although not a guarantee against HIV infection, are a key consideration in prevention of HIV transmission.
Courtesy of CDC.

I felt weird when Karen insisted that we go to the doctor together before we had sex. I guess I was afraid that one of us would have something. But we didn't and, you know, I think that our relationship is stronger because she insisted. I respect her for having the courage it took to do that. I wish that it had been my idea.

—**22-year-old man**

When to Get Tested or Treated

People who experience potential symptoms of STIs, or who may have been exposed, should make the choice to get tested. Deciding to get tested and then actually making and following through with an appointment is often a difficult process, but some form of treatment is available for all STIs. Many STIs can be cured easily with proper antibiotic regimens. Others can be treated to alleviate symptoms and reduce or prevent harm to the body. Women (and men) may visit a trusted clinician for testing, but health departments and Planned Parenthood facilities also offer confidential, low-cost testing and treatment for most STIs (see **It's Your Health** on where to get tested).

Symptoms for STIs may be painful and obvious, entirely absent, or mistaken for other conditions. If you think that you or your partner has a chance of being

Self-Assessment 7.1
Assessing Sexual Practices—Safety First for Sexual Health

Answer each of the following questions:

1.	I avoid having multiple or anonymous sex partners.	yes	no
2.	I avoid exchanging sex for money or drugs.	yes	no
3.	I use latex condoms, female condoms, or dental dams each time I have oral, anal, or vaginal sex with an untested partner.	yes	no
4.	I avoid sex with someone whom I don't know well or in situations where I may be in physical danger.	yes	no
5.	I avoid using intravenous drugs.	yes	no
6.	I avoid sex with anyone who has genital sores, lesions, or other obvious symptoms.	yes	no
7.	If I am having sexual contact with men, I take precautions to prevent unwanted pregnancy.	yes	no
8.	I avoid sexual activity while under the influence of drugs or alcohol.	yes	no
9.	I get regular Pap tests or have been tested for HPV.	yes	no

If you answered any of these questions with a "no," reconsider the risks involved with your personal sex behaviors and think about being tested for STIs.

infected, both you and your partner should curtail sexual activity and seek testing. Even if symptoms disappear, the disease may still be present, transmissible, and causing harm to the body. Treating one partner and not the other often results in a back-and-forth cycle of infection and reinfection. In addition, sharing one antibiotic prescription between two people usually means that neither partner receives adequate treatment and can contribute to antibiotic resistance. Using leftover antibiotics from previous infections is also ineffective because supplies are usually inappropriate and inadequate, and may serve merely to mask the symptoms, complicating an accurate diagnosis later. Curtail sexual activity or use latex condoms for every sexual encounter until both partners are certain of a cure.

Women are often embarrassed to mention their fears about STIs to a clinician. If you (or a friend or partner) have a risk of infection, discuss this possibility with a

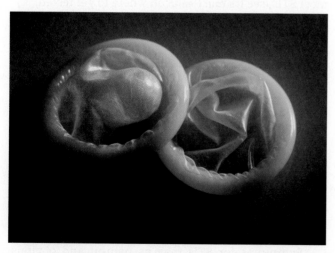

Latex condoms, although not a guarantee against infection, are a key component of risk reduction for STIs.
Courtesy of CDC

clinician. Although no one wants to find out that she has an STI, it is always better to know than not to know: STIs can be spread and do serious biological damage even in the absence of symptoms. Clinicians may not routinely test for STIs or look for them in a routine gynecological examination. If you or a partner has had a possible exposure through oral or anal sex, discuss that possibility with a clinician so that a comprehensive examination may be conducted. Finally, it helps to be prepared. Writing down a list of questions to ask a clinician and practicing questions to ask with a friend beforehand are two strategies women can use to make sure they get all the information they need without making additional visits.

A physical examination for STIs is often like a routine gynecological examination, but it is not limited to the genital area. An examination of the mouth, throat, and lymph nodes usually precedes the genital examination. The genital examination is conducted in a lithotomy position, which requires that the woman lie on her back with her legs spread and positioned in stirrups. This position enables the healthcare provider to examine the perineal area. The examination begins with a careful visual inspection by the clinician. A speculum is inserted into the vagina for an internal examination. The clinician then examines the vagina for discharge, odor, ulcerations, or inflammation.

If a woman has douched before the visit, the clinician may not be able to diagnose the condition accurately. A bimanual examination follows the internal examination.

Over spring break my boyfriend went skiing and he said he "slept around a little." So what should I do about protecting myself? I'm on the pill, but should we get tested or use a condom? I really am confused.

—22-year-old woman

(See Chapter 4 for details of the gynecological examination.) Any suspicious lesion in the perineal area is cultured, and a rectal culture is obtained if the woman has had anal intercourse.

Treatment Concerns

Treatment regimens for STIs vary according to the specific pathogen involved, severity of infection, location of infection, previous infections, and personal medical history. If you are being tested or receiving treatment for an STI, inform your clinician if you are taking any prescriptions or over-the-counter medications, or if you have had reactions to certain drugs in the past. If you think you are pregnant, advise the clinician of that possibility as well. Pregnant women should avoid some antibiotics because they can stain the permanent teeth of the developing fetus or cause other side effects.

Several STIs require follow-up examinations to ensure that the treatment regimen was successful. Failure to comply with follow-up guidelines may result in unsuccessful treatment and continued disease transmission and damage.

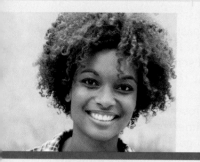
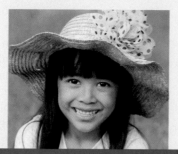
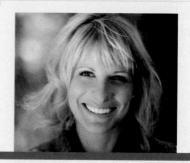
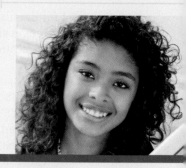

CASE STUDY

Christina and Marie are young women who have been going out together for some time. They have both had partners in the past—Christina has had male and female partners and Marie has only been with other women. Wanting to be safe and responsible, they got tested for STIs before engaging together in any sexual activity more risky than hugs and kisses. They were both negative for all the tests available at the local health department: HIV, gonorrhea, chlamydia, and syphilis.

Christina sometimes gets cold sores, and when she does, she makes sure she only kisses Marie on the cheek or on other unbroken skin, and does not perform oral sex on her partner until the sore has completely healed. However, 6 months into their relationship, Marie notices blister-like sores around her labia. She has never noticed anything like this in the past. Her doctor diagnoses her with herpes simplex virus. She feels very distressed.

Questions

1. Is there anything else that this couple should consider before starting sexual activity that will include oral sex and genital-to-genital touching?

2. How could Marie have acquired herpes? (Hint: there are multiple possibilities.)

3. What can Marie do to cope with her current outbreak?

4. How might she discuss this situation with Christina?

■ Summary

Sexually transmitted infections, which have been present throughout human history, are now at epidemic levels. Today, most people who are sexually active will be exposed to an STI during some point in their lives. STIs can be caused by bacteria, viruses, or parasites (**Table 7.3**). They can cause harm or permanent damage to the body even in the absence of symptoms and are a leading cause of infertility among women. Women (and men) who are

sexually active should take steps to reduce their risk, learn about STIs, and have themselves and their partners tested.

At the same time, it is also possible to overstate the dangers of STIs. All STIs can be treated in some fashion, and many STIs, if found early, can be cured completely. Most cases of HPV, the most common STI in the United

Profiles of Remarkable Women

Felicia Hance Stewart, MD (1943–2006)

Felicia Hance Stewart was an obstetrician/gynecologist who was also a distinguished clinician and researcher. Following her time as a practicing physician, Stewart served as deputy assistant secretary for population affairs in the Department of Health and Human Services, making her the most senior official in the United States responsible for domestic and international policies on family planning and population issues. In this position, she had direct responsibility for management of the National Family Planning Program (Title X) and the Adolescent Family Life Program (Title XX).

In 1996, Stewart was appointed as the director of reproductive health programs for the Henry J. Kaiser Family Foundation, where she focused on improving services for low-income women and preventing unintended pregnancy. In 1999, she joined the Center for Reproductive Health Research and Policy at the University of California, San Francisco. As a co-director of the center, Stewart conducted U.S. and international projects that spanned the disciplines of contraception, abortion, and sexually transmitted infections.

Stewart served as the principal investigator on many research projects and published numerous articles and textbooks on contraception and family planning. She contributed greatly to issues concerning reproductive health and, consequently, served on many national scientific and professional advisory and review committees. Stewart authored *Understanding Your Body: The Concerned Woman's Guide to Gynecology and Health,* a nontechnical reference book, and coauthored *Contraceptive Technology,* a professional reference for family planning. Stewart may be most remembered for her leading role in the research establishing that the emergency contraceptive known as Plan B is both safe and effective when sold without a physician's prescription. Her published research led to the availability of over-the-counter Plan B in a number of states, including California.

Table 7.3   Basic Information About the Major Sexually Transmitted Infections

AIDS (Acquired Immune Deficiency Syndrome)

Organism	Viral—HIV (human immunodeficiency virus)
Transmission	Blood or sexual fluids entering the body, usually through sexual intercourse, sharing needles, or from mother to child before or during birth
Symptoms	Flu-like symptoms such as fever, weight loss, fatigue, and enlarged lymph nodes may appear and disappear shortly after infection; identifiable opportunistic infections may take years to appear.
Diagnosis	AIDS diagnoses are made based on T-cell counts or the presence of opportunistic infections; HIV can easily be identified with antibody tests.
Treatment	No treatment will prevent HIV infection or rid the body of HIV; however, antiviral medications, when used properly, can delay the onset of AIDS and improve quality of life.
Special concerns for women	Increased reproductive health problems; possible perinatal (mother-to-child) transmission (can be dramatically reduced with treatment)
Potential long-term consequences	If AIDS goes untreated, opportunistic infections can cause grave illness or death.

Chlamydia

Organism	Bacteria—*Chlamydia trachomatis*
Transmission	Direct contact with infected mucosal membrane or sexual fluids
Symptoms	Most women are asymptomatic; symptoms may include vaginal discharge and excessive urination, pelvic pain, fever, and nausea.
Diagnosis	Urine tests or culture of symptoms or discharge; alternatively, a diagnosis may be made by examining symptoms and ruling out gonorrhea.
Treatment	Antibiotics will stop infection but may not be able to repair damage from long-term infection.
Special concerns for women	Pelvic inflammatory disease (see PID), possible coinfection with gonorrhea; reinfection with an untreated partner; perinatal (mother-to-child) transmission
Potential long-term consequences	Infertility, ectopic pregnancy, chronic pelvic pain, possibility of systemic infection

Gonorrhea

Organism	Bacteria—*Neisseria gonorrhoeae*
Transmission	Direct contact with infected mucosal membrane or sexual fluids
Symptoms	Most women are asymptomatic; symptoms may include vaginal discharge and excessive urination, pelvic pain, fever, and nausea.
Diagnosis	Urine tests or culture of discharge or the infected area
Treatment	Antibiotics will stop infection but may not be able to repair damage from long-term infection.
Special concerns for women	Pelvic inflammatory disease (PID); possible coinfection with chlamydia; reinfection with an untreated partner; perinatal transmission
Potential long-term consequences	Infertility, ectopic pregnancy, chronic pelvic pain, possibility of systemic infection

Hepatitis B (HBV)

Organism	Virus—hepatitis B virus
Transmission	Entrance of blood or sexual fluids into the body; most cases occur through unprotected sexual contact or shared needles.
Symptoms	Often asymptomatic; symptoms include nausea, fever, dark urine, jaundice (yellowing of the skin and eyes), and abdominal discomfort.

(continues)

Table 7.3   Basic Information About the Major Sexually Transmitted Infections (continued)

Diagnosis	Blood tests to identify virus or antibodies; liver tests and symptoms may also be used in diagnosis.
Treatment	No cure for hepatitis B exists, but antiviral medications may help in some chronic cases; a three-shot vaccine will prevent hepatitis B infection; most infants born in the United States after 1982 have received this vaccine.
Special concerns for women	Perinatal transmission
Potential long-term consequences	Possible liver disease or liver cancer in chronic cases; most infections eventually resolve on their own.

Herpes Simplex Virus (HSV)

Organism	Virus—herpes simplex (two types—1 and 2)
Transmission	Direct contact with symptoms; contact with the infected area carries a low but real risk even without symptoms.
Symptoms	Painful sores, blisters, or rashes on the genital area, rectum, or mouth that appear and disappear periodically; women may be asymptomatic or have symptoms in the cervical area that go unnoticed.
Diagnosis	Examination or culture of symptoms; blood tests can identify herpes antibodies.
Treatment	No cure or vaccine available; some antiviral medications can reduce duration or number of outbreaks.
Special concerns for women	Possible perinatal transmission, especially if herpes infection takes place during pregnancy; herpes sores may increase the likelihood of receiving HIV or other STIs if exposed.
Potential long-term consequences	Rare in otherwise healthy adults; severity, duration, and frequency of symptoms usually diminish over time.

HPV (Human Papillomavirus)

Organism	Virus—human papillomavirus (almost 100 strains, about a dozen of which are sexually transmitted)
Transmission	Genital skin-to-genital skin contact
Symptoms	"High-risk" strains of HPV can cause abnormal cell growth on the cervix; if untreated, this cell growth (dysplasia) can sometimes advance to cervical cancer. Other, "low-risk" strains can cause warts to appear on the external genital or anal areas in men or women.
Diagnosis	Warts may be diagnosed by physical examination; cervical dysplasia may be diagnosed with biopsy; DNA testing of the virus can identify the presence of HPV.
Treatment	Abnormal cell changes in the cervix may be treated by cryotherapy, loop electrosurgical excision procedure (LEEP), cone biopsy, or laser surgery. Treatment for genital warts revolves around removing symptoms, not eliminating the virus, and consists of topical caustic agents, electrocautery, cryotherapy, and laser surgery.
Special concerns for women	Cervical changes, if untreated, may develop into cervical cancer; warts may interfere with pregnancy in rare cases.
Potential long-term consequences	Cervical dysplasia can lead to cervical cancer if undiagnosed or untreated; most cases of HPV go away on their own eventually.

Pelvic Inflammatory Disease (PID)

Organism	Bacteria—usually *Chlamydia trachomatis* (chlamydia) or *Neisseria gonorrhoeae* (gonorrhea)
Transmission	PID itself is not transmitted but usually develops as a complication of gonorrhea or chlamydia.
Symptoms	Cases may be asymptomatic; abdominal pain or pain during intercourse, unusual vaginal discharge or bleeding, fever, and nausea.
Diagnosis	Clinical evaluation based on symptoms and possible presence of a causative bacterial agent
Treatment	Antibiotics; surgery may be necessary in advanced cases.
Special concerns for women	Reinfection of bacterial infection from untreated or undertreated partners; possible perinatal transmission of bacterial agent
Potential long-term consequences	Infertility, ectopic pregnancy, recurrent infection, chronic pelvic pain

Table 7.3	**Basic Information About the Major Sexually Transmitted Infections (continued)**
Syphilis	
Organism	Bacteria—*Treponema pallidum*
Transmission	Skin-to-skin contact with infected area or symptoms; perinatal transmission
Symptoms	Primary stage: painless sore (chancre)
	Secondary stage: rash, hair loss, enlarged lymph nodes
	Tertiary stage: systemic damage
Diagnosis	Blood test; microscopic verification of organism; examination of symptoms
Treatment	Antibiotics will stop infection but cannot undo systemic damage.
Special concerns for women	Perinatal transmission; possible reinfection from untreated or undertreated partners; sores may increase likelihood of receiving HIV or other STIs if exposed.
Potential long-term consequences	Untreated infections can cause permanent damage to all major body systems or even death.
Trichomoniasis	
Organism	Single-celled protozoan—*Trichomonas vaginalis*
Transmission	Direct sexual contact; less likely through contaminated wet objects (towels, swimming suits)
Symptoms	Many women and most men are asymptomatic; symptoms may include white or greenish yellow discharge, vaginal itching, or painful urination.
Diagnosis	Examination of symptoms or culture of infected area
Treatment	Oral antibiotics
Special concerns for women	Reinfection from untreated or undertreated partners
Potential long-term consequences	Rare for otherwise healthy women

States, resolve on their own without causing any harm. In the right environment, and with the right partner, sexual activity is an enjoyable part of the human experience. Practices such as monogamy, using latex condoms, and having one's sexual partners tested for STIs offer the chance to reduce the risk for STIs and enjoy sex in a healthy relationship.

◼ Topics for Discussion

1. From a biological perspective, how do STIs affect women more than they affect men? What are some cultural or psychological factors that make STIs more difficult for women? Are there any cultural or psychological factors that make STIs more difficult for men?

2. Infection rates for many STIs continue to be highest among young people (typically defined as around 15–24 years old). What are some reasons for this? What would you recommend to increase prevention or encourage testing or treatment among this group?

3. What challenges do global HIV/AIDS treatment efforts face? How do these challenges compare to those facing HIV/AIDS treatment efforts based in the United States?

4. Imagine that you are in a relationship and that you have an infection with HSV or HPV. How and when would you begin discussing your infection? How would you feel if the situation were reversed?

5. What are some productive ways to begin a conversation with a potential partner about STIs? How and where would you begin such a conversation?

6. In spite of the knowledge base about AIDS, people still report a strong fear of AIDS. Why? What myths or rumors have you heard about HIV?

7. How does the HIV testing process work? What should a woman do upon learning of a positive HIV antibody test?

8. Herpes and HPV are similar to HIV in that they are sexually transmitted viruses without a cure. How are they different from HIV?

9. What would you tell a friend or loved one who suspected that she might have an STI but was afraid to get tested?

10. Balancing STI risk reduction with flexibility and intimacy in sexual relationships is a difficult task for many people. How do you balance these two needs? Are these two needs always in opposition to each other?

■ Key Terms

AIDS (acquired immune deficiency syndrome)

Asymptomatic viral shedding

Bacteria

Bacterial vaginosis (BV)

Chlamydia

Ectoparasitic infections

Enzyme-linked immunosorbent assay (ELISA)

Gonorrhea

Hepatitis

Herpes simplex virus (HSV)

HIV (human immunodeficiency virus)

Human papillomavirus (HPV)

Immune system

Jaundice

Opportunistic infections

Pelvic inflammatory disease (PID)

Prodrome

Pus

Retrovirus

Sexually transmitted infections (STIs)

Sitz baths

Syphilis

Toxic shock syndrome (TSS)

Trichomoniasis

Viruses

Western blot test

Yeast infection

■ References

1. Satterwhite, C., Torrone, E., Meites, E., et al. (2013). Sexually transmitted infections among US women and men. *Sexually Transmitted Diseases* 40(3): 187–193.

2. Hanson, J., Ponser, S., Hassig, S., et al. (2005). Assessment of sexually transmitted diseases as a risk factor for seroconversion in a New Orleans sexually transmitted disease clinic, 1990–1998. *Annals of Epidemiology* 15(1): 13–20.

3. Centers for Disease Control and Prevention (CDC). (2010). Sexually transmitted disease treatment guidelines. *Morbidity and Mortality Weekly Report* 59: 1–109.

4. CDC. (2014). *Sexually transmitted diseases surveillance 2012.* Atlanta, GA: U.S. Department of Health and Human Services. Available at: http://www.cdc.gov/std/stats12/

5. Chesson, H., Blandford, J., Thomas, L., et al. (2004). The estimated direct medical costs of sexually transmitted disease among American youth, 2000. *Perspectives on Sexual and Reproductive Health* 36(1): 11–19.

6. World Health Organization. (2014). *Fact Sheet: HIV/AIDS.* Available at: http://www.who.int/mediacentre/factsheets/fs360/en/

7. Rietmejer, C., Van Bemmelen, R., Judson, F., et al. (2002). Incidence and repeat infection rates of *Chlamydia trachomatis* infections among male and female patients in an STD clinic: Implications for screening and rescreening. *Sexually Transmitted Diseases* 29: 65–72.

8. Adderley-Kelly, B., & Stephens, E. (2005). Chlamydia—A major threat to adolescents and young adults. *Association of Black Nursing Faculty* May/June: 52–55.

9. Sweet, R., & Gibbs, R. (2012). Infectious diseases of the female genital tract. Philadelphia, PA: Lippincott Williams & Wilkins.

10. Schwebke, J., & Desmond, R. (2005). Risk factors for bacterial vaginosis in women at high risk for sexually transmitted diseases. *Sexually Transmitted Diseases* 32(11): 654–658.

11. Esber, A., Vicetti, M., Cherpes, T., et al. (2015). Risk of bacterial vaginosis among women with herpes simplex virus type 2 infection: A systematic review and meta-analysis. *Journal of Infectious Diseases.* 212(1): 8–17.

12. Klebanoff, M., Schwebke, J., Zhang, J., et al. (2004). Vulvo-vaginal symptoms in women with bacterial vaginosis. *Obstetrics and Gynecology* 104: 267.

13. Zhang, J., Hatch, M., Zhang, D., et al. (2004). Frequency of douching and risk of bacterial vaginosis in African-American women. *Obstetrics and Gynecology* 104: 756–760.

14. Schiffman, M., & Castle, P. (2005). The promise of global cervical-cancer prevention. *New England Journal of Medicine* 353(20): 2101–2104.

15. Bradley, H., Markowitz, L., Gibson, T., et al. (2013). Seroprevalence of herpes simplex virus types 1 and 2—United States, 1999–2010. *Journal of Infectious Diseases* 209(3): 325–333.

16. Dungan, J. (2009). Single-day, patient-initiated famciclovir therapy versus 3-day valacyclovir regimen for recurrent genital herpes: A randomized, double-blind, comparative trial. *Yearbook of Obstetrics, Gynecology and Women's Health* 2009: 193–194.

17. Holmes, K., Levine, R., & Weaver, M. (2004). Effectiveness of condoms in preventing sexually transmitted diseases. *Bulletin of the World Health Organization* 82(6): 454–461.

18. CDC. (2013). *Viral hepatitis surveillance, 2012.* Atlanta, GA: U.S. Department of Health and Human Services.

19. Prejean, J., Song, R., Hernandez, A., et al. (2011). Estimated HIV incidence in the United States, 2006–2009. *PLoS ONE.* 6(8): e17502. doi:10.1371/journal.pone.0017502

20. HIV outbreak began decades earlier than thought. (October 1, 2008). *Washington Post.* Available at: http://www.washingtonpost.com/wp-dyn/content/article/2008/10/01/AR2008100101660.html

21. Joint U.N. Programme on AIDS. (2010). *2008 report on the global AIDS epidemic.* Geneva: UNAIDS.

22. CDC. (2012). Estimated HIV incidence in the United States, 2007–2010. *HIV Surveillance Supplemental Report* 2012 17(4).

23. Bunders, M., Bekker, V., Scherpbier, H., et al. (2005). Haematological parameters of HIV-1 uninfected infants born to HIV-1 infected mothers. *Acta Paediatrica* 94(11): 1571–1577.

24. CDC. (2013). *Condom effectiveness: Fact sheet for public health personnel.* Available at: http://www.cdc.gov/condomeffectiveness/latex.html

CHAPTER 8

Menopause and Hormone Therapy

Learning Objectives

On completion of this chapter, the student should be able to discuss:

1. Menopause as a biological event, as well as physiological changes that occur before, during, and after menopause.

2. How social, cultural, and demographic changes over the past 100 years have affected how women experience and think about menopause.

3. The biology of natural menopause, as well as factors that can cause early menopause.

4. Symptoms and complications of menopause.

5. The concept of "medicalization" and how medicalization has affected women's experiences during midlife.

6. Both major forms of hormone replacement, as well as their potential benefits and health risks.

7. The history of hormone use for menopause management.

8. How the Women's Health Initiative and Million Women Study have advanced our understanding of hormone therapy.

9. Medical and nonmedical options for managing menopause.

10. Concerns with "bio-identical" hormone products.

11. Informed decision-making strategies for women about menopause.

INTRODUCTION

As they reach midlife, women experience menopause, the end of their menstrual cycles. Menopause is not synonymous with midlife; it is a biological event that brings both physical and emotional changes. Menopause, a topic that was once not discussed in public, is now recognized as an important women's health issue. While women now are better informed about menopause than before, many women continue to lack basic information, such as its effects on the body, the potential benefits and drawbacks to hormone therapy, and other forms of menopause management.

This chapter reviews how cultural and social attitudes about aging and medicine have influenced attitudes about menopause, the negative and positive effects that menopause can have on a woman's life, the basic biology of menopause, how and when menopause occurs, and the health effects of menopause. In addition, the chapter discusses the medicalization of menopause, the history of hormone use to manage menopause, and the two major studies about menopause and their results. The chapter concludes with informed decision-making guidance for women and the special caution to be exercised with popular "bio-identical" menopausal therapies.

SOCIAL AND CULTURAL REFLECTIONS ON MENOPAUSE

Because menopause is a natural aging process, all women who live to enjoy their later years will experience it. However, it was not until the 20th century that the life expectancy reached a point where most women lived much beyond menopause. Today most women will live one-third or more of their lives postmenopausally. As the median age of the population continues to increase (see **Figure 8.1**), a growing proportion of women will have experienced, or will be experiencing, menopause. Nearly a million women—about 18% of the total female population—are currently between the ages of 45 and 54, the age group at which menopause most often begins.[1]

Over the past century, the medical and public health research has furthered our understanding of the clinical and demographical dimensions of menopause. However, the media coverage and public discussions of this emerging research, along with alternative management options, have often been inaccurate, misunderstood, or exaggerated. As a result, many women remain unsure about how to best manage many of the natural symptoms associated with menopause.

In the United States, where society values and media emphasis are on youthful behaviors and appearance in women, menopause has often been viewed as a negative event. This trend is not universal. In many Asian countries, for example, women have traditionally gained respect and influence, often becoming the head of the household, as

they reached middle age. In the United States, popular culture has portrayed menopause as a difficult time for women, focusing on experiences of uncontrollable moodiness, irritability, and depression. In the 1800s and early 1900s, popular myths and stereotypes, often encouraged by the medical community, depicted menopause as a tragedy that caused hypochondria, hysteria, and irritability. This view implied that solace from these conditions could be found only in a physician's office with pharmacological remedies or surgical intervention. In the 1940s and 1950s, treatment for menopause often focused on psychiatric conditions of depression and melancholy.

Popular culture depicted menopausal women as burdens to themselves, to their families, and, if they were married, to their suffering husbands. In subsequent decades, menopause was examined as a "disease," with clinical concern focused on women reporting symptoms and seeking medical intervention for specific symptom relief. An explosion of commercial pharmacological options and the heavy marketing of them to clinicians and women made the situation even more complicated.

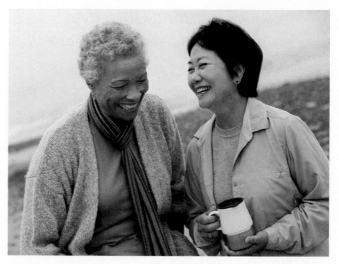

Women today are more open in their discussions about all aspects of their sexual well-being, including menopause.
© IPGGutenbergUKLtd/Getty Images

Now menopause is understood as a natural, predictable biological process, not a medical illness or a disease. Open discussions about sexuality and life issues have allowed women to talk about menopause and aging without fear, embarrassment, or stigmatization. Many women either welcome menopause or do not fear it. The cessation of menses frees them from contraceptive concerns, in some cases leading to increased sexual satisfaction. Other women appreciate the freedom from menstrual periods, which may have been inconvenient or uncomfortable. Menopause may be a time of fewer family obligations, accompanied by increased opportunities in the workforce. For some, this life stage is more flexible in terms of leisure time and financial resources, increasing the opportunities for new forms of activity and self-expression. For others, it is merely the continuation of intense work, with many

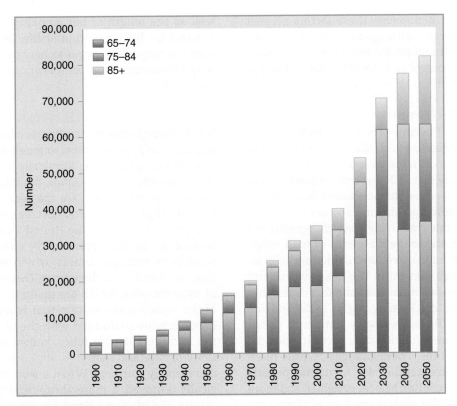

Figure 8.1   **Older population by age, 1900–2050.**

Source: U.S. Census Bureau. (2000).

women taking on childcare responsibilities for grandchildren or caring for their own parents.

While the symptoms of menopause, as well as how those symptoms are perceived, vary from woman to woman, all women should understand the biological and psychological factors associated with this important and inevitable life change. A survey found significant information gaps remain about menopause in all age groups. In fact, almost one in four women (24%) said they have more information about symptoms and treatments for erectile dysfunction for men than they have about menopause for women.[2]

MENOPAUSE

Also known as the climacterium or "change of life," menopause marks the end of menstruation and childbearing capability. Menopause is the permanent end of menstruation and fertility, officially occurring 12 months after a woman's last menstrual period. The transitional stage immediately before menopause is called **perimenopause**. During this period, physical changes begin to accelerate and women are most likely to experience perceptible physical changes as production of estrogen and other hormones diminishes. These symptoms usually last about 1 year after a woman's last menstrual period. **Postmenopause** follows menopause and lasts the rest of a woman's life.

Like the onset of a girl's first period, the age of onset of menopause varies. Most women enter and complete menopause between the ages of 45 and 55, with the average age of natural menopause being 51.[3] Many factors influence the age at which a woman has her last period, including family history, environmental factors, personal behaviors, and genetics.[4] Menopause is considered "late" when it occurs after age 55. Late menopause may provide a moderate protective effect for premature death.[5] Early or premature menopause, typically defined as menopause that occurs before age 40, may also occur as the result of hysterectomy—surgical removal of the uterus (sometimes including the ovaries)—exposure to some types of chemotherapy, naturally occurring ovary failure, or other circumstances. Early menopause is a potential risk factor for cardiovascular disease.[6] Women who smoke, have not graduated from college, or are unemployed, or have had heart disease all reach natural menopause sooner than other women. Although it is hard to determine the

I was diagnosed with breast cancer at age 27. I went through a couple of months of chemotherapy, which was effective in eliminating the cancer. I know I'm very lucky, and I'm glad the treatment worked, but as a side effect I'm going through menopause, with hot flashes and all the other symptoms. It's a lot to go through, both intellectually and emotionally. I'm still trying to wrap my head around it.

—33-year-old woman

exact causes of early menopause, these factors suggest that poor health may reduce the age at which menopause naturally occurs. Late menopausal women are more likely to have taken birth control pills, be ethnically Japanese, and to have given birth.[7]

Biology of Natural Menopause

Natural menopause occurs when the ovaries stop responding to the luteinizing and follicle-stimulating hormones that are produced in the anterior pituitary gland.[8] As a woman reaches her late 30s, her ovaries produce less **estrogen** and **progesterone**, the hormones that regulate menstruation. As a result, ovulation becomes somewhat erratic. The mechanisms underlying these changes are not fully understood. Whatever the reasons, a woman entering menopause will have more luteinizing and follicle-stimulating hormones present in the bloodstream and less estrogen and progesterone than she had during her regular menstrual cycling. Fertility begins to decline due to these hormonal effects. Pregnancy remains a possibility, however, because ovulation may occur in sporadic intervals during this time. These changes become more pronounced as women enter their 40s. Menstrual periods may become longer or shorter, heavier or lighter, and more or less frequent until the ovaries cease to produce eggs and periods end. Early in the transition process, many women experience 2-week cycles. Further into the process, women may skip periods for months at a time, with skipped periods often followed by a heavier period. The number of consecutively skipped periods increases as the time of the last period approaches. Natural menopause occurs when the ovaries fail to respond to the luteinizing and follicle-stimulating hormones produced in the anterior pituitary, which is under the control of the hypothalamus. Menopause is considered complete once monthly periods have ceased altogether for at least 12 months.

> *I guess that I was one of the lucky ones. My menopause was fairly short and easy. One of my friends had severe hot flashes and another friend was moody. Menopause has been different for each of us, but we all got through it in one piece.*
>
> **—55-year-old woman**

After menopause, women continue to produce estrogen, mostly through the adrenal glands, which makes precursors of estrogen that stored fat converts to estrogen. Far less estrogen, however, is produced in this manner than was produced in the ovaries before menopause.

Smoking can also influence the biology of menopause. Women who smoke produce less estrogen and tend to experience menopause earlier than nonsmoking women. In addition, women who smoke, or who were exposed to secondhand smoke, are also at increased risk for some complications associated with menopause, such as osteoporosis. The number of cigarettes a woman smokes, as well as the length of her smoking habit both increase her risk for fractures in later life. In addition, smokers with fractures take longer to heal than nonsmokers and may experience more complications during the healing process.[9]

Menopause and Hysterectomies

While menopause most often occurs as a natural consequence of aging, it can also result as the consequence of a medical procedure. "Surgically induced menopause" happens with **hysterectomies**, the surgical removal of the uterus. Hysterectomies are the second most frequently performed procedure, after cesarean sections, on women of reproductive age in the United States.[10] They are performed for certain reproductive cancers and for other conditions such as fibroids, which are benign growths that can develop on the uterus. There are different types of hysterectomy, which are distinguished by the extent of the reproductive system that is removed (**Figure 8.2**). Hysterectomy performed with the removal of both ovaries and the fallopian tubes, known as a **total hysterectomy** or **bilateral salpingo-oophorectomy**, has become increasingly common. When a woman's ovaries are surgically removed, a more abrupt and earlier menopause results. The pituitary gland continues to produce luteinizing and follicle-stimulating hormones, but the ovaries are not present to respond with ovulation. The body no longer produces estrogen and progesterone at the same level as it did before the removal of the ovaries. Women who have had both ovaries removed before the onset of menopause experience more severe menopausal symptoms.[11] Hysterectomy in women aged 50 years or younger increases the risk for cardiovascular disease later in life; oophorectomy appears to increase the risk of both coronary heart disease and stroke.[12]

This high prevalence of surgical procedures continues to be controversial. Hysterectomies can have serious, lifelong consequences for women, yet women often either receive little information about these consequences or have little chance to consider them. Close to 500,000 hysterectomies are performed annually in the United States, and approximately 20 million U.S. women have had a hysterectomy.[13] More than one-third (37%) of hysterectomies with oophorectomy are performed on women aged 15 to 44 years; the majority of these procedures are performed for benign (noncancerous) conditions.[10] The frequency of hysterectomy also varies greatly by geography and race. Hysterectomies are more common in the Midwest and South than in the comparatively more well off Northeast or Western regions of the United States (**Figure 8.3**); they are also about four times more likely to be performed on Black, as opposed to White, women.[10] These differences may be due in part to differences in medical need (Black women are more likely than White women to develop fibroids, a common underlying reason for hysterectomy). However, it is likely that socioeconomic and cultural factors, including cultural beliefs, geographic/

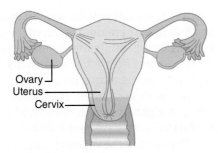

Partial hysterectomy: only the uterus is removed.

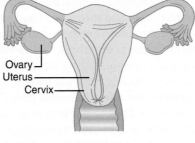

Total hysterectomy: both the uterus and cervix are removed.

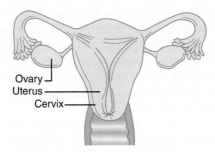

Total hysterectomy with bilateral salpingo-oophorectomy: both ovaries, the fallopian tubes, the uterus, and the cervix are removed.

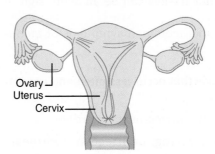

Radical hysterectomy: both ovaries, the fallopian tubes, the uterus, the cervix, and the lymph nodes are removed.

Figure 8.2   Four types of hysterectomy.

racial differences in patient–physician communication, and physician preference, play a larger role.[10] In addition to being more likely to undergo hysterectomy, minority women and women living in the South and Midwest are also more likely to undergo hysterectomies that are more

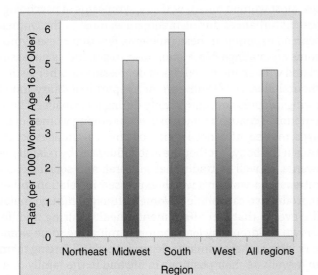

Figure 8.3   Hysterectomy rates by geographic region: United States.

Source: Wu, J., Wechter M., Geller E., et al. (2007). Hysterectomy rates in the United States, 2003.

invasive and require additional recovery time.[13] Further study is needed to investigate the reasons behind these differences and to make sure that all women have access to care and the ability to make fully informed decisions about their health.

In addition to hysterectomies, chemotherapy and/or radiation therapy, which are common cancer treatments, can induce menopause. Menopausal symptoms such as hot flashes often present during the course of treatment or within 3 to 6 months.

Primary ovarian insufficiency is another condition that results in early menopause. Approximately 1% of women experience menopause before the age of 40.[14] This condition may result from failure of the ovaries to produce normal levels of reproductive hormones. The condition may be due to genetic factors or autoimmune disorders, but for many women, the primary cause is not known.

Menopause Symptoms

Hormonal changes during menopause affect women physically and emotionally (Figure 8.2). Studies examining menopause show considerable variance in the prevalence of symptoms, especially severe symptoms. The duration and severity of symptoms for any individual woman cannot be predicted in advance.

The most frequently reported physical symptom is the vascular response or instability due to hormonal fluctuations, also known as **hot flashes** or hot flushes. Hot flashes are uncomfortable sensations of internally generated heat, beginning in the chest and moving to the neck and head, or spreading throughout the body. Increased heart rate and temperature, shallow breathing, and sweating followed by chills are all common during hot flashes. In some women, hot flashes actually raise the body temperature by a few degrees in just a few minutes. Despite the discomfort they cause, hot flashes are generally not considered harmful to a woman's health. In addition, a significant number of women do not find them disturbing.[15] Hot flashes often begin before a woman has stopped menstruating, and then continue for several years after menopause. Early hot flashes can be an acute sign of estrogen deficiency.

Besides hot flashes, common symptoms of menopause include:[16,17]

- Menstrual periods that occur less often and eventually stop
- Decreased fertility, progressing to infertility
- Heart pounding, racing, or irregular heartbeats (palpitations)
- Night sweats
- Skin flushing
- Sleep disturbances
- Decreased interest in sex and decreased response to sexual stimulation
- Forgetfulness
- Increased abdominal fat
- Thinning hair
- Loss of breast fullness
- Headaches
- Mood swings including irritability, depression, and anxiety
- Urine leakage
- Vaginal dryness and painful sexual intercourse
- Vaginal infections
- Joint aches and pains

Menopausal symptoms also vary depending on the woman's lifestyle, menstrual status, race/ethnicity, and socioeconomic status.[18] Cross-cultural studies suggest that there are significant ethnic differences in the frequency and severity of the total physical, psychological, and psychosomatic symptoms, as well as in how women interpret and report these symptoms.[19,20] African American women often present with menopausal symptoms earlier than White women, while Asian American women seem to have the fewest symptoms.[18] Symptoms such as mood changes, fatigue, and vaginal dryness tend to be more common and more severe for Hispanic women.[17,20]

It is often difficult for women to directly connect any or all of these symptoms with menopause. Other factors such as aging, family life, health issues, work, and home stresses can affect what symptoms women experience and how women interpret them. Symptoms can also interact with each other. Hot flashes, for example, often occur at night, disrupting sleep and contributing to much of the insomnia associated with menopause.

Thinning of the vaginal lining, known as **vaginal atrophy,** also sometimes occurs after menopause. As estrogen levels decline, layers of the vaginal surface become drier and more sensitive. The vaginal wall becomes thinner, less elastic, and more vulnerable to infection. Some women experience pain or burning during intercourse, vaginal discharge, and more frequent vaginal infections. Physiological changes that affect the vaginal tract may affect a woman's sexual response as well. For example, lack of vaginal lubricant may affect sexual arousal. A change in hormone levels—specifically androgen production—may diminish libido.

Other symptoms associated with menopause include breast changes, changes in hair growth, and changes in skin. As estrogen levels decrease during menopause, a rapid loss of collagen occurs, causing the skin to become thinner and less elastic. In addition, the cycling levels of hormones may cause a change in the prevalence or intensity of headaches.[21]

The medical community has associated a variety of psychiatric and mental health conditions either with menopause or the physical symptoms it causes. These conditions include postpartum psychosis and depression, premenstrual syndrome, post-hysterectomy depression, and menopausal psychiatric syndromes. Many of these associations have been based on myths, stereotypes, unwarranted assumptions, and methodically flawed studies. Most women have few, if any, symptoms of psychological disturbances during menopause; most of the women who do experience these problems feel that these symptoms are manageable. Menopause, in general, is not associated with an increased risk of depression or other lasting mental illnesses.[22] Some women report irritability, mood swings, depression, and anxiety during menopause. These emotional changes, which also occur among women of all ages, may be influenced in part by physical changes occurring in the body, but they are also influenced by related life events, as well as traditional, cultural, and social expectations of a woman's worth expressed in relation to her reproductive capabilities. Women often go through major life events that can affect mental health during midlife. Grown children may leave home, eliminating some women's view of their primary role as mother and forcing them to reevaluate their positions in life and in the family unit. A menopausal woman's parents may die or need chronic care, causing grief, stress, and additional work.

Medication or counseling may help women who experience severe symptoms. Estrogen has been correlated with a positive effect on mood and overall sense of well-being, and it appears to be important for memory and mental functioning. As with all hormone-related issues, sensitivity and validation by a woman's physician is an important component of any treatment.

Menopause Complications

The dramatic reduction in estrogen production that occurs after menopause is associated with three major chronic complications: cardiovascular disease, osteoporosis, and urinary incontinence. Of these, cardiovascular disease, the leading cause of death in women and men (see Chapter 10), is by far the most serious. During a woman's reproductive years, the regular doses of estrogen produced by the ovaries may provide a protective effect against cardiovascular disease. While the average risk for heart attack begins to increase around age 45 for men, this risk does not increase until around age 50 for women. As estrogen levels drop during menopause, however, this protective effect wears off. A woman's risk for a heart attack, which begins to rise in the perimenopausal years, continues to increase after menopause. Lower-than-usual levels of estrogen after menopause also increase the risk for developing cardiovascular disease in the smaller blood vessels.[15,20]

Osteoporosis, the loss of bone mass or bone density that leads to brittle bones that are more likely to fracture, and **osteopenia**, a related but less severe condition (see Chapter 11), are also serious concerns for many postmenopausal women. Osteoporosis is far more prevalent in women than men, and smaller and thinner women are at more risk than larger women. Osteoporosis tends to present in individuals with a family history of the disease.[21] It is a serious problem for many elderly women; falls resulting from or leading to bone fractures are a major cause of death and disability in older women. Postmenopausal women are especially susceptible to fractures of their hips, wrists, and spine.[15] Bone loss is particularly rapid in the first few years following menopause. During this time, the spine may also lose flexibility and begin to curve. The prevalence of reduced bone density in older women varies by race and ethnicity. Low bone density and osteoporosis are most common among non-Hispanic White and Asian women.[22]

Urinary incontinence is another possible complication of menopause. As the vagina and urethra lose their elasticity, some women may also experience atrophy of the urinary tract. Diminished muscle tone may result in urinary incontinence. Some women also experience longer or more frequent urinary tract infections.

Many women gain weight after menopause. Estrogen appears to help regulate body weight; with lower estrogen levels, metabolic rates drop and it is easier to gain weight. However, other factors also influence weight gain during this time. Some women become less active and exercise less as they age. Physical inactivity leads to lost muscle mass, which also decreases resting metabolism, making it easier to gain weight. In addition, aerobic capacity declines with age, so for women to use the same energy as in the past and lose weight, they need to increase the amount and intensity of their physical exercise.

Some researchers have hypothesized a connection between menopause and dementia, but the evidence for these associations has generally been weak. They speculated that the loss of estrogen in older women might affect the development of **Alzheimer's disease**, because more women than men have the disease and almost two-thirds of all Americans living with Alzheimer's are women.[23] However, studies examining the association of hormones and menopause have found conflicting results.[24] A more likely explanation for the larger proportion of older women with Alzheimer's disease or other dementia appears to be the fact that women live longer than men. Experts now conclude that women are *not* more likely than men to develop dementia at any given age.[23]

MEDICALIZATION OF MENOPAUSE

"Medicalization" is a process in which societies or individuals define and treat basic human conditions as medical problems to be solved or cured. These conditions thus become the subjects of medical study, diagnosis, prevention, or treatment. Medicalization may begin as a legitimate attempt to help individuals with severe symptoms or as part of a scientific effort to better understand a condition. However, medicalization can also have other harmful effects. When a topic becomes medicalized, education to consumers and clinicians often becomes framed in medical jargon and in "solutions" that typically earn profits for the medical community. Once a significant proportion of society accepts a condition as a medical problem, this model dominates other social models for management and understanding. Individuals with medicalized conditions, especially women, have often been encouraged to cede their authority and responsibility for self-care to doctors and medical professionals (who are often men), who "know best."

In the United States, both childbirth and menopause have been heavily medicalized. Many have suggested that menopause in the United States became medicalized during the middle of the 20th century when it was promoted as an estrogen-deficiency disease. Proponents of medicalizing menopause assert that all (or at least many) dimensions of a woman's aging are directly linked to the shutdown of her estrogen production. By providing an outside source of estrogen to the body through the use of hormone therapy, these experts argue, many of the negative effects of menopause can be avoided or delayed. This line of reasoning has been behind the use of hormone therapy.

Hormone Therapy

Hormone therapy has been the standard treatment for symptoms of menopause for the past 70 years. The idea behind these therapies has been to replace or supplement the hormone levels that fall during menopause. While hormone therapy primarily has been used to treat symptoms of menopause, it has also been studied extensively for potential harmful and beneficial effects on health. These studies have produced conflicting results. In 2002, the Women's Health Initiative (WHI), a major clinical trial, found increased risks for breast cancer and heart disease associated with hormone therapy, but also slightly reduced risks for colorectal cancer and fractures. While millions of women stopped taking hormone therapy as a result, hormone therapy remains a common treatment today.

Modern hormone therapy comes in two primary forms: estrogen alone or estrogen and either progesterone or progestin (a synthetic form of progesterone). Estrogen alone is usually prescribed for women who do not have a uterus. If a woman's uterus is intact, her hormone therapy is typically a combination of estrogen and progesterone: The addition of progesterone to the therapy prevents estrogen from raising the woman's risk for uterine cancer. The ideal regimen, if any, for a woman will depend on her own symptoms, risks, and feelings; flexibility and discussion with a healthcare provider are key to determining the correct dose and form of hormone therapy for each individual.

The FDA has approved many hormone products for use in hormone therapy; these products have received extensive testing, are manufactured under precise criteria for uniformity, and are only available with a medical prescription (**Table 8.1**). The prescriptions are available as pills, patches (transdermally), creams, gels, or sprays. Vaginal creams, suppositories, tablets, or rings that release hormones within the vagina are also available. Oral preparations are prescribed most frequently. Women can take hormone therapy daily, or only on certain days of the month. Each of these methods has dose options that can be tailored to a woman's preferences and symptoms. Hormone therapy delivered through the skin and low-dose oral estrogen may have lower risks of blood clots

and strokes than standard doses of oral estrogen. Vaginal creams containing estrogen can help women whose only symptom is vaginal dryness, but they do not appear to provide other benefits, such as relief from hot flashes. Transdermal application of hormone therapy can benefit women whose livers respond to oral doses of estrogen by deactivating it with enzymes that raise triglyceride levels, which contributes to heart disease. However, oral doses of estrogen increase levels of HDL cholesterol ("good" cholesterol) for some women. Long-term studies are under way to evaluate these newer hormone delivery options and their associated risks and benefits.[25] Despite recent controversy and negative study results, the hormone therapy market continues to grow and is estimated to reach $3.04 billion in 2017.[26]

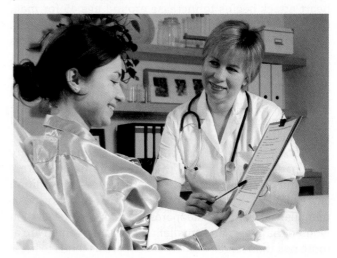

Menopausal hormone therapy is available in a variety of preparations, routes of administration, and dosages.
© Alexander Ratha/Shutterstock

Hormone therapy may be especially useful for women who experience menopause or who have lost normal ovarian function, called premature ovarian failure, before age 40. These women have a different set of health risks compared to women who reach menopause near the average age of 50, including a higher risk of coronary heart disease (CHD). In these special, younger populations of women, hormone therapy appears to actually reduce their risk of CHD.[27]

Hormone therapy carries potential risks and benefits to health. Hormone therapy appears to be a higher health risk for some groups of women, such as older women and smokers. At the same time, used properly, and by women in low-risk groups, hormone therapy is usually a safe product that can provide relief for women with severe symptoms associated with menopause.

History of Hormone Use in the United States

For the latter half of the 20th century, millions of women received hormone therapy to treat symptoms of menopause and protect their long-term health (see **Table 8.2** for a timeline view of hormone therapy use over the past 100 years). Large pharmaceutical companies have used

Table 8.1   Types of Menopause Treatments and Drugs

Menopause is unique to each woman. These treatments and drugs are often used to address specific symptoms:

- Hot flashes
  - Hormone therapy
    - Estrogen
    - Estrogen plus progesterone
  - Low-dose antidepressants
  - Other drugs
- Bone loss
  - Bisphosphonates
  - Selective estrogen receptor modulators (SERMs)
- Vaginal dryness
  - Tablets, rings, and creams

Table 8.2   Hormone Therapy Timeline

1890s	Experiments of hormone therapy (HT) with testicular extracts for aged men
1920s	Estrogen distilled from urine of pregnant women
1930s	Pharmaceutical companies manufacture purified and synthesized hormones
1938	DES, a powerful synthetic, nonsteroidal estrogen formula published
1939	*Journal of the American Medical Association (JAMA)* publishes "Estrogen therapy—A Warning" cautioning against use of DES, a possible carcinogen.
1940	Thirteen drug companies apply to FDA to market DES, but FDA does not approve their applications. The companies band together and form an aggressive campaign to gain approval.
1941	As a result of the campaign, FDA approves DES for use in menopausal symptoms and menstrual disorders. Physicians began to use it "off-label" for preventing miscarriages—later shown to be the most harmful use of DES.
1942	FDA approves Premarin, made from urine of pregnant horses.
1950s	William Masters promotes expansion of short-term HT to long-term, describing "ovarian failure as the Achilles heel" for women.
1960	FDA approves oral contraceptives, beginning long-term hormonal use by many women.
1960s	Large-scale manufacturing and marketing of psychotropic drugs and hormones
1966	Robert Wilson writes the best-selling book *Feminine Forever*, promoting the prevention of menopause with HT.
1970s	Premarin one of top five prescribed medications in the United States
1971	Studies show DES used to prevent miscarriage during pregnancy causes vaginal cancer in their daughters.
1971	National Institutes of Health (NIH) conference examines use of estrogen therapy for menopause; deplores lack of data and concerns.
1975	Retrospective studies find that estrogen use caused endometrial cancer.
1976	FDA mandates patient labeling for estrogen.
1977	NIH Consensus Development Conference to assess estrogen use and provide guidance for clinicians
1980	Synthetic progesterone, progestin, added to HT as "opposed therapy or combo."
1980s	Studies find protective effect of estrogen on bone loss and osteoporosis in women who had surgical menopause; hormones were promoted for osteoporosis protection for all women; some studies show small elevations of breast cancer risk in long-term hormone users.
1984	NIH Consensus Conference warns against widespread use of hormone therapies but also notes estrogen to be effective against osteoporosis. Messaging to women begins to emphasize osteoporosis prevention and minimize cancer risk.
1985	Nurses' Study shows estrogen users had reduced risk of CHD.
1986	FDA approves estrogen as treatment for postmenopausal osteoporosis.
1980–1990	Opposed therapy becomes one of the most prescribed drugs in America, used by nearly 40% postmenopausal women.
1987	PEPI (Postmenopausal Estrogen/Progestin Interventions) Trial started to assess HT on CVD risk factors.
1990s	Studies find decreased risk of heart disease in women on HT.
1991	WHI started. Four components to study were: (1) estrogen-progestin vs. placebo, (2) conjugated estrogen vs. placebo, (3) calcium and vitamin D vs. placebo, and (4) nonintervention cohort
1992	Premarin ranks number 1 in prescribed U.S. drugs—promoted to prevent heart attacks and osteoporosis.
1992	Nurses' Study shows increased risk of breast cancer among hormone therapy users; contradictory findings in Framingham study show increased risk, but study participants were older and had received higher doses.
1993	HERS study begins to see if combination hormone therapy alters the risk for CHD in women with established coronary disease.

(continues)

Table 8.2	Hormone Therapy Timeline (continued)
1995	PEPI Trial results find combination hormone therapy better than estrogen for protection against uterine cancer; progesterone found to interfere with the beneficial effect of estrogen on cholesterol.
1996	PEPI Trial results find estrogen alone greater risk for hyperplasia than placebo.
1997	Premarin sales reach $1 billion.
1998	HERS study finds that hormone therapy does not protect women with heart disease against further progression of heart disease. The use of hormone therapy nearly triples the participant risk of having a blood clot.
1999	Studies confirm elevated risk of breast cancer in long-term hormone therapy users.
2002	HERS II study finds no CVD prevention benefit to combination hormone therapy but does find an increased risk of stroke, clots, and need for gallbladder surgery.
2002	WHI component (1) trial ended early due to greater incidence of CHD, breast cancer, stroke, and blood clots in treatment group vs. placebo. Findings also show decreased risk of colorectal cancer and fewer fractures in the treatment group. As a result, authors publish an article in *JAMA* saying estrogen-progestin should not be used for the prevention of heart disease.
2003	Five articles in *JAMA* find: (1) Combination hormone therapy did not improve women's quality of life, vitality, mental health, depressive symptoms, or sexual satisfaction; (2) Hormone users had a two-fold increased risk of developing dementia; (3) An increased risk of stroke in the hormone therapy treatment group; (4) An increased risk of breast cancer with hormone therapy, and cancers in hormone users are diagnosed at a more advanced stage than placebo users; and (5) The longer women used combined HT, the greater their risk of developing breast cancer.
2003	FDA strengthens warning label requirements for hormone products. Products have to highlight increased risks for heart disease, heart attacks, strokes, and breast cancer and have to state that products have not been approved for prevention of heart disease or memory loss.
2003	Results of the Million Women Study show women taking hormones are at higher risk of breast cancer. Women taking estrogen alone had an increased risk of uterine and breast cancers.
2004	WHI component (2) terminated 1 year early because estrogen alone did not reduce risk of heart disease; however, it did decrease risk for colon cancer and hip fracture.
2005	NIH State-of-the-Science Conference changes "hormone replacement therapy" to its current name—menopausal hormone therapy—shifting emphasis away from the concept of "replacing" hormones.
2003–present	FDA recommends hormone therapy for postmenopausal women be at the lowest doses for the shortest amount of time needed to reach treatment goals.

Data from: Rothenberg, C. J. (2005) *The rise and fall of estrogen therapy: The history of HRT*. Harvard Law School. Paper submitted in satisfaction of the Food and Drug Law course and the third year written work requirement. Available at: http://leda.law.harvard.edu; Watkins, E. S. (2007). *The estrogen elixir: A history of hormone replacement therapy in America*. Baltimore, MD: The Johns Hopkins University Press; *Project MUSE*. (2012). Available at: http://muse.jhu.edu/

their influence to shape public policy and national education campaigns. Commercial emphasis on positive attributes of therapies has misled women and clinicians, while risks were minimized or ignored.[28] At the same time, many of the supposed negative effects of current hormonal products for menopause have been exaggerated, misunderstood, or falsely inferred.

The Food and Drug Administration (FDA) approved the first product for use in menopausal symptoms in 1941. Diethylstilbestrol (DES), a synthetic form of estrogen, became used both for symptoms of menopause and for the prevention of miscarriage. For the next 40 years, various hormonal combinations were positioned as a cure for many afflictions of aging. In addition, doctors often prescribed these products as preventive drugs for chronic conditions such as heart disease, osteoporosis, and dementia. Over the years, many observational and case studies supported these positive attributes of hormones, and a billion-dollar business system evolved. The pathway to widespread adoption became more complicated in the 1970s. During this decade, studies found increased rates of vaginal cancers in women whose mothers used DES during pregnancy. In addition, research also found a link between estrogen and uterine cancer, with the suggestion of possible links with hormone therapies and other cancers. However, until large-scale studies provided clearer insight, American women continued to routinely receive hormones for menopausal symptom treatment and chronic disease prevention.

Major Studies

In 1991, the federal government embarked on an expansive, rigorous set of clinical studies to better understand life after menopause. The Women's Health Initiative

(WHI) was a 15-year research program aimed at learning more about cardiovascular disease, cancer, and osteoporosis, the most frequent causes of death, disability, and low quality of life in postmenopausal women. The clinical trials also examined the effects of two major postmenopausal hormone therapies, estrogen alone and estrogen plus progestin, compared to placebo. Additional studies examined the effects of diet modification: calcium and vitamin D supplements, on heart disease, fractures, and breast and colorectal cancers. The WHI studies were the largest studies ever conducted in the United States. The trials and an observational study recruited more than 161,000 generally healthy postmenopausal women. The studies were complex, and the interpretation of the findings has been the subject of hundreds of professional papers and medical presentations.

In 2002, the estrogen plus progestin portion of the WHI was stopped early. Preliminary data indicated that women faced an increased risk of breast cancer and heart disease. Women in this group also had a slightly lower risk of developing hip fractures and colon cancers, but the increased risk for other diseases outweighed these benefits. The effects that estrogen plus progestin had on these conditions, although statistically significant, were still small for any individual woman. For example, the study found that for every 10,000 women taking estrogen pills:

- 38 developed breast cancer each year, compared to 30 breast cancers seen in every 10,000 women taking the placebo.

- 37 had a heart attack, compared to 30 out of every 10,000 women taking the placebo.

- 10 had hip fractures, compared to 15 out of every 10,000 women taking the placebo.

- 10 developed colon cancer, compared to 16 out of every 10,000 women taking the placebo.

Women in the estrogen-alone portion of the WHI continued taking pills until 2004, when researchers concluded that estrogen alone did not appear to affect the risk for heart disease or stroke. **Table 8.3** presents the major findings from these two studies in greater detail.

Another important study for hormone therapy was the Million Women Study, which was conducted in the United Kingdom and completed in 2003. The Million Women Study, the largest observational study of all time, showed that women taking hormones had a higher risk of developing breast cancer than the women not taking hormones. The study also confirmed the increased risk for uterine cancer in women who had their uterus and were taking estrogen alone. Consistent with other studies, the findings showed that prior use of hormones did not seem to affect the current risk of developing breast cancer, suggesting that the effects of the hormones on breast cancer risk diminished within 2 years of stopping them.[29]

Table 8.3	Results from the Estrogen Plus Progestin Study Compared to the Results from the Estrogen-Alone Study
Results from the Estrogen Plus Progestin Study	**Results from the Estrogen-Alone Study**
Compared with the placebo, the estrogen plus progestin resulted in:	Compared with the placebo, estrogen alone resulted in:
Increased risk of heart attack	No difference in risk for heart attack
Increased risk of stroke	
Increased risk of blood clots	Increased risk of stroke
Increased risk of breast cancer	Increased risk of blood clots
Reduced risk of colorectal cancer	Uncertain effect for breast cancer
Reduced risk of fractures	No difference in risk for colorectal cancer
No protection against mild cognitive impairment and increased risk of dementia (study included only women aged 65 and older)	Reduced risk of fractures

Data from Heiss, G., Wallace, R., Anderson, G., et al. (2008). Health risks and benefits 3 years after stopping randomized treatment with estrogen and progestin. *Journal of the American Medical Association, 299*(9), 1036–1045.

While the findings of the WHI and Million Women Study are important, they have still not answered all of the questions about menopause and hormone therapy. Today, experts continue to debate the merit of the studies and the interpretations of the data.[30]

Current Medical Menopause Management Options

Hormone therapy continues to be prescribed for women who want relief from menopausal symptoms. The absolute risk of heart disease or breast cancer to an individual woman taking hormones is low. For a woman who has severe symptoms such as intense hot flashes, the benefits of hormonal therapy may outweigh the risks. Many clinical studies have provided evidence that estrogen with or without progesterone effectively helps such conditions such as hot flashes, vaginal dryness, night sweats, and bone loss. These benefits can lead to improved sleep, sexual relations, and quality of life. Hormone therapy does not "cure" any disease; rather, hormone therapy helps to reduce symptoms associated with the hormone changes that result from menopause. Some women may face only mild symptoms of menopause or are not bothered by them. Others may opt for healthful, nonmedical methods of coping with symptoms. Women most often take hormone therapy during menopause and perimenopause. The consensus guidance for hormones today is to take the lowest possible dose for the shortest amount of time possible for menopausal symptom relief.

Current Nonmedical Menopause Management Options

The question of whether menopause should be medically treated, and if so, how, remains a controversial and misunderstood topic. Some experts are concerned that providers and women now consider menopause, a natural and normal life process, as something to be cured with medical treatment rather than experienced or managed through behavior change or nonmedical options. These choices can be at least as effective as medical procedures for reducing unwanted symptoms of menopause, while also improving overall health. Regular exercise; avoiding smoking; a balanced, healthful diet; a thorough, honest examination of one's position in life; and if warranted, counseling, can help women cope with many of the symptoms associated with menopause and aging. These options also allow women to take an active role in maintaining health, rather than relying on prescribed medications that imply illness or disease. Women can also take actions to avoid specific symptoms: for example, wearing less restrictive clothing or lowering the temperature to deal with hot flashes, or reducing stress and eliminating caffeine to cope with insomnia.

Regular physical activity is critical in the menopausal years, a time when a woman is at increased risk for osteoporosis and osteoporosis-related fractures, heart disease, and chronic diseases such as diabetes. Weight-bearing exercise can increase bone density and improve balance and flexibility to decrease falls, thereby reducing fractures. Aerobic exercise can reduce a woman's risk for cardiovascular disease by improving cardiac function, decreasing high body weight, and lowering LDL ("bad") cholesterol levels. In addition to its many other benefits, exercise also may reduce the incidence and severity of hot flashes. Other symptoms associated with hormonal changes of menopause, such as insomnia, depression or other mood changes, weight gain, and headache, all may improve with exercise.[31]

"Bio-Identical" Hormones

In recent years, large marketing campaigns have promoted "bio-identical" hormones as alternative therapies to prescriptive medical hormones. Fueled by the controversy associated with hormone research studies and preying on the fears of women with menopausal symptoms, these products claim to be identical to natural female hormones. The FDA has expressed concern that these products pose a potentially serious risk to women. "Bio-identical" hormones are not sanctioned by the FDA. Sellers of these products often claim that they are safe, "all natural," and free of the risks that present with the FDA-approved drugs for hormone therapy. The "bio-identical" products have not been subjected to the rigorous testing required by the FDA for drugs. FDA-approved drugs for hormone therapy are sold by prescription only.

"Bio-identical drugs" are compounded in pharmacies where practices do not always conform to FDA standards, and these drugs have not been systematically evaluated to ensure safety and effectiveness. Often the manufacturers claim that estriol, the weak form of estrogen in their products, offers a safe alternative to hormone therapy. However, the FDA has not reviewed any data on these products. In addition, claims from companies that "create a personal drug" based on a saliva test have not been validated.

Millions of women have tried custom-compounded hormones or herbal supplements like black cohosh and red clover to cope with symptoms of menopause. Alternative remedies such as these often appeal to women who like to research and find their own solutions to medical problems. However, instead of a safer option, they are getting products of unknown risk that still contain the estrogen many of them fear.

In summary, the nonprescriptive option of a risk-free hormonal product is appealing to many women. However, products that have not been evaluated by the FDA have inherent risks. To date, the FDA is not aware of any credible scientific evidence to support claims made regarding the safety and effectiveness of compounded

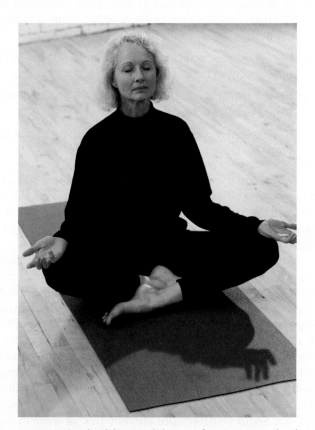

Symptoms associated with hormonal changes of menopause, such as hot flashes, may improve with regular exercise.
© Photodisc

> *I am approaching menopause and I feel very frustrated with the lack of clear information about menopause and hormone therapies. First, hormone therapy was supposed to be a cure-all; now, everyone seems to think you're risking your life if you choose to take it. Haven't we been using this stuff for decades? Why is there so much we still don't know?*
>
> **—46-year-old woman**

> *I started exercising when menopause started and it helped me in many ways, just not the ones I was expecting. In terms of symptoms, it really only helped me sleep a bit better, but it certainly helped me feel healthier, stronger, and more relaxed. I am glad that exercise is now a regular part of my daily routine.*
>
> **—57-year-old woman**

"bio-identical" products, and they urge women to consult with their healthcare provider before consuming them.[32]

INFORMED DECISION MAKING

As they reach menopause, women will face questions about if and how to take hormone therapy, as well as what other strategies to take to cope with symptoms of menopause. A woman can make the decision that is right for her by learning about hormone therapy and the aging process from unbiased sources and by carefully considering her own feelings, preferences, and symptoms. Family history, personal medical history, and the lifestyle choices made before menopause may also influence these decisions. A person who stopped having periods before 40 or lost her normal ovarian function before 40 has a different set of health risks compared to women who reached menopause at age 50.

Women who decide to take hormone therapy can take three main strategies to reduce their risk:[27]

- Start hormone therapy early. HT does not appear to significantly increase the risk of heart disease in women younger than age 60. Some studies suggest that estrogen may protect against heart disease when taken early in the menopausal years.

- Minimize the amount of medication. Use the lowest effective dose for the shortest amount of time needed to alleviate symptoms.

- Try a form of hormone therapy that provides limited rather than systemic effects, such as patches, gels, creams, or suppositories.

Although many women believe that health problems that occur during midlife are an unavoidable consequence of aging, many of these problems can actually be prevented or controlled. Healthy behavior changes, such as quitting tobacco, eating a healthful diet, and getting regular physical exercise, can improve both the quality and the quantity of life at any age and reduce the risk of age-related diseases such as heart disease or osteoporosis. For some women, menopause is a time for reflection and renewed determination to engage in these healthier behaviors. For many women, finding someone to talk to is another important coping mechanism. Menopause, something that all women go through, is no longer a dirty word. Being able to share experiences, finding (and acting as) a sympathetic ear, and asking for advice about how to cope with symptoms or other life events are all healthful and effective ways of coping with changes that come with aging.

Staying informed about health research and new treatment options is also important. Unfortunately, many women are uninformed about their health and about the steps they can take to become and remain healthy. The confusing and complicated historical reality of hormone therapy, as well as the lack of in-depth, nuanced coverage of the subject, has not helped. One study found that most women discontinued hormone therapy after the WHI results were published. Given their experience with therapy, some women, particularly non-Whites, are now less trusting of medical recommendations and less likely to take drugs for cardiovascular disease prevention.[27]

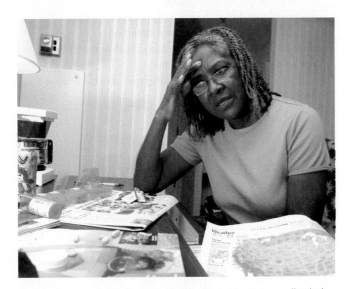

Seemingly contradictory findings about hormone therapy, as well as lack of nuanced media coverage of the subject, has made it difficult for many women to decide whether hormone therapy is right for them.
© Jones and Bartlett Publishers. Courtesy of MIEMSS.

> *I started hormone therapy but with all the contradictory news I decided that I preferred to not take "medicine" to get through a normal transition. Yes, I did have hot flashes, but they were manageable. I got through it.*
>
> **—61-year-old woman**

The decision about whether to take hormone therapy is a personal one. No two women respond exactly the same way to the same therapy. Hormone therapy may provide relief for some women while not making much of a difference for others. Factors such as a woman's age at menopause, cultural background, and ethnicity may affect either how women experience symptoms of menopause, how they interpret those symptoms, or both. Many women choose to live with symptoms because they consider them signs of normal developmental transition and aging. Women who decide to take hormone therapy may need to work with a healthcare provider to find the dose, product, and regimen that work for them. Women with difficult menopause symptoms; who have thin bones, as measured by a bone density test; or who are at high risk of heart disease are possible candidates for hormone therapy. Women who have a history of liver disease, who are prone to blood clots, or who have had breast cancer are generally considered to be at too high a risk to begin hormone therapy (**Table 8.4**). Women should carefully weigh the potential benefits and risks of any treatment before making a decision (see **Self-Assessment 8.1**).

Table 8.4 Conditions That May Preclude the Use of Hormone Therapy

- Personal history of breast cancer
- History of blood clots in legs, lungs, or eyes
- Undiagnosed or abnormal vaginal bleeding
- Preexisting cardiovascular conditions, such as blood clots, stroke, or uncontrolled hypertension
- History of liver, gallbladder, or pancreatic disease; impaired liver function

---

Self-Assessment 8.1
Strategies for Hormone Therapy Decision Making

The decision to use hormone therapy is a personal and private one.

Women should consider several factors when making the decision:

1. Personal and family medical history
   - History of breast cancer
   - Blood clots in the legs, lungs, or eyes
   - Abnormal vaginal bleeding
   - Preexisting cardiovascular conditions, such as blood clots, stroke, or uncontrolled high blood pressure
   - Liver, gallbladder, or pancreatic disease
2. Menopausal symptoms and their severity
   - Hot flashes
   - Vaginal irritation and discomfort
   - Urinary tract problems
   - Emotional and mood changes
3. Review risks and benefits
4. Reevaluate decision periodically

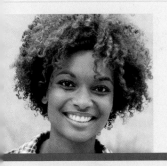
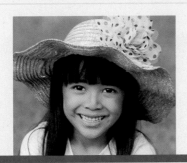
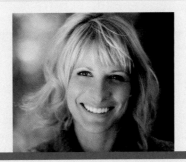
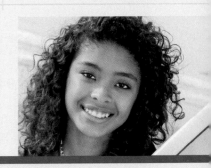

CASE STUDY

Cecilia was 44 years old when her periods started to become erratic. Usually they had been reliable "like clockwork," but now they started to last for 2 weeks at a time and come every 6 to 8 weeks. These symptoms were often accompanied by splitting headaches. Cecilia also started to feel distressingly hot for hours on end. At work and at home, it was impossible to concentrate. Normally one to sleep under a down comforter, Cecilia kicked off all her sheets and rolled from side to side at night, unable to sleep. After enduring these symptoms for several months, Cecilia made an appointment with her gynecologist.

Questions

1. Given Cecilia's background and experiences, what is a likely explanation for her symptoms?

2. What are some helpful questions Cecilia can ask her gynecologist about these symptoms?

3. Why would it be hard for her gynecologist to give her a definitive answer on the subject?

4. In addition to hormone therapy, what are some other ways that Cecilia can cope with her symptoms?

■ Summary

Once considered "the beginning of the end of life," menopause should instead be seen as the beginning of a new life phase, where women are no longer confined or defined by procreative abilities. Fears about aging and the myths and misconceptions about the aging process should be replaced with better knowledge and insight into the myriad opportunities that exist in the second half of a woman's life. In addition to causing physical symptoms, menopause often inspires questions about a woman's role and place in life. Menopause management—especially hormone therapy—remains a complex area that deserves continuing research and requires individual choices by women and their physicians. For some women, this therapy is a solution to distressing symptoms associated with menopause. For other women, hormone therapy may cause more health problems than it solves. Women should learn all they can about emerging options and consult with their providers to understand the best course of action for themselves as it relates to menopause and their individual process of aging.

Profiles of Remarkable Women

Lynn Johnston (1947–)

Lynn Johnston is a cartoonist and the creator of the comic strip *For Better or For Worse*. The strip has been a staple in North American newspapers since its debut in 1979. Johnston grew up in British Columbia, where she studied art and began her career as an illustrator. She spent the early 1970s as a commercial artist. In 1975 she developed *For Better or For Worse*, a comic strip set in Canada and loosely based on her own family experiences. The strip is a perennial favorite and appears internationally in several languages. Johnston is the first woman to receive a Rueben Award for Cartoonist of the Year by the National Cartoonist Society, in 1985. She has also received the Order of Canada and claims a star on Canada's Walk of Fame.

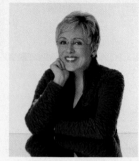

Courtesy of Lynn Johnston

Johnston's characters, loosely based on her own family members and friends, aged together more than 30 years over the course of the comic strip, which ended in 2007. She humorously depicted social, cultural, and physical realities of women, families, work, and relationships. While focusing on the daily life of a typical middle-class household, Johnston has not been afraid to tackle controversial issues, such as menopause, gay marriage, and child abuse. Johnston has been candid about her personal experiences with abuse and her own doubts about childrearing during her lifetime. Many of her strips captured real dimensions of her own thoughts and experiences during menopause. Her humor and honesty have been inspirational to her readers and she is a model for women around the world.

Additional information about Lynn and her work can be found at: www.fbofw.com.

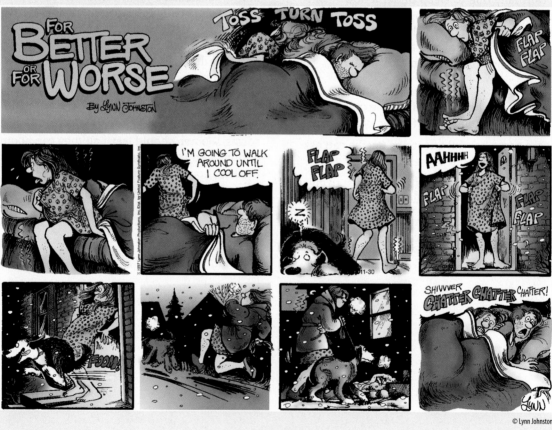

© Lynn Johnston

Topics for Discussion

1. How has our medical understanding of menopause changed over the past 50 years? What areas still need improvement?

2. Can you think of any depictions of menopause or women going through life issues associated with menopause in popular culture? How does this compare to popular depictions of men going through midlife crises or other events at a similar age?

3. Imagine that you are going through menopause. What questions would you want to have answered? How would you choose to manage your symptoms?

4. What can a woman do to maximize the effectiveness of her decision making about menopausal symptom management?

5. What are some of the physical, emotional, and social dimensions of menopause?

6. What are some new areas that merit research in the arena of midlife and maturity for a woman?

Key Terms

Alzheimer's disease

Bilateral salpingo-oophorectomy

Estrogen

Hormone

Hot flash

Hysterectomy

Natural menopause

Osteopenia

Osteoporosis

Perimenopause

Postmenopause

Progesterone

Total hysterectomy

Vaginal atrophy

References

1. U.S. Census Bureau. (2013). *Age and sex composition in the United States: 2012.* Available at: http://www.census.gov/population/age/data/2012comp.html

2. OWL—The Voice of Midlife and Older Women. (2012). *OWL releases menopause survey findings.* Available at: http://www.owl-national.org/blog/owl-releases-menopause-survey-findings

3. National Institute on Aging. (2015). *Health and aging. Age page: Menopause.* Available at: https://www.nia.nih.gov/health/publication/menopause

4. Stolk, L., Perry, J. R. B., Chasman, D. I., et al. (2011). Meta-analysis identifies 13 loci associated with age at menopause and highlight DNA repair and immune pathways. *Nature Genetics* 44: 260–268. Available at: http://www.nature.com/ng/journal/v44/h3/full/ng.1051.html

5. Jacobson, B. K., Heuch, I., & Kvale, G. (2002). Age at natural menopause and all-cause mortality: A 37-year follow-up of 19,731 Norwegian women. *American Journal of Epidemiology* 157(10): 923–929.

6. Wellons, M., Ouyang, P., Schreiner, P., et al. (2012). Early menopause predicts future coronary heart disease and stroke. *Menopause: The Journal of the North American Menopause Society* 19(10): 1081–1087.

7. Guttmacher Perspectives. (2001). Multiple factors, including genetic and environmental components, influence when menopause begins. *Family Planning Perspectives* 33(5). Available at: http://www.guttmacher.org/pubs/journals/3323601.html

8. Burger, H. (2008). The menopause transition—endocrinology. *Journal of Sexual Medicine* 5(10): 2266–2273.

9. NIH Osteoporosis and Related Bone Diseases National Resource Center. (2012). *Smoking and bone health.* Available at: http://www.niams.nih.gov/health_info/bone/Osteoporosis/Conditions_Behaviors/bone_smoking.asp

10. Whiteman, M. K., Hillis, S. D., Jamieson, D. J., et al. (2008). Inpatient hysterectomy surveillance in the United States. *American Journal Obstetrics and Gynecology* 198(1): 34.e1–7.

11. Hunter, M. S., Gentry-Maharaj, A., Burnell, M., et al. (2012). Prevalence, frequency and problem rating of hot flashes persist in older postmenopausal women: Impact of age, body mass index, hysterectomy, hormone therapy use, lifestyle and mood in a cross-sectional cohort study of 10,418 British women aged 54–65. *British Journal of Gynecology* 119(1): 40–50.

12. Ingelsson, E., Lundholm, C., Johansson, A. L. V., et al. (2010). Hysterectomy and risk of cardiovascular disease: A population based cohort study. *European Heart Journal* 32(6): 745–750.

13. Cohen, S., Vitonis, A., & Einarsson, J. (2014). Updated hysterectomy surveillance and factors associated with minimally invasive hysterectomy. *JSLS: Journal of the Society of Laparoendoscopic Surgeons* 18(3): e2014.00096.

14. Beck-Peccoz, P., & Persani, L. (2006). Premature ovarian failure. *Orphanet Journal of Rare Diseases* 1: 9. Available at: http://www.ojrd.com/content/1/1/9

15. Luoto, R. (2009). Hot flashes and quality of life during menopause. *BMC Women's Health* 9: 13. Available at: http://www.biomedcentral.com/1472-6874/9/13

16. National Institutes of Health (NIH), National Library of Medicine. (2013). Menopause. *MedlinePlus Medical Encyclopedia.* Available at: http://www.nlm.nih.gov/medlineplus/ency/article/000894.htm

17. Mayo Clinic. (2015). *Menopause.* Available at: http://www.mayoclinic.com/health/menopause/DS00119

18. Gold, E. B., Sternfeld, B., Kelsey, J. L., et al. (2000). Relation of demographic and lifestyle factors to symptoms in a multi-racial/ethnic population of women 40–55 years of age. *American Journal of Epidemiology* 152(5): 463–473.

19. NIH. (2005). *NIH State-of-the-Science Conference on Management of Menopause-Related Symptoms.* Available at: http://consensus.nih.gov/2005/menopausestatement.htm

20. Im, E., Lee, B., Chee, W., et al. (2010). Menopausal symptoms among four major ethnic groups in the U.S. *Western Journal of Nursing Research* 32(4): 540–565.

21. Geweke, L. O. (2007). Menopause and migrane. *Menopause Management.* Available at: http://www.menopause mgmt.com/issues/16-05/MM0910_feature.pdf

22. National Institute of Mental Health. (2007). *Women and depression.* Available at: http://psychcentral.com/lib/2007/women-and-depression/all/1

23. Alzheimer's Association. (2015). *Alzheimer's disease facts and figures.* Available at: http://www.alz.org/alzheimers_disease_facts_and_figures.asp

24. Shumaker, S. A., Legault, C., Rapp, S. R., et al. (2003). Estrogen plus progestin and the incidence of dementia and mild cognitive impairment in postmenopausal women. *Journal of the American Medical Association* 289(20): 2651–2662.

25. The North American Menopause Society. (2012). *Hormone therapy for women in 2012.* Available at: http://www.menopause.org/psht12patient.pdf

26. Global Industry Analysts, Inc. (2011). Global hormone replacement therapy (HRT) market to reach US$3.04 billion by 2016. *PRWeb.* Available at: http://www.prweb.com/releases/hormone_replacement/therapy_HRT/prweb8853368.htm

27. Mayo Clinic. (2015). *Hormone replacement therapy and your heart.* Available at: http://www.mayoclinic.com/health/hormone-replacement-therapy/WO00131

28. Rothenberg, C. J. (2005). *The rise and fall of estrogen therapy: The history of HRT.* Harvard Law School. Paper submitted in satisfaction of the Food and Drug Law course and the third year written work requirement. Available at: http://leda.law.harvard.edu

29. Narod, S. A. (2011). Hormone replacement therapy and the risk of breast cancer. *Nature Reviews Clinical Oncology* 8(11): 669–676.

30. Chlebowski, R. T., & Anderson, G. L. (2012). Changing concepts: Menopausal hormone therapy and breast cancer. *Journal of the National Cancer Institute* 104(7): 517–527.

31. National Cancer Institute. (2011). *Menopausal hormone therapy and cancer fact sheet.* Available at: http://www.cancer.gov/cancertopics/factsheet/Risk/menopausal-hormones

32. Food and Drug Administration (FDA). (2008). *Consumer health information. Bio-identicals: Sorting myths from facts.* Available at: http://www.fda.gov/forconsumers/consumerupdates/ucm049311.htm

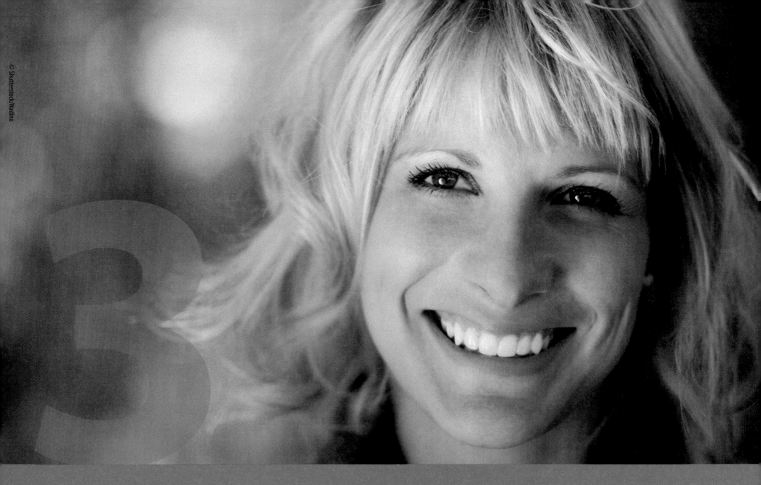

PART THREE

Physical and Life Span Dimensions of Women's Health

© Shutterstock/Nadino

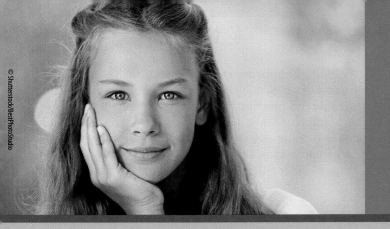

CHAPTER 9

Nutrition, Exercise, and Weight Management

Learning Objectives

On completion of this chapter, the student should be able to discuss:

1. How a balanced diet and an active lifestyle improve health and lower the risk for disease.

2. Basic elements of nutrition.

3. The six major nutrients and how they fit into a nutritious diet.

4. How to choose and eat a nutritious diet.

5. Factors contributing toward unbalanced diets and sedentary lifestyles, as well as ways to overcome those challenges.

6. How physical activity and exercise improve health.

7. The complementary benefits of aerobic exercise and strength training.

8. How to calculate one's body mass index (BMI) and maximum and target-range heart rates.

9. Physical fitness concerns specific to women.

10. Myths and facts about exercise and fitness.

11. Reasons why women should maintain a healthy weight.

12. Biological, cultural, and economic factors contributing to weight gain.

13. The effects of obesity and overweight on health.

14. Effective ways that women can reach or maintain a healthful weight.

15. Sociocultural influences on body image.

16. Hunger and malnutrition as global and national public health problems.

INTRODUCTION

Healthful eating and regular exercise are two of the simplest, most effective ways that women (and men) can improve their health. These behaviors improve mental and physical health in the present, prevent disease, and help people live longer, healthier, happier lives in the future.

A balanced, nutritious diet lowers the risk of cardiovascular disease, cancer, diabetes, hypertension, and other chronic conditions. Eating enough calories to supply, but not exceed, the body's needs helps maintain a healthy weight and extends the quality and length of life. Regular physical activity offers numerous benefits, including improving cardiovascular health, mood, and quality of sleep; reducing stress; and helping older adults to maintain function and preserve independence.

Unfortunately, 21st-century American living has made it extremely easy to adopt unhealthful eating patterns and lead sedentary lives. These two behaviors are responsible for 400,000 deaths each year. Unhealthy eating habits and a sedentary lifestyle either cause or exacerbate chronic conditions, such as cardiovascular disease, type 2 diabetes, hypertension, or some forms of cancer, in almost 120 million Americans—about half of the adult population.[1] Together, poor nutrition and a sedentary lifestyle are the second-leading preventable cause of death in the United States, just behind tobacco use.[2]

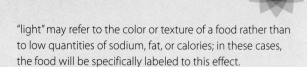

It's Your Health

Food manufacturers use a variety of claims to get consumers to purchase their products. Many claims focus on nutritional aspects of a product, drawing attention to the fact that it is low in calories, sugar, or fat. Always evaluate these claims with a critical eye. Food manufacturers often make misleading claims about food products to make them sound healthier than they actually are. A candy made almost entirely out of sugar may be advertised as being "fat free" while a bag of corn chips loaded with saturated fat, sodium, and extra calories may proclaim that it has almost no sugar. Some nutrition-related terms, such as "low fat," are strictly regulated by the FDA and have a set meaning, while others, such as "natural," can be used in almost any situation.

Other food-related claims provide information about the conditions in which the food is grown or raised. These claims may focus on the absence of antibiotics or harmful chemicals used during farming, the environmental impact of farming practices, whether the business model justly compensates farmers and workers, the living conditions of farmed animals, or a combination of these factors. In many cases, these conditions may work together naturally: A farm that operates without pesticides may add fewer toxins to nearby rivers, while also causing less harm to the environment and its laborers.

Be aware of the definition of the following food-label phrases and terms to be a more knowledgeable and responsible consumer.

Nutritional Claims

- *Enriched*: The replacement of nutrients in a product that may have been lost during processing; for example, bread may be enriched with iron, niacin, thiamine, and riboflavin. The nutrients added during enrichment usually replace only a small portion of the nutrients removed by processing.

- *Fortified*: The addition of vitamins and minerals that were not originally present in a food product; for example, orange juice may be fortified with calcium.

- *Light*: A food that is labeled "light" meets the definition for "low calorie" or "low fat." "Light in sodium" means the sodium content has been reduced by at least 50%. In some cases, "light" may refer to the color or texture of a food rather than to low quantities of sodium, fat, or calories; in these cases, the food will be specifically labeled to this effect.

- *Low-calorie*: Food that has fewer than 40 calories per serving and less than 0.4 calorie per gram.

- *Low-fat*: Food that has 3 grams or fewer of fat per serving. Food manufacturers sometimes add large amounts of sugar to low-fat foods to compensate for the taste.

- *Low-sodium*: Food that has 140 mg or less of sodium per serving; food labeled as "very low sodium" has 35 mg or less per serving.

- *Natural*: Meat, poultry, and egg products labeled as "natural" have no artificial ingredients and are minimally processed. For other types of food, the term may be used without any specific requirements (and thus has little guaranteed meaning). "Natural" does not mean nutritious; many foods labeled as natural are highly processed, high in fat or sugar, or loaded with preservatives.

- **Recommended Dietary Allowance (RDA)**, or the estimated amount of various nutrients needed each day to maintain good health. The guidelines were developed to address dietary needs for large populations; individual needs may vary owing to genetic, personal, and demographic factors.

- *Reduced*: A food that has at least 25% less of a given characteristic (such as calories, fat, cholesterol, sodium, or sugar) than a regular preparation of a given product. The product label must display the nutritional comparison.

- *Sugarless and sugar-free*: Contains less than 0.5 grams of sugar per serving.

Ethical/Responsibility Terms

- *Biodynamic*: A stricter method of organic farming that focuses on reducing environmental impact and using sustainable methods (see terms below).

It's Your Health (continued)

- *Cage-free*: Poultry and egg products with this label are farmed in a common area with unlimited access to food and water. Caged birds often live their lives in a small cage with several other birds; "cage-free" birds may still live in crowded conditions but at least have the freedom to move around.

- *Fair Trade*: Foods with the Fair Trade logo are grown on farms that meet set standards for farmer's compensation and working conditions. Some products without this label, such as chocolate, coffee, or sugar, are often produced in conditions where laborers and farmers work in dangerous conditions and receive little of the products' net profit.

- *Free-range*: Farmers may label poultry and egg products as "free-range" if the birds have access to the outdoors. Because of the flexibility of this definition, conditions found on different "free-range" farms may vary widely, from a crowded pen where thousands of chickens share access to a single ledge, to an open farm where animals can roam freely.

- *Grass-fed*: Beef, lamb, and other animal meat with this label come from animals that get most of their nutrients from grass, rather than from grain. Grass-based diets are more natural and healthy for cows and sheep than grain-based diets. Grass-fed meat may also be more nutritious, environmentally friendly, and less likely to contain harmful bacteria than grain-fed meat.

- *Humane, or humanely raised*: This term implies that farm animals are raised within certain basic living standards. It may refer to an animal's shelter, access to food and water, or the absence of hormones and antibiotics used to raise animals. In the absence of a standard definition, what this label means often varies from company to company.

- *Locally grown or raised*: Food that is either grown or raised within a certain distance of where it is sold, often within the same or a neighboring state. Locally grown food supports local agriculture and reduces the greenhouse gases needed for transportation. Food referred to as regionally grown or raised may be produced at a slightly farther, but relatively moderate, distance.

- *Organic*: Food produced using renewable resources and without traditional pesticides or artificial fertilizers. Animals that produce organic products, meat, and eggs receive no antibiotics (which helps to reduce the spread of antibiotic-resistant bacteria) or growth hormones. Organically grown food may be marginally more nutritious than conventionally grown food, but the extent of this difference is still being researched.

- *Pasture-raised*: Pasture-raised animals live and grow up on open grazing fields, with a diet focusing on grass, rather than grain.

- *Sustainable*: A method of raising food that does not cause lasting harm to the environment, provides just compensation for farmers and workers, and uses a variety of plant and animal species.

HEALTHFUL EATING AND NUTRITION

Nutrition is the science that investigates the need for food and the role of food in nourishing the body and fostering good health. To survive and stay healthy, the human body needs six basic **nutrients**, which fall into three types:

- *Macronutrients*, which include carbohydrates, proteins, and fats, are needed in large amounts.

- *Micronutrients*, which include vitamins and minerals, are needed in smaller amounts.

- *Water*, a substance often overlooked as a nutrient, is indispensable for virtually every bodily function.

Components of a Healthy Diet

Decades of health research have found several basic guidelines that should be part of any diet:

- A primary focus on fruits, vegetables, and whole grains, as well as low-fat dairy products, seafood, legumes (beans, peas, and lentils), and nuts

- Reduced amounts of red and processed meats and fatty dairy products

- Small amounts of refined grains, sweetened foods, and drinks

- For adults who drink, moderate amounts of alcohol[1]

A variety of more detailed eating plans exist for individuals who want guidance beyond these basic rules. When considering an eating plan, think about how well the plan follows the guidelines listed above, as well as how well the plan fits your needs, and how likely you think you will be able to follow the plan.

The U.S. Department of Agriculture (USDA) has issued dietary guidelines for Americans that offer rough estimates of how much of each basic food group to eat to maintain a balanced, nutritious diet. The most recent guidelines use a plate as a basic visual metaphor (see **Figure 9.1**). Fruits and vegetables make up the left side of the plate, with vegetables taking up a slightly larger share than fruit. Grains and protein foods (meat, poultry, seafood, beans and peas, and nuts and seeds) make up the right half of the plate, with each taking up a roughly equal amount. Each of these plate "halves" corresponds to just under half of a balanced diet. Dairy products, represented by a cup next to the plate, make up the remaining portion

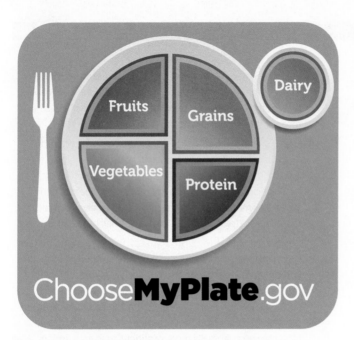

Figure 9.1   MyPlate: The 2010 USDA food plate.

Reproduced from U.S. Department of Agriculture. http://www.choosemyplate .gov/

three-fourths (78%) of American high school students do not get enough fruits and vegetables each day; a higher percentage drinks at least one can of soda or soft drinks on a daily basis.[3] Poor eating habits that begin during childhood and adolescence typically carry into adulthood and become harder to break.[4]

Other food guide pyramids challenge or complement the USDA's food guide. The Harvard School of Public Health also offers a healthy plate eating guide, with a reduced emphasis on dairy products compared to the USDA's but similar proportions of other food types. Food guides exist for special populations, such as people older than 70 years of age and vegetarians. Healthy, balanced eating plans also exist based on traditional Arabic, Southern African American, Chinese, Indian, Russian, and Mexican cuisines.

Over the past decade, the so-called Mediterranean diet has emerged as one model for healthful eating. This diet is based on the traditional eating habits of Greece, Italy, and southern Spain. In that region, rates of chronic diseases, such as heart disease and stroke, are consistently lower than they are in many other regions, while life expectancy remains high. The Mediterranean diet is based on the following basic rules:

- An abundance of food from plant sources, including fruits and vegetables, bread and grains, beans, nuts, and seeds
- Emphasis on fresh, locally grown foods
- Olive oil as the principal fat

of the diet. The USDA also has recommendations within each food group. **It's Your Health**: Dietary Guidelines for Americans summarizes these recommendations.

The typical American diet includes too much saturated fat, sugar, salt, and "empty calories" as well as too few fruits, vegetables, and whole grains.[1] More than

---

It's Your Health

Dietary Guidelines for Americans

The USDA makes the following recommendations for the five food groups as part of a balanced, 2000-calorie per day diet:

Vegetables

- Vary the vegetables you eat. Try to eat at least two different colors of vegetables every day.
- Try to eat 2.5 cups of vegetables a day.
- Especially nutritious vegetables include:
  - Dark green vegetables like spinach and broccoli.
  - Orange vegetables like carrots and sweet potatoes.
  - Dry beans and peas like kidney beans, pinto beans, and lentils.

Fruits

- Eat a variety of fruit.
- Try to eat 2 cups of fruit every day.
- Whenever possible, eat whole fruit rather than drinking juice.

Grains

Eat 6 ounces of grains every day (1 ounce equals one 1 cup of cereal, ½ cup of cooked rice or pasta, or 1 slice of bread).

- Make at least half of the grains you eat whole rather than refined grains.

Dairy Products

- Consume about 3 cups of low-fat or nonfat dairy products or other calcium-rich foods every day.
- Calcium-fortified soy products are a nutritious alternative to dairy foods.

Proteins

- Aim for about 5.5 ounces of protein-rich foods every day.
- Consume baked, broiled, or grilled meat products when possible.
- Eat seafood as a protein source twice a week (roughly 8 ounces per week).
- Make beans and peas a regular protein source.
- Limit consumption of processed meats such as sausage, luncheon meats, and hot dogs.

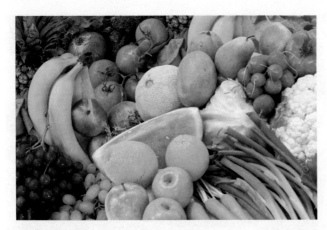

Fruits and vegetables should make up roughly half of a balanced diet.
© Denis Pepin/Shutterstock

- Moderate amounts of fish, poultry, cheese, and yogurt
- Moderate consumption of wine
- Limited consumption of red meat, dairy products, and sweets

Other food guides attempt to correct what some experts see as the excesses of a Western diet. Author and food expert Michael Pollan summarized one approach with seven words: "Eat food, not too much, mostly plants."[5] The first part, "eat food," refers to avoiding processed foods—food with long ingredient lists, artificial ingredients, or ingredients that a person would not have recognized as food 100 years ago. The second part, "not too much," encourages people to reduce snacking and to stop eating just before they feel full. The third part, "mostly plants," encourages people to make fruits, vegetables, and grains the bulk of their diet, with meat and dairy products acting as supplementary, not primary, sources of energy.

Nutrition Facts Label

The Nutrition Facts label is designed to help people make balanced food choices and compare the nutritional quality of foods. The food label lists information on a packaged food's serving size, calories, nutrients, and vitamin and mineral content (**Figure 9.2**). The Daily Value (%DV) section indicates the amount of each of the major nutrients (expressed as a percentage of a person's daily requirement of that nutrient) in a serving of food. These values are based on recommendations for a 2000-calorie daily diet. A woman under doctor's orders to eat a higher- or lower-calorie diet will need to recalculate these numbers to fit her own needs.[1]

Carbohydrates

Carbohydrates provide the basic fuel for the body and are available in two forms: simple carbohydrates (sugars) and complex carbohydrates (starches). Complex

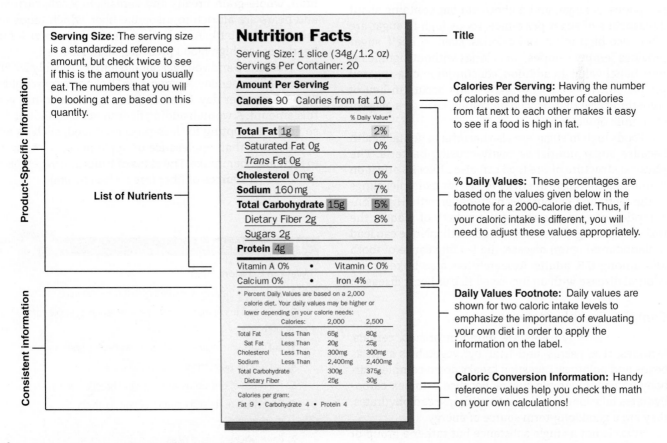

Figure 9.2   Example of the Nutrition Facts label.

carbohydrates are almost always more nutritious than simple carbohydrates. Simple carbohydrates often provide little more than a quick burst of energy (fruit is a notable exception). Foods rich in complex carbohydrates are more likely to contain vitamins, minerals, and other nutrients than sugar-rich foods.

During digestion, the body breaks down all carbohydrates into sugar (glucose). The body breaks down simple carbohydrates quickly, making them little more than a quick energy source. Starches are broken down at a slower pace, providing energy at a steadier rate. Whether it comes from simple or complex carbohydrates, glucose enters the blood, where cells throughout the body use it for energy. The pancreas makes a hormone called insulin, which allows cells to absorb sugar from the blood. A diet rich in complex carbohydrates allows the body to make insulin at a comparatively steady pace, while a diet rich in simple sugars creates rapid swings in blood sugar, forcing irregular insulin production that can overwork the pancreas and contribute to type 2 diabetes.

Simple Carbohydrates

Simple carbohydrates, or sugars, have four virtually identical forms: sucrose, glucose, fructose, and lactose. They are present in many foods, from fruit to ice cream to ketchup. Processed foods often have much more sugar than unprocessed foods from the same food group. A typical 12-ounce soft drink contains the equivalent of 8 teaspoons of sugar, and a chocolate bar contains about 3 teaspoons of sugar per ounce. Foods high in sugar are often also high in fat and calories. Even by itself, sugar provides "empty calories," or calories without significant nutritional value. In addition, consumption of a sugared product, such as a soft drink, usually occurs in lieu of something else that may be nutritious, such as a glass of skim milk or water.

Foods high in sugar are also harmful to dental health because sugar nourishes cavity-causing bacteria. The physical structure of the food can also affect its effect on dental health. Sugar in sticky foods, for example, clings to the teeth and encourages bacterial growth. High consumption of sugar promotes the growth of plaque, the toxin-producing film that forms on teeth; plaque can lead to periodontal (gum) disease, the leading cause of tooth loss among U.S. adults. Research has also linked periodontal disease with an increased risk of heart disease.[6]

Complex Carbohydrates

Complex carbohydrates are found in breads, cereals, legumes, rice, pastas, and "starchy" vegetables such as beans and potatoes. Digestion breaks down complex carbohydrates into simple sugars. Because complex carbohydrates take longer to digest than simple carbohydrates, they are a good long-term source of energy.

Fiber is not a single substance but rather a group of substances with varied physical properties. Fiber comes

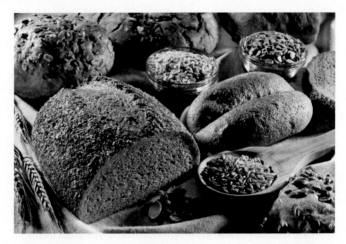

Complex carbohydrates are a good source of minerals, vitamins, and fiber.
© DUSAN ZIDAR/Shutterstock

from the parts of plants that cannot be broken down by enzymes in the human digestive tract. It is essential to digestion and helps improve overall health.

There are two kinds of fiber: soluble and insoluble. Both kinds benefit the body. Soluble fiber absorbs water in the digestive tract and is easily fermented by bacteria in the large intestine. Oats, for example, are rich in soluble fiber, which helps lower blood cholesterol and manage blood sugar levels. In contrast, most insoluble fiber remains essentially unchanged during digestion. Wheat bran, whole-grain breads and cereals, broccoli, carrots, and pears are all rich in insoluble fiber, which tends to increase stool bulk. A high-fiber diet lowers the risk for heart disease, high blood pressure, and diabetes.[7]

Women 50 and younger should aim for roughly 25–28 grams of fiber per day; women over 50 can aim for roughly 20–25 grams per day. Most women, however, do not get this amount. A woman adding fiber to her diet should do so gradually. Opting for less-processed food, such as an apple rather than applesauce or apple juice, is one way to increase fiber intake. The skins of fruits and vegetables are also rich sources of fiber (see **It's Your Health**).

It's Your Health

Ways to Eat More Fiber

1. Eat whole fresh fruit instead of just drinking juice.
2. Eat the skins of fruits and vegetables, such as apples and potatoes.
3. Eat fruits with edible seeds, such as berries and kiwis.
4. Eat whole-grain foods.
5. Eat more of the stems when having broccoli or asparagus.
6. Peel citrus fruits and eat the sections with their membranes.
7. Eat more beans and peas.

Glycemic Index

The **glycemic index** measures how quickly glucose enters the bloodstream after a carbohydrate is eaten and thus how quickly the carbohydrate increases a person's blood sugar. In general, foods that are mostly simple sugars, are highly processed, or contain refined sugars have a high glycemic index. This group includes refined breakfast cereals, white bread, white rice, white spaghetti, soft drinks, and sugar. Some complex carbohydrates, such as potatoes, behave just as simple carbohydrates do, elevating blood sugar to an excessive level. These complex carbohydrates have a high glycemic index, while complex carbohydrates that are high in fiber tend to have a lower glycemic index. Fiber slows digestion, so sugars in high-fiber foods take longer to be absorbed into the bloodstream.

The rationale for avoiding high-glycemic-index foods relates to the resulting production of insulin. Avoiding high-glycemic-index foods and eating only low-glycemic-index foods may facilitate fat loss by reducing excess insulin. However, a food's glycemic index is only one part of the larger picture. Many fruits, for example, have very high glycemic indexes but are high in desirable fiber and vitamins.[8]

Proteins

Protein provides the framework for muscles, bones, blood, hair, and fingernails. It is the main supply of amino acids—the building blocks that construct, repair, and maintain body tissues. There are nine "essential" amino acids that the body cannot manufacture itself and must receive from dietary sources. Complete sources of protein contain all of the essential amino acids in their required proportions; incomplete sources of protein lack one or more of the essential amino acids. Complete proteins include meat, fish, poultry, and dairy products. Incomplete sources include beans, peas, peanuts, and grains. Complementary proteins are protein sources that, when eaten together, supply the necessary amounts of all the essential amino acids; for example, black or pinto beans with rice has complementary proteins. One difficulty for vegetarians, vegans, or even people eating a diet low in animal proteins is that the body cannot store amino acids. To benefit the body, a person must consume all of the essential amino acids at the same meal.

The Food and Drug Administration (FDA) recommends that women between the ages of 19 and 30 eat 5.5 ounces of protein-rich foods per day. For a nutritious diet, vary protein sources to include beans, peas, fish, seafood, and only eat limited amounts of red meat (pork, beef, and lamb).

Some high-protein diets focus on obtaining a majority of daily calories from protein. These diets often inadvertently encourage consumption of proteins high in saturated fat, such as red meat and cheese, while discouraging consumption of healthy carbohydrates such

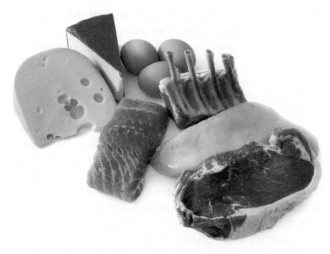

With the exception of fish and shellfish, all animal-based sources of protein contain saturated fat.
© Robyn Mackenzie/Shutterstock

as fruit, vegetables, and fiber. Diets high in saturated fat increase a person's risk for heart disease and certain types of cancer. The average American already gets enough protein to meet the body's needs. Extra protein consumed beyond this need provides no benefit and is simply converted into fat. Finally, high-protein diets may increase a woman's risk for osteoporosis, because excess dietary protein increases calcium loss in the urine.

Soy is another vegetarian-based protein source. Soy-based products have no saturated fat, and they can be a low-fat source of calcium, protein, and other nutrients. Excessive consumption of soy isoflavones, a product found in soy, may be harmful to women because isoflavones can act like estrogen in the human body. However, when consumed in moderation, the benefits of soy-based foods likely vastly outweigh these risks.[8]

Fats

Fats perform many essential bodily functions. They store energy, maintain healthy hair and skin, carry **fat-soluble vitamins**, supply essential fatty acids, affect levels of blood cholesterol, and create a feeling of "fullness." **Cholesterol** is a type of fat produced by the liver. It is a vital constituent of cell membranes and nerve fibers and serves as a building block for estrogen, testosterone, vitamin D, and bile. Cholesterol is transported in the bloodstream in protein packages called lipoproteins, which are assembled in the intestinal tract and liver. There are two main forms of cholesterol in the body. **Low-density lipoproteins (LDLs)**—called the "bad" cholesterol—carry the cholesterol through the blood, dropping it off where it is needed for cell building and leaving any excess in arterial walls and other tissues. This excess accumulates inside the arterial walls, where it contributes to plaque buildup in arteries. **High-density lipoproteins (HDLs)**—known as the "good" cholesterol—pick up cholesterol deposits and bring them to the liver for reprocessing or excretion.

Higher levels of LDLs are associated with an increased risk of heart disease. Increased levels of HDLs reduce the risk for heart disease, though some studies suggest they may simply be a marker of other factors that lower the risk for heart disease.

In addition to HDL and LDL cholesterol, another form of cholesterol, called "dietary cholesterol," is found in foods such as eggs, seafood, and liver. Whereas the body assembles HDL and LDL cholesterol from fats in the diet, dietary cholesterol is cholesterol that is fully formed in foods. Although nutritionists had previously recommended limiting the daily consumption of this dietary cholesterol, recent scientific evidence has found that dietary cholesterol, by itself, does not appear to be a health risk.

There are three types of fats:

1. **Saturated fats** come primarily from animal sources such as meat, poultry, milk, cheese, and butter. Some vegetable oils, such as coconut, palm kernel, and palm oil, are also saturated fats. At the molecular level, saturated fats are "saturated" with hydrogen atoms; each molecule holds as many as it can possibly carry. Saturated fats are generally solid at room temperature. They raise both LDL and HDL cholesterol, thereby increasing the risk of heart disease.

2. **Unsaturated fats** come from plants and include most vegetable oils. Carbon atoms in unsaturated fats have multiple bonds with each other, which prevents them from carrying the maximum number of hydrogen atoms they can carry (hence the name "unsaturated"). In turn, this configuration gives the molecules "kinks" that prevent unsaturated fat molecules from solidifying. They include two types:
   - **Monounsaturated fats**, such as those in olive, peanut, grapeseed, and canola oils
   - **Polyunsaturated fats**, such as those in safflower, sunflower, corn, and flaxseed oils

   Like saturated fats, unsaturated fats are high in calories. In all other respects, however, unsaturated fats are a much more healthful nutrient. Both types of unsaturated fats lower LDL cholesterol and raise HDL cholesterol, which has a positive effect on overall blood cholesterol levels and can therefore lower the risk of heart disease.

3. **Trans fats** form when vegetable oils are processed into margarine or shortening. They are found in snack foods such as potato chips, commercial baked goods with "partially hydrogenated vegetable oil" or "vegetable shortening," many types of fast foods (french fries and onion rings), stick margarine, and some dairy products. These fats are especially harmful to health, raising LDL cholesterol and lowering HDL cholesterol.[9] Whereas small amounts of saturated fats are part of a healthy diet, even small amounts of trans fats can be harmful to health. Trans fats have been found so harmful to health that the FDA has ordered food manufacturers to remove trans fats from all foods by 2018. This move is expected to prevent about 7000 deaths from heart disease and 20,000 heart attacks per year.[10]

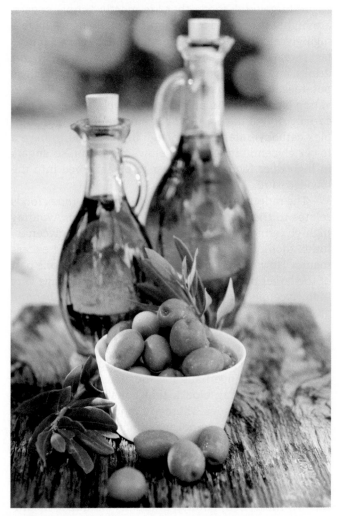

Monounsaturated fats like olive oil are more nutritious choices than saturated fats (coconut oil and fats found in meat, chicken, and dairy products).
© Christian Jung/Shutterstock

Lowering one's intake of saturated fat and trans fat is one of the major modifiable risk factors for coronary heart disease.[10]

Fat should be a part of any balanced diet. However, most Americans get more fat than they need. Most women should obtain 30% or less of their daily calories from fat, with unsaturated fats making up the majority of their fat intake. Try to make 10% of average daily calories come from saturated fat (**Table 9.1**).[1] If possible, avoid eating any trans fats, because any amount of these fats appears to be harmful.[11] How well these guidelines fit a person's diet as a whole is more important than how well they fit on any given day. These guidelines, which parallel the dietary guidelines endorsed by the USDA and the U.S. Department of Health and Human Services, emphasize careful eating patterns from early childhood to old age.

Table 9.1	Differences in Saturated Fat and Calorie Content of Common Foods

This table compares the saturated fat content of different forms of common foods. Even foods that are similar in nature (such as regular cheddar cheese and low-fat cheddar cheese) may have significantly different amounts of fat and saturated fat.

Food Category	Portion	Saturated Fat Content (grams)	Calories
Cheese			
Regular cheddar cheese	1 oz	6.0	114
Low-fat cheddar cheese	1 oz	1.2	49
Ground beef			
Regular ground beef (25% fat)	3 oz (cooked)	6.1	236
Extra lean ground beef (5% fat)	3 oz (cooked)	2.6	148
Milk			
Whole milk (3.24%)	1 cup	4.6	146
Low-fat (1%) milk	1 cup	1.5	102
Breads			
Croissant	1 medium	6.6	231
Bagel, oat bran	1 medium (4-inch)	0.2	227
Frozen desserts			
Regular ice cream	1/2 cup	4.9	145
Frozen yogurt, low-fat	1/2 cup	2.0	110
Table spreads			
Butter	1 tsp	2.4	34
Soft margarine with zero trans fat	1 tsp	0.7	25
Chicken			
Fried chicken (leg with skin)	3 oz (cooked)	3.3	212
Roasted chicken (breast, no skin)	3 oz (cooked)	0.9	140
Fish			
Fried fish	3 oz	2.8	195
Baked fish	3 oz	1.5	129

Data from U.S. Department of Agriculture, U.S. Department of Health and Human Services. (2015). *Scientific report of the Dietary Guidelines Advisory Committee.*

Currently, few American women meet these standards (see **Table 9.2**). **Self-Assessment 9.1** reviews the method for calculating daily fat intake.

Vitamins

Vitamins are organic substances that perform a variety of functions and are needed by the body in very small amounts. Vitamins promote good vision, form normal blood cells, help maintain strong bones and teeth, prevent certain diseases, and ensure proper functioning of the heart and nervous system. There are 13 essential vitamins: A, C, D, E, K, and eight types of B vitamin. Each vitamin carries out specific functions. **Table 9.3** summarizes facts known for each of the essential vitamins.

Vitamins can either be fat soluble or water soluble. The body can store fat-soluble vitamins (A, D, E, and K)

in fat cells in the liver, so the body does not need them every day. **Water-soluble vitamins**, B-complex vitamins and vitamin C, are needed every day (these vitamins also tend to be more delicate and are thus more easily lost during cooking).

Supplements pose a dilemma for people looking to get the vitamins and minerals they need. Most Americans do not get their daily recommended amount of vitamins—particularly A, D, C, E, and folate (B9), and supplements offer a convenient way to get these nutrients.[2] However, the body is much better at absorbing or using the vitamins found naturally in foods than it is at using vitamins found in supplements. In addition, only a certain amount of vitamins provide benefit for the body. Taking much more than the body needs (such as through multiple vitamin supplements) will either result in waste, as

Table 9.2 Typical American Diets Compared to Recommended Intake Levels

Foods to Eat More of:	Average American Intake
Whole Grains	15% of recommended levels
Seafood	44% of recommended levels
Dairy Products	52% of recommended levels
Fruits	42% of recommended levels
Vegetables	59% of recommended levels
Healthful Oils	61% of recommended levels
Foods to Eat Less of:	
Refined Grains	200% of recommended levels
Sodium	149% of recommended levels
Saturated Fat	110% of recommended levels
Calories from added sugar and solid fats	280% of recommended levels

Data from U.S. Department of Agriculture, U.S. Department of Health and Human Services. (2015). *Scientific report of the 2015 Dietary Guidelines Advisory Committee.*

Self-Assessment 9.1
Calculating Daily Fat Limits

To determine the maximum number of daily grams of fat:

1. Calculate approximately how many calories are consumed on a daily basis.
2. Divide the answer total by 33.

Women who find that they are eating more grams of fat than the calculated number should work on achieving this desired amount. Women with an intake of greater than 30% of calories from fat are at greater risk for many chronic diseases as well as obesity.

the body excretes the excess vitamins, or may actively harm one's health.

A single daily (or even occasional) multivitamin may provide some health benefits, both by ensuring the body has enough vitamin B9 (folic acid), which is important in preventing fetal neural tube development, as well as vitamins underrepresented in the typical American diet (such as vitamin D). Larger doses of vitamin supplements are

Table 9.3 Facts About Vitamins

Vitamin	Women's RDA*	Sources	What It Does
Vitamin A	700 mg	Liver, eggs, dairy products, carrots, bell peppers, green leafy vegetables, squash	Promotes good vision; helps form and maintain healthy skin and mucous membranes; helps fight infections
Vitamin B1 (thiamin)	1.1 mg	Whole grains, dried beans, lean red meats, fish, sunflower seeds	Helps release energy from carbohydrates; necessary for healthy brain and nerve cells and for functioning of heart
Vitamin B2 (riboflavin)	1.1 mg	Dairy products, liver, whole grains, spinach, broccoli	Aids in the release of energy from food; helps form antibodies and red blood cells
Vitamin B3 (niacin)	14 mg	Nuts, dairy products, liver, enriched grains, poultry	Aids in the release of energy from food; involved in the synthesis of DNA; maintains normal function of skin, nerves, and digestive system
Vitamin B5 (pantothenic acid)	5 mg	Whole grains, dried beans, eggs, nuts	Aids in the release of energy from food; essential for synthesis of numerous body materials
Vitamin B6 (pyridoxine)	1.3 mg	Fortified breakfast cereals, meat, nuts, beans	Important in chemical reactions of proteins and amino acids; involved in normal functioning of brain and formation of red blood cells
Vitamin B12 (cobalamin)	2.4 mg	Liver, beef, eggs, milk, shellfish	Necessary for development of red blood cells; maintains normal functioning of nervous system
Biotin	30 mg	Yeast, liver, eggs, milk	Important in the formation of fatty acids; helps metabolize amino acids and carbohydrates
Vitamin C† (ascorbic acid)	75 mg	Citrus fruits and juices, bell peppers, tomatoes, spinach, broccoli	Promotes healthy gums, capillaries, and teeth; aids iron absorption; maintains normal connective tissue; aids in healing wounds

Table 9.3   Facts About Vitamins (continued)

Vitamin	Women's RDA*	Sources	What It Does
Choline	425 mg	Whole grains, egg yolks, legumes, liver, soybeans, green leafy vegetables	Manages cholesterol in body; important for brain function; involved in production of hormones; necessary for functioning of folic acid
Vitamin D (calciferol)	15 mg	Dairy products, mackerel, sardines, salmon and other cold-water fish	Promotes strong bones and teeth; necessary for absorption of calcium
Vitamin E (tocopherol)	15 mg	Nuts, vegetable oils, whole grains, margarine, dark green vegetables	Protects tissue against oxidation; important in formation of red blood cells; helps body use vitamin K
Folate (folic acid/folacin)	400 mg	Liver, fortified breakfast cereals, lentils, chickpeas, spinach, beans	Important in the synthesis of DNA; acts together with vitamin B12 in the production of hemoglobin; vital to healthy fetal development
Vitamin K	90 mg	Leafy green vegetables, soybeans, broccoli, cauliflower	Aids in the clotting of blood

*Pregnant or breastfeeding women need additional levels of these vitamins.

†Smokers should consume an additional 35 mg daily of vitamin C.

Data from U.S. Department of Agriculture, U.S. Department of Health and Human Services. (2010). *Dietary guidelines for Americans;* Willet, W. C. (2002). *Eat, drink and be healthy: The Harvard Medical School guide to healthy eating.* New York, NY: Simon and Schuster.

probably not beneficial for health unless a woman has an identified shortage or deficiency.

Folic Acid

Folate, or vitamin B9, is found in chickpeas, spinach, strawberries, kidney beans, and citrus fruits and juices. It is vital for cell growth and function and for the development of healthy neural tubes in fetuses. Folic acid, a synthetic form of folate, is used to fortify grain-based foods, such as bread, flour, rice, pasta, and cereal. Folic acid and folate are also present in prenatal vitamins. Neural tube defects, including spina bifida, are birth defects affecting the brain and spinal cord. Since fortification of cereal grains with folic acid began in the United States in 1998, the incidence of neural tube disorders has decreased by 20 to 30%. All women of childbearing age should include 400–600 micrograms (0.4–0.6 mg) of folate or folic acid in their daily diet. However, on average, women of childbearing age consume an average of 200 micrograms per day, only half of the recommended amount.[12] Folate also helps maintain levels of homocysteine, an amino acid that builds and maintains tissues, but it can increase the risk of cardiovascular disease if consumed at excessive levels. Fortification with folic acid (a synthetic form of folate) in processed foods is a public health intervention that, like immunization, actually saves money; one economic analysis concluded that folic acid fortification in the United States saves $88 million to $145 million annually and is associated with an overall economic benefit of $312 million to $425 million per year.[13]

Antioxidants and Phytochemicals

Antioxidants, which include vitamins E and C, are substances that can neutralize oxidants, harmful molecules that can build up in the body. Antioxidants and **phytochemicals** (substances such as carotenoids and flavonoids that appear to act as antioxidants) have been widely studied for their roles in disease prevention and health promotion. Diets rich in fruits, vegetables, and grains—all of which are sources of antioxidants—are associated with a decreased risk of cardiovascular disease and cancer. Damage to cells from oxidation is associated with an increased risk of various diseases. Antioxidants appear to block some of the oxygen-induced cell damage by stabilizing and neutralizing the effects of free radicals (toxic particles) in the body.

Vitamin E may protect against damage in the artery lining, thereby decreasing the risk of coronary artery disease. Eating fruits and vegetables rich in vitamin C and beta-carotene (the carotenoid that is the precursor of vitamin A) may reduce the risk for many cancers. Carotenoids and flavonoids, found in foods such as onions, broccoli, red wine, green tea, and black tea, also reduce the risk for heart disease.

To stay healthy, eat foods high in carotenoids, such as red, orange, and deep yellow fruits and vegetables (e.g., tomatoes, carrots, sweet potatoes) and dark green leafy vegetables (e.g., spinach, broccoli); vitamin E (e.g., vegetable oils, salad dressings, margarine, whole grains, peanut butter); and vitamin C (e.g., citrus fruits, strawberries, broccoli). Eating a variety of fruits and vegetables supplies the body with vitamins, fiber, and antioxidants that may reduce the risk of heart disease and some kinds of cancer.[8]

Minerals

Minerals are inorganic substances essential to bone formation (calcium), enzyme synthesis (iron), blood pressure maintenance (sodium), and normal functioning of the digestive process (potassium). As components of the body, minerals are present in small amounts. Six minerals (calcium, chloride, magnesium, phosphorus, potassium, and sodium) are generally designated as macrominerals, or major minerals; other nutrients, which are equally essential but needed in smaller amounts, are referred to as microminerals. **Table 9.4** summarizes facts about each of the essential minerals. Calcium and iron are especially important for women's health.

Like vitamins, minerals can be consumed naturally through the diet or through pill-like supplements. Minerals appear to be absorbed more efficiently, and to provide greater health benefits, when eaten naturally through a balanced diet rather than by supplements. Mineral supplements also offer the potential for overdoses that are harmful to health. For years, healthcare providers have recommended that women take calcium and vitamin D supplements to improve their long-term bone health. However, recent research indicates that calcium and vitamin D supplements do not appear to prevent cancer or reduce the risk of bone fractures; in addition, women who take the equivalent of their RDA of calcium and vitamin D as supplements every day may have a slightly increased risk for kidney stones.[14] The risk for supplements appears to be the greatest when women take the equivalent of more than one RDA of calcium per day. Supplements may

Table 9.4 Facts About Minerals			
Mineral	**Adult RDA***	**Sources**	**What It Does**
Calcium	1000–1200 mg*	Milk and milk products, sardines and salmon eaten with bones, dark green leafy vegetables, certain types of tofu and soy milk, fortified orange juice	Builds bones and teeth and maintains bone density and strength; helps prevent osteoporosis; helps regulate heartbeat, blood clotting, muscle contraction, and nerve conduction; helps prevent hypertension
Chloride	700 mg	Table salt, fish, pickled and smoked foods	Maintains normal fluid shifts; balances pH of the blood; forms hydrochloric acid to aid digestion
Magnesium	310–320 mg*	Whole grains, raw leafy green vegetables, nuts (especially almonds and cashews), soybeans, tofu, hard water	Aids in bone growth; assists function of nerves and muscles, including regulation of normal heart rhythm; important in energy metabolism
Phosphorus	700 mg*	Meats, poultry, fish, egg yolks, dried peas and beans, milk and milk products, nuts; present in almost all foods	Aids bone growth and strengthening of teeth; important in energy metabolism
Potassium	4700 mg†	Oranges and orange juice, melons, bananas, dried fruits, dried peas and beans, potatoes	Promotes regular heartbeat; active in muscle contraction; regulates transfer of nutrients to cells; controls water balance in body tissues and cells; contributes to regulation of blood pressure
Sodium	500–2300 mg (estimated safe amount for dietary intake)	All from salt and foods containing salt	Helps regulate water balance in body; helps maintain blood pressure; excess sodium may raise blood pressure to unhealthful levels
Chromium	50–200 mg†	Meat, cheese, mushrooms, oysters, peanuts, brewer's yeast, potatoes	Important for glucose metabolism; may be a cofactor for insulin; regulates cholesterol production in liver; aids in digestion of protein
Copper	900–1000 mg†	Wheat, peanuts, shellfish (especially oysters), nuts, beef and pork liver, dried beans	Formation of red blood cells; cofactor in absorbing iron into blood cells; assists in production of several enzymes involved in respiration; interacts with zinc
Fluorine (fluoride)	3.1 mg†	Fluoridated water, foods cooked with or grown in fluoridated water, fish, tea, gelatin	Contributes to solid bone and tooth formation; prevents dental cavities; may help prevent osteoporosis

Mineral	Adult RDA*	Sources	What It Does
Iodine	0.15 mg*	Primarily from iodized salt, but also seafood, seaweed food products, vegetables grown in iodine-rich areas, eggs, certain cheeses, whole milk	Necessary for normal function of the thyroid gland; essential for normal cell function; keeps skin, hair, and nails healthy; prevents goiter
Iron	18 mg*	Liver (especially pork liver), kidneys, red meats, egg yolks, peas, beans, nuts, dried fruits, green leafy vegetables, enriched grain products, blackstrap molasses	Essential to formation of hemoglobin, the oxygen-carrying factor in the blood; part of several enzymes and proteins in the blood
Manganese	320–350 mg†	Nuts, whole grains, vegetables, fruits, instant coffee, tea, cocoa powder, beets, egg yolks	Required for normal bone growth; helps maintain healthy skin; important for metabolism of glucose and fatty acids
Molybdenum	75–250 mg	Peas, beans, cereal grains, organ meats, some dark green vegetables	Important for normal cell function
Selenium	50–55 mg	Fish, shellfish, red meat, egg yolks, chicken, legumes, whole grains	Protects cells against effects of free radicals that can damage cells; essential for normal functioning of the immune system and thyroid gland
Zinc	8 mg	Meat, liver, eggs, oysters, legumes, whole grain cereals, nuts	Essential for growth and skeletal development; important for immune system; assists in production of DNA and RNA

Table 9.4   Facts About Minerals (continued)

*These figures are not applicable to pregnant or breastfeeding women, who need additional minerals.

†Although there is no RDA for these minerals, the Food and Nutrition Board recommends this value as an average healthy intake.

Data from U.S. Department of Agriculture, U.S. Department of Health and Human Services. (2010). *Dietary guidelines for Americans*; Willet, W. C. (2002). *Eat, drink and be healthy: The Harvard Medical School Guide to healthy eating*. New York, NY: Simon and Schuster.

be less of a risk when used in smaller doses, such as taking daily supplements to provide 50% or less of the RDA, or taking the RDA on an irregular basis to supplement dietary calcium. Getting calcium through the diet, however, is the ideal choice.

Calcium

Calcium is a mineral of special concern to women. It is an integral component of bones and teeth, and calcium deficiency is a major contributor to osteoporosis. Calcium helps regulate heartbeat, blood clotting, muscle contraction, and nerve conduction. This mineral also helps prevent high blood pressure, is essential in the development of the fetus during pregnancy, and may reduce the risk for colon cancer. When calcium levels in the blood fall too low, the body draws the mineral from the supply in the bones to meet its needs elsewhere. This process accelerates the gradual bone loss that occurs most dramatically in postmenopausal women.

The NIH's **Recommended Dietary Allowance** (RDA) recommendation that women receive 1000 mg of calcium per day is deceptive. Adolescents, young women (ages 11 to 24), nursing mothers, and postmenopausal women are advised to consume 1200–1300 mg daily. Three to five cups of milk or servings of other calcium-rich foods such as

collard greens, cheese, tofu, cornbread, or sardines can supply the daily recommended amount. (See **It's Your Health**.)

The 2010 "MyPlate" food guide continues to emphasize dairy products as an important part of a healthy diet. Dairy foods are an excellent source of calcium as well as protein, vitamin D, and other nutrients; however, they often contain large amounts of saturated fat and calories, and they are not an option for lactose-intolerant individuals. Women do not have to rely on dairy products for their calcium. A cup of collard greens, for example, has virtually the same amount of calcium as a cup of skim milk (see **It's Your Health**).

Iron

Iron is necessary to produce **hemoglobin**, a key component of red blood cells and the oxygen-carrying protein that gives blood its red color. Iron is also stored in the liver, spleen, bone marrow, and other tissues. The body only needs small amounts of iron each day—about 18 mg each day for an average adult—but without iron the body becomes fatigued and weak. Reduced levels of hemoglobin result in anemia, a serious risk for women whose diets are chronically deficient in iron. Symptoms of iron-deficiency anemia include headaches, fatigue, general

It's Your Health

Calcium Sources

Food	Amount	mg Calcium	Percentage of RDA 1000 mg/day	1200 mg/day
Plain yogurt	1 cup	415	41%	35%
Sardines with bones	3 oz	372	37%	31%
Skim milk	1 cup	302	30%	25%
Collard greens	1 cup	290	29%	24%
Swiss cheese	1 oz	262	26%	22%
Cheddar cheese	1 oz	213	21%	18%
Canned salmon, with bones	3 oz	167	17%	14%
Low-fat cottage cheese	1 cup	154	15%	12%
Blackstrap molasses	1 tbsp	137	14%	12%
Cooked broccoli	1 cup	136	14%	12%
Dried and cooked beans	1 cup	90	9%	7%
Orange	1 (medium)	54	5%	4%

weakness, and pallor. In severe cases, anemia can lead to an irregular or increased heart rate. Iron-deficiency anemia is relatively common in the United States, with 12% of women ages 12 to 49 experiencing some form of iron deficiency.[15]

Iron absorption is a complex process that varies with the types and combination of foods consumed and the body's needs. Lean red meats (particularly liver—one 4-ounce serving contains almost 150% of the RDA) are a good source of iron. Chicken and fish are another alternative; they provide one-third to one-half the iron of red meat but also tend to have less saturated fat. Vegetarian sources of iron include chickpeas, soybeans, kidney beans, and lentils. Some breads, cereals, and pasta labeled "enriched" or "fortified" and unrefined whole grains, such as whole-wheat bread, supply a fair amount of iron. Eating foods high in vitamin C facilitates the body's absorption of iron. For vegetarians and vegans, consuming vitamin C with meals is a must. Cooking in cast-iron cookware also helps to increase the iron content of foods. The more acidic the food (such as spaghetti sauce) and the longer it cooks, the more iron will be absorbed. Other compounds, such as coffee, tea, and dietary fiber, block the body's ability to absorb iron; women attempting to increase their iron intake may wish to avoid eating foods with these compounds in the same meal as iron-rich foods.

Sodium

Sodium, which comes into the body primarily through salt, is another macromineral necessary for human health. Unlike other macrominerals, however, the main health concern in the United States (and other developed countries) is not too little sodium, but too much. The main health concern regarding excessive sodium intake is sodium's effects on blood pressure. Excess sodium intake is associated with hypertension, which raises the risk for heart disease, stroke, and other conditions. However, not everyone is affected by that risk. About half of Americans appear to be "salt sensitive," meaning that their blood pressure rises in response to extra sodium intake. The blood pressure of people who are not salt sensitive is mostly unchanged by sodium intake. African Americans, people over the age of 60, and people of Chinese descent are most likely to be salt sensitive.[16]

Processed and restaurant foods are the biggest contributors to excess salt in the American diet. Women can reduce their sodium consumption by cutting back on processed foods, such as rolls, cold cuts, and luncheon meats; eating fewer fast food and other high-sodium meals at restaurants; and paying attention to the sodium content on the nutrition facts label of foods purchased at the grocery store.

Water

The human body is approximately 50 to 70% water. Every system in the body depends on water to function: Water regulates body temperature and chemical actions, disposes of waste, lubricates joints, cushions the fetus during pregnancy, transports nutrients, prevents bowel problems, and helps enzymes function properly.

Water is so essential that the human body can survive only 3 days without it, even though the body can be denied food for several weeks and still recover. The average female requires 8 to 9 cups of fluid per day; pregnant women need slightly more. As little as 2 to 5% loss of body weight from water loss results in symptoms of dehydration, including headache, fatigue, flushed skin, and excessive thirst. Greater need for fluids occurs during exercise and conditions of high temperature, high altitude, and low humidity, and when it is necessary to counter the effects of high intakes of caffeine and alcohol, which promote fluid loss.

Sweetened sodas and sports drinks have become a daily part of life for millions of Americans. These drinks add sugar and calories to the diet while offering no additional nutritional benefit. Although diet or unsweetened sodas typically contain almost no sugar or calories, water still appears to be a more beneficial choice. Saving these drinks for special occasions, or eliminating them entirely, is a simple way to improve one's diet and improve one's overall health.

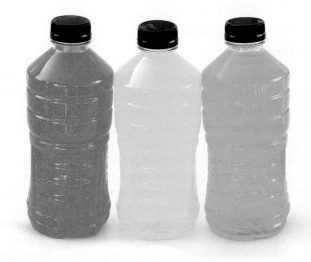

Sports and energy drinks may claim to "replenish" body fluids but often contain large amounts of sugar. Water alone is almost always a better (and cheaper) option.
© Chuck Wagner/Shutterstock

PHYSICAL ACTIVITY AND FITNESS

Regular physical activity is one of the best ways to improve one's health. However, physical inactivity remains a serious national problem. Each year, physical inactivity contributes to more than 300,000 deaths in the United States and more than 5 million deaths worldwide.[2] Only about one out of six (16.6%) women in the United States gets the government-recommended levels of physical activity—2.5 hours per week of moderate physical activity.[17] More than one-half of U.S. adults do not get enough physical activity to provide even basic health benefits. Physical

activity decreases with age and is less common among those with lower incomes, less education, and non-White ethnicity/race (see **Table 9.5**).[17]

> I've made a real effort to incorporate exercise into my daily routine this semester. On Mondays, Wednesdays, and Fridays I go straight to the gym after class, and I go running Tuesdays, Thursdays, and Saturdays, taking Sunday off. It's funny, because I never really thought about exercise much until this year, but now it's a normal part of my life.
>
> **—20-year-old student**

Benefits of Physical Activity

Adults and children of all age groups and body types, including people with disabilities, benefit greatly from regular physical activity. Being active reduces a person's estimated chances of coronary artery disease by 45%, stroke by 60%, osteoporosis by 59%, and hypertension by 30%.[2] Being active also reduces the chances of developing diabetes, depression, and breast, lung, and colon cancer; for women with depression or diabetes, physical activity makes the conditions less severe.[2] Finally, regular physical activity has numerous benefits in day-to-day life, from improving the quality of sleep to controlling stress, to maintaining a healthy weight, to improving independence and daily functioning later in life (**Table 9.6**). Substantial

Table 9.5	Percentage of U.S. Women Engaging in Adequate Aerobic Activity, 2013
Total	**43.9%**
Education Level	
Less than high school	25.9%
High school or equivalent	34.7%
Some college	45.6%
College degree	59.3%
Race/Ethnicity	
White*	48.5%
Black *	32.9%
Hispanic	33.6%
Native American/American Indian*	41.0%
Asian*	40.0%
Multiple race*	48.2%

*Non-Hispanic

Data from U.S. Department of Health and Human Services. (2013). *Women's health USA 2013*. Rockville, MD: U.S. Department of Health and Human Services.

Table 9.6   Benefits of Regular Physical Activity

Long-term:

Reduces the risk of early death

Reduces the risk of developing coronary heart disease and stroke

Lowers the risk of breast, lung, colon, and other cancers

Reduces the risk of developing type 2 diabetes, osteoporosis, and depression; for people with these conditions, reduces the severity of symptoms

Lowers high blood pressure and cholesterol

For older adults, improves ability to complete day-to-day tasks, reduces the risk of falls, and improves mental cognition

Short-term:

Improves aerobic capacity, muscle strength, and muscle endurance

Helps maintain healthy muscles, joints, and bones

Can improve mood

Can reduce symptoms of depression and increase cognitive functioning

Helps control weight, build muscle, and reduce body fat

Can promote better sleep and increase energy

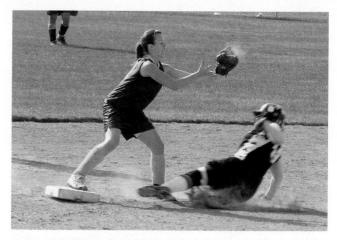

Organized sports are one form of exercise.
© Wendy Nero/Shutterstock

health benefits occur if a person gets at least 150 minutes (2.5 hours) of moderate-intensity activity (such as brisk walking) a week, or 75 minutes (1 hour and 15 minutes) of high-intensity exercise (such as fast running) a week. Alternatively, women can combine high- and moderate-intensity exercise to reach the total of 150 minutes, with every minute of high-intensity exercise counting for 2 minutes of moderate-intensity exercise. Greater health benefits occur with twice that amount or more (300 minutes a week of moderate-intensity activity, 150 minutes of high-intensity activity, or a combination of both).[18] However, even small amounts of physical activity are better than none at all. Women who get 1 hour or more of moderate physical activity per week or more are 33% less likely to die from cancer, 50% less likely to die from cardiovascular disease, and 66% less likely to die early than women who do not excercise.[19]

Studies have confirmed the potential value of aerobic exercise, along with medication if necessary, as a complementary therapy for depression.[20] People who exercise regularly report being happier and feeling better about themselves, and in general experience a better quality of life than people who do not. Regular exercise may also reduce anxiety and depression that can appear during pregnancy.[21] Other psychological benefits from exercise include decreased stress, increased sense of well-being, and improvements in cognitive function and mood. Proper exercise during pregnancy also has many benefits, including improved psychological well-being, shorter labor, and speedier recovery after childbirth. (See Chapter 6.)

Components of Physical Fitness

Exercise physiologists usually define fitness in four major areas:

- Cardiovascular endurance
- Muscular strength
- Muscular endurance
- Flexibility

Modern lifestyles do not require much physical movement, and today few women are naturally fit as a result of daily activities. Most women who wish to become fit in today's society will need to commit time and energy to exercise.

Cardiovascular endurance, the ability to carry on vigorous physical activity for an extended period of time, is the most vital element of fitness. It measures the heart's ability to pump blood efficiently through the body. Developing cardiovascular endurance enhances the ability of the heart, blood vessels, and blood to deliver oxygen to the body's cells and to remove waste products. Although muscles are able to draw on quick sources of energy for short-term exertion, the muscles require oxygen from the blood when exercise lasts more than a minute or two. Such physical activity is called aerobic exercise. With repeated regular exercise, the heart becomes able to pump blood and deliver oxygen more efficiently. Aerobic exercise also improves the muscles' capacity to use this oxygen. The coupled events are referred to as the "training effect." The heart rate, both at rest and exertion, decreases as a result of this regular exercise, and the heart becomes able to recover from the stress of exercise more quickly.

Muscular strength is the total force that muscle groups produce in one effort, such as a lift, jump, or heave. Strength training with free weights, weight machines, or other equipment is the best way to increase muscle strength. Strength gains come most quickly from heavy resistance and few repetitions.

Muscular endurance is the ability to perform repeated muscular contractions over time without tiring. Although muscle endurance requires strength, it is not a single, all-out effort. The keys to increasing endurance are repetition, working at a moderate level, and building up to a specified goal. Women can build both muscle strength and endurance by varying the amount of weight lifted and the number of repetitions per workout.

Flexibility is the ability of the joints to move through their full range of motion. Natural flexibility varies from person to person and from joint to joint. Women tend to be more flexible than men because of differences in their skeletons, muscle mass, and body composition. Good flexibility protects the muscles against pulls and tears because short, tight muscles may be more likely to be overstretched. Stretching the major body areas (legs, shoulders, arms, neck, and back) for 15–30 seconds at a time, at least three times a week, is the best way to improve and maintain flexibility.[22] Some women find that stretching certain muscle groups helps relieve or prevent pain. Stretching hamstring and lower back muscles may alleviate lower back pain, and calf stretches may help prevent leg cramps. To lower the chances of injury and receive the most benefit, stretch after rather than before a workout.

Body composition refers to the ratio of lean body weight (muscle and bone) to fat weight. Exercise affects body composition in two major ways: by reducing excess body weight through energy expenditure and by increasing the body's overall metabolism rate. The body burns extra calories during both the period of physical exercise and for several hours after exercise ends (known as afterburn). The longer and more intense the exercise, the longer the **basal metabolic rate (BMR)** remains elevated. Regular exercise improves overall muscle tone, contributing to a trimmer appearance. Exercise can also improve balance, coordination (the ability to skillfully use different body parts and the senses together), and agility (the ability to coordinate multiple movements and to react quickly and safely).

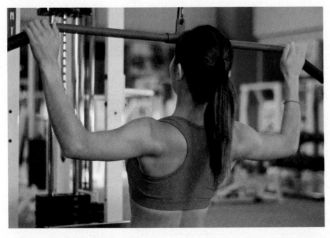

Maintaining a strong back through strength training protects it from injury.
© Philip Date/Shutterstock

Physical Activity and Exercise

Physical activity consists of any movement of moderate intensity that lasts a few minutes or more. Many day-to-day activities, such as climbing a flight of stairs or walking for an extended period, count as physical activity. **Exercise** refers to a deliberate session of physical activity for the purpose of improving health. Exercise tends to fall into two rough categories: aerobic training and strength training. Both types of exercise provide benefits. Aerobic training increases the body's ability to use oxygen, strengthens the heart and blood vessels, and improves the general health of the body. Strength training strengthens specific muscle groups, improves the health of bones, and helps with everyday living, such as carrying groceries. Together, aerobic and strength training provide better benefits than either form of exercise alone. Although a healthy diet with a reduced calorie intake plays the primary role in weight loss, exercise can contribute to weight loss in a secondary role and also help prevent the regaining of lost weight.

Aerobic Exercise

Aerobic exercise significantly raises the heart rate for a sustained period of time and is the form of physical activity most important for general health. Aerobic exercise improves blood cholesterol levels and blood pressure more than strength training. It also improves the ability of the heart and lungs to supply the muscles with oxygen; strength training generally does not provide this benefit.

Components of Aerobic Exercise   Health experts generally measure three important parts of an aerobic workout: intensity, duration, and frequency. Intensity, duration, and frequency all affect the amount of health benefit any exercise program provides; no one of these variables is more important than the others.

Exercise intensity is the work per unit of time. It can be monitored by measuring the target heart rate—the exercise heart rate needed to produce a training effect—for 20 to 30 minutes during each workout. See **Table 9.7** for examples of moderate- and high-intensity activities.

Exercise duration is the length of one exercise session. To benefit the heart, aerobic exercise must be intense enough to increase the heart rate and must continue for a minimum amount of time depending on the intensity of the workout. Aerobic activity provides the most benefit when performed for 30 minutes or more, but sessions as short as 10 minutes can still strengthen the heart and body.[18]

Exercise frequency measures the number of exercise sessions over the long term. Engaging in regular periods of exercise is essential for any exercise program. Exercising in three to five half-hour periods per week builds muscle and improves fitness faster and more safely than a single two-hour workout.

Table 9.7	Examples of Moderate- and High-Intensity Activities
Moderate-Intensity Activities	
Walking briskly (3 mph or more)	
Ballroom dancing	
Playing tennis, doubles	
Bicycling 5 to 9 mph, level terrain	
Weight-lifting	
High-Intensity Activities	
Swimming laps	
Hiking with a heavy backpack or on hilly terrain	
Aerobic dancing	
Playing tennis, singles	
Jumping rope	

Data from Department of Health and Human Services. (2008). *2008 physical activity guidelines for Americans.*

Self-Assessment 9.2
How to Check Your Pulse

Each "pulse" you feel when you put your fingers on an artery represents the blood pushed by one pump of a person's heart. The easiest way to measure your pulse is to place your fingers on the carotid artery in your neck or the radial artery in your wrist.

1. To find the radial artery, place your first two or three fingers on the thumb side of your inner wrist. To find the carotid artery, place your fingers just below the edge of the jaw bone. Apply gentle pressure. Do not use your thumb.
2. Using a stopwatch or clock with a second hand, count the number of pulses in 30 seconds. Multiply by two to get the number of beats per minute.

Maximum and Target Range Heart Rates   No aerobic exercise program will be beneficial unless it forces the heart to pump beyond its normal output. To determine this ideal pace, check whether the heart is beating fast enough to ensure that the activity pushes the heart muscle to the point of improving fitness, but not so fast that it will become quickly exhausted or cause physical harm. (See **Figure 9.3** to determine maximum and target heart rates.) Checking the pulse during or immediately after exercise is one way to determine the intensity level of a workout (see **Self-Assessment 9.2**). An exercise program should keep

the heart rate within the target range. If the heart does not reach the lower limit of the target heart range during an exercise activity, increase the intensity by exercising more vigorously. If the heart rate exceeds the upper limit of the target heart range, particularly in the early phases of an exercise program, reduce the intensity to stay within the range.

Forms of Aerobic Exercise   Regular exercise is important. The form it takes is of secondary importance. Some women enjoy sticking with a single form of exercise. Others keep their interest in exercise by changing their physical activity on a regular basis. Seasonal variations, changes in schedules, and access to equipment and facilities also influence women's exercise habits.

The *2008 Physical Activity Guidelines for Americans* distinguish between moderate and intense forms of aerobic

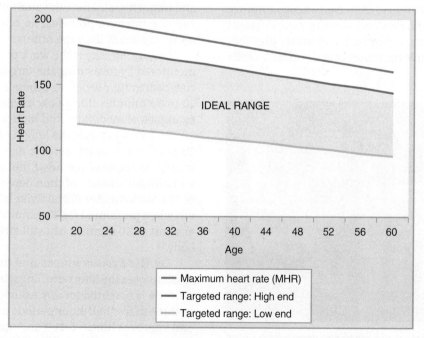

Figure 9.3   Maximum and target heart rates.

exercise. Both forms raise the heart rate and improve overall health; however, intense aerobic activity provides roughly the same benefits as moderate aerobic activities in about half the time. A woman can reach the recommended guidelines by performing 2 hours and 30 minutes (150 minutes) of moderate aerobic activity per week, 1 hour and 15 minutes (75 minutes) of intense activities, or a combination of the two. Moderate forms of aerobic exercise include brisk walking, bicycling at a slow pace, dancing, water aerobics, gardening, doubles tennis, and using a manual wheelchair. Intense forms of aerobic exercise include aerobic dance or cardio-kickboxing classes, playing soccer or basketball, fast or hilly riding on a bicycle, singles tennis, and swimming laps.[17]

Moderate- to brisk-paced walking is an easy, safe, and enjoyable way to stay healthy. Walking for 30 to 45 minutes per day provides excellent health benefits and burns as many calories as running or jogging the same distance. Walking is also an activity in which people of most abilities and body types can participate. Most problems with walking can be avoided by simply paying attention to one's surroundings and wearing good walking shoes.

Jogging is aerobic exercise somewhere between a fast walk and a run, usually defined as moving at a pace slower than a 9-minute mile, with running defined as a 9-minute mile or faster. Both activities count as intense forms of aerobic exercise. Although running and jogging are excellent forms of aerobic exercise, women (and men) should be careful not to put too much stress on their knees, ankles, and other joints. Ways to reduce joint stress while running or jogging include using good running shoes; running on grass, dirt, or asphalt rather than concrete; limiting average weekly distance to 12 to 15 miles per week; and alternating between running or jogging and other forms of aerobic exercise.

Bicycling, whether on a stationary bike or outdoors, can be an excellent cardiovascular conditioner. Stationary biking in aerobic settings, often referred to as "spinning," offers a variety of speed resistances to simulate biking a hilly course or race.

Stair climbing, either in buildings or on stair machines, is another form of aerobic exercise that involves less impact on the joints and feet than high-impact forms of aerobic exercise. Step aerobics is another form of this exercise. Stair climbing and bicycling can each act as moderate or intense forms of aerobic exercise, depending on the pace.

Swimming is an excellent way to strengthen and tone muscles as well as promote aerobic fitness. Swimming has the advantage of not placing excess stress on the joints, as do many other forms of aerobic exercise.

Aerobic dance is exercise that combines music with kicking, stretching, bending, and jumping, to deliver the same benefits as running, cycling, or swimming. Aerobic classes based on kickboxing or other martial arts are another form of exercise. These intense classes combine punches, kicks, and other activities with an aerobic

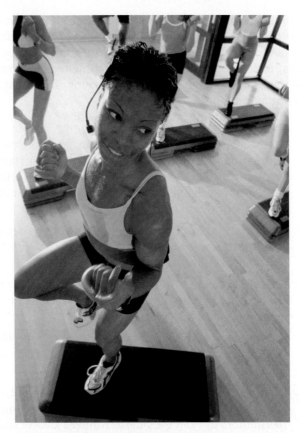

Aerobic exercise can take many forms. It is not limited to running or exercise classes.

workout to provide excellent benefits in strength, coordination, balance, speed, flexibility, and agility.

> *Tennis was a big part of my life when I was in high school. Our school's women's tennis team was one of the best in the state, but we were always a second priority to the men's team, which was pretty mediocre. The female players weren't even allowed to wear our letters on our school jackets. My younger daughter plays soccer, and I love seeing her play. It's nice to see the women's teams getting some recognition!*
>
> **—55-year-old doctor**

Strength Training

Strength training is another essential component of a well-balanced exercise program. Like aerobic exercise, strength training helps prevent or delay many of the declines associated with aging or inactivity. The *2008 Physical Activity Guidelines for Americans* recommend two or more sessions of strength training exercises per week. A good strength training workout should involve all the major muscle groups and should use enough weight that a person can just barely do 8 to 12 repetitions.

Strength training is not just a tool for bodybuilders and muscle enthusiasts. An equally valid term for strength training could be "body conditioning." Strength training helps to tone the body, build bone strength, and improve overall health in addition to increasing muscle mass. A woman can use free weights, dumbbells, barbells, resistance bands, weight machines, or her own body weight (through push-ups, chin-ups, and sit-ups) for strength training.

Strength training offers many benefits:

■ Well-toned muscles help maintain good posture. Maintaining a strong back through strength training reduces the risk of injury. Lower back pain often results from weakness of back and abdominal muscles, both of which help support the back.

■ Muscle strength produces benefits in daily living, from lifting items to engaging in physical activity, by increasing stamina and self-confidence.

■ Strength training can help prevent or delay many of the declines in everyday functioning associated with aging or inactivity.

■ Strength training increases bone density, thereby helping to delay or minimize osteoporosis and vulnerability to fractures.

■ Injury prevention is another important benefit of strength training, especially for musculoskeletal injuries induced by exercise, such as runner's knee or shin splints. These injuries are due in part to muscle weakness and imbalances as well as joint instability. Such conditions are often corrected with strength training.

Women tend to have less muscle mass than men, especially in the upper body. Gender differences in size, hormones, and normal activity levels contribute to this discrepancy. Women who work out, however, gain strength at the same rate as men. Many women have avoided strength training out of fear of becoming "muscle bound." A moderate program will not create obvious muscle bulk in men or women but will instead result in a firmer, trimmer physique.

Physical Fitness and Women

Psychological, social, historical, and cultural factors all affect how women think about fitness and exercise. Historically, women were labeled "the weaker sex" and were not encouraged to become as fit as their male counterparts. Prejudices have traditionally limited women's access to and full participation in sports. Self-esteem and self-confidence with physical activity are developmental tasks of childhood. Because young girls were not encouraged to excel or compete in the physical arena, they often lacked the self-esteem and confidence necessary to participate in sports as they grew older. It was not until 1978 that legislation known as **Title IX** mandated that public schools provide equal funding for girls' sports. However, even since its passage, opportunities, resources, and, perhaps most importantly, encouragement for physical fitness have not been equally distributed to children,

regardless of gender. Groups like the Women's National Basketball Association and a new generation of popular women's sports stars are revising the societal rule that says only male athletes can be admired.

Traditionally, men have excelled in physical competition against women. In general, men are able to run longer and faster, jump higher and farther, lift more and longer, and so forth. Over the past 30 years, however, women have become more competitive in all athletic arenas. Despite these advances, young girls and boys are still often raised with different levels of emphasis, encouragement, and training in physical fitness.

The fact that men are stronger than women reflects the larger absolute quantity of their muscle mass. Individual muscle fibers do not appear to be different, and women's bodies respond to training as quickly as do men's. Women are typically about half as strong as men in the upper body areas of the shoulders, arms, and back and two-thirds as strong in the legs and lower body, primarily because men have larger muscle fiber areas and greater lean body weight (total weight minus body fat). Women's naturally higher percentage of body fat, essential for reproduction and general health, may have more of an effect on their physical performance than any other factor. Typically about 25% of a woman's body weight is fat, compared with 15% for men. Women's extra body fat may be a hindrance in sports such as running but an advantage in sports such as swimming. In general, women also have a lower blood volume, about 5% less hemoglobin, smaller hearts, and less lung capacity than men.

Women's performances in endurance sports have dramatically increased over the past 30 years. Over the same period, the gender gap in biking, swimming, and other sports has been gradually shrinking. Female professional athletes may not reach the same levels of absolute performance as their male counterparts for every sport, but women should not let prejudice or feelings of inferiority prevent them from reaching their own optimal fitness levels.

Exercise Myths and Facts

Fear and misinformation about fitness, workouts, or muscles cause many women to avoid exercise or to exercise inappropriately. These fears are usually unfounded and may prevent women from engaging in healthful behaviors.

Myth: Exercise increases the appetite.
Fact: Many factors affect the appetite more than exercise. Depending on the circumstance, exercise may increase, decrease, or have no noticeable effect on the appetite. Women who do eat more when they exercise usually add fewer calories than they burn in their workouts. Exercise raises the basal metabolic rate, which remains elevated not only for the exercise period but also for an extended time after the physical activity ends. Calories are thus burned at a higher rate for an extended period of time.

Myth: I am too out of shape or old to exercise.

Fact: People of all ages and body types benefit from physical activity. Exercise programs can begin with a few minutes of activity per day, such as walking or climbing a flight of stairs, and then gradually increase the amount of activity. This will help a person get in better shape and prepare him or her for additional activity. Any amount of physical activity provides some health benefits.

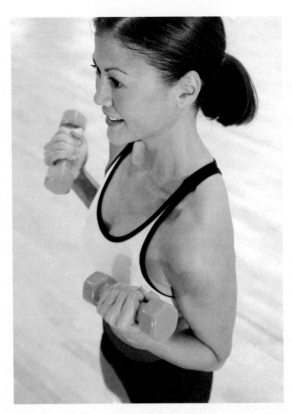

It is a common myth that a woman will develop bulging muscles if she lifts weights.
© Photodisc

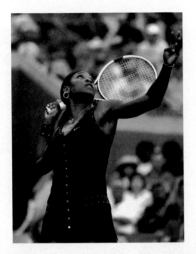

Women are increasingly being recognized as proficient athletes, whether in competition with one another or in mixed sports.
© Philip Date/Shutterstock

Myth: Exercising special spots will reduce local fat.

Fact: There is no such thing as effective "spot reduction." Fat tissue cannot be converted into muscle. When a woman exercises, she uses energy produced by burning fat in all parts of the body—not just around the muscles that are doing the most work. Sit-ups will not take fat off the abdomen any faster than any other body area. Strengthening the abdominal muscles through exercise may improve posture, however, and help hold the abdomen in more.

Myth: No pain, no gain.

Fact: Exercise does not have to hurt to provide benefits. If a person is beginning or intensifying an exercise program, some muscle discomfort is probable. However, this discomfort should not extend beyond the feeling of a slight ache into actual pain. Avoid pain during and after exercise by intensifying workouts slowly and by beginning each session with a warm-up and ending it with a cooldown.

Myth: Lifting weights gives women a bulky, masculine physique.

Fact: The bulky image of male bodybuilders often seen in popular culture is only possible through a deliberate, dedicated workout routine consisting of hours of daily exercise. Strength training offers as many benefits to bone strength and general health as it does to major muscle groups.

Myth: The more sweat produced, the more fat (or weight) lost.

Fact: Exercising in extreme heat or while wearing a plastic suit will, indeed, cause a person to sweat and lose weight, but sweat reflects the loss of water, not fat. Normal consumption of food and water will soon cause the weight to return. An individual who sweats too much during exercise without replenishing essential liquids runs the risk of developing heat exhaustion or

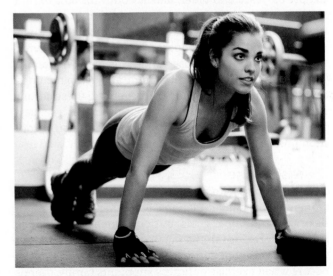

Strength training can help prevent or delay many of the declines associated with aging or inactivity.
© antoniodiaz/Shutterstock

dehydration. The amount of sweat produced is not a measure of energy expended. Sweating depends more on temperature, humidity, lack of conditioning, body weight, and individual variability.

Myth: Exercise is not good for weight loss because weight is gained in muscle.

Fact: Aerobic exercises burn more fat than they add muscle. With exercises such as weight lifting, muscle gain may indeed weigh more than burned-off fat. Usually, however, this tradeoff results in increased trimness because the added muscle is less dense and bulky than the lost fat. One added benefit is that the few extra pounds of muscle do not carry the health risks of excess fat. Another is that the body burns 15 to 20 times the calories to maintain a pound of muscle than it burns to maintain the same amount of fat.

Myth: Women cannot perform well athletically while menstruating.

Fact: Most women can perform physical activities consistently throughout their menstrual cycles. Researchers have found no significant differences in physical capabilities, such as oxygen intake, throughout the menstrual cycle. In fact, exercising during menstruation helps relieve pain and discomfort associated with the menstrual cycle.

Exercise and Aging

Exercise becomes more important with age. Many problems commonly associated with aging, such as increased body fat, decreased lean body weight (muscle mass), decreased muscle strength and flexibility, loss of bone mass, lower metabolism, and slower reaction times, are often signs of inactivity that can be minimized or even prevented by exercise. Reduced muscle strength is a major cause of physical disability in the elderly. Muscle strength and flexibility are critical components of maintaining the ability to walk and remain independent. For people 65 years and older, falls account for 80% of injuries requiring a hospital visit.[23] In addition to improving physical fitness, exercise reduces the risk of developing type 2 diabetes and osteoporosis and can reduce symptoms for people with these conditions (see Chapter 11). The combination of strength training and aerobic exercise seems to be the best method for preventing these chronic debilitating conditions. Exercise also promotes a sense of well-being and reduces symptoms of depression, a common problem among aging women.

Exercise Abuse

Pressure to be svelte and physically attractive bombards women from many directions. Being healthy and fit are desirable and noble goals, but occasionally individuals become so zealous in the pursuit of fitness or the desire to be attractive that injury or harm results. Exercise abuse occurs when exercise or fitness supplants family, friends, work, and education in importance; when the body is pushed beyond healthful limits; or when athletic injuries

are ignored. A body part or the entire body is considered overused if it is exercised beyond its biological limit to the point of injury. Common overuse injuries affect the muscles, tendons, ligaments, joints, and skin. Excessive exercise, faulty technique, and poor equipment are all common causes of overuse injuries. Pushing beyond discomfort into pain is dangerous because the pain of overexertion is the body's message indicating that something is wrong; such a problem should be addressed, not ignored.

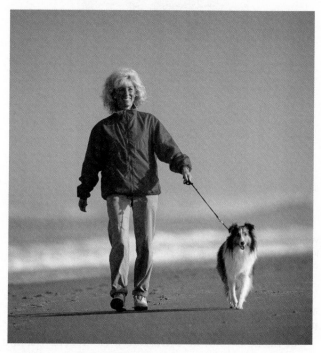

Exercise throughout the life span can reduce or prevent many of the health problems associated with aging.
© Photodisc

Some women may exercise so much that they stop menstruating. This condition, known as athletic amenorrhea, usually is the direct result of excessive exercise and an abnormally low ratio of body fat to body weight. The long-term consequences of prolonged athletic amenorrhea include the early onset of osteoporosis and its resultant risk for injury and debilitation. Athletic amenorrhea often affects adolescent female athletes who train in sports that emphasize slenderness, such as long-distance running, gymnastics, figure skating, and ballet, or women who are endurance athletes, such as distance swimmers and runners.[24] The **female athlete triad** is the relationship among disordered eating, amenorrhea, and osteoporosis. This problem usually begins with disordered eating. The combination of poor nutrition and intense athletic training causes weight loss and a decrease in or shutdown of estrogen production. Consequently, amenorrhea occurs. The final condition in the triad, osteoporosis, may follow if estrogen levels remain low and the woman's diet continues to lack calcium and vitamin D.

Anabolic steroid use is another form of exercise abuse. Anabolic steroids are synthetic derivatives of the male hormone testosterone. Although steroid use is most common among teenage males, women use these drugs as well. Men and women who take steroids with heavy resistance training increase their muscle and lean body mass but also experience severe physical and psychological side effects. Documented adverse physical effects of steroid use in women include enlargement of the clitoris, growth of facial hair, changes in or cessation of the menstrual cycle, deepened voice, and breast diminution. Other potential side effects include increased risk of heart disease and stroke, increased aggression, liver tumors and jaundice, aching joints, bad breath, and acne.

In adolescents, steroid use can halt growth prematurely. The AIDS epidemic has introduced another liability from steroid use: increased risk of human immunodeficiency virus (HIV) transmission from sharing needles. The psychological effects of long-term, high-dose anabolic steroid use may lead to addiction, drug cravings, and withdrawal symptoms when use of the drugs is stopped.[25] Hepatitis B and C, two diseases that can seriously damage the liver, are also easily spread by needle sharing. Clearly, anabolic steroids should be totally avoided.

MAINTAINING A HEALTHY WEIGHT

To maintain a healthful weight, a woman should balance the calories she consumes as part of a balanced diet with the calories she burns through daily physical activities. Most women who do not live active lifestyles need about 1600–2000 calories per day; for physically active women, this number increases to about 2000–2400 calories per day. In most cases, weight loss requires substantial, but not excessive calorie reduction; physical activity can play a secondary role by burning additional calories. A good rough estimate for moderate weight loss is a combination of calorie reduction and exercise to burn 500–1000 calories per day, which will typically produce a weight loss of 1–2 pounds per week.[26]

For a rough estimate of ideal weight, adults can evaluate their weight-for-height ratio, or **body mass index (BMI)**. (See **It's Your Health** and **Self-Assessment 9.3**.) A BMI of between 25 and 29.9 indicates overweight and a BMI of 30 or higher indicates obesity in adults. Although it is a useful tool, the BMI is only effective for certain body types. A person who has a lot of muscle, a large body frame, and little fat may have a BMI above the healthy range but may still be healthy; similarly, a person who has a lot of fat and little muscle may have a BMI in the healthy range but may not be at his or her ideal weight. Another way to define overweight is to measure the proportion of fat in the body, though it is a difficult measurement to perform accurately, even with professional training.

In addition to total weight, weight distribution is an important consideration. Women whose body-fat

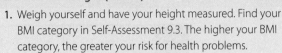

It's Your Health

Evaluate Your Weight (Adults)

1. Weigh yourself and have your height measured. Find your BMI category in Self-Assessment 9.3. The higher your BMI category, the greater your risk for health problems.

2. Measure around your waist while standing, just above your hip bones. If this measurement is greater than 35 inches for women or 40 inches for men, you probably have excess abdominal fat. This excess fat may place you at greater risk of health problems, even if your BMI is about right.

3. The higher your BMI and waist measurement, the more you are likely to benefit from weight loss.

distribution favors the upper body ("apples") rather than the hips and thighs ("pears") are at higher risk of developing type 2 diabetes, coronary artery disease, hypertension, gallbladder disease, and polycystic ovarian syndrome.[27] Consequently, waist measurement has been used as a loose measure of one's chance of developing heart disease, cancer, or other chronic diseases. A waist larger than 35 inches for a woman and 40 inches for a man is considered to be a risk factor for the aforementioned diseases.

What Causes Weight Gain

Many factors influence weight loss and gain. In most cases, overweight and obesity result from excess calorie consumption and/or inadequate physical activity. A small percentage of people may have a genetic predisposition to gain weight or a genetic need to eat more than they need for energy; a larger percentage may simply have a body that tends to store extra fat, making it harder for them to lose weight (and keep weight off).

Weight gain occurs when a person consumes more calories than she or he burns. Beneath this simple truth, however, lies a more complex reality. Today, most Americans work, study, and relax in environments that require little physical activity and have easy access to processed foods that are cheap; high in calories, fats, and sugars; and lacking in healthful nutrients. Women still have responsibility for taking care of their health, but these realities of modern living make getting adequate physical activity and eating a balanced diet difficult.

People who are overweight or obese are often blamed for overindulging or overeating, whereas people who lose weight or stay at a healthy weight are praised for their discipline. It is not only discipline and a desire to be fit that influence whether a person chooses to exercise—it is also how much free time a woman has; whether she was encouraged to exercise as a child and had opportunities for doing so; whether she lives in a neighborhood with safe and satisfying places to walk, run, or play sports; and whether her work schedule allows her to visit a health club while it is open.

Self-Assessment 9.3
Are You at a Healthy Weight?

Body Mass Index Table

	Normal						Overweight					Obese										Extreme Obesity														
BMI	19	20	21	22	23	24	25	26	27	28	29	30	31	32	33	34	35	36	37	38	39	40	41	42	43	44	45	46	47	48	49	50	51	52	53	54
Height (inches)													Body Weight (pounds)																							
58	91	96	100	105	110	115	119	124	129	134	138	143	148	153	158	162	167	172	177	181	186	191	196	201	205	210	215	220	224	229	234	239	244	248	253	258
59	94	99	104	109	114	119	124	128	133	138	143	148	153	158	163	168	173	178	183	188	193	198	203	208	212	217	222	227	232	237	242	247	252	257	262	267
60	97	102	107	112	118	123	128	133	138	143	148	153	158	163	168	174	179	184	189	194	199	204	209	215	220	225	230	235	240	245	250	255	261	266	271	276
61	100	106	111	116	122	127	132	137	143	148	153	158	164	169	174	180	185	190	195	201	206	211	217	222	227	232	238	243	248	254	259	264	269	275	280	285
62	104	109	115	120	126	131	136	142	147	153	158	164	169	175	180	186	191	196	202	207	213	218	224	229	235	240	246	251	256	262	267	273	278	284	289	295
63	107	113	118	124	130	135	141	146	152	158	163	169	175	180	186	191	197	203	208	214	220	225	231	237	242	248	254	259	265	270	278	282	287	293	299	304
64	110	116	122	128	134	140	145	151	157	163	169	174	180	186	192	197	204	209	215	221	227	232	238	244	250	256	262	267	273	279	285	291	296	302	308	314
65	114	120	126	132	138	144	150	156	162	168	174	180	186	192	198	204	210	216	222	228	234	240	246	252	258	264	270	276	282	288	294	300	306	312	318	324
66	118	124	130	136	142	148	155	161	167	173	179	186	192	198	204	210	216	223	229	235	241	247	253	260	266	272	278	284	291	297	303	309	315	322	328	334
67	121	127	134	140	146	153	159	166	172	178	185	191	198	204	211	217	223	230	236	242	249	255	261	268	274	280	287	293	299	306	312	319	325	331	338	344
68	125	131	138	144	151	158	164	171	177	184	190	197	203	210	216	223	230	236	243	249	256	262	269	276	282	289	295	302	308	315	322	328	335	341	348	354
69	128	135	142	149	155	162	169	176	182	189	196	203	209	216	223	230	236	243	250	257	263	270	277	284	291	297	304	311	318	324	331	338	345	351	358	365
70	132	139	146	153	160	167	174	181	188	195	202	209	216	222	229	236	243	250	257	264	271	278	285	292	299	306	313	320	327	334	341	348	355	362	369	376
71	136	143	150	157	165	172	179	186	193	200	208	215	222	229	236	243	250	257	265	272	279	286	293	301	308	315	322	329	338	343	351	358	365	372	379	386
72	140	147	154	162	169	177	184	191	199	206	213	221	228	235	242	250	258	265	272	279	287	294	302	309	316	324	331	338	346	353	361	368	375	383	390	397
73	144	151	159	166	174	182	189	197	204	212	219	227	235	242	250	257	265	272	280	288	295	302	310	318	325	333	340	348	355	363	371	378	386	393	401	408
74	148	155	163	171	179	186	194	202	210	218	225	233	241	249	256	264	272	280	287	295	303	311	319	326	334	342	350	358	365	373	381	389	396	404	412	420
75	152	160	168	176	184	192	200	208	216	224	232	240	248	256	264	272	279	287	295	303	311	319	327	335	343	351	359	367	375	383	391	399	407	415	423	431
76	156	164	172	180	189	197	205	213	221	230	238	246	254	263	271	279	287	295	304	312	320	328	336	344	353	361	369	377	385	394	402	410	418	426	435	443

Source: Adapted from *Clinical Guidelines on the Identification, Evaluation, and Treatment of Overweight and Obesity in Adults: The Evidence Report.*

BMI measures weight in relation to height. The BMI ranges shown here are for adults. They are not exact ranges of healthy and unhealthy weights but rather show that health risk increases at higher levels of overweight and obesity. Even within the healthy BMI range, weight gain can carry health risks for adults.

Directions: Find your weight on the bottom of the graph. Go straight up from that point until you come to the line that matches your height. Then look to find your weight group.

Healthy Weight: BMI from 18.5 to 24

Overweight: BMI from 25 to 29

Obese: BMI 30 or higher

Source: Adapted from *Clinical guidelines on the identification, evaluation, and treatment of overweight and obesity in adults: The evidence report.*

Similarly, if a woman lives in an area where nutritious foods are unavailable, inconvenient, or considerably more expensive than processed foods high in fats and sugars, she is less likely to eat a well-balanced diet than if she lives in an area where nutritious foods are easier to find or purchase. The processed food industry uses a variety of tactics to sell its products and to maximize its sales. Companies use deceptive advertising methods to portray their products as being nutritious, such as emphasizing that a product is low in sugar even as it is high in fat and salt (or vice versa). Another tactic has been to increase portion sizes to market the idea of customers getting a "better deal." These tactics have earned hundreds of millions of dollars for the fast-food and carbonated-beverage industries in particular. Unfortunately, these same tactics have also resulted in millions of people consuming extra, unneeded calories without adding nutrients to their diet. **Table 9.8** provides examples of changes in portion size over the past 20 years.

Overweight and Obesity

Although the word "overweight" is often used subjectively or with judgmental overtones, the word also has a medical definition, meaning that a person weighs more than is generally healthy for a certain height. A person is considered to be **overweight** if he or she has a BMI of 25 to 29.9. **Obesity** defines people with additional unhealthful weight beyond the overweight range, with a BMI of 30 or greater. Obesity is a complex, multifactorial chronic disease. The proportion of people who are overweight and obese has increased among genders and among all population groups over the past 100 years. Today, more than one-third of U.S. adults are obese, and about one-third are overweight.[28] The prevalence of obesity is higher among African American women and Hispanic women than among White and Asian American women. Obesity and overweight are also more common among people with low incomes and low education. These associations exist for many reasons, in part because people of color or those living in poverty have reduced access to nutritious foods and opportunities to exercise. People living in poverty are also more likely to be exposed to high-calorie, energy-dense foods and sweetened beverages, either through greater exposure to advertising or directly in terms of availability in local food and grocery stores.

Obesity and overweight among children are also a growing public health problem. Approximately one out of five U.S. children is overweight, and one-third of those who are at a healthy weight are at risk of soon becoming overweight.[28] Children who are overweight or obese are likely to stay that way as they grow up. They also often develop health problems before they reach adulthood, from unhealthy cholesterol levels and high blood pressure, to impaired blood glucose tolerance (a precursor to type 2 diabetes), to breathing problems such as asthma and sleep apnea. The shame and stigmatization associated with childhood obesity or overweight can also have lasting cascading effects, from reduced mental health, to impaired social functioning, to reduced academic achievement.[29]

One important factor behind this increase in rates of obesity has been the jump in average calorie intake over the past 30 years. Today, the average daily calorie consumption is over 300 calories more than the average consumption in 1980. Refined grains, added fats, and added sugars account for most of this increase.[28]

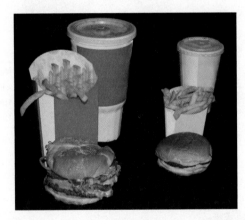

Food portions have become noticeably larger in the past 20 years. Single portions now often provide enough food for at least two people.

Overweight and obesity are the second leading preventable causes of death in the United States, just behind tobacco use. Obesity increases the risk for heart disease,

Table 9.8	Portion Distortion		
Food Item	**Size and Calories**		**Ways to Burn the Extra**
	20 Years Ago	**Today**	
Bagel	3-inch diameter/140 calories	6-inch diameter/350 calories	Rake leaves for 50 minutes to burn an extra 210 calories
French fries	2.4 ounces/210 calories	6.9 ounces/610 calories	Walk 2 hours, 20 minutes to burn an extra 400 calories
Soda	6.5 ounces/85 calories	20 ounces/250 calories	Garden for 35 minutes to burn an extra 165 calories
Turkey sandwich	320 calories	820 calories	Bike for 1 hour, 25 minutes to burn an extra 500 calories

Data from National Heart, Lung, and Blood Institute. *Stay young at heart.*

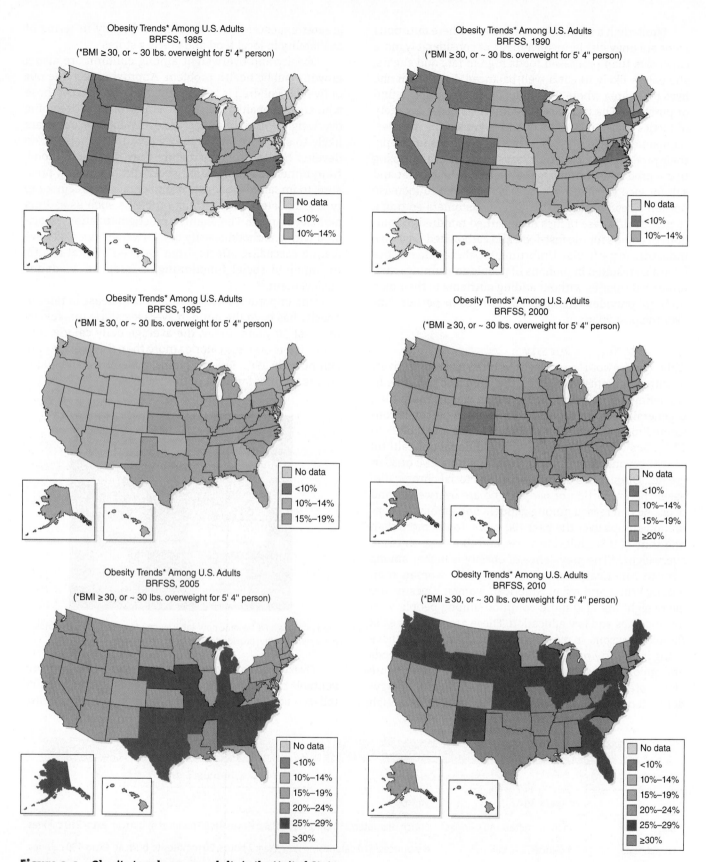

Figure 9.4   Obesity trends among adults in the United States.

Reproduced from the Centers for Disease Control and Prevention. Obesity trends among U.S. adults. *Behavioral Risk Factor Surveillance System.* 1985, 1990, 1995, 2000, 2005, 2010.

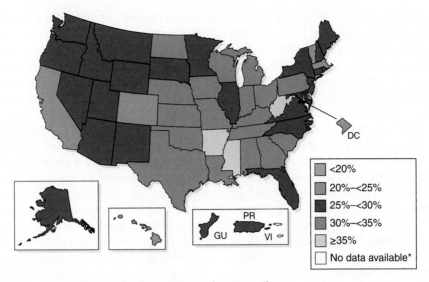

Figure 9.4   **Obesity trends among adults in the United States. (continued)**

stroke, many forms of cancer, hypertension, diabetes, and other conditions. Every year, about 50,500 cases of cancer among women (about 7% of total cancers in women) occur as a direct result of obesity.[30] Cancers of the thyroid, esophagus, colon, endometrium (uterine lining), kidney, pancreas, gallbladder, and other areas are more likely to develop in people who are overweight or obese. Being 30 pounds overweight can increase a woman's risk of endometrial cancer threefold and being 50 pounds overweight can increase her risk tenfold.[31] People who are obese also are subject to discrimination and social stigmatization, and consequently they may suffer from low self-esteem and depression.

Being overweight or obese can lead to many health problems, including adult-onset diabetes, hypertension, coronary heart disease, gout, gallbladder disease, and arthritic conditions. Women suffer from additional obesity-related problems, including irregular menstrual cycles, amenorrhea, infertility, and polycystic ovarian syndrome. Studies show that the risk of death rises with increasing weight.

Moderate excess weight (10 to 20 pounds for a person of average height), even for women who exercise, increases the risk of death, particularly among adults ages 30 to 64 years. At the same time, even moderate weight loss can reduce a woman's risk for heart disease, diabetes, and cancer: The National Cancer Institute estimates that reducing the country's average BMI by 1% (about 2 pounds of weight loss per person) would prevent about 100,000 cases of cancer.[32]

Obesity was only recognized as a major health issue in the latter half of the 20th century. Discussions of obesity as a potential public health concern began in the 1970s, but not until 1985 at the NIH Consensus Development Conference was it acknowledged that obesity leads to increased morbidity and mortality. Concern over the subject has increased as the proportion of people who are obese or overweight has grown.

Although the development of obesity is complex, the benefits of treatment are certain. The ideal goal is to return a person to a healthful weight. However, even a small loss of weight (such as 5–10% of a person's body weight), if maintained, has significant health benefits. Obesity treatments often begin with weight loss, employing reduced-calorie diets along with physical activity, behavior therapy, medications, and weight-loss surgery for people who are severely obese (BMIs equal to or greater than 40).

Economic Dimensions of Obesity and Overweight

The medical costs for obesity in the United States are more than $150 billion a year.[33] This figure includes the direct medical costs to treat diseases associated with obesity such as diabetes, joint problems, and heart disease and the indirect costs of injuries associated with the condition. In addition, overweight and obesity incur indirect costs from lost productivity, premature disability, and early death. Healthcare costs and the likelihood of complications from surgery for obese and overweight people are higher than those for people of healthful weight. Individuals and families face additional costs, such as specially designed chairs and beds to support an obese frame, specialty clothes, and higher-than-average numbers of medications. Together, these items can create a significant cost burden to families.

Weight Loss

Millions of Americans who are overweight or obese are aware that they weigh more than a healthy amount and want to lose weight (and stay at a healthy weight). Most of them, however, are unable to do so. At the population level, many factors contribute to unhealthy weight gain.

Millions of Americans have limited opportunities to exercise. Cities and suburbs are often designed with cars, not pedestrians, in mind, making walking unpleasant or dangerous; for people living in some neighborhoods, being outside for an extended period can be a safety risk. Leaders of weight-loss, fast-food, soft-drink, and other processed food industries all expect continued growth and billions of dollars per year in profits. To reach these goals, these industries create advertising and promotional campaigns to make processed foods appear everywhere and appear healthy. Advertisements and commercials constantly tout ways that their methods or products can help people lose weight, but their claims are often biased, exaggerated, or inaccurate. Advertisements for weight-loss programs, meanwhile, promise quick, easy, and dramatic results.

Americans spend more than $60 billion every year, most of it unsuccessfully, addressing weight concerns. This money includes health-club memberships, home gym equipment, diet books, and participation in weight-loss programs. About 70 million people—almost one out of four people in the United States—attempt to lose weight every year. Only about 5% of these people are ultimately successful.[34]

These statements are not intended to cause anyone to lose hope. Achieving and maintaining a healthful weight can be done and is a worthwhile goal. For millions of Americans, however, reaching this goal will require acknowledging the obstacles in one's path, making significant lifestyle changes, and setting realistic goals for weight loss.

Losing weight depends on burning more calories than the body ingests. The body takes in calories through food and drinks (other than water) and burns calories both through normal daily living activities as well as through physical activity. If a woman consumes the same number of calories that she ingests, she will maintain her current weight.

Calorie and portion control should be the primary component of a successful weight loss program. Physical activity can play a secondary role, by burning some calories and helping to prevent the regaining of weight that has been lost. For weight loss, however, exercise by itself may be difficult or impossible in most practical situations: Reducing one's daily calorie intake by 600 calories, for example, would take about an hour of vigorous jogging per day. Regardless of its direct effects on weight and body fat, exercise improves overall health by lowering blood pressure, improving cholesterol levels, strengthening the cardiovascular system, helping to prevent type 2 diabetes and other conditions, and reducing stress.

Keeping a food and exercise diary may help some women identify their eating and exercising patterns. All meals, snacks, drinks, and all forms of physical activity should recorded in the diary. After a review of a few days of diary notes, objectively examine your own eating habits and set realistic goals that rely on a diet based on healthy foods and regular exercise. Women can monitor their progress through the food diary and weekly (not daily) checks with the scale. Once a reasonable desired weight loss is achieved, focus on maintaining that weight through sensible eating and exercise.

Ways Not to Lose Weight

Women (and, increasingly, men) spend countless hours worrying, thinking, and obsessing over weight loss. Diet books, programs, and plans make enormous profits by preying on women's insecurities about their weight, and then offering their new product as an easy solution to this "problem." When women do not lose weight, or lose weight but gain it back, they often blame themselves, even if the diets themselves are flawed, ineffective, or unrealistic.

Starvation, hunger, or eliminating fats (or another food group) is not a healthy or even effective way to lose weight. Food substitution, such as replacing simple carbohydrates with complex ones, or replacing empty calories, high-calorie proteins, or carbohydrates with vegetables, is far better than food restriction.

Alcohol should also be avoided or consumed sparingly in any weight-loss effort. Alcohol provides empty calories that contribute to weight gain without providing any nutritional benefit. Alcohol may also promote the storage of body fat by causing the body to burn fat more slowly in its presence.

Yo-yo dieting is a term that characterizes the repeated, chronic pattern of dieting and then regaining weight that describes most dieters' behavior. In addition

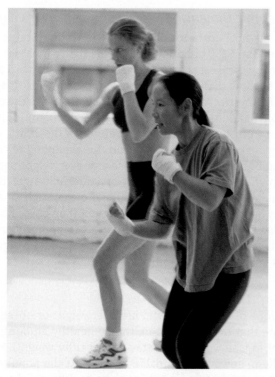

Regular exercise is an essential component of any weight-control program.
© Photodisc

It's Your Health

Helpful and Unhelpful Weight-Loss Strategies

Helpful

Allow occasional treats or servings of favorite foods.

Develop realistic, long-term goals that can be maintained.

Reduce but do not eliminate fat from the diet.

Use monounsaturated oils like olive oil more than other sources of fat.

Stick with the program even if there are lapses.

Plan meals and snacks to include more complex carbohydrates, fruits, and vegetables.

Limit intake of fatty foods, oils, and dressings.

Avoid packaged snack foods.

Develop new interests that do not involve food.

Vary sources of protein to include fish and seafood and peas and beans in addition to meat and poultry.

Eat foods slowly.

Exercise regularly.

Drink water rather than carbonated beverages or sports drinks.

Reduce sugar intake—look for levels of simple carbohydrates.

Join a support group or share the process with a friend.

Clean the pantry—give away foods that are not part of the new healthy eating plan.

Try a new nutritious recipe each week.

Eat small meals throughout the day to keep from getting too hungry.

Unhelpful

Setting unrealistic expectations for dramatic, near-instant results.

Focusing solely on short-term goals.

Choosing a program that makes eating unpleasant.

Adopting unconventional theories to explain how food combinations add or decrease body weight.

Following a diet that omits any one food group or focuses on one particular food, such as grapefruit or yogurt.

Maintaining a daily caloric intake of less than 1200 calories, unless under medical supervision.

Using any diet that promotes megadoses of vitamins to make up for nutritional deficits.

Fasting or starvation diets.

Taking any pill or potion that "melts fat."

Using appetite-suppressant drugs.

Giving up all sweets or breads.

Using muscle stimulators or body wraps.

---

to being frustrating, yo-yo dieting may be hazardous to health, because it may increase the risk for coronary heart disease, although separating the direct physiological effects of the behavior and the resulting stress that comes with trying and failing to lose weight is difficult.[35] Yo-yo dieting may also weaken the immune system, making dieters more likely to become and stay sick.[35] Yo-yo dieters may store more and more fat in the abdominal area with each failed diet; abdominal fat is more harmful to one's health than fat in other places.

Diet supplements are another unhealthful way to lose weight. Weight-loss supplements often contain stimulants, which in high amounts may lead to an increased heart rate, heart attacks, nervousness, insomnia, headaches, seizures, or death. Many women have used supplements such as ephedra, which has been linked to adverse health outcomes and even death. Because these products are not subjected to the same testing standards as substances regulated by the FDA, supplements may have a higher rate of contamination or contraindications not stated on warning labels. Other weight-loss products may also be harmful or simply ineffective.

Other Weight-Loss Strategies

Many popular diets encourage specific eating regimens to attain maximum weight loss. In the 1990s, diets typically focused on high-carbohydrate/very-low-fat daily regimens. Later, the high-protein, high-fat, low-carbohydrate (Atkins) diet reemerged as a popular weight-loss strategy. Many people were not able to lose weight on these diets because they mistakenly believed that they could eat unlimited amounts of certain foods. In reality, excessive calories from any food source cause weight gain. Low-fat foods are often packed with sugar to make up for the loss of flavor when fat is removed. Several high-profile diets, including the Atkins diet and the Zone diet, identify high-protein/low-carbohydrate meals as being optimal. These diets have become financial empires, with books, snacks, prepared meals, and energy drinks all being sold to the millions of people who are subscribing to them. A *Consumer Reports* analysis found that people in Atkins and the Zone weight-loss programs were at least as

---

I have tried every diet in the book. I have had times where I have eaten only grapefruit, only rice, or only salads. I have also tried all the gimmicks—pills, liquids, body wraps. You name it, I've tried it. But nothing has really worked. I quickly gain the weight back, sometimes more, within a short time after I lose it. I always swear I won't try another stupid method, but as soon as I read an ad or see a new product, I feel that I have to give it a try.

—22-year-old woman

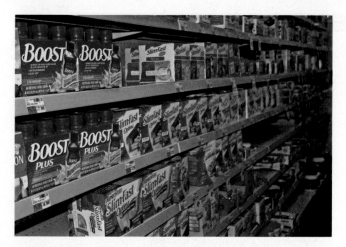

Weight-loss products should be used only when prescribed by a health-care provider; in these selected patients, the products should be used in combination with lifestyle changes to increase the success of long-term weight loss.

likely as people in other top-rated weight-loss programs to lose weight in the short term but were more likely to drop out in less than a year. They were also more likely to eat too much saturated fat and not enough fruits and vegetables.[36]

Weight-loss surgery has emerged as a tool for people who are severely overweight or obese. Gastrointestinal surgery for obesity, also called **bariatric surgery**, alters the digestive process. The operation promotes weight loss by closing off parts of the stomach to make it smaller. Operations that only reduce stomach size are known as "restrictive operations" because they restrict the amount of food the stomach can hold. Other operations, known as malabsorptive operations, combine stomach restriction with a partial bypass of the small intestine. These procedures create a direct connection from the stomach to the lower segment of the small intestine, bypassing portions of the digestive tract that absorb calories and nutrients. These operations often make eating and swallowing food extremely painful. These procedures are typically appropriate only for severely obese individuals who have not been able to control their weight with diet, exercise, and appropriate pharmaceutical interventions.

BODY IMAGE AND SHAPE

Body image is a result of a complex interrelationship among self-perception, family attitudes toward bodies and food, social norms, and individual experiences. Standards for beauty and desirability are not absolute; they vary over time and from culture to culture. Today, popular culture is filled with young, underweight women who do not represent what the typical American woman looks like. In Greek and Roman representations of Aphrodite and Venus as well as in paintings by Titian, Rubens, and Rembrandt, "ideal" women often had ample thighs, hips,

waists, and abdomens. The Venus de Milo, considered by many to be one of the most beautiful of the classical female torsos, is muscular and rounded. Contemporary society is weight conscious, fashion conscious, exercise conscious, diet conscious, and intolerant of perceived physical imperfection. Almost all women depicted in popular culture are naturally beautiful, young, and digitally enhanced; women who are over the age of 35, not conventionally attractive, or not airbrushed and wearing makeup are relegated to the sidelines or left out entirely. Modern Western society trains women to believe that their physical attractiveness determines their social value.

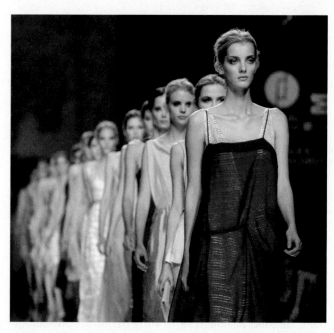

Women have been socialized to believe that an ultra-thin body shape is desirable.
© catwalker/Shutterstock

These images, which appear on commercials, Internet advertisements, magazines, movies, and other locations, have serious unconscious psychological effects. A study examining physical measurements of Miss America contestants, models, and Playboy Playmates over the course of the 20th century found that women in all three groups were likely to be underweight and were often thin enough to meet the World Health Organization's (WHO's) definition of anorexic. The weight and BMI of all three groups of women have also fallen, even as the weight of the average American woman has increased over the past 50 years.[37]

The gulf between what women see in the media and what they see in the mirror results in excessive dieting, eating disorders, a perceived need for plastic or cosmetic surgery, and feelings of self-loathing and inadequacy in many women, as seen in the following statistics:

- A national poll found that 24% of the people who said they would try any diet to lose weight were obese women, whereas only 9% were obese men. Obese women were also much more likely than men to feel guilty about eating.[38]

- Females account for more than 70% of the estimated 8 million sufferers of eating disorders.[39]

- Nearly 11 million surgical and nonsurgical cosmetic procedures were performed in the United States in 2014, according to the American Society for Aesthetic Plastic Surgery (ASAPS). This represents an increase of roughly 430% over the past 20 years. Although the number of surgical procedures, such as liposuction, breast augmentation, and eyelid or nose surgery grew, the biggest increase has been in procedures that do not require actual surgery, such as Botox injections and laser hair removal.[40]

Unhealthy body images begin early, with inappropriate eating habits and high anxiety about being overweight prevalent among adolescent girls. A large U.S. school-based study found that more than one-third of adolescent girls believed they were overweight, and more than 60% of female adolescents were trying to lose weight.[3] High school girls use starvation, fad diets, and purging methods, which can result in disordered eating behaviors, to lose weight. This finding is especially disturbing given the importance of high calcium intake for building healthy bones and developing critical bone mass, as well as the need for dietary fat to ensure healthy breast development in adolescents. Once established, an unhealthy preoccupation with body image and discontent with body shape during adolescence may persist for years, if not for life.

Excessive dieting and bodily preoccupation increase the likelihood that a person will have or will develop an eating disorder. New research findings and growing numbers of activists are seeking to influence the women and girls who are alienated from their bodies and obsessed with dieting (**Table 9.9**).

> I guess when I look in the mirror I see only the things that I feel are wrong. I wish I was thinner and taller, with a flatter stomach and a bigger chest. When I think about it, I realize that there are many things I actually like about myself but I can't seem to focus on them. When I look at other women, I notice their positive attributes. I wonder why I can't do that with myself.
>
> **—26-year-old woman**

> It's taken me most of my life, but I've finally gotten comfortable with my body. I'm not skinny. But you know what? I'm not overweight or out of shape, either. I exercise, I eat a good diet, and I don't smoke. And guess what? I can stay out dancing at a club hours after most of the skinny girls are wiped out.
>
> **—24-year-old woman**

Table 9.9   Comparing the Body Proportions of a Barbie Doll and the Average U.S. Woman

The popular "Barbie" doll is just one of many unrealistic body images that women face from childhood. If enlarged to the size of a real woman, a Barbie doll would have the following body proportions that are clearly impossible to emulate:

	Size, Average U.S. Woman	Size, Life-Sized Barbie Doll
Head:	21-22"	22"
Neck:	12-13"	9"
Biceps:	10-11"	7"
Forearms:	9-10"	6"
Wrists:	6-7"	3.5"
Bust:	35-36"	32"
Hips:	37-38"	29"
Thighs:	21-22"	16"
Calves:	14-15"	11"
Ankles:	8-9"	6"

Data from *Health* magazine, September 1997; NEDIC, a Canadian eating disorders advocacy group; Anorexia Nervosa and Related Eating Disorders, Inc., 2003.

Sociocultural Perspectives on Body Image

Women who grew up in largely African American communities often have different perspectives on body ideals than women who grow up in White-dominated communities. Similarly, girls who grow up in families where their mothers had their own disordered eating habits or poor body images are more likely to internalize those signals and adopt similar attitudes. Religion also can influence a girl's or woman's concept of her body, through doctrines of self-restraint, hard work, negative viewpoints on sloth, or in other ways. Even when these attitudes are not specifically directed toward body size, these messages can translate into feelings of blame for girls and women who struggle to control their weight. Cultural norms significantly influence weight management. A woman who wishes to change her eating habits may have to rebel against the traditions of her family or community.

Millions of women suffer from eating disorders, illnesses that develop around harmful, unusual eating habits. Eating disorders are most common among young, educated White and Hispanic females from middle to upper social classes, with new cases peaking at age 18. Eating disorders can have roots in social, emotional, and even biological factors in women's lives: pressure to "fit in" with popular cliques or peers; desire to avoid consumption as a way of dealing with strong emotions or maintaining control over one's life; and even feelings of euphoria that can occur when a person skips meals can

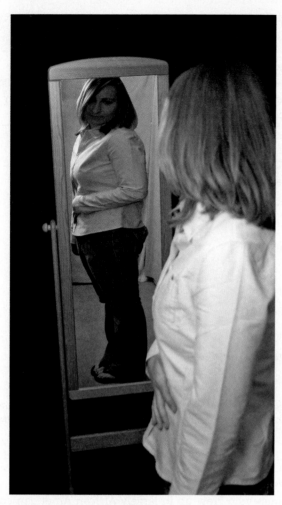

Women's perceptions about their bodies often are inaccurate.

all encourage a woman (or man) to adopt or continue an eating disorder. At the same time, these behaviors undermine one's health, self-esteem, and sense of competency. (For more on eating disorders, see Chapter 12.)

HUNGER

Hunger is the painful or uneasy feeling and biological harm caused by the continuous, unwanted lack of food. Hunger continues to be one of the world's greatest health risks, affecting almost 800 million people—about one out of nine people on the planet.[41] Most of these people live in the developing world, particularly in poorer countries in Asia and sub-Saharan Africa. Chronic hunger results when a person's daily calorie intake is not enough to lead an active, healthy life. **Malnutrition** refers to an imbalance between the body's nutritional needs and the intake or digestion of nutrients. Malnutrition may result in disease or death; it can be caused by an unbalanced diet or from problems in digesting or absorbing food.

Young children under the age of 5 are particularly vulnerable to the effects of hunger and malnutrition. Hunger and malnutrition are responsible for half of the global deaths in this age group—more than 3 million young children every year. Millions of other children become seriously sickened or injured as the result of not getting enough to eat. Malnourishment magnifies the effects of every disease. On average, malnourished children are ill about 160 days each year. Many factors contribute to hunger: artificially low global food prices that make it hard for local farmers to compete with large farms in the developed world, global warming, increased demands for energy, and the lingering effects of the recent global financial crisis.[42]

Although most people think of malnutrition as **undernutrition**, this term also includes **overnutrition**, which results from overeating, insufficient exercise, or excessive intake of vitamins and minerals. Overnutrition can lead to overweight and obesity, epidemics that are growing around the world. For people living in hunger, finding and preparing food typically takes more time, resources, and effort than for people who do not live in hunger.

Poverty is also a major contributing factor to hunger. Today, one out of five people in the world lives on less than $1 a day; twice that population lives on less than $2 a day. Another one out of five people around the world lacks access to clean water, and twice that number lack access to sanitation.[43] Providing these simple services could save millions of lives per year and prevent much pain and suffering.

In addition to young children, other populations especially affected by hunger include women who are pregnant or breastfeeding, the elderly, vegetarians, fad dieters, alcoholics or substance abusers, and people with certain chronic diseases. The most destructive form of malnutrition, which mainly affects infants and young children, is **protein-energy malnutrition (PEM)**. Children have high energy and protein needs, and therefore they suffer most when protein is lacking in their diets. Protein-energy malnutrition affects more than one-fourth of the world's children. More than 70% of PEM-afflicted children live in Asia, 26% in Africa, and 4% in Latin America and the Caribbean.[44]

Other nutrients that are extremely important for health include the following:

- *Vitamin A.* Vitamin A deficiency (VAD) is the leading cause of preventable blindness. It also reduces the body's resistance to disease and infection, and it can cause growth retardation in children. An estimated 250,000 to 500,000 children lose their sight every year due to VAD. Half of these children die within 12 months after becoming blind. VAD also harms pregnant women and their fetuses, causing night blindness (the inability to see well under low light conditions), increased risk of maternal mortality,

GENDER DIMENSIONS: Health Differences Between Men and Women

Extreme Dieting

Many women who try restrictive or long-term diets experience troublesome changes in the way they think, feel, and act. These women may feel cold, listless, and tired; have recurring, obsessive thoughts about food; grow anxious or afraid; and feel a reduced sex drive. Society has often designated these feelings as being somehow feminine in nature. But the results of a landmark study conducted more than 50 years ago found that these symptoms are not unique but instead reflect the body's reaction to starvation. This same study also found that diets that severely restrict calorie intake are ultimately unproductive in producing lasting weight loss.

In 1944, researcher Ancel Keys enrolled 36 male volunteers in what would be known as the Minnesota starvation experiment. This experiment was designed to examine the effects of a "semi-starvation diet" that many Europeans had been forced to adopt during World War II, with the goal of learning how to best help such people. The results of the experiment, first published in 1950, are still cited by scientists studying the thought and behavioral patterns of people with eating disorders.

All of the participating men were young, healthy, tested to be emotionally stable, and of normal weight. The requirements of the semi-starvation diet were actually less restrictive than the diets many women put themselves through today. Participants received a low-fat, low-protein diet of 1,800 calories a day over a 6-month period, with the goal of losing about 25% of their body weight. The men also were required to walk about 3 miles a day.

Physical symptoms appeared soon after the men started the diet and increased as time progressed. They became gaunt, lost hair, and broke out in rashes. The men reported feeling dizzy, tired, slow, clumsy, and cold. Participants slept under layers of blankets during the warm summer weather, and their sex drive plummeted.

But the researchers were even more surprised by the psychological changes that occurred. The men became withdrawn and irritable. Several men who were taking classes at the university had to withdraw because they couldn't concentrate. The men also became increasingly obsessed with food: They developed rituals, such as chewing food slowly, watering down meals, or drinking cup after cup of tea, that today are associated with eating disorders.

Even after the 6-month period of food restriction was over, the men's metabolisms continued to be affected by the diet restrictions. Symptoms continued for weeks after the restrictions were lifted. Many men did not feel full, no matter how much they ate; several men gorged themselves in attempts to do so. Most of the weight they gained back returned as fat, not muscle. Although the men eventually made full recoveries, the process was painful, difficult, and slow. The study found that vitamins and minerals weren't enough—participants also needed to consume a diet containing 4,000 calories per day for weeks to fully recover.

Interviewed more than 50 years later, the surviving study participants said they would do the experiment again because of the beneficial research it produced. Nevertheless, they all cited the study as the most difficult part of their lives.

Now that the risks of severely limiting calorie intake are known, the Minnesota starvation experiment would never be allowed today. The participants of the study enrolled because they believed their results could help victims of war. Women (or men) who are considering a similar diet plan today may want to ask themselves if their sacrifice is worth the effort.

Data from Kalm, L., & Semba, R. (2005). They starved so that others might be better fed: Remembering Ancel Keys and the Minnesota experiment. *Journal of Nutrition* 135: 1347–1352.

---

premature birth, low birth weight, and infection. Breastfeeding is the best way to protect babies from VAD, because breast milk is a natural source of vitamin A.

- *Iron.* Iron deficiency is the principal cause of anemia, which affects one-fourth of the world's population[44] Iron deficiency and anemia impose a heavy economic burden on society, because affected individuals are less able to work and be productive members of a community. In many developing countries, malaria and worm infections leech additional iron from the body, making problems caused by iron deficiency even worse. Health consequences for pregnant women and their fetuses include premature birth, low birth weight, and increased risk of maternal death. Twenty percent of all global maternal deaths have been attributed to anemia.

- *Iodine.* Iodine deficiency is primarily known for causing goiters (enlarged thyroid glands), a condition that can be dramatically disfiguring. Iodine deficiency disorders (IDDs) threaten the mental health of children, representing the world's most prevalent cause of brain damage. Iodine deficiency during pregnancy may result in stillbirth, miscarriage, congenital abnormalities, and mental impairment in the baby. More than 13% of the world's population (740 million people) is affected by this problem. Salt iodization has improved iodine status in many countries.

Hunger is also a serious concern in the United States. Along with poverty, hunger increased in the United States as a result of the global financial crisis. In 2013, 49 million people in the United States, or almost one in seven Americans, did not have consistent access to a varied diet throughout the year, compared to 36 million in 2006. Considerable variety existed within these households. About 6% of households (about 7 million households) had very low food security: People in these homes went hungry from time to time and had to make serious changes to their eating habits at some point during the year. A similar number of people faced low food security, a lesser but still serious problem in which food shortages cause individuals to reduce the variety in their diets, obtain food from emergency kitchens, or participate in federal food programs.[45] People at greatest risk of food insecurity are more likely to:

- Have children and be in households headed by a single woman
- Be Hispanic or Black
- Live in the South
- Be located in large cities or rural areas[46]

INFORMED DECISION MAKING

Nutrition

Healthful eating is essential to health promotion and disease prevention. A balanced diet should derive the bulk of its calories from fruits, vegetables, and whole grains. Protein should be a regular but limited part of the diet, with fish, shellfish, poultry, beans, and nuts playing a larger role than red meats such as beef or pork. When possible, avoid processed foods and sources of empty calories. Following these rules will help to supply the vitamins, minerals, and macronutrients necessary for healthy living, while reducing exposure to saturated fats and added sugars.

Maintaining a Personal Exercise Program

Exercise provides enormous benefits to health and disease prevention. Exercise should be not just a means to an end, such as "losing another 5 pounds," but a permanent part of life. The most health benefits come from at least 150 minutes (2.5 hours) per week of moderate-intensity physical activity. High-intensity physical activity (activity that, when you are performing it, works you hard enough that conversation is difficult) can be included in this total, with every 1 minute of high-intensity activity counting for 2 minutes of moderate-intensity activity. The ideal exercise program should include both aerobic and strength training activity. Additional exercise beyond 150 minutes per week provides additional benefits, but any amount of exercise is better than none at all.

Common perceived barriers to exercise for women include lack of time to exercise, lack of encouragement from family and friends, not wanting to exercise alone, the desire to avoid exertion or soreness, and a fear of looking silly.[46] Staying committed to exercise can also be a challenge: About 50% of people who start structured exercise programs drop out in 6 to 12 months. Habits that can make sticking with an exercise program easier include:

- Keeping an exercise log
- Recording total calories burned in a workout, distance traveled, or improvements in performance
- Exercising with a friend or in a class
- Choosing activities that are personally enjoyable
- Switching to new programs or rotating between programs to maintain interest
- Giving oneself periodic rewards for continuing to exercise

Imagining exercise as a normal part of one's routine maintenance (like brushing one's teeth) can also help a woman stay on a program: A woman who misses an exercise session or who forgets to brush her teeth before going to bed one night should not give up on either activity but should continue both habits the next day as if nothing unusual had happened.

Body Image and Weight Management

Some women want to lose weight to improve their health, others to improve their physical appearance. Many women feel a combination of both desires. However, women who feel an especially powerful desire to lose weight may want to reflect on their own body image. Society places enormous pressure on women to be thin and to conform to artificial body types that may be unhealthy or impossible to achieve. Developing a healthy body image, with the help of a medical professional if necessary, may benefit some women more than an Olympian-level fitness program.

Extra weight neither accumulates nor disappears overnight. Weight-loss programs that focus on slow but steady weight loss are healthier and more likely to keep weight off than programs that focus on dramatic short-term results. An average weekly loss of 1 pound is a realistic, safe goal for weight loss. Joining a group or making a serious arrangement for support with a friend can help sustain a long-term commitment.

A woman who adopts a healthful diet or starts an exercise program should not stop either activity once she reaches her initial weight-loss goal. A balanced diet and exercise continue to provide benefits only for as long as they are practiced. Reverting to unhealthy habits not only harms the body but also is likely to result in the return of lost weight.

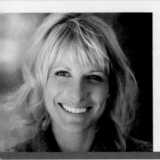
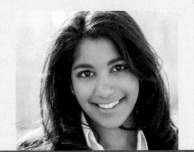
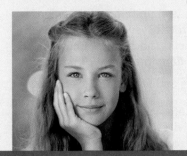
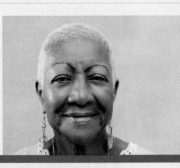

◾ Summary

The human body needs six nutrients to function and stay healthy:

- *Carbohydrates*, which can be simple (sugars) or complex (starches), provide fuel for the body.

- *Proteins* supply amino acids, which construct, repair, and maintain body tissues.

- *Fats* store energy and perform many other functions. Many Americans consume too much fat; however, no diet should eliminate this vital nutrient.

- *Vitamins*, which the body uses for nearly all aspects of function, are needed in small but regular amounts.

- *Minerals* are inorganic substances that help with bone formation, enzyme synthesis, maintaining blood pressure, and digestive function. Calcium and iron are especially important minerals for young women.

- *Water* is required for all of the body's actions. Women should consume 8 to 9 cups of water per day.

There are many ways to eat a nutritious diet and supply these nutrients to the body; however, there are some core guidelines to balanced eating:

- Focusing on fruits and vegetables (a good rough estimate to shoot for is to make about half the food you eat fruits and vegetables; if this is difficult try to make them at least one-third of your diet).

- Eating more complex carbohydrates than simple carbohydrates (whole rather than refined grains).

Profiles of Remarkable Women

Michelle Obama (1964–)

Michelle Obama is a lawyer, community activist, a mother of two, and the husband of the 44th U.S. President, Barack Obama. Since becoming the First Lady of the United States in 2008, she has been a strong advocate for a balanced diet and physical fitness. In 2010, she launched a national initiative called *Let's Move!* to reduce and prevent childhood obesity and improve the health of American children. The *Let's Move!* program improves access to nutritious, affordable foods; increases children's physical activity; provides balanced meals in school; and educates and empowers parents and guardians to improve their children's physical activity.

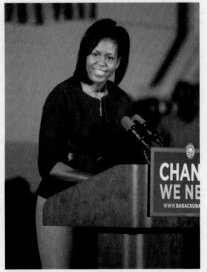

© spirit of america/Shutterstock

Mrs. Obama was born and raised in Chicago as the second of two children of Marian and Fraser Robinson. She was an excellent student and went on to study sociology at Princeton University and then law at Harvard Law School. She joined Sidley Austin, a Chicago law firm and met her future husband when she was assigned to be his mentor. Mrs. Obama left Sidley Austin in 1991 to work for the government of Chicago and to direct a Chicago nonprofit that encouraged young people to become socially active and participate in public service. Mr. and Mrs. Obama were married in 1992.

From 1996 to 2002, Mrs. Obama worked for the University of Chicago, where she helped build the university's community service center. She later worked for the University of Chicago hospitals and the University of Chicago Medical Center. Mrs. Obama continued to work part-time while she raised their two daughters, Sasha and Malia, and helped with her husband's Senate, and later, presidential campaigns.

In addition to working to improve children's physical fitness, Mrs. Obama works to help support military families, promote national service, help women balance career goals and family aspirations, and encourage education in the arts.

- Eating moderate amounts of protein and dairy foods, with an emphasis on proteins, such as chicken, fish, seafood, and soy products, and reduced amounts of red meats and high-fat dairy products.

- Eating more "real" foods and fewer processed foods.

Women in the United States spend most of their waking hours in sedentary activity. By incorporating physical activity into their daily routine, women can become more fit, improve their quality of life, and reduce their risk of chronic disease and premature death. These dramatic benefits to activity can also be pleasurable.

Around the world and in the United States, both hunger, and obesity and overweight are serious public health concerns. Hunger affects about one in seven people in the United States and around the world, causing a variety of health problems, including anemia, protein-energy deficiency, and death. Obesity and overweight cause a variety of health problems and raise the risk of developing cancer, heart disease, and other conditions.

■ Topics for Discussion

1. How well do your eating habits compare to those outlined in the 2010 *Dietary Guidelines for Americans*? What patterns are healthful? What are one or two ways that you can sustainably improve your eating habits?

2. How does the modern American lifestyle make getting regular physical activity and a balanced diet difficult? What are some ways to overcome these challenges?

3. Women who are physically active are healthier and therefore at lower risk of chronic disease and early mortality than those who are inactive. Should they have to pay the same insurance rates as those women whose lifestyles place them at greater risk for illness? If so, how should insurance policies be implemented to be fair and accurate?

4. Some believe that the physical fitness craze has been detrimental to the women's movement because it has added another layer of pressure to conform to an "ideal" body shape or size. How valid is this argument? How can efforts to improve physical fitness avoid alienating and discouraging women?

5. What can be done to improve women's attitudes toward exercise and physical fitness?

6. In an effort to curb obesity, the government of New York City recently proposed banning the sale of sodas and soft drinks of larger than 16 ounces at restaurants and stadiums. Is this concern about public health, personal freedom, or both? Is the ability to purchase soft drinks of a certain serving size comparable to freedom of speech?

7. What are the biggest challenges to regular exercise and a healthy diet that you face? How are these challenges going to change over the next 5 years? How do they differ from the challenges your female friends have in these areas?

8. How do the problems of hunger and malnutrition compare at the national and global levels? What are some realistic ways to reduce hunger and malnutrition in the United States and around the world?

CASE STUDY

By the midpoint of her junior year, Karen had gained her "freshman fifteen" and then some; at 163 pounds she weighed 21 pounds more than she did when she started college. Although Karen had gained a few pounds when she was introduced to a 24-hour, all-you-can-eat cafeteria, most of this weight gain had occurred over the most recent year and a half, when she began taking extra courses to allow for a double major in economics and theater. As Karen looked back at how her living situation had changed, it was not hard to pinpoint why. Although she had been fairly active during her freshman year, Karen found little time to exercise in the past year and a half. She had dropped out of her school's rugby team to allow more time for another course. She had also been rewarding herself, first with snacks and then with a second dinner of comfort food, during her late-night study sessions and drinking multiple caffeinated soft drinks per day to stay awake.

After trying on yet another set of pants that no longer fit, Karen is determined to improve her health and lose weight.

Questions

1. What are some productive ways that Karen can improve her diet and eating habits, given her busy schedule?

2. At 5 feet 6 inches tall, what weight category does Karen have according to her BMI (feel free to use a BMI chart or calculator)? How much of a health concern should this be for her?

(Karen's story has been drawn from the experiences of multiple women; her name and other identifying information have been changed to preserve anonymity.)

■ Key Terms

Anabolic steroid

Antioxidant

Bariatric surgery

Basal metabolic rate (BMR)

Body composition

Body mass index (BMI)

Calcium

Carbohydrate

Cardiovascular endurance

Cholesterol

Complex carbohydrate

Exercise

Fat

Fat-soluble vitamin

Female athlete triad

Fiber

Flexibility

Folate

Glycemic index

Hemoglobin

High-density lipoprotein (HDL)

Hunger

Iron

Low-density lipoprotein (LDL)

Malnutrition

Mineral

Monounsaturated fat

Muscular endurance

Muscular strength

Nutrient

Nutrition

Obesity

Overnutrition

Overweight

Phytochemical

Polyunsaturated fat

Protein

Protein-energy malnutrition (PEM)

Recommended Dietary Allowance (RDA)

Saturated fat

Simple carbohydrate

Sodium

Title IX

Trans fat

Undernutrition

Unsaturated fat

Vitamin

Water-soluble vitamin

Yo-yo dieting

■ References

1. United States Department of Agriculture, Department of Health and Human Services. (2015). *Scientific report of the 2015 Dietary Guidelines Advisory Committee.* Available at: http://health.gov /dietaryguidelines/2015-scientific-report/

2. Kraus, W., Bittner, V., Appel, L., et al. (2015). The National Physical Activity Plan: A call to action from the American Heart Association: A science advisory from the American Heart Association. *Circulation* 131(21): 1932–1940.

3. Kann, L., Kinchen, S., Shanklin, S., et al. (2014). *Youth Risk Behavior Surveillance—United States, 2013.* Atlanta, GA: Centers for Disease Control and Prevention.

4. Lowry, R., Galuska, D. A., Fulton, J. E., et al. (2002). Weight management goals and practices among U.S. high school students: Associations with physical activity, diet, and smoking. *Journal of Adolescent Health* 31(2): 133–144.

5. Pollan, M. (2009). *Food rules: An eater's manual.* New York, NY: Penguin Books.

6. Rufail, M. L., Schenkein, H. A., Barbour, S. E., et al. (2005). Altered lipoprotein subclass distribution and PAF-AH activity in subjects with generalized aggressive periodontitis. *Journal of Lipid Research* 46: 2752–2760.

7. James, S. L., Muir, J. G., Curtis, S. L., et al. (2003). Dietary fibre: A roughage guide. *Internal Medicine Journal* 33(7): 291–296.

8. Willet, W. C. (2005). *Eat, drink and be healthy: The Harvard Medical School guide to healthy eating.* New York, NY: Simon and Schuster.

9. Centers for Disease Control and Prevention (CDC). (2010). *Trans fat: The facts.* Available at: http://www.cdc.gov/nutrition /everyone/basics/fat/transfat.html

10. Dietz, W., & Scanlon, K. (2012). Eliminating the use of partially hydrogenated oil in food production and preparation. *Journal of the American Medical Association* 308(2): 143.

11. Lichtenstein, A. (2014). Dietary trans fatty acids and cardiovascular disease risk: Past and present. *Current Atherosclerosis Reports* 16(8): 433.

12. Egen, V., & Hasford, J. (2003). Prevention of neural tube defects: Effect of an intervention aimed at implementing the official recommendations. *Soz Praventivmed* 48(1): 24–32.

13. Grosse, S. D., Waitzman, N. J., Romano, P. S., et al. (2005). Reevaluating the benefits of folic acid fortification in the United States: Economic analysis, regulation, and public health. *American Journal of Public Health* 95: 1917–1922.

14. U.S. Preventive Services Task Force. (2012). *Vitamin D and calcium supplementation to prevent cancer and osteoporotic fractures in adults: U.S. Preventive Services Task Force recommendation statement.* Available at: http://www.uspreventiveservicestaskforce.org/draftrec3 .htm

15. CDC. (2002). Iron deficiency: United States, 1999–2000. *Morbidity and Mortality Weekly Report* 51(40): 897–899.

16. Li, Y. (2012). α-Adducin Gly460Trp gene mutation and essential hypertension in a Chinese population: A meta-analysis including 10960 subjects. *PLoS ONE* 7(1): e30214.

17. U.S. Department of Health and Human Services (DHHS). (2013). *Women's health USA 2013.* Rockville, Maryland: U.S. Department of Health and Human Services

18. DHHS. (2008). *2008 physical activity guidelines for Americans.* Available at: http://www.health.gov/PAGuidelines/

19. Hu, F. B., Willet, W. C., Li, T., et al. (2004). Adiposity as compared with physical activity in predicting mortality among women. *New England Journal of Medicine* 351(26): 2694–2703.

20. Elavsky, S., McAuley, E., Motl, R. W., et al. (2005). Physical activity enhances long-term quality of life in older adults: Efficacy, esteem, and affective influences. *Annals of Behavioral Medicine* 30(2): 138–145.

21. Da Costa, D., Rippen, N., Drista, M., et al. (2003). Self-reported leisure-time physical activity during pregnancy and relationship to psychological well-being. *Journal of Psychosomatic Obstetrics and Gynaecology* 24(2): 111–119.

22. Page, P. (2012). Current concepts in muscle stretching for exercise and rehabilitation. *International Journal of Sports Physical Therapy* 7(1): 109–119.

23. Kannus, P., Sievanen, H., Palvenen, M., et al. (2005). Prevention of falls and injuries in elderly people. *Lancet* 366(9500): 1885–1893.

24. Warren, M. P., & Goodman, L. R. (2003). Exercise-induced endocrine pathologies. *Journal of Endocrinological Investigation* 26(9): 873–878.

25. Quaglio, G., Fornasiero, A., Mezzelani, P., et al. (2009). Anabolic steroids: Dependence and complications of chronic use. *Internal Emergency Medicine* 4(4): 289–296.

26. DHHS. (2010). Maintaining a healthy weight on the go: A pocket guide. Available at: http://www.nhlbi.nih.gov/files/docs/public/heart/AIM_Pocket_Guide_tagged.pdf

27. Savard, M., & Svec, C. (2005). *The body shape solution to weight loss and wellness.* New York, NY: Atria.

28. CDC. (2008). *Obesity and overweight: U.S. obesity trends.* Available at: http://www.cdc.gov/nccdphp/dnpa/obesity/trend/maps/

29. Freedman, D. S., Mei, Z., Srinivasan, S. R., et al. (2007). Cardiovascular risk factors and excess adiposity among overweight children and adolescents: The Bogalusa Heart Study. *Journal of Pediatrics* 150(1): 12–17.e2.

30. Polednak, A. (2008). Estimating the number of U.S. incident cancers attributable to obesity and the impact on temporal trends in incidence rates for obesity-related cancers. *Cancer Detection and Prevention* 32(3): 190–199.

31. Calle, D., Rodriguez, C., Walker-Turmond, K., et al. (2003). Overweight, obesity, and mortality from cancer in a prospectively studied cohort of U.S. adults. *New England Journal of Medicine* 348: 1625–1638.

32. National Cancer Institute. (2012). *Obesity and cancer risk.* Available at: http://www.cancer.gov/cancertopics/factsheet/Risk/obesity

33. Finkelstein, E., Trogdon, J., Cohen, J., et al. (2009). Annual medical spending attributable to obesity: Payer and service-specific estimates. *Health Affairs* 28(5): 822–831.

34. Palmer, H. (May 30, 2007). *Our loss, diet industry's gain.* American Public Media [radio broadcast]. Available at: http://marketplace.publicradio.org/display/web/2007/05/30/our_loss_diet_industrys_gain/

35. Dulloo, A., & Montani, J. (2015). Pathways from dieting to weight regain, to obesity and to the metabolic syndrome: An overview. *Obesity Review* 16: 1–6.

36. Rating the diets from A to Z. (2005). *Consumer Reports* 70(6): 18–22.

37. Byrd-Bredbenner, C., Murray, J., & Schlussel, Y. (2005). Temporal changes in anthropometric measurements of idealized females and young women in general. *Women and Health* 41(2): 13–20.

38. Yin, S. (2004). Size and gender. *American Demographics* 26(2): 14.

39. National Institute of Mental Health. (2014). *What are eating disorders?* Available at: http://www.nimh.nih.gov/health/publications/eating-disorders-new-trifold/index.shtml

40. American Society for Aesthetic Plastic Surgery. (2015). *Cosmetic surgery national databank statistics.* Available at: http://www.surgery.org/sites/default/files/2014-Stats.pdf

41. World Food Programme. (2015). *Hunger statistics.* Available at: https://www.wfp.org/hunger/stats

42. Food and Agriculture Organization of the United Nations. (2008). *Clinton at UN: Food, energy, financial woes linked.* Available at: http://www.fao.org/newsroom/en/news/2008/1000945/index.html

43. UNICEF. (2007). *State of the world's children, 2008.* New York, NY: United Nations.

44. World Health Organization. (2003). *Nutrition.* Available at: http://www.who.int/nutrition/index.htm

45. Feeding America. (2015). *Hunger & poverty statistics.* Available at: http://feedingamerica.org/hunger-in-america/hunger-facts/hunger-and-poverty-statistics.aspx

46. Harne, A. J., & Bixby, W. R. (2005). The benefits and barriers of strength training among college-age women. *Journal of Sport Behavior* 28(2): 151–166.

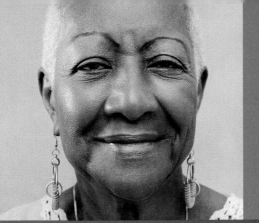

CHAPTER 10

Understanding and Preventing Cardiovascular Disease and Cancer

Learning Objectives

On completion of this chapter, the student should be able to discuss:

1. The main components and functions of the circulatory system and blood.

2. The processes leading to atherosclerosis and myocardial infarction.

3. The conditions that contribute to congestive heart failure.

4. Types of congenital heart disease and their associated prevalence and mortality rates.

5. The cause and effects of rheumatic heart disease.

6. The significance of angina pectoris.

7. Conditions that lead to peripheral artery disease.

8. The major causes of cerebrovascular accidents.

9. The major modifiable risk factors for cardiovascular disease (CVD).

10. Cardiovascular disease from an epidemiological perspective, including sex/gender, race/ethnicity, and socioeconomics.

11. The process of cancer development and metastasis.

12. Cancer from an epidemiological perspective, including sex/gender, race/ethnicity, and socioeconomics.

13. Types of benign conditions of the breast, cervix, uterus, and ovaries.

14. Risk factors, screening methods, and treatment modalities for breast, cervical, uterine, and ovarian cancer.

15. Pap smears and HPV tests and how they relate to benign cervical conditions as well as cervical cancer.

16. Risk factors, screening methods, and treatment modalities for lung cancer, colorectal cancer, and skin cancer.

17. Prevention of CVD and cancer through lifestyle changes and health screening.

INTRODUCTION

Cardiovascular disease and cancer are the greatest causes of death in the United States. These chronic conditions are rarely caused by infectious diseases but primarily by genetics and lifestyle factors, which play a major role in who gets the disease(s) and who dies from them. Genetics clearly influences who is at greatest risk for both cardiovascular disease and cancer. Lifestyle alone cannot overcome a strong genetic loading for either condition. However, behavior can greatly reduce the risk of developing the disease and help limit the effects of the disease. This chapter addresses cardiovascular disease and cancer and presents them in several modalities: epidemiology, risk factors, screening, treatment, and personal decision making to reduce the risk of disease.

CARDIOVASCULAR DISEASE

Cardiovascular disease (CVD) comprises a group of diseases that affect the heart and blood vessels. This includes **stroke**, a condition that affects the brain's blood vessels. The major cardiovascular diseases include coronary heart disease, cerebrovascular disease, peripheral artery disease, rheumatic heart disease, congenital heart disease, and deep vein thrombosis and pulmonary embolism. In the United States, estimates show that about 610,000 million people die of heart disease annually.[1] Of those, one in four are women.[2,3] Stroke accounted for over 75,000 deaths in women (see **Figure 10.1**).[4] Annually, cardiovascular disease is estimated to cost over $300 billion in healthcare costs and lost productivity the United States.[5] And the threats and costs from cardiovascular disease are only predicted to rise.

Cardiovascular deaths usually occur in later years when women are beset with a variety of comorbid conditions such a high blood pressure, diabetes, and others. **Table 10.1** illustrates the death rates from cardiovascular disease among women and men by age.

Perspectives on Cardiovascular Disease

Epidemiology

Cardiovascular disease is the leading cause of death for women regardless of racial or ethnic group. Of the various forms of CVD, coronary heart disease (CHD), or diseases of the heart in which the coronary arteries that supply blood to the heart become narrowed or blocked, is number one. Among those women who died, nearly two-thirds died with no previous history of chest pain.[6] Because the symptoms of a heart attack can be different in women and men, women often wait longer to seek care than do men. Stroke, the third leading cause of death among women (after heart disease and cancer), killed over 75,000.[4] Compared with men, approximately 55,000 more women than men suffer a stroke annually.[7] Deaths from stroke are greatest among African American/Black and White women beginning around age 60 and older.[8]

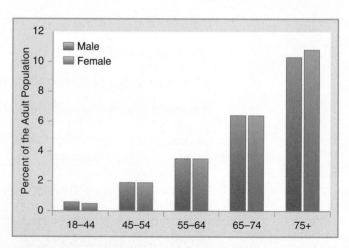

Figure 10.1 Prevalence of cardiovascular disease in adults by age and sex, 2011–2012.

Reproduced from Miniño AM, Klein RJ. (2010). Health mortality from major cardiovascular diseases: United States, 2007. Health E-Stats. National Center for Health Statistics.

Table 10.1   Death Rates* for Diseases of the Heart and Cerebrovascular Disease by Sex, Race, Hispanic Origin, 2013

Race/Ethnicity	Heart Disease		Cerebrovascular Disease	
	Male	Female	Male	Female
African American/Black	262.8	172.1	54.1	44.7
American Indian/Alaska Native	152.3	93.9	22.7	25.5
Asian/Pacific Islander	118.4	73.3	31.2	27.9
Hispanic	151.5	97.0	31.8	27.6
White	213.0	132.0	35.0	34.2

*Deaths per 100,000 resident population.

Data from Centers for Disease Control and Prevention. *Health, United States, 2014.* Tables 24 and 25. Available at: http://www.cdc.gov/nchs/hus/contents2014.htm#024; http://www.cdc.gov/nchs/hus/contents2014.htm#025

Although some cardiovascular diseases occur among children and adolescents, they typically occur among men and women who are at least 50 years of age and older. The incidence of CHD begins to rise for women between the ages of 55 and 60, about 10 years later than it does for men. The incidence of stroke begins to sharply rise in both women and men after the age of 55.[9]

Economic Dimensions of Cardiovascular Disease

Cardiovascular disease imposes a heavy burden on the healthcare system in the United States, particularly on emergency medical departments and hospitals. Clinical care of CVD patients is costly and often prolonged. The direct cost of cardiovascular disease and stroke in the United States in 2011 was $215 billion.[10]

- Direct costs include present health expenditures, including those for physicians and other health professionals, hospital and nursing home services, medications, home health care, and other medical durables.

- Indirect costs include lost productivity resulting from morbidity and mortality.[10]

Cardiovascular disease often affects individuals during their peak productive work years, causing significant disruption to families who depend on the person's support and income. The high rate of CVD also influences the national economy by killing or disabling otherwise productive workers. In addition, the emotional cost to the individual and his or her family, friends, and coworkers is incalculable.

Global Dimensions

Over the past century, cardiovascular disease has surpassed infectious diseases to become the leading cause of death and disability globally. With an ever-increasing life expectancy, countries that were once overwhelmed with infectious and communicable diseases, maternal and infant deaths, and malnutrition are now besieged with CVD. Cardiovascular disease is the leading cause of death among women worldwide and, according to the World Heart Federation, kills more women than cancers, tuberculosis, HIV/AIDS, and malaria combined.[11]

The growing convenience and lower prices of high-fat, high-calorie processed foods, a decrease in physical exercise, and high rates of cigarette smoking have all contributed to this problem worldwide. **Figure 10.2** presents obesity worldwide, with the United States having some of the highest rates internationally. Of the top 10 industrialized countries in the world, the United States ranks number 1 in obesity.[12]

In the United States, smoking rates among women have begun to plateau or decline, in part because of strong and widespread public health education and intervention. Yet marketing that targets women, especially young women, remains quite unsuccessful and many continue to smoke, use smokeless tobacco, or use electronic cigarettes. In some countries, predominantly in Asia, women may use smokeless forms such as chewing tobacco.[13] In addition, women often have more difficulty quitting. According to the American Lung Association, while the number of lung cancer deaths associated with smoking in men appears to have plateaued, the rates continue to rise among women.[14] Some interventions may not be as successful in women compared to in men, in part because many programs were initially designed for male audiences. **Table 10.2** presents smoking trends among women and men in the United States from 1990 to 2013.[15] Note that these numbers vary by poverty level and education. Those who are below the poverty level and those who have less education smoke more.

Cultural attitudes affect lifestyle habits. Women in many countries have moved from rural to urban areas—from physically active lifestyles such as farming to more

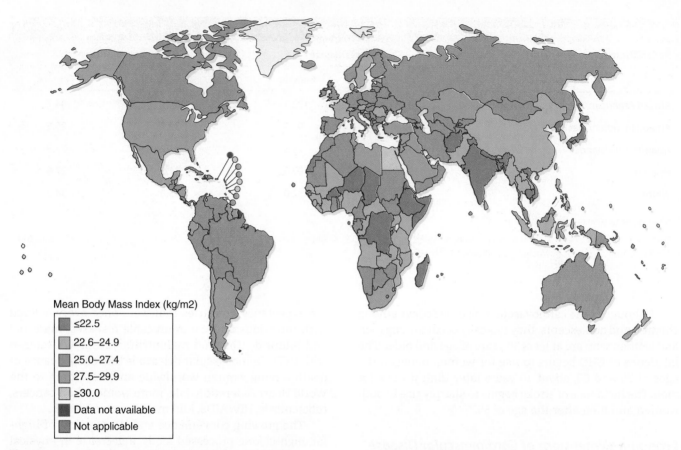

Figure 10.2   Female mean body mass index worldwide.

Mean Body Mass Index (kg/m2)

- ≤22.5
- 22.6–24.9
- 25.0–27.4
- 27.5–29.9
- ≥30.0
- Data not available
- Not applicable

sedentary work in offices and industry. Another concern is the "migration" effect that occurs among women who migrate from developing to developed countries. As with migration from rural to urban, women who migrate to more developed countries are exposed to different cultures and styles of living. Unhealthy foods may be convenient, cheap, and present in greater quantities, whereas nutritious foods and opportunities for physical activities may be more difficult to access. These lifestyles put women emigrating from rural areas to cities

and from other countries at particularly high risk for obesity, high blood pressure, high blood cholesterol, and diabetes—all risk factors for CVD. Unfortunately, in many countries and for many women migrants to the United States, disease prevention and health care remain fragmented.

The Heart

Cardiovascular disease cannot be understood without an appreciation of the heart as a vital organ. The heart

Table 10.2   Percentage of Persons Aged 18 Years or Older Who Were Current Cigarette Smokers

	Male			Female		
Race	1990–1992	1999–2001	2011–2013	1990–1992	1999–2001	2011–2013
White	27.4	25.1	20.9	24.3	22.2	17.0
Black/AA	33.9	27.2	22.3	23.1	19.7	14.8
AI/AN	34.2	30.3	25.6	36.7	34.7	19.1
Asian	24.8	20.3	14.8	6.3	6.7	5.2
Hispanic	25.7	22.2	16.7	15.8	12.1	7.5

AA = African American; AI/AN = American Indian/Alaska Native

Data from Centers for Disease Control and Prevention. *Health, United States, 2014.* Table 53. Available at: http://www.cdc.gov/nchs/hus/contents2014.htm#053

relentlessly pumps blood throughout the body 24 hours a day without stopping, throughout a person's life.

The heart is located in the chest behind the **sternum**, also known as the breastbone located in the center of the chest. The **cardiovascular system** consists of the heart, arteries, veins, and capillaries. The heart has four major chambers: the **right atrium**, the **right ventricle**, the **left atrium**, and the **left ventricle** (see **Figure 10.3**).[16] The right and left atria are the upper blood-receiving chambers and the right and left ventricles are the lower blood-pumping chambers. The right atrium and ventricle and the left atrium and ventricle are each separated by a valve. The right atrium and ventricle are separated by the **tricuspid valve**. The left atrium and ventricle are separated by the **bicuspid valve** Blood flows from the atrium through the valve to the ventricle below. A thick muscular wall known as the **septum** separates the right and left sides of the heart.

Oxygen-poor blood from throughout the body travels to the heart so that it can be pumped to the lungs for oxygenation. The oxygen-poor blood enters the right atrium of the heart from the **inferior** and **superior vena cava** (major veins). From the right atrium, blood flows through the tricuspid valve into the right ventricle, where it is pumped to the lungs via the **pulmonary arteries**.

In the lungs, carbon dioxide and waste products are removed from the blood and exchanged for fresh oxygen. The newly oxygen-rich blood leaves the lungs via the **pulmonary veins** and flows into the left atrium. From the left atrium, it passes through the **mitral valve** into the left ventricle. The left ventricle contracts and forces the oxygen-rich blood through the **aortic valve** into the **aorta** (the main artery) and from there throughout the major **arteries** flowing gradually into smaller and smaller arteries, **arterioles**, and finally **capillaries** throughout the body.

The capillaries—microscopic vessels with thin walls—are the sites where the nutrients and oxygen in the blood are exchanged for waste and carbon dioxide at the cellular level. From the capillaries, the oxygen-poor but carbon dioxide-rich flows into the **venules** and veins as it makes it way back to the heart. Then the cycle begins again.[17]

For this system to function properly, the pump—the heart—must remain strong and forceful. It must contract powerfully and quickly when a woman runs a marathon, yet it must slow for rest during sleep. The heart is activated to perform its pumping function by electrical stimuli from specialized tissues called nodes buried in the cardiac muscle. This electrical stimulation can be detected by a special device known as an **electrocardiograph (ECG)**, sometimes known as an EKG. An ECG can detect a normal heart rhythm or abnormalities such as a heart attack or congenitally damaged tricuspid valve (see **Figure 10.4**).[18]

Similar to the heart, the arteries have muscles that must expand and contract vigorously to meet the demands placed on the body, yet remain supple and open. Veins, although they remain supple and open, do not have muscles and therefore must rely on surrounding muscles to move the blood along through the venous system to its destination.

Blood is the vehicle for transporting food and waste throughout the body. An average woman circulates about 6 quarts of blood per day. Blood consists of many critical components that are all suspended in plasma, the liquid in which the different components of the blood travel. The primary components are:

- **Red Blood Cells (Erythrocytes)** carry oxygen and carbon dioxide. **Hemoglobin** is an important protein in red blood cells that carries oxygen from the lungs throughout the body. It also gives blood its red color.

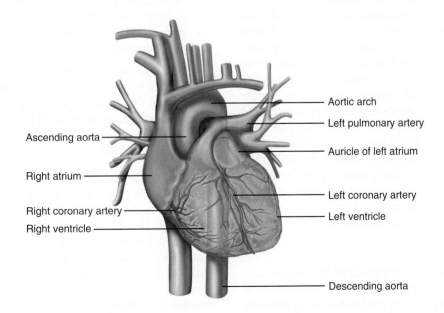

Aortic arch
Left pulmonary artery
Ascending aorta
Auricle of left atrium
Right atrium
Left coronary artery
Right coronary artery
Left ventricle
Right ventricle
Descending aorta

Figure 10.3 Illustration of a heart.

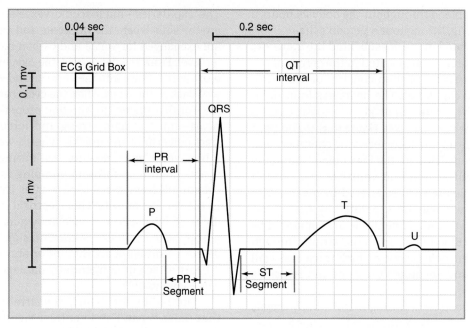

Figure 10.4 Electrocardiogram (ECG/EKG).

- **White Blood Cells (Leukocytes)** act as scavengers to rid the blood and body of bacteria and waste. Several types of white blood cells exist, each of which has a role in fighting bacterial, viral, fungal, and parasitic infections.
- **Platelets (Thrombocytes)** cause the blood to clot.[19]

If the heart's electrical signal loses its regular pattern, the heart can begin to beat irregularly and less effectively—a condition called **arrhythmia**. Arrhythmias are very common and can occur in an otherwise healthy heart. In some cases, however, they may indicate a serious problem and can lead to heart disease.

When atria emit uncoordinated electrical signals, the condition is called **atrial fibrillation** (AF or AFib). When disordered electrical activity causes rapid, uncoordinated contractions of the ventricle, the condition is called **ventricular fibrillation** (VF). Atrial fibrillation is not usually life threatening, but it can lead to other more serious conditions. For example, when the atrium does not pump blood evenly, some blood may remain in the atrium and form a clot. If this clot enters the bloodstream, it can travel to the brain and cause a stroke. In VF, little or no blood may be pumped from the heart, which results in collapse and sudden death. Physicians can detect heart abnormalities and will first determine the origins of the arrhythmia and its severity before considering treatment.[20]

Pathophysiology of the Heart

Cardiovascular disease encompasses heart disease (coronary heart disease, congestive heart failure, rheumatic heart disease, angina pectoris, peripheral artery disease), hypertension, and cerebrovascular disease (stroke). Many of these diseases can be prevented or controlled with lifestyle modifications and/or medications.

Coronary Heart Disease

Coronary heart disease is the result of narrowed or clogged arteries. **Atherosclerosis**, a form of arteriosclerosis, is a major culprit in CHD. It causes the heart vessels to become clogged, thereby impairing a woman's heart from functioning properly (see **Figure 10.5**).[21] This can happen in a variety of ways:

- The arteries can become clogged with waste, usually fat deposits (**plaques**). Low-density lipoprotein (LDL), or "bad" cholesterol, and other waste deposits penetrate the inner lining of the arteries. There they build up over time, impeding the flow of blood.
- The arteries can become stiff with age or disease, rendering them less able to respond to the demands placed on them. If the blood flow is compromised, the area being fed by that particular artery or arteries does not receive proper nutrition and can become damaged or die.

When arteries surrounding the heart become twisted and tortuous, they are particularly prone to developing atherosclerosis. When that occurs a woman is at increased risk of suffering a **heart attack (myocardial infarction)**. A heart attack, or death of a portion of the heart, occurs when one or more of the coronary arteries in the heart becomes damaged or clogged. Consequently, the arteries close off. Such blockages can occur from a circulating blood clot called an **embolus**. As an embolus moves through the bloodstream, it can become

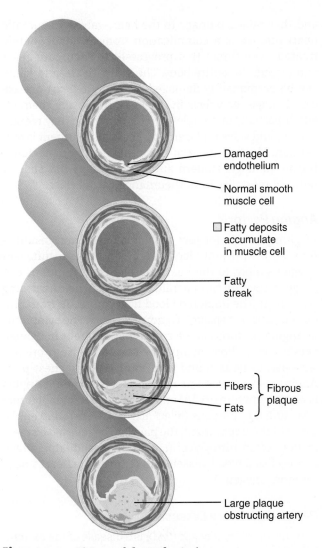

Damaged endothelium

Normal smooth muscle cell

☐ Fatty deposits accumulate in muscle cell

Fatty streak

Fibers } Fibrous
Fats } plaque

Large plaque obstructing artery

Figure 10.5   **Picture of clogged arteries.**

lodged in an artery, further blocking any blood from getting through. The resulting blockage is called a **thrombus** (stationary blood clot). A clot can also form as a result of plaque (cholesterol) buildup within the inner arterial wall. Whatever the cause, the blood cannot flow downstream from the blockage. As a result, the part of the body fed by the blocked artery does not receive blood, carrying oxygen and nutrients, and becomes severely impaired or dies. Blockages within different coronary arteries create different problems. For example, if the blockage occurs within the major artery feeding the left ventricle (the main pump of the heart), the entire ventricle can cease to pump. This stops blood flow to the rest of the body. If this situation is not reversed immediately, the woman can die or suffer irreversible brain damage from lack of oxygen to the brain.

The heart can also become damaged from other diseases or conditions, such as rheumatic heart disease, or from injury, such as a heart attack, which can lead to heart failure in which the heart is impaired and cannot pump effectively. Atherosclerosis cannot be cured, but its

progression can be slowed. Treatment often depends on which organs are involved.[21]

For heart conditions, cholesterol-lowering medications, which can control high cholesterol levels, are a critical factor in treatment. Surgical procedures, such as **balloon angioplasty**, can be performed. Balloon angioplasty is a procedure used to open narrowed or blocked coronary arteries. A surgeon inserts a small hollow tube called a catheter into an artery near the blockage. The surgeon then inflates the balloon near the end of the catheter. This action widens the vessel and allows blood to flow more freely. The surgeon often places a wire mesh, a **stent**, at the site of the blockage to keep the artery open. Alternately, **coronary artery bypass graft (CABG) surgery** creates a new passage around the blocked part of the coronary artery to restore blood flow to the heart muscle.

When the brain is affected, antiplatelet medications, including aspirin, and anticoagulant medications, such as warfarin and heparin, may help prevent strokes. When atherosclerosis narrows arteries that supply an area, balloon angioplasty may be used or a bypass arterial graft may be performed. Some of these treatments may also be useful in treating a patient after a heart attack. The ultimate goal of treatment is to minimize the damage by restoring blood flow to the affected area of the heart.[22]

Acute Coronary Syndrome

Acute coronary syndrome (ACS) describes a condition in which an individual presents with specific cardiac symptoms: myocardial infarction (heart attack) or unstable angina (chest pain) that is unexpected or unusual and may be more severe than usual. The important diagnostic category identifies individuals when they are moving toward a heart attack (unstable angina) or are in the early stages of a heart attack. The goal is to intervene before serious damage occurs. However, heart attack signs may present differently in women than they do in men (see **Table 10.3**).[23,24]

Congestive Heart Failure

Congestive heart failure (CHF) occurs when heart muscles are weak and cannot pump with strength. In such a case, the heart loses its ability to contract properly or

Table 10.3   Warning Signs of Heart Attack
■ Pain or discomfort in the chest: Heart attacks often involve pain or discomfort in the chest. The pain can be intense, mild, or in-between. Discomfort can feel like a sense of squeezing, pressure, or fullness.
■ Pain or aching in other parts of the upper body. A heart attack can cause pain or uncomfortable feelings in the back, neck, jaw, one or both arms, or stomach.
■ Unexplained feelings of nausea, dizziness, or shortness of breath, or feeling lightheaded, that last a few minutes or more.

sufficiently to meet the demands placed on it. Even if the arteries remain open, without a strong pumping action from the heart, the nutrient-rich and oxygen-rich blood may not be able to reach the cells. The cells can suffer damage or die. In addition, the heart muscle itself depends on a rich blood supply from the coronary arteries, which must remain open and supple if the heart is to perform properly. As a result, circulation suffers and fluids begin to accumulate in veins, causing breathing problems, kidney problems, and swelling in the extremities, especially the legs.

Congestive heart failure may have many causes, but it is often a disease of older women who have suffered heart damage from high blood pressure, atherosclerosis, arteriosclerosis, or a heart attack. In some cases, CHF occurs because of a congenital heart defect or damage to the heart from a bacterial disease such as rheumatic heart disease.

Congestive heart failure can often be prevented or minimized by controlling high blood pressure, treating underlying bacterial infections, and following lifestyle modifications that prevent other forms of CVD. Medication, reducing salt intake, and possibly surgery to alleviate blockages in coronary arteries may help improve heart function once CHF has been diagnosed.[25]

Congenital Heart Disease

Congenital heart disease is an abnormality of the heart that is present at birth. It can include one or more of the following:

- Hole in the septum
- Imperfectly formed blood vessels
- Valvular damage
- Left ventricular imperfections

Patent ductus arteriosis is a congenital condition in which the ductus arteriosis (passageway between the pulmonary artery and aorta) does not close. It is a common condition in premature babies. Another congenital heart disease, called **pulmonary stenosis**, occurs when the valve between the ventricle and the pulmonary artery is defective and does not open properly. Atrial or ventricular septal defects occur when an opening appears between the two upper or lower chambers of the heart. Most of these imperfections can be corrected with surgery.[26]

Nearly, 40,000 babies are born each year with congenital heart defects. The majority of congenital heart defect deaths occur in children younger than 1 year of age.[27] Mortality associated with congenital defects has declined due to advances in diagnosis and surgical treatment.[28,29]

Rheumatic Heart Disease

Rheumatic heart disease results from a bacterial infection (*Streptococcus*) that has been inadequately treated and that causes damage to the heart valves. Rheumatic heart disease is a complication from an inadequately treated strep throat that progresses to rheumatic fever and affects the entire body. The brain, heart, and joints can be permanently damaged. Rheumatic heart disease can damage the valves in the heart by closing them off either partially or completely. This condition may require surgery and valve replacement. The best treatment is prevention. The treatment of the initial infection precludes further damage. Modern antibiotic therapy has sharply reduced mortality from rheumatic heart disease.[30]

Angina Pectoris

Angina pectoris (or just *angina*) is chest pain resulting from an insufficient blood supply, and thus insufficient oxygen supply, to the heart muscle. The symptoms can range in severity from a mild cramping ache to crushing chest pain. The impaired blood flow can result from atherosclerosis or a spasm of a normal artery. The symptoms of angina pectoris can be somewhat different in women versus men. Those symptoms can range from breathlessness, to nausea and vomiting, to sharp chest pain. Angina is as common in women as it is in men.[25] Angina is also a symptom of CVD and may be a predictor of future myocardial infarctions (heart attacks). Depending on the cause of the impairment, the pain can be relieved by medication, often nitroglycerin, a strong vasodilator, which opens closed blood vessels and reduces the heart's need for more oxygen.[31]

Peripheral Artery Disease

Peripheral artery disease (PAD) is a disease of the extremities (hands, arms, or, most commonly, legs and feet) in which the blood supply is diminished. As such, sufficient oxygen and nutrients do not reach these areas properly and waste products accumulate. A woman with PAD can experience symptoms ranging from cramping and numbness to gangrene (tissue death), which may require amputation of the extremity. The cause of PAD is related to atherosclerosis and arteriosclerosis and is particularly associated with diabetes, smoking, and hypertension. Of all the known risk factors, smoking and diabetes are the most strongly related to PAD. Treatment options include lifestyle modification such a smoking cessation, increased exercise, anticoagulant and/or antiplatelet medications, angioplasty, or bypass surgery. Although women may know about PAD, many do not understand the risk factors for it, especially smoking and diabetes.[32]

Metabolic Syndrome

Metabolic syndrome is a group of diseases that can occur together and increase the risk for CVD. The National Heart, Lung, and Blood Institute and the American Heart Association note that the presence of three or more of the following risk factors or diseases predisposes a person to an increased risk for metabolic syndrome.

- Elevated waist circumference
  - Men: Equal to or greater than 40 inches (102 cm)
  - Women: Equal to or greater than 35 inches (88 cm)
- Elevated triglycerides
  - Equal to or greater than 150 mg/dL
- Reduced HDL ("good") cholesterol
  - Men: Less than 40 mg/dL
  - Women: Less than 50 mg/dL
- Elevated blood pressure
  - Equal to or greater than 130/85 mm Hg
- Elevated fasting glucose
  - Equal to or greater than 100 mg/dL[33]

The principal factors contributing to metabolic syndrome appear to be central obesity (fat collected around the person's midsection) and insulin resistance—factors that are increasingly common among women.[34] Prevalence of the disease is estimated at 30.4% in individuals 20 to 59 years of age. The Fruge study showed that metabolic syndrome was most prevalent in Black women and White men.[35] Another study by Beltran-Sanchez and colleagues also confirmed that metabolic syndrome, especially with increasing obesity levels, is a major risk factor, particularly in women.[31] Preventive actions to address metabolic syndrome are weight loss and control, healthy eating, and increased physical activity.[36]

Cerebrovascular Accident (Stroke)

Cerebrovascular accident, commonly called a stroke, is a condition in which blood vessels leading to and within the brain become damaged. The process of blood flow blockage that occurs in the coronary vessels of the heart is similar to that which occurs in the brain. The other major process involved in stroke is vessel rupture, often occurring from atherosclerotic vessels. When a blood vessel is blocked or bursts, that part of the brain cannot obtain blood and, therefore, oxygen, which it needs to survive. The most common type of stroke, **ischemic stroke**, is caused by blockage. The clot in such cases is called a *cerebral thrombus* or *cerebral* **embolism**. **Hemorrhagic strokes** are cause by ruptured blood vessels (see **Figure 10.6**).[37,38]

An **aneurysm** is one type of weakened blood vessel that can cause a stroke. It involves ballooning of a weakened region of a blood vessel and results from several possible factors: congenital defect, hypertension, or any of the previously mentioned injuries to the brain. If left untreated, the aneurysm will continue to weaken until it ruptures and bleeds into the brain.

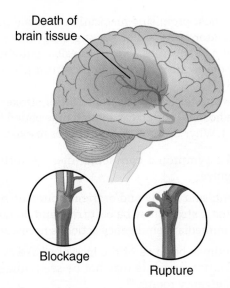

Figure 10.6   Cerebrovascular accident.

A variety of tests can diagnose a stroke by examining the brain and outlining the brain injured area:

- Imaging tests, such as a computed tomography (CT) or computed axial tomography (CAT) scan, produce a picture of the brain similar to an X-ray.
- Electrical tests, such as electroencephalogram (EEG) or an evoked response test, record the impulses of the brain.
- Blood flow tests, such a B-mode imaging, Doppler testing, duplex scanning, and angiography (arteriogram or arteriography), show problems that may cause change in blood flow to the brain.[38]

As described by the National Heart, Lung, and Blood Institute, the signs and symptoms of a stroke may include:[38]

- Sudden weakness
- Paralysis (an inability to move) or numbness of the face, arms, or legs, especially on only one side of the body
- Trouble speaking or understanding speech
- Trouble seeing in one or both eyes
- Problems breathing
- Dizziness, trouble walking, loss of balance or coordination, and unexplained falls
- Loss of consciousness
- Sudden and severe headaches

Stroke therapies include surgery, drugs, acute hospital care, and rehabilitation. Treatment of ischemic stroke involves removing the obstruction and restoring blood flow. The most promising medication is tissue plasminogen activator (tPA), a clot-busting drug. This medication should be given as soon as possible but absolutely within 4 hours after symptoms present if it is to work effectively.[39]

Unfortunately, only about 3 to 5% of stroke victims reach the hospital within the allotted time period for such treatment. Why? Several reasons appear to exist:

- Stroke symptoms can sometimes be difficult to recognize.

- Patients and family and/or friends often do not realize that a stroke may be occurring and do not know that immediate emergency action is necessary.

- Sometimes because of the lack of stroke symptom recognition, patients may not be seen immediately in emergency rooms.[40]

If tPA cannot be administered, then antiplatelet medications, such as aspirin, may be used to block blood clotting. Anticoagulants, also known as "blood thinners," can be used to help reduce clotting.

Other interventions may be used, such as carotid endarterectomy, balloon angioplasty, or implantable stents, that can open blocked arteries. Current research is exploring intra-arterial thrombolysis in which a catheter (a tube) is inserted into an artery and pushed up to the brain. Anticlotting medications can be delivered through this process and clots broken up.

To treat a hemorrhagic stroke, an obstruction needs to be introduced to prevent rupture and bleeding of the affected blood vessel. Surgical treatment may involve placing a metal clip at the base of the aneurysm (rupture) or removing the affected vessel.[41]

After a stroke, rehabilitation is often necessary to help survivors relearn skills that may be lost when part of the brain is damaged. They may learn new ways to compensate for the disabilities. Therapy usually begins in the acute-care hospital after the patient's condition has been stabilized—often within 24–48 hours after the stroke. Post-stroke rehabilitation requires the services of physicians, rehabilitation nurses, and selected rehabilitation therapists, such as physical, recreational, speech-language, and vocational, as well as mental health professionals.[42]

The types and degrees of disabilities that follow a stroke depend on which areas of the brain have been damaged. Generally, stroke can cause the following disabilities:

- Paralysis is one of the most common disabilities. It usually appears on the side of the body opposite the side of the brain damaged by the stroke. It may affect the face, an arm, a leg, or the entire side of the body.

- Stroke patients may lose the ability to sense touch, pain, temperature, or position. Some experience pain, numbness, or odd sensations such as tingling or prickling in the paralyzed or weakened limbs. Urinary incontinence or loss of bowel control is relatively common after a stroke and often results from a combination of sensory or motor deficits.

- At least one-fourth of all stroke survivors experience language impairments involving the ability to speak, write, and/or understand written and spoken language. There are also sex-related differences in language impairments depending on which section of the brain is affected. Functional MRI scans have shown that males predominantly rely on areas of the left hemisphere of the brain, whereas females activate both the left and right regions for certain aspects of language. A stroke that occurs in the left hemisphere, therefore, can have disastrous results for men in terms of speech, whereas women can use the other, unaffected side to regain speech. This knowledge helps to explain why women are more resilient to the effects of such injury and are more likely to recover language ability after suffering a left-hemisphere stroke.[43]

- Stroke can damage parts of the brain responsible for memory, learning, and awareness. Stroke survivors may have dramatically shortened attention span or may lose their ability to make plans, comprehend meaning, learn new tasks, or engage in complex mental activities.

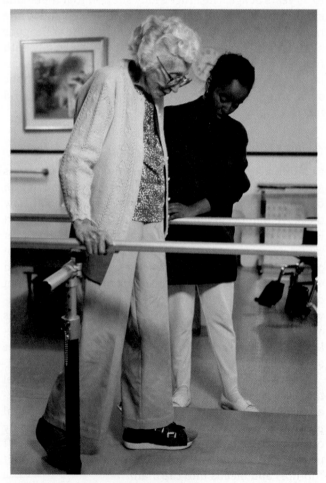

Recovery from a stroke can be very difficult.
@ Photodisc

■ Survivors of stroke often feel fear, anxiety, frustration, anger, sadness, and a sense of grief for their physical and mental impairments. The physical effects of brain damage are responsible for some of these emotional disturbances and personality changes. Clinical depression appears to be the emotional disorder most commonly experienced by stroke survivors.[43]

Whatever the cause of the stroke, the damage to the artery prevents oxygen and nutrients from reaching a particular area of the brain. As a result, that portion of the brain dies. Depending on where the stroke occurs in the brain, speech, memory, thought, and movement can be diminished or lost. Stroke is the leading cause of severe long-term disability. Recovery depends on many factors, a number of which stem from the individual's pre-stroke status: age, mental status, physical abilities, economic support, and cultural perceptions. Often women are older when they experience a stroke and frequently do less well compared to men in recovering physical and mental function.

Although a stroke can happen at any time to anyone, it generally occurs in older individuals. The risk of stroke substantially increases for those over 55 years of age. Women and men are about equal in terms of dying of stroke. Stroke death rates are highest in African American women followed by White, then Asian/Pacific Islander and Hispanic, with the lowest rates among American Indian/Alaska Native women; however, it can occur at any age.[37] Please see "I had a mini-stroke at 24."[44]

Stroke death rates are highest in the southern United States. The following states—called the "stroke belt"—include North and South Carolina, Georgia, Mississippi, Tennessee, Louisiana, Arkansas, and Alabama (see **Figure 10.7**).[45,46]

Risk Factors for Cardiovascular Disease

Cardiovascular diseases result from a complex interaction of genetics, lifestyle, and environmental factors that lead to different pathological conditions of the cardiovascular system. The major risk factors for CVD that can be modified or controlled include tobacco use, high blood pressure, high blood cholesterol, diabetes, obesity, and sedentary lifestyle. Risk factors that cannot be changed or controlled include increasing age, family history of CVD, and race. Although these factors can contribute to a person's risk of disease, they are not perfect predictors of disease development. A woman with normal cholesterol levels, for example, may have heart disease. Conversely, a woman with high cholesterol levels may not

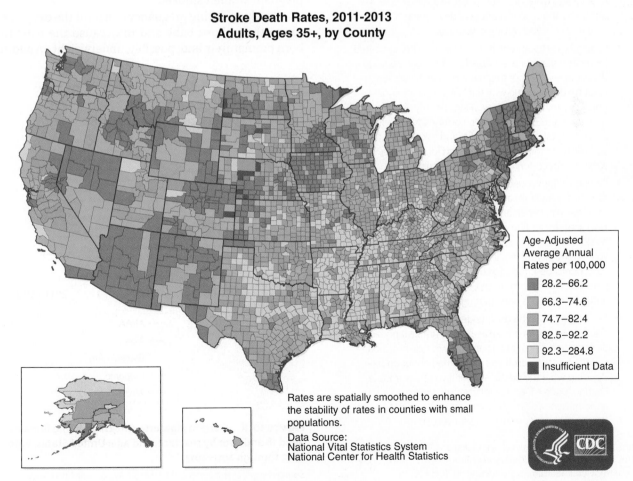

Stroke Death Rates, 2011-2013
Adults, Ages 35+, by County

Age-Adjusted Average Annual Rates per 100,000

- 28.2–66.2
- 66.3–74.6
- 74.7–82.4
- 82.5–92.2
- 92.3–284.8
- Insufficient Data

Rates are spatially smoothed to enhance the stability of rates in counties with small populations.

Data Source:
National Vital Statistics System
National Center for Health Statistics

Figure 10.7   Stroke death rates: Adults, ages 35-plus by county, 2008–2010.
Courtesy of CDC.

have heart disease even though she does have a factor that puts her at risk. The important action here is to talk with your health provider and be forthright and honest about your health behaviors.

Self Assessment 10.1
Heart Disease

The first step toward heart health is becoming aware of your own personal risk for heart disease. Some risks, such as smoking cigarettes, are obvious: Every woman knows whether or not she smokes. But other risk factors, such as high blood pressure or high blood cholesterol, generally do not have obvious signs or symptoms. So you will need to gather some information to create your personal "heart profile."

You and Your Doctor: A Heart Healthy Partnership
A crucial step in determining your risk is to see your doctor for a thorough checkup. Your doctor can be an important partner in helping you set and reach goals for heart health. But don't wait for your doctor to mention heart disease or its risk factors: Many doctors do not routinely bring up the subject with women patients. Here are some tips for establishing good, clear communication between you and your doctor:

- Speak up. Tell your doctor you want to keep your heart healthy and would like help in achieving that goal. Ask questions about your chances of developing heart disease and how you can lower your risk.

- Keep tabs on treatment. If you already are being treated for heart disease or heart disease risk factors, ask your doctor to review your treatment plan with you. Ask: Is what I'm doing in line with the latest recommendations? Are my treatments working? Are my risk factors under control? If your doctor recommends a medical procedure, ask about its benefits and risks. Find out if you will need to be hospitalized and for how long, and what to expect during the recovery period.

- Be open. When your doctor asks you questions, answer as honestly and fully as you can. While certain topics may seem quite personal, discussing them openly can help your doctor find out your chances of developing heart disease. It can also help your doctor work with you to reduce your risk. If you already have heart disease, briefly describe each of your symptoms. Include when each symptom started, how often it happens, and whether it has been getting worse.

- Keep it simple. If you don't understand something your doctor says, ask for an explanation in simple language. Be certain that you understand how to take any medication you are given. If you are worried about understanding what the doctor says, or if you have trouble hearing, bring a friend or relative with you to your appointment. You may want to ask that person to write down the doctor's instructions for you.

Source: Reproduced from National Heart, Lung, and Blood Institute. (2010). *The healthy heart handbook for women.* Available at: http://www.nhlbi.nih.gov/educational/hearttruth/lower-risk/find-out.htm

Tobacco Use

Tobacco use is one of the greatest preventable causes of death in the United States. Tobacco use increases the risk of several kinds of cancer and also sharply increases the risk of heart attack (especially sudden death from heart attack), stroke, and PAD. Although smoking rates have declined sharply since 1960, about 15.8% of women still smoke. Smoking among women varies by race and ethnicity (see **Figure 10.8**).

Furthermore, smoking is more prevalent among women with little education and lowest among women with a college education or higher. Yet smoking still exists among some pregnant women.[47]

> *I started smoking last year. It's helped me lose weight, and gives us something cool to do before school. I'm not worried about getting cancer—that takes years to develop, and I can quit any time I want.*
> **—15-year-old female student**

Pregnant women were less likely to smoke than nonpregnant women. Indeed, the number of women who smoke during pregnancy has dropped sharply to an estimated 9% in 2012 since 1989, when approximately 20% of pregnant women smoked.[48]

Smoking during pregnancy can limit the oxygen supply to the unborn baby and may cause the baby to be born prematurely and, possibly, underweight. In addition,

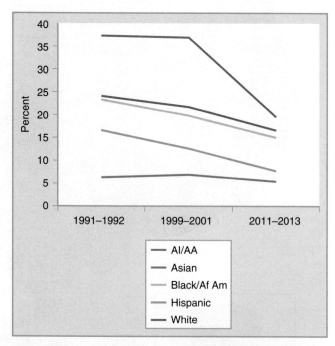

Figure 10.8   Current cigarette smoking among females aged 18 and over by sex, race, and age: United States, 1990–1992 through 2011–2013.

Source: *Health, United States, 2014.* Table 54. Available at: http://www.cdc.gov/nchs/hus/contents2014.htm#054

babies whose mothers smoked during and after pregnancy may be more susceptible to sudden infant death syndrome (SIDS).[48]

Certain components in cigarette smoke act as **vasoconstrictors**, meaning that they narrow the blood vessels. One such compound is carbon monoxide, a gas that reduces the amount of oxygen that red blood cells can carry. This poor oxygen-carrying ability reduces the amount of oxygen available to the heart, brain, muscles, and every organ of the body. Nicotine is another vasoconstrictor. By narrowing the blood vessels, it increases the likelihood of blood clot formation. Over time, vasoconstriction contributes to the increased fragility and brittleness of the arteries, which, in turn, contributes to atherosclerosis. The good news is that when a woman stops smoking her risk for heart disease and other risks begin to decline within 1 month.[49]

Secondhand smoke, also known as **environmental tobacco smoke (ETS)**, comes from nearby tobacco products that are burning. The toxins contained in secondhand smoke include more than 60 cancer-causing agents, including nicotine and carbon monoxide. Secondhand smoke is associated with a number of potentially lethal conditions: lung cancer, sinus cancer, lung conditions (such as asthma or impaired lung function—especially in young children), heart disease, low birth weight in babies (especially when the mother smoked during pregnancy), and others. Repeated exposure to secondhand smoke almost doubles the risk of heart disease.[50]

Relatively recently a new form of "smoking" has emerged—electronic cigarettes. Electronic cigarettes have not been fully studied and research continues into the effects of using such devices. However, early evidence shows that while e-cigarettes are promoted as "safe" they still deliver a substantial number of toxic chemicals. Users heat up the liquid that produces a substance that the user "vapes," or inhales. No smoke is released. Early studies indicate that e-cigarettes contain chemicals that are irritants to lungs. Furthermore, some of the substances may create an environment in which germs are harder to destroy. These new "cigarettes" do not appear to offer any better situation than regular cigarettes and may, in the long term, be even more deadly.[51–55]

Hypertension

Blood pressure is the pressure exerted against the walls of the arteries when the heart pumps, specifically when the left ventricle pumps. This pressure is crucial in maintaining equilibrium throughout the vascular system as different forces affect this system. For example, when an athlete runs a race, the heart must pump faster and harder to meet the demands of the cells for oxygen. As part of this process, the arteries must constrict to keep the pressure constant to accomplish the task of running.[56]

Blood pressure is measured with a **sphygmomanometer**—a device that consists of a cuff that is connected

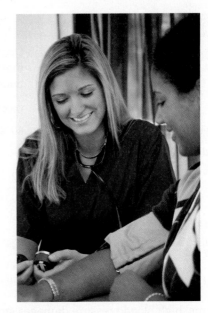

All women should know their personal risk for hypertension and regularly monitor their blood pressure.
© Rob Marmion/Shutterstock

to a measuring device. The cuff is wrapped around the woman's upper arm (or in rare instances, the leg) and the health professional then places a stethoscope over the individual's artery in the arm or leg. The cuff is then inflated, thereby constricting the underlying artery and stopping the blood flow—and with it, the sound of the heartbeat. Gradually the pressure in the cuff is released and the blood begins to flow back through the artery and the sound of the heartbeat returns. The first number that the health professional sees on the measuring device represents the **systolic** pressure—the amount of force that the blood exerts against the wall of the artery when the heart contracts. The second number, which appears at the end of the measurement, is the **diastolic** pressure, which represents the amount of pressure the blood exerts against the wall of the artery when the heart rests between beats.[57]

Hypertension, also known as high blood pressure, is a blood pressure that remains elevated above what is considered a safe level. Hypertension is not the same as excessive stress or tension, as some individuals mistakenly imagine. Although the numbers such as 120/80 mm Hg have been noted over the years as "normal" blood pressure, blood pressure measurements vary throughout the day and activities. A young woman may have a blood pressure of 90/70 mm Hg during a visit to the doctor, whereas an older woman may have a blood pressure of 138/80 mm Hg during her doctor visit. Both may be considered within healthy limits.[56]

Table 10.4 presents the blood pressure measurement levels for normal blood pressure levels, followed by prehypertension and hypertension (high blood pressure) recommended by the National Heart, Lung, and Blood Institute of the National Institutes of Health.[56]

Table 10.4 Categories for Blood Pressure Levels* in Adults

Category	Systolic (top number)		Diastolic (bottom number)
Normal	Less than 120	*and*	Less than 80
Prehypertension	120–139	*or*	80–89
High blood pressure			
Stage 1	140–159	*or*	90–99
Stage 2	160 or higher	*or*	100 or higher

*Measured in millimeters of mercury, or mm Hg

Data from http://www.nhlbi.nih.gov/health/health-topics/topics/hbp

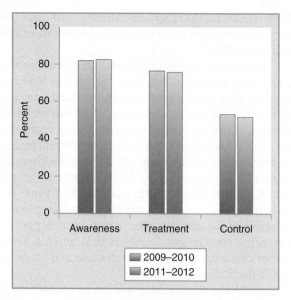

Figure 10.9 Age-adjusted awareness, treatment, and control of hypertension among adults with hypertension: United States, 2009–2012.

Over time, high blood pressure damages small arteries, known as arterioles. Arterioles become thicker and less elastic, resulting in **arteriosclerosis**. This condition, coupled with the effects from atherosclerosis, greatly increases a person's risk for a cardiovascular event. When faced with the demands of heavy exertion (such a running, shoveling heavy snow, lifting heavy items), arterioles, particularly in the brain, heart, or kidneys, can close, rupture, or leak, causing a stroke, heart attack, or renal accident (in the kidneys). Clearly, high blood pressure affects individuals of all racial/ethnic groups (see **Table 10.5**).[56]

In many cases, high blood pressure can be controlled by diet, weight loss, and weight control. In some women, especially African American women, salt sensitivity appears to affect the development and control of high blood pressure. People who are salt sensitive have blood pressure that rises depending on the amount of salt that they consume. For those individuals, consistently restricting salt intake can help lower and control high blood pressure. A woman with high blood pressure should be under the supervision of a healthcare provider. Blood pressure should be checked periodically, especially as a woman ages.[57]

Awareness of high blood pressure is rising, but treatment and control still need attention if individuals are to maintain their health and well-being (see **Figure 10.9**).

Table 10.5 High Blood Pressure Among Women and Men by Race/Ethnicity, 2013

Race/Ethnicity	Men (%)	Women (%)
African American	43	45.7
Mexican American	27.8	28.9
White	33.9	31.3

Data from the Centers for Disease Control and Prevention, *High Blood Pressure Facts*. http://www.cdc.gov/bloodpressure/facts.htm

High Blood Cholesterol

Cholesterol is a waxy substance that is essential for cell manufacture and maintenance as well as the production of sex hormones and nerves throughout the body. Although cholesterol may be obtained through diet, the body, on its own, manufactures enough cholesterol to serve its needs. In some individuals, however, blood cholesterol levels may be excessively high because of obesity, poor diet, or genetic abnormalities. Blood cholesterol levels of greater than 240 mm/dL are associated with an increased risk of morbidity and mortality.[58]

When excessive cholesterol is present, the body can become overwhelmed and deposit unused cholesterol on the inner walls of the arteries. Over time, usually decades, these deposits penetrate the inner lining of the arteries and, accumulating slowly, narrow the space for blood to flow (see **Figure 10.10**).

The inner walls of the artery become brittle and clogged and pieces of the artery tear, leaving jagged edges.

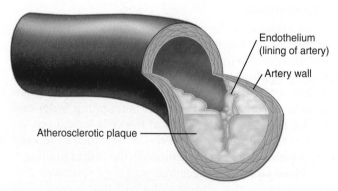

Figure 10.10 Plaque buildup in arteries.

These jagged edges stick up and catch materials that flow by in the bloodstream, thereby adding more waste deposits to the inner lining. The arteries are gradually closed off either by a fatty plaque, a clot, or some other blockage that becomes lodged in the narrowed arteries. Another type of plaque, called an unstable plaque, also may cause blood to clot. If the plaque bursts within the artery wall, its contents are released into the bloodstream and can trigger a blockage. In any case, the blood does not reach a part of the body that depends on it and that part will die unless the artery is once again opened.[59]

The liver and small intestine manufacture cholesterol, which moves throughout the body in a **lipoprotein**. Lipoproteins consist of fats and protein bound together in a chemical structure that enables them to be transported in the blood. They are made up of the following elements: low-density lipoprotein (LDL), high-density lipoprotein (HDL), very-low-density lipoprotein (VLDL), and triglycerides. Everyone has each of these substances in varying amounts of each lipoprotein molecule.

- LDL (low-density lipoprotein) cholesterol is often referred to as "bad" cholesterol because of its affinity for sticking to the wall of the artery and lodging there.

- HDL (high-density lipoprotein**)** cholesterol has often been referred to as "good" cholesterol because it appears to function somewhat like a trash collector, removing cholesterol from various sites, including blood vessel walls where it accumulates.

- **VLDL (very-low-density lipoprotein)** cholesterol is associated with the transport of fats known as triglycerides.

- **Triglycerides** are a form of fat that comes from food and is also made in the body. High triglycerides are often a sign of high total cholesterol.

When discussing cholesterol levels in the blood, health professionals generally either refer to the total cholesterol level or to the LDL or HDL cholesterol and triglyceride levels (see **Table 10.6**). Cholesterol levels are measured from a small amount of blood (about one teaspoonful) drawn from a vein. To obtain an accurate measurement, the individual should be fasting for at least 12 hours prior to the sample being drawn. The measurement is shown in milligrams per deciliter (mg/dL).[60]

Low levels of HDL cholesterol ("good" cholesterol) are a predictor of mortality from CHD in both young and older women. They are a stronger predictor in women than in men.[60–64] Women, particularly those who are fit and slender and who have not experienced menopause, tend to have slightly elevated HDL cholesterol levels compared with men and postmenopausal women.[63,64] Elevated HDL cholesterol levels either protect against heart disease or indicate the presence of other factors that reduce the risk of heart disease. Around menopause, a woman's hormone levels begin to change, and so do her cholesterol levels.

Table 10.6	Categories for Blood Cholesterol and Triglyceride Levels
Cholesterol	**Status**
Total Cholesterol	
Less than 200 mg/dL	Ideal
200–239 mg/dL	Borderline High
240 or more	High
LDL (Bad) Cholesterol	
Less than 100 mg/dL	Ideal
100–129 md/dL	Near optimal/above optimal
130–159 mg/dL	Borderline High
160–189 mg/dL	High
190 mg/dL and higher	Very High
HDL (Good) Cholesterol	
Less than 40 mg/dL	Major risk factor
40–59 mg/dL	The higher, the better
60 mg/dL and higher	Considered protective
Triglyceride Levels	
Less than 150 mg/dL	Normal
150–199 md/dL	Borderline
200–499 mg/dL	High
500 mg/dL or above	Very high

Modified from National Heart, Lung, and Blood Institute. http://www.nhlbi.nih.gov/health/health-topics/topics/hbc/printall-index.html; Data from U.S. National Library of Medicine. National Institutes of Health. Available at: http://www.nlm.nih.gov/medlineplus/ency/ar-ticle/003493.htm

Total cholesterol, especially LDL cholesterol and triglyceride levels, tends to increase and with that a woman's risk for heart disease.[65]

As with other health threats, managing cholesterol levels varies with sex and race. **Table 10.7** demonstrates the difference in high blood cholesterol by sex and age. Among women aged 20 years and older, White women had the highest levels of total cholesterol, followed by African American and Mexican American women.[66]

A person's diet influences his or her cholesterol levels. A diet low in cholesterol and saturated fat is essential in maintaining a low overall total cholesterol level. Eating saturated fats increases the total blood cholesterol, particularly the LDL cholesterol. This means that a woman should limit both the dietary cholesterol and the dietary saturated fats that she eats. Although diets vary by culture, they can be modified to maintain their cultural richness while limiting the dietary fat involved. Daily consumption of essential nutrients remains crucial.

Table 10.7	Percentage of Population with High Cholesterol*	
Age	Male	Female
20–44	12.6	9.4
45–64	39.8	42.4
65–74	50.7	57.7
75 and above	51.2	53.3

*Greater than or equal to 240 mg/dL

Data from Centers for Disease Control and Prevention. *Health, United States, 2014.* Table 61. Available at: http://www.cdc.gov/nchs/hus/contents2014.htm#061

Other substances in the blood may also contribute to cardiovascular disease.

C-Reactive Protein

Even though cholesterol acts as a strong predictor of potential heart attack or stroke, almost half of the people who have heart attacks have normal levels of cholesterol. Studies have shown that **C-reactive protein** (CRP), a protein found in the blood when inflammation is present, may actually be a stronger predictor of potential cardiovascular disease than cholesterol levels. CRP levels can be measured by a simple blood test. The American Heart Association and the Centers for Disease Control and Prevention (CDC) guidelines recommend that CRP screening should be reserved for people with moderate cardiovascular risk and that it should not replace assessment for major risk factors.[67]

If CRP levels are high, treatments to lower cholesterol—such as exercise, aspirin, and **statins** (a medication to lower cholesterol)—can also be used to lower CRP. Although CRP can be useful as a predictor, high levels of this protein can indicate other acute and chronic conditions, including arthritis, tuberculosis, cancer, pneumonia, or the common cold.

Whether CRP should be used as a screening mechanism for elevated cardiovascular risk remains unclear. Even when controlling for other risk factors, CRP levels are generally higher in women of all racial and ethnic groups compared with men.[68]

Homocysteine

Another substance found in the blood is **homocysteine**, an essential amino acid. Increased levels harm the arterial lining and increase the risk for heart disease. Folic acid and vitamins B6 and B12 can lower homocysteine levels, though whether such efforts reduce the risk of heart disease is not yet clear. Until the evidence is stronger, women at high risk for heart disease should make certain their diet is rich in folic acid and vitamins B6 and B12 (fruits and green leafy vegetables).[69]

Diabetes

Diabetes is a disorder of the pancreas in which naturally occurring insulin—a hormone that controls the level of glucose in the blood—is either insufficient or because the body's cells do not respond appropriately to insulin, or both. The most common form of diabetes is type 2 diabetes. Untreated, diabetes can cause many serious problems and can lead to life-threatening conditions.[70] The number of women with diabetes is rising, most often in those who are overweight or obese. Indeed, the rate of physician-diagnosed diabetes has risen among women from 8.7% in 1988–1994 to 10.1% in 2007–2010. The prevalence rates are highest among African American women, followed by Mexican American and White women (see **Table 10.8**).[71] Women who develop diabetes during pregnancy (gestational diabetes) are at high risk of developing the disease later in life.[72]

The presence of diabetes increases the risk for heart disease and stroke. The reasons for this greater prevalence are not entirely clear, although higher rates of overweight and obesity certainly contribute to the risk. High levels of glucose in the blood may also accelerate damage to the blood vessels, increasing the rate of plaque development. The role of genetic predisposition to the disease among certain racial and ethnic groups continues to be explored. In addition, poverty levels often contribute to poor dietary conditions, thereby increasing the risk for diabetes.[71]

The critical issue for people with diabetes is to understand the disease and its effects on health and well-being and to ensure that they maintain proper nutrition, exercise habits, and medication.

The way fat is distributed on a woman's body may also affect her risk for heart disease. Truncal distribution of fat (around the stomach and upper body), as opposed to hip and thigh distribution, appears to be more risky. The truncal distribution has been referred to as an "apple" shape, and the hip and thigh distribution has been referred to as the "pear" shape.[73]

Overweight and Obesity

Overweight and obesity are major risk factors for many chronic diseases, especially for heart disease. Overweight is defined as having a body mass index (BMI) of 25 or greater; obesity is defined as having a BMI of 30 or greater (see **Table 10.9**).[73] Perhaps one of the most troubling issues

Table 10.8	Diabetes Prevalence by Race and Hispanic Origin, 2007–2010
White	9.1
African American	17.9
Mexican American	10.7

Data from Centers for Disease Control and Prevention. *Health, United States, 2014.* Table 44. Available at: http://www.cdc.gov/nchs/hus/contents2014.htm#044

Table 10.9	Percentage of Overweight and Obesity Among Females and Males Aged 20 to 74 Years (Age Adjusted)			
Race/Ethnicity	Overweight		Obesity	
	Male	Female	Male	Female
Black/African American	70.2	81.8	38.1	57.5
Mexican	81.9	78.3	40.2	46.3
White	73.2	60.9	34.3	32.3

Data from Centers for Disease Control and Prevention. *Health, United States, 2014.* Table 64. Available at: http://www.cdc.gov/nchs/hus/contents2014.htm#064

is the number of children who are overweight or obese (see **Figure 10.11**). Developed in childhood and adolescence, this can carry over into adulthood and be very difficult to change.[74]

> *I know I'm overweight. In fact, our whole family could probably stand to lose a few pounds. But after work, I'm usually too tired to cook healthy meals or to get out to the health club. The thought of getting back into shape seems like so much work that I just want to give up.*
>
> **—35-year-old mother**

This condition is a major risk factor for the development of CHD through the heightened risk of developing high blood pressure, high blood cholesterol, and diabetes. Overweight and obesity are also correlated with poor

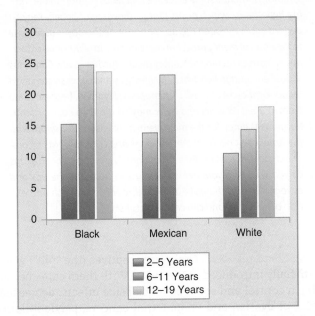

Figure 10.11   Obesity among children and adolescents aged 2 to 19 years by race/ethnicity, 2009–2012.

nutrition and sedentary lifestyles—other CHD risk factors. Sitting in front of a computer or television for long periods and not exercising reduces the need to "burn" calories. Eating a diet rich in saturated fats and cholesterol can lead to clogged arteries. This compromises blood flow, especially to the heart, and can lead to a heart attack or stroke. A person can calculate her BMI by doing the calculation found in **Figure 10.12**, or one can go online to a website such as the National Heart, Lung, and Blood Institute and have it calculated automatically. The website information is located at the end of this chapter.

Physical Inactivity

Physical inactivity, or sedentary lifestyle, is another important modifiable risk factor for cardiovascular disease. Physical inactivity simply means that a woman is not getting enough regular aerobic exercise—any movement that raises the heart rate significantly for an extended period of time. The latest data show that aerobic activity wanes over the years from a high of 60% for the 18- to 44-year age group, to 24.3% in the 75 years and older group.[75] Of course, those 75 years of age and older who do participate should be commended for engaging in such important actions. For all races, women participate less often than men.

Aerobic exercise is a critical factor in keeping the heart and other muscles strong and in good working condition. Regular exercise also aids in controlling weight, helping to raise HDL cholesterol, and both controlling and reducing the risk of developing diabetes.[76] The Nurses' Health Study, a large, ongoing study observing female nurses, showed similar protective effects against coronary heart disease for brisk walking and vigorous exercise.[77]

Other Factors Affecting CVD Risk

Intrauterine Environment   This is a critically important factor in a child's development both in the womb (uterus) and in his or her subsequent development throughout life. If the mother does not have a healthy lifestyle and diet while she is pregnant, the metabolic and endocrine status of the baby may be severely compromised throughout life.[78]

This is particularly challenging if the child develops intrauterine growth restriction (IUGR), a condition in which the fetus grows more slowly than usual. As a result, when the child is born, many exhibit a "catch-up" period in which excess consumption occurs and often leads to increased fat (adipose tissue). This deregulation can lead to obesity, type 2 diabetes, and ultimately cardiovascular disease. Thus, it is critically important for women to maintain a healthy lifestyle during pregnancy so that their babies have the best environment in which to develop.[79]

Menopause   After menopause (cessation of menses or "periods") the risk for heart disease and stroke increases

BMI = weight (in pounds) divided by height (in inches) times height (in inches) × 703

$$\frac{\text{Weight}}{\text{Height} \times \text{Height}} \times 703 =$$

Example: For a 5' 5" woman weighing 146 lbs

$$\frac{146 \text{ lbs}}{65 \times 65} = \frac{146}{4,225} = 0.034 \times 703 = 24.9$$

Alternately, you can go to one of many websites and have it calculated for you. One such website is the National Institutes of Health's National Heart, Lung, and Blood Institute: www.nhlbisupport.com/bmi/

Figure 10.12   BMI calculation.

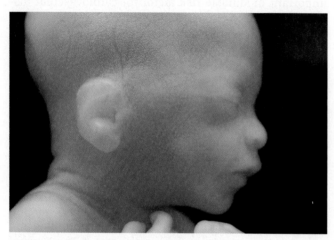

The lifestyle choices a woman makes during pregnancy affect not only her health, but also the health of her developing child.
Chris Downey/Stockphoto/Thinkstock

significantly for women. Coronary heart disease rates in women after menopause are two to three times higher than for women of the same age who have not yet reached menopause. One reason appears to be related to the loss of natural estrogen. Scientists believe that during and after menopause, women experience a decrease in HDL cholesterol and an increase in LDL cholesterol and triglycerides. Increased plaque appears in the arteries, and heart attacks and strokes increase. The decrease in estrogen as a result of natural or surgical menopause is associated with these changes in serum lipid profiles (blood cholesterol levels).[80]

Estrogen loss during menopause and the use of hormone therapy (HT) have inspired tremendous debate in the last several decades. Observational studies in both animals and humans, carried out largely in the 1970s and 1980s, showed that HT could be beneficial in slowing the onset of heart disease. More recent trials in the 1990s and early 2000s, however, showed that HT had no effect or was dangerous. Recent examination of some of those clinical trials has shown where some of the differences may exist. The increased risk appears to be greatest in women who started HT after they had been menopausal for several years or more and those with established heart disease, especially women on a particular regimen of HT. Women who started HT during or immediately after cessation of menstrual periods generally did not show an increased risk.[81] In addition, different types of medication, dosage, and routes of administration clearly affect how a woman responds. As of 2013, the American College of Obstetricians and Gynecologists recommends the following:

Menopausal hormone therapy should not be used for the primary or secondary prevention of coronary heart disease at the present time. Evidence is insufficient to conclude that long-term estrogen therapy or hormone therapy use improves cardiovascular outcomes. Nevertheless, recent evidence suggests that women in early menopause who are in good cardiovascular health are at low risk of adverse cardiovascular outcomes and should be considered candidates for the use of estrogen therapy or conjugated equine estrogen plus a progestin for relief of menopausal symptoms. There is some evidence that lends support to the "timing hypothesis," which posits that cardiovascular benefit may be derived when estrogen therapy or hormone therapy is used close to the onset of menopause, but the relationship of duration of therapy to cardiovascular outcomes awaits further study. Clinicians should encourage heart-healthy lifestyles and other strategies to reduce cardiovascular risk in menopausal women. Because some women aged 65 years and older may continue to need systemic hormone therapy for the management of vasomotor symptoms, the American College of Obstetricians and Gynecologists recommends against routine discontinuation of systemic estrogen at age 65 years. As with younger women, use of hormone therapy and estrogen therapy should be individualized based on each woman's risk–benefit ratio and clinical presentation.[82]

Oral Contraceptives   Oral contraceptives (the "pill") were officially introduced in the 1960s. With them came better birth control and some beneficial side effects: decreased risk of ovarian and endometrial cancers, pelvic inflammatory disease, and dysmenorrhea (painful menstrual periods). However, birth control pills also increased the risk for cardiovascular disease, especially in women who had risk factors for CVD. Over time, scientists and drug manufacturers changed the formulation of oral contraceptives, significantly lowering dosages of estrogen and progestin—key hormonal agents. The question remained, however, as to whether the changed dosage would change the CVD risks. Studies examining the risks associated with oral contraceptives, especially the lower dosage medications, and CVD have shown that changing the dosage did reduce the risks for CVD, especially heart attack and stroke, but did not eliminate them. The risk of heart attack and stroke are uncommon in women of childbearing age. However, for women who are at risk of CVD, such as women who smoke or have high blood pressure, taking oral contraceptives can pose a risk. Older women and obese women have the highest risk of increased blood pressure from oral contraceptives.[83,84]

Oral contraceptive users with a history of migraines are two to four times more likely to have an ischemic stroke compared with women who suffer migraines but do not use oral contraceptives.[77] Studies suggest that the risk is greater among women who have severe migraine headaches with "aura"—focal neurologic symptoms such as blurred vision, temporary loss of vision, seeing flashing lights or zigzag lines, or trouble speaking or moving. Experts now recommend that a woman who has migraine headaches with focal neurologic symptoms should not start combined oral contraceptives. A woman 35 years of age or older without focal neurologic symptoms should also consider another method of birth control. Mild or severe headaches that are not migraine-related do not rule out use of birth control pills.[85] Because the risk of CVD increases in oral contraceptive users with other risk factors, women should have a complete medical checkup before choosing oral contraceptives as their method of birth control.

Alcohol and Illicit Drugs   Consuming modest levels of wine or other alcohol (no more than one drink per day) can reduce the risk of coronary heart disease in women. There is, however, an increased risk of stroke and other causes of morbidity and mortality with moderate-to-heavy consumption of alcohol. Therefore, nondrinkers should not take this as a recommendation to begin drinking, and those who are drinking more than the recommended amount should cut back.[86] **Figure 10.13** demonstrates what is considered a "standard" drink.

Illicit drugs, such as cocaine, lysergic acid diethylamide (LSD or acid), and heroin, may cause short-term cardiovascular effects as well as long-term cardiovascular complications. Cocaine and LSD both increase heart rate and blood pressure while constricting the blood vessels. Cocaine can lead to medical complications such as heart attack, stroke, heart failure, and irregular heartbeats. Cocaine-related deaths are often the result of cardiac arrest. Heroin slows down cardiac function during use. Its long-term effects include scarring and collapsing of veins and bacterial infections of the blood vessels and heart valves, often leading to death. These drugs, and many others, are also associated with many other short- and long-term negative effects.[87]

Stress   Stress is a normal part of everyday life and, in fact, is essential to proper functioning of the body. External stimulation can push a person to study for a test or to sprint the final lap in a race. A kiss from a loved one can also create stress, but most would not want to do without it. Stress also has negative side effects. The extent to which these negative side effects influence a person's sense of self and well-being differ greatly. However, continual exposure to psychological stress can damage the cardiovascular system. Studies have associated heart disease with work-related stress, defined as low job control and high job demands. Researchers are also investigating the link between anger in stressful situations and increased risk of premature cardiovascular disease. Whether women manifest stress differently from men requires additional study. What does seem clear is that

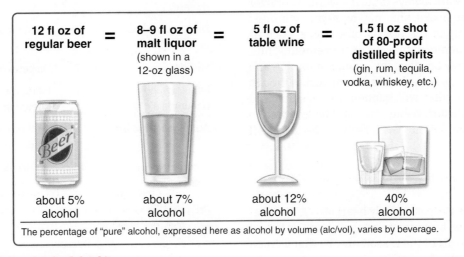

Figure 10.13   What is a standard drink?

stress makes both women and men more susceptible to heart disease and stroke.[88]

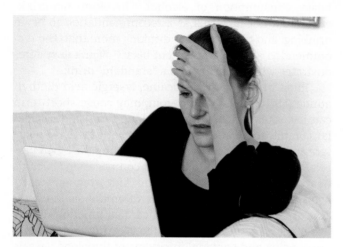

Chronic stress increases a woman's chances of heart disease, stroke, and other conditions.
© Dwaschnig/Shutterstock

Compounding Risk Factors

Many risk factors affect a person's likelihood of developing CVD. Together, multiple risk factors have a cumulative effect. For example, consumption of a diet high in saturated fats and cholesterol leads to high blood cholesterol and deposition of fatty plaques in the arteries. That same diet, which also is often high in calories, leads to overweight and obesity, which strains the heart and arteries and contributes to high blood pressure and diabetes. These factors place additional strain on arteries already carrying increasing amounts of plaque. The addition of cigarette smoking compounds the problem by making arteries fragile and more constricted. Arteries become clogged with waste and the supreme pump—the heart—becomes sluggish and weak. In short, the combination of these risk factors produces a scenario for disaster: heart attack, stroke, CHF, and PAD.

Such events are not always fatal. If a woman survives the heart attack or stroke, she may be severely limited by a damaged heart or the effects of a stroke, such as impaired vision, memory, speech, or movement. Thus, even though she may be alive, the quality of her life and that of her family may be seriously diminished. Although no one can predict what will happen, establishing and maintaining good health habits early in life reduces the likelihood of CVD and limits the effects of the disease if it occurs.

Sex/Gender Differences in Cardiovascular Disease

Cardiovascular disease, particularly heart attack, is sometimes not considered by women and their families to be a disease of women. Part of the reason may be that women often present with signs and symptoms of the disease some 10 to 15 years later than men. Between the ages of 20 and 49, CVD is prevalent in men compared with women. From ages 60 to 79 the prevalence is about equal, and from 80 onward, women surpass men. These differences may, in part, stem from estrogen loss as women age. Estrogen appears to have a positive effect on the cardiovascular system. As women begin to age and estrogen levels diminish, CVD rates rise.[89,90]

Overall, more women than men die from cardiovascular diseases. Fifty-one percent of women die from cardiovascular disease compared with men.[90] Of course, those numbers vary by racial/ethnic group. Heart disease and cerebrovascular disease are the first and third leading causes of death in women; whereas in men, heart disease is the leading cause of death and cerebrovascular disease is fifth. That does not imply that men are in better cardiovascular health than women. It simply means that other diseases, conditions, and behaviors affect men and their health differently than they do women. For example, the third leading cause of death among men is unintentional injury (traffic and other accidents), while it is the sixth leading cause of death in women (see **Table 10.10**). On a more positive note, data from the CDC (**Figure 10.14**)

Table 10.10	Leading Causes of Death by Sex, 2013		
Male	**Rank**	**Female**	**Rank**
Diseases of the heart	1	Diseases of the heart	1
Malignant neoplasms	2	Malignant neoplasms	2
Unintentional injuries	3	Chronic lower respiratory disease	3
Chronic lower respiratory disease	4	Cerebrovascular disease	4
Cerebrovascular disease	5	Alzheimer's disease	5
Diabetes mellitus	6	Unintentional injuries	6
Suicide	7	Diabetes mellitus	7
Influenza and pneumonia	8	Influenza and pneumonia	8
Alzheimer's disease	9	Nephritis, nephrotic syndrome, nephrosis	9
Chronic liver disease and cirrhosis	10	Septicemia	10

Data from Centers for Disease Control and Prevention. *Health, United States,* 2014. Table 20. Available at: http://www.cdc.gov/nchs/hus/contents2014 .htm#020

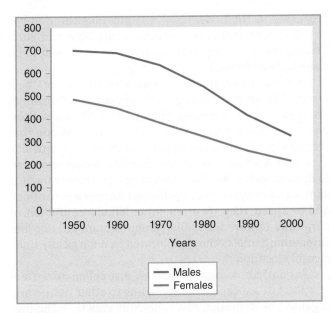

Figure 10.14 **Heart disease mortality trends for males and females, 1970–2013.**

indicate that cardiovascular disease mortality is declining in both women and men.

The signs and symptoms of myocardial infarction (heart attack) also underscore sex differences. Both men and women may experience the following symptoms:

- Pain or discomfort in the chest region
- Pain or discomfort in the upper torso (trunk and arms)
- Shortness of breath
- Cold sweats, nausea, or dizziness

However, women often do not have the well-known severe pain or discomfort in the chest region. Instead, they may more commonly experience shortness of breath, dizziness, nausea, and fatigue. Women may not even be aware that they are having a heart attack. These symptoms often present a challenge not only to family, friends, and coworkers but also to health professionals. In addition, cultural beliefs can affect a woman's perception of the symptoms.[91] Rather than a heart attack, a woman may believe that she is experiencing gastrointestinal symptoms (gas, upset stomach) and thus not act quickly.

Immediate action is essential at the first signs and symptoms of a heart attack. The sooner the person gets to treatment, preferably within the first 3 hours of symptom onset, the sooner treatment can be administered and the effects of the attack minimized. Unfortunately, many do not heed the warnings.[91,92]

Further complicating the issue is that some women experience a "silent" heart attack, in which there are few, if any, signs or symptoms. As such, a woman may choose to ignore the signs and proceed with her routine. About 64% of women who die suddenly may have no symptoms.[93]

The reasons for these sex-related differences are not entirely clear. One key factor may be the age difference between women and men at the time of the event. Women are generally older and have more compromising risk factors. Scientists are exploring these differences, but such studies take time because it is important to follow groups of individuals over decades to obtain accurate and reliable data. Such long-term studies, which have already provided important CVD data on women and men, include the Framingham Heart Study, the Nurses' Health Study, the Bogalusa Heart Study, the Rancho Bernardo Study, the Women's Health Initiative, and a number of others.

Racial/Ethnic Differences in Cardiovascular Disease

The age-adjusted death rates for heart disease and stroke vary significantly among women in the major United States designated racial and ethnic groups. Rates are highest among African American, White, and Hispanic women. The lowest rates are among Asian American/Pacific Islander and American Indian/Alaska Native women.[85]

Of particular concern is the number of children and youth who are at elevated risk for CVD earlier in life because of these and related risk factors. Overweight is increasing among girls from 2 to 19 years. This translates into a considerable increase in risk factors among girls as they mature and age (see **Table 10.11**).[94]

On a positive note, participation in workout activities (aerobic and muscle strengthening activities) has increased among women from 35% in 1998 to 46.6% in 2012. It is interesting to note that these increases occurred among women ages 18 to 75-plus years.[95]

Social Determinants

Social factors also play a critical role in the development of cardiovascular disease. Numerous factors affect these determinants: the environment in which the individual lives, the economy, resources, the healthcare system, health inequities, discrimination, and cultural beliefs.

A woman living under challenging economic and social conditions in an area that does not have easily accessible health care and that has limited resources (healthy food sources, safe drinking water, safe air quality)

Table 10.11	Children and Adolescent Risk Factor Percentages, 1988–2012	
Risk Factor	**1988–1994**	**2009–2012**
Diabetes	8.7	10.1
High cholesterol (240 mg/dL and above)	24	27.5
Obesity	14.7	18.4
Smoking	23.7*	16.7*

*Dates for smoking are from 1990–1992 and 2010–2012.

Data from Centers for Disease Control and Prevention. *Health, United States, 2013*. Tables 46, 59, 69, and 70. Available at: http://www.cdc.gov/nchs/data/hus/hus13.pdf

and who has not been educated about health and staying healthy is at greatly increased risk for CVD and its risk factors. Furthermore, the force of a community or culture can have an important effect on how a woman sees herself—fat, thin, just right—and what she eats, how she behaves, and how she maintains her health.

CANCER

Cancer is a disease characterized by uncontrolled cellular growth and reproduction. It is not a new phenomenon. Hippocrates, in the 4th century BCE, coined the term **carcinoma**, meaning a cancerous growth. More than 100 different diseases are categorized as "cancer." **Table 10.12** summarizes the number of new cases of cancer by race and ethnicity in women and men. **Figure 10.15** summarizes the cancer incidence rates by race and ethnicity in women. Many distinctions may be made among these types of cancers, although they all follow similar basic

Table 10.12	Number of New Cancer Cases per 100,000 by Race, Ethnicity, and Sex, 2008–2012	
Male		**Female**
516.6	All races	411.2
519.8	White	423.9
590.1	Black	401.2
325.4	Asian/Pacific Islander	297.5
340.8	American Indian/Alaska Native	308.8
395.0	Hispanic	322.2
534.5	Non-Hispanic	425.4

Data from National Cancer Institute. SEER stat fact sheets: All cancer sites. Available at: http://seer.cancer.gov/statfacts/html/all.html

processes in the body. **Table 10.13** provides the number of U.S. cancer deaths between the years 2008 and 2012. Clearly, there are important differences that need to be more fully addressed.

A **tumor**, also referred to as a **neoplasm** or "new growth," is an abnormal growth of cells. Some tumors are solid, whereas others, known as **cysts**, are a thin-walled sac filled with fluid. A **benign tumor** is one that remains localized and confined to its original growth site, that is, it does not invade surrounding tissue or spread to distant body sites. Examples of benign tumors include skin warts or cysts. Because benign tumors are confined and localized, they are often either left alone, drained, or surgically removed. Usually benign tumors are not life-threatening unless they are located in a surgically inaccessible location.[96]

In contrast, **malignant tumors**, also called **malignant neoplasms**, are capable of spreading to other tissues and organs—the definition of a cancerous growth.[96] The process of cancer cell invasion and spreading is known as **metastasis**. Cancer cells circulate through the blood or lymphatic system and can invade healthy cells in other parts of the body. These circulating cells often become trapped in the first network of capillaries that they encounter, usually the lungs. Blood leaving every organ other than the intestines travels to the lungs for oxygenation, so the lungs are a common site for metastasis. Blood leaving the intestines goes to the liver, the second most common site of metastasis. Some cancer cells have an affinity for other receptors and, therefore, may metastasize to certain types of tissue. Once metastasis has occurred, local surgical treatment is often impossible.[97,98]

There are two main types of **carcinogens**: those that damage genes that control cell reproduction and migration and those that enhance the growth of tumor cells. Many agents, including chemical substances, viral or bacterial carcinogens, physical agents, and natural substances in the blood, can cause **carcinogensis**. As noted by the American Cancer Society:

Carcinogens do not cause cancer in every case, all the time. Substances labeled as carcinogens may have different levels of cancer-causing potential. Some may cause cancer only after prolonged, high levels of exposure. And for any particular person, the risk of developing cancer depends on many factors, including how they are exposed to a carcinogen, the length and intensity of the exposure, and the person's genetic makeup.[98]

Tobacco use is one of the major causes of carcinogenesis. Smoking cigarettes is associated with increased risk for cancers of the lung, mouth, nasal cavities, pharynx, esophagus, pancreas, liver, cervix, kidney, and bladder. The frequency of smoking, tar content, and duration of the habit all influence the initiation and promotion of cancer-cell growth.

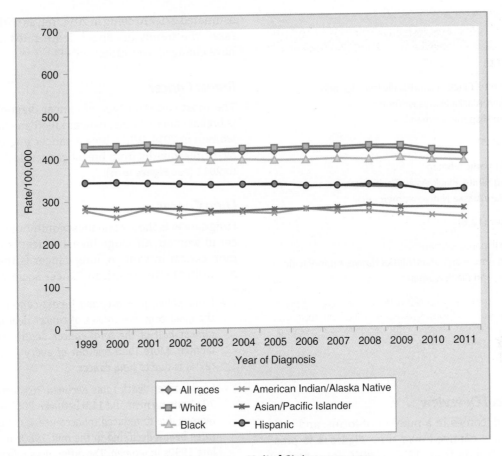

Figure 10.15 Trends in cancer incidence rates among women: United States, 1999–2012.

What about electronic cigarettes? It is not yet clear the extent to which such cigarettes may cause or contribute to cancer. While many e-cigarette manufacturers state that they are "safe," sufficient studies over time have not been done to demonstrate such "safety." What has been noted is that a number of substances used in e-cigarettes are indeed carcinogenic. An important factor is that these cigarettes contain and deliver nicotine—a toxic substance found in tobacco.[99,100]

Dietary factors are also related to carcinogenesis. What a woman consumes is as important as what she avoids. Saturated fats and non-nutrient food additives such as salt, nitrites, and alcohol have been associated with an increased risk of cancer. In contrast, fruits and vegetables containing phytochemicals may reduce the risk for cancer.[101,102] Phytochemicals are plant compounds that may also be known as antioxidants, flavonoids, and by a number of other names.[103] Radiation, occupational carcinogens such as asbestos, and even certain drugs or medications can cause cancer. Viral carcinogens have also been recognized as contributing to cancer. For example, human papillomavirus (HPV) causes cervical cancer and some cases of anogenital cancer.[104]

Perspectives on Cancer

Cancer is the second leading cause of death for women in the United States, with an estimated 275,710 deaths from all cancers in 2014.[104,105] Cancer was the second leading cause of death among both Black and White women but was the first leading cause of death among Hispanic, Asian/Pacific Islander, and American Indian/Alaska Native women (see **Table 10.14**).[106]

Table 10.13	Number of Cancer Deaths per 100,000 Persons by Race, Ethnicity, and Sex, 2008–2012 (Age-Adjusted)	
Male		**Female**
207.9	All races	145.4
206.4	White	145.6
261.5	Black	166.3
128.4	Asian/Pacific Islander	91.2
186.7	American Indian/Alaska Native	133.9
148.0	Hispanic	99.4
212.9	Non-Hispanic	149.4

Data from National Cancer Institute. SEER stat fact sheets: All cancer sites. Available at: http://seer.cancer.gov/statfacts/html/all.html

Table 10.14	Leading Causes of Cancer Death Among Women

Lung cancer (37.0)

- First among White, Black, Asian/Pacific Islander, and American Indian/Alaska Native women
- Second among Hispanic women

Breast cancer (21.5)

- First among Hispanic women
- Second among White, Black, Asian/Pacific Islander, and American Indian/Alaska Native women

Colorectal cancer (12.8)

- Third among Hispanic women
- Fourth among American Indian/Alaska Native, Asian/Pacific Islander, White, and Black women

U.S. Cancer Statistics Working Group. (2014). *United States cancer statistics: 1999–2011 incidence and mortality web-based report.* Atlanta, GA: Department of Health and Human Services, Centers for Disease Control and Prevention, and National Cancer Institute.

Epidemiological Overview

Cancer, as noted, comes in a number of forms, and incidence trends have changed over time. **Figure 10.16** presents incidence trends from 1930 to 2010 for a variety of cancers in women. Unfortunately, the appearance of cancer in women seems to remain relatively stable over years.

The incidence rates then trend into death rates for those who do not survive the diagnosis. Cancer is a major cause of death for women in the United States, with an estimated 275,710 dying in 2014. Yet, as with the incidence rates, the trends in cancer death rates among women have changed over time.[106,107,108]

Breast Cancer

The most common type of cancer diagnosed in women is breast cancer. Breast cancer killed an estimated 40,000 women in 2014. While breast cancer numbers have risen over time, deaths from breast cancer declined from 1999 to 2011 (see **Figure 10.17**).

Lung Cancer

Lung cancer is the second most commonly diagnosed cancer in women. Although breast cancer is the most common cancer in women, lung cancer is the most deadly. According to the American Cancer Society:

- *Lung, colon, prostate, and breast cancers continue to be the most common causes of cancer death, accounting for almost half of the total cancer deaths among men and women. More than one out of every four cancer deaths (27%) is due to lung cancer.*

- *Lung cancer death rates declined 36% between 1990 and 2011 among men and 11% between 2002 and 2011 among women due to reduced tobacco use. Lung cancer incidence rates began declining in the mid-1980s in men and in the late 1990s in women. The differences reflect historical patterns in tobacco use, where women began smoking in large numbers about 20 years later than men.*

- *Death rates for breast cancer are down more than one-third (35%) from peak rates, while prostate and colon cancer death rates are each down by nearly half (47%) as a result of improvements in early detection and treatments.*

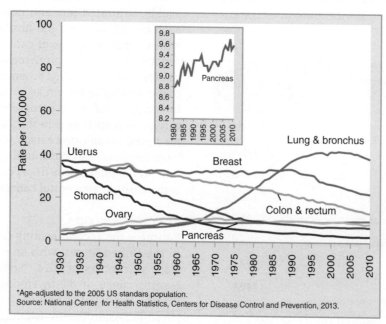

*Age-adjusted to the 2005 US standars population.
Source: National Center for Health Statistics, Centers for Disease Control and Prevention, 2013.

Figure 10.16   Trends in cancer death rates from 1930 to 2010 for a variety of cancers among women.

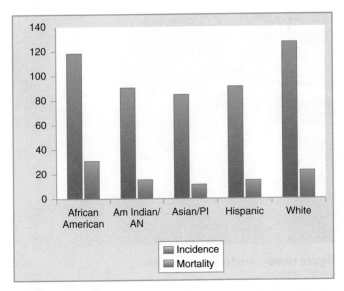

Figure 10.17 Breast cancer incidence and mortality rates by race/ethnicity, 2006–2010.

- *The three most commonly diagnosed types of cancer among women in 2015 are expected to be breast, lung, and colon cancer, accounting for one-half of all cases in women. Breast cancer alone is expected to account for 29% of all new cancers among women in the U.S.[109]*

Smoking is a major risk factor for lung and associated cancers. According to the CDC, national estimates show:

- 15.8% of women smoke, compared to 20.5% of men
- Highest ages of cigarette consumption: between the ages of 25 and 64 years
- Among different racial/ethnic groups, those who smoke include
  - American Indian/Alaska Natives: 21.8%
  - Whites: 19.7%
  - African Americans: 18.1%

- Hispanics: 12.5%
- Asians (excludes Native Hawaiians and Pacific Islanders): 10.7%
- Smoking varies by education
  - Adults with 12 years or less of education: 24.7%
  - Adults with GED diploma: 41.9%
  - Adults with a high school diploma: 23.1%
  - Adults with an undergraduate college degree: 9.1%
  - Adults with a postgraduate college degree: 5.9%
- Smoking varies by income status
  - Adults who live below the poverty level: 27.9%
  - Adults who live at or above the poverty level: 17.0%[110]

In addition, smoking rates vary by state, with the highest levels in the Midwest and South, compared with the Northeast and West (see **Figure 10.18**). It is interesting to note that the cost of cigarettes may influence smoking rates. Here are some examples of the cost of a pack of cigarettes:

- Kentucky: $4.96
- West Virginia: $5.07
- Delaware: $6.00
- Maine: $7.12
- DC: $7.89
- New York: $14.50[111]

The smoking death rates by state appear to be largely higher in states where cigarettes are cheaper—Kentucky, West Virginia, Oklahoma, Missouri—as opposed to states where they are more expensive—New York, Hawaii, Arizona, New Mexico. Estimates indicate that over 108,210 women will have died from lung cancer during the 2014 time period.[109]

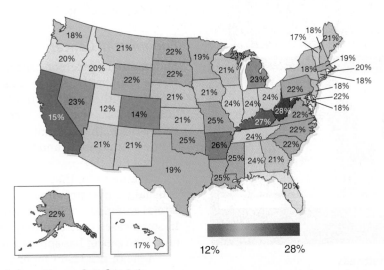

Figure 10.18 Percentage of cigarette smokers by state.

Women have a number of reasons for smoking. Some say that it helps them maintain a lower weight, while others feel that it makes them appear sophisticated. Cigarette advertising, which has been in place for decades, has been very clever in marketing (see **Figure 10.19**). Marketing continues and it remains a major issue in smoking rates, often targeting adolescents with messages presented at retail outlets and signs located near schools (see **Figure 10.20**). Once smoking is initiated, it can be very difficult to quit as one ages. In addition, YouTube has numerous cigarette ads available and targeted toward specific age groups.

Colorectal Cancer

Colorectal cancer is the third leading cause of cancer deaths among all women. However, it remains the second leading cause of death among Asian/Pacific Islander

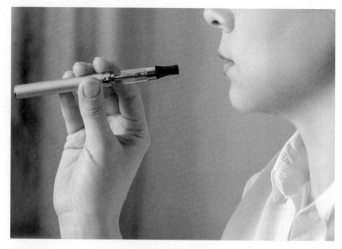

Figure 10.20   **Modern cigarette ads.**
© Alex Shalamov/Shutterstock

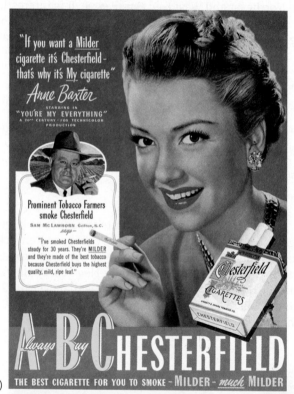

(A)

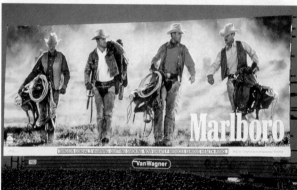

(B)

Figure 10.19   **Vintage cigarette ads.**
(A) © APIC/Getty Images, (B) © Gilles Mingasson/Hulton Archive/Getty Images

and Hispanic women and third for American Indian/Alaska Native, Black, and White women.[99] Men appear to be more prone to the disease than women. Nevertheless, the most recent death figures available, 2014, show that 24,040 women died of the disease. Death rates rise as women age.[112]

When diagnosed early in the cancer's development, the death rates are low. Early diagnosis through regular screening can serve as an important prevention measure. In addition, several other factors play an important role in prevention:

- Maintaining a healthy diet: limiting consumption of red and processed meats and enhancing intake of fruits and vegetables as well as whole grain products

- Limiting alcohol and tobacco use

Although colorectal cancer death rates are declining, they are still a threat and they are more frequently diagnosed as people age, with the highest rates among those 65 to 74 years of age.[112]

Endometrial Cancer

Endometrial cancer, or cancer of the uterine lining (see **Figure 10.21**), is the fourth most common cancer among women, with an estimated 52,630 cases diagnosed in 2014 and 8590 deaths.[113] According to the National Cancer Institute, this accounts for 6% of all cancers affecting women. If diagnosed and treated early, there is a very high survival rate.[113]

Treatment for those whose cancer is diagnosed early is usually a hysterectomy (removal of the uterus) and bilateral salpingo-oophorectomy (removal of the ovaries). In some cases radiation may be utilized. In severe cases and if the cancer has spread, medications may be used.[114]

A major risk factor for endometrial cancer is estrogen exposure, which can occur in several ways: obesity (estrogen

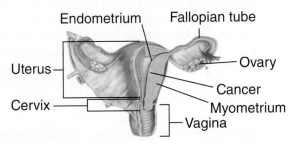

Stage IA Endometrial cancer

Endometrium — Fallopian tube

Uterus —

Cervix —

Ovary

Cancer

Myometrium

Vagina

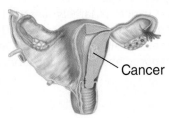

Stage IB Endometrial cancer

Cancer

Figure 10.21   Endometrial cancer.

is contained in fat cells), estrogen therapy for postmenopausal women, late menopause, a history of polycystic ovary syndrome, breast or ovarian cancer, and diabetes.

Ovarian Cancer

There are three types of cells that are part of the ovaries: epithelial cells, germ cells, and stromal cells. Each of these cells can morph into a tumor. Although most are benign, epithelial malignancies (carcinomas) represent approximately 85–90% of ovarian cancers. These cancerous cells metastasize and frequently spread to the abdomen and pelvis linings and organs. The latest figures posit that an estimated 21,290 women will be diagnosed with the disease in 2015 and approximately 14,180 will die.[115] The highest death rates for ovarian cancer are among White women (see **Figure 10.22**).[116]

Cervical Cancer

Cervical cancer is another important form of reproductive organ cancer in women. This form of cancer is caused by certain "high-risk" strains of human papillomavirus (HPV). Women who begin having sex at an early age or who have many sexual partners are at a much greater risk for HPV. However, as has been noted, women who have had only one sexual partner can still develop the disease. Studies point out that cigarette smoking and long-term use of oral contraceptives has also influenced the rise in cervical cancer.[117]

Screening is very important in detecting cervical cancer. The Pap test is the commonly used detection device. Although this is an important test, doctors note that it is not perfect. The critical message here is that a woman should be screened regularly. Among different racial/ethnic

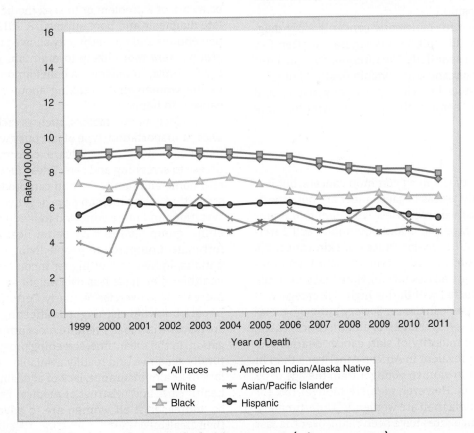

Figure 10.22   Ovarian cancer death rates by race and ethnicity, 1999–2011 (rates per 100,000).

groups, cervical cancer is diagnosed in earlier stages in White women, followed by Black women, and usually in women younger than 50 years of age.

Treatment for cervical cancer is largely laser ablation (removal of the tissue), cryotherapy (freezing the affected area), or surgery at the site. Survival rates are quite high for women diagnosed and treated for cervical cancer.[117]

Pancreatic Cancer

The pancreas is an organ located in the abdomen and serves as producer of enzymes that assist in digesting food.

Pancreatic cancer is a challenging and deadly disease, often because it is difficult to diagnose early. In 2014, the American Cancer Society estimates that 22,890 women will be diagnosed with pancreatic cancer and 19,420 will die. The number of deaths per 100,000 are: Black 12.4, White 9.4, American Indian/Alaska Native 8.0, Hispanic 7.7, and Asian/Pacific Islander 7.2.[118]

There are two major types of pancreatic cancers: exocrine tumors and endocrine tumors. The exocrine tumors are the more common malignant tumors, making up the majority of pancreatic tumors. Risk factors for developing pancreatic cancer include tobacco use, being overweight, and workplace exposure to certain chemicals such as pesticides and dyes. In addition, people with excessive alcohol intake may be more likely to develop cirrhosis of the liver. People with cirrhosis of the liver seem to be more prone to developing pancreatic cancer. There is also a genetic predisposition.[119]

A major issue with pancreatic cancer is early diagnosis. This is very difficult because there are often few symptoms that present early. This frequently translates into a late diagnosis and unavoidable death. Maintaining a healthy lifestyle, knowing your family history, and being very aware of some of the signs and symptoms are critical.

Skin Cancer

Skin cancer is one of the most common cancers, but it is difficult to properly assess because most are not reportable diseases by cancer registries. There are two major types: basal cell carcinoma and squamous cell carcinoma.[120,121] One of the major causes of skin cancers is exposure to the sun. Tanning, severe sunburn, and lifetime sun exposure are all risk factors. Note that sun lamps and tanning booths fall within this high-risk category.[122] According to the American Cancer Society, although melanoma is estimated at less than 2% of all skin cancer cases, it accounts for the majority of skin cancer deaths. The disease is far less prevalent in African Americans than in Whites and higher in women younger than the age of 45 compared with men. However, men are more at risk for dying from melanoma than are women.[123] Unfortunately, melanoma incidence rates have been rising over the last several decades, in part due to the focus on tanning beds and suntans. This is an area that is particularly troubling, especially among young White women. The CDC notes that indoor tanning provides high levels of UV radiation and, over time, will contribute to prematurely aging the skin with wrinkles and spots and a much higher risk for melanoma.[122,123] MedicineNet provides a slide show of the different presentations of skin cancers.

Racial/Ethnic and Socioeconomic Dimensions

The rates of disease and death from cancer vary by race/ethnicity as well as geography. Interestingly, cancer incidence rates also vary by state. For example, the highest incidence rates for lung cancer are in the following states: Alaska, Delaware, Illinois, Indiana, Kentucky, and West Virginia. The highest incidence rates for breast cancer are in Connecticut, Massachusetts, Vermont, and Washington. Death rates for breast cancer were among the highest in the District of Columbia, New Jersey, Louisiana, Maryland, and Ohio. For pancreatic cancer, the death rates were among the highest in the District of Columbia, Louisiana, Massachusetts, and New Hampshire.[124,125]

Because cancer risk is strongly associated with lifestyle and behavior, differences in key factors can play a critical role in an individual's health and well-being. Cultural values and belief systems can affect a person's willingness and ability to understand the need for preventive action and to seek medical care. Poor health knowledge and literacy can also make a person less likely to be aware of a problem or to seek medical care, leading to late diagnosis and poor survival. A 2013 study on cancer perceptions and race/ethnicity showed that some cultural groups were more likely to maintain a fatalistic belief. For example, "fatalismo," a belief among some Hispanic/Latina women that speaking about breast cancer can cause it to happen.[125–127]

Socioeconomic factors, such as lack of health insurance, transportation, type of job, busy work schedule, low income, or need for childcare, can impede a woman's access to screening and care. These factors affect a women's home and family life and can produce high levels of stress that, over time, can have negative effects on health. Wealthier and more educated individuals of any racial or ethnic group tend to have better health than those less fortunate. Compared to people living in low-income situations, individuals of higher income smoke less, eat a healthier diet, have less overweight and obesity, and are more likely to exercise regularly. Certainly income has an impact, but what else might be affecting behaviors? These are issues that clearly require more attention and investigation. In the meantime, screening programs must be culturally sensitive and readily available. Language barriers, lack of health insurance, lack of availability and access to health care, and mistrust of medical professionals must be addressed if all women are to advance and protect their health.[125,126,128]

Economic Dimensions

The Agency for Healthcare Research and Quality (AHRQ) estimates that in 2011 cancer cost $88.7 billion in the United States. Of that sum, "50 percent were for hospital outpatient or doctor visits, 35 percent for in patient hospital stays, and 11 percent for prescription drugs."[129] As stated by the American Cancer Society: "Uninsured patients and those from ethnic minorities are substantially more likely to be diagnosed with cancer at a later stage, when treatment can be more extensive and more costly."[129] Cancer patients and their families also face burdens in terms of time, reduced employment opportunities, payments for cancer treatments not covered by insurance, and the emotional costs of pain and suffering.

Global Perspective

Cancer knows no boundaries, and it is estimated to be responsible for 14 million new cases and 8.2 million deaths in 2012, the latest year for World Health Organization (WHO) statistics.[130] The WHO estimates that those numbers will rise substantially over the next 20 years. Economically evolving countries bear the greatest burden with 60% of cases presenting in Africa, Asia, and Central and South America. Why? Early diagnosis and limited access to the latest and most effective treatments may be severely limited. Furthermore, the cost of the most highly beneficial treatments is rising and is a burden on even the most financially sound countries.[131] One of the most challenging aspects of cancer prevention is helping individuals to avoid the Western lifestyle: cigarette smoking, high-fat diets, and less physical exercise.[132]

Breast Conditions

More than half of all women go through the frightening experience of finding a lump in a breast. In the majority of cases, the lump is benign and needs no treatment. However being able to understand the issues and concerns about breast conditions is a vitally important dimension of women's health.

Benign Breast Diseases

There are several types of benign breast conditions.

- **Hyperplasia:** This condition is an overgrowth of cells and usually occurs inside the milk ducts in the breast. Hyperplasia can increase the risk of breast cancer.

- **Cysts:** These are sacs filled with fluid. They are more common in premenopausal women. The cause of these cysts is not entirely clear.

- **Fibroadenomas:** These are solid tumors that are benign and are most commonly present in younger women. Most do not increase breast cancer risk.

- **Intraductal papillomas:** These papillomas present in the breast milk ducts and may cause discharge from the nipples. Again, these are more common among younger women (35–55 years of age). They can be surgically removed. They are not a serious risk factor for breast cancer unless they have abnormal cells.

- **Sclerosing adenosis:** These are small breast lumps that often can be felt. They are usually recognizable on mammograms and can be painful. If they appear on mammograms, the woman may need to undergo a biopsy to rule out breast cancer. Whether they increase the risk of breast cancer is not clear.

- **Radial scars:** These have a core of connective tissue fiber and are also known as "complex sclerosing lesions." As with sclerosing adenosis, they can be mistaken for cancer on mammograms and therefore usually require a biopsy.[132,133]

Breast Cancer

Breast cancer is a frightening, conflicting, and sometimes misleading condition for women. Understanding breast cancer is important for all women, because the disease is one of the most treatable cancers if detected early. The classification for breast cancer consists of five levels:

- **Stage 0:** This is a noninvasive form of breast cancer where there are no cancer cells or noncancerous abnormal cells metastasizing to other areas of the body.

- **Stage I:** This is an invasive breast cancer that is largely contained in the breast tissue and no lymph nodes are involved. Tumors are usually 2 centimeters or smaller.

- **Stage II:** These tumors are generally 2–5 cm in size and may have spread to axillary lymph nodes.

- **Stage III:** These tumors are usually larger than 5 cm or have grown into the chest wall, skin, or distant lymph nodes.

- **Stage IV:** These are tumors that have spread to other parts of the body. Stage IV breast cancer is sometimes referred to as "advanced" or "metastatic."[133]

Risk Factors Several factors can increase a woman's chance of getting breast cancer.

Genetics: Women with mothers or sisters (first-degree relatives) who have breast cancer are generally at higher risk of developing the disease. Some 5–10% of cases are thought to be hereditary. Most of the hereditary cases result from mutations in two breast cancer genes: *BRCA1* and *BRCA2*. These genes reduce the risk for breast cancer by manufacturing a protein that prevents abnormal cell growth. However, if the gene is mutated, it increases a woman's risk for breast cancer, ovarian cancer, and pancreatic cancer. Although *BRCA1* and *BRCA2* are generally the most common gene defects leading to breast cancer in women, other mutations also exist.

Although many women can have such mutated genes, they are most common in women of Ashkenazi Jewish (generally of Eastern European origin), Norwegian, Icelandic, or Dutch ancestry. The increased frequency of mutated genes may be more common in these groups because of shared ancestry.[134]

In addition, there is also a type of breast cancer known as "triple-negative." These tumors lack receptors for estrogen and/or progesterone and a protein called human epidermal growth factor (HER2). Women of African descent may have a great risk for developing this type of breast cancer.[135,136]

However genetics are not the only factor. Whereas White women are more likely to develop breast cancer, African American women are more likely to die from breast cancer; often this is because they have less access to early detection and treatment.[136]

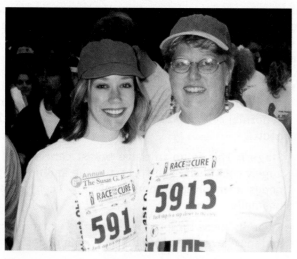

Breast cancer survivors and advocates have raised awareness and billions of dollars for research.
Courtesy of David Emanuel

Hormones: Exposure to two hormones, estrogen and progesterone, influence a woman's development and her ability to become pregnant and bear children. These hormones can also create some increased risk, depending on a woman's lifetime exposure, the type of medication used, and how it is administered. Some examples follow:

- *Early onset menstruation*: Women who have early onset menstruation (less than 12 years of age) or later menopause (after 50 years of age) have a somewhat greater risk. Part of the reason may be the longer exposure to the naturally occurring hormones estrogen and progesterone.[137–139]

- *Pregnancy*: Never having had a child or having a child later in life (after 30 years of age) may present an increased risk. These hormones play a crucial role in pregnancy.

- *Overweight and obesity*: Estrogen is made largely in the ovaries. It is also manufactured in fat cells. After menopause, the estrogen in a woman's body largely comes from fat cells. The heavier the woman, the greater the exposure.

- *Hormone replacement therapy (HRT)*: Studies from the late 1990s have suggested that the use of estrogen alone or estrogen and progesterone together increases the risk of breast cancer. However, more recent meta-analyses do not support these findings. Short-term use does not appear to pose a threat in most women. The threat of developing breast cancer with long-term use of estrogen plus progesterone is not entirely clear.

- *Oral contraceptives*: Whereas oral contraceptives are safe for most women, some women at risk for breast cancer should not use them. They include women older than 35 who smoke and/or have high blood pressure, women who have had or are at risk for heart disease or stroke, women who have migraines, women who have breast or estrogen-dependent cancers, and women who have liver disease. On the positive side, oral contraceptives can reduce risks for the following diseases: pelvic inflammatory disease, ovarian and endometrial cancers, colorectal cancer, and bone loss (osteopenia).[140–142]

> *My aunt was diagnosed with breast cancer when I was in high school. I couldn't believe it—she's only 10 years older than me, and has always been more like a big sister than an aunt. She had to have a lumpectomy and was really worried for a while. But almost four years later there's no sign of the cancer returning, and she just completed a marathon!*
>
> **—18-year-old woman**

Screening and Diagnosis Many risk factors for breast cancer cannot be modified by lifestyle behaviors. Early detection of breast cancer, however, can be lifesaving. Indeed, the prognosis for breast cancer strongly depends on the stage at which it is diagnosed. There are three basic methods for early detection of breast cancer, all of which are important to prevention and detection.

- **Breast self-examination (BSE)** consists of the systematic palpation of the breast tissue of each breast while lying on one's back. The most common sign of breast cancer is a new lump or mass in the breast, although other signs, such as swelling of the breast, skin dimpling, or nipple changes, may present as well. The American Cancer Society recommends that women 20 years of age and older examine their breasts monthly, after menses and at the same time each month. For women who have reached menopause,

BSE should also be done on a regular monthly schedule. In addition to examining for lumps, women should also check for breast discharge. **Figure 10.23** provides detailed guidance on the BSE procedure. Monthly BSE should always include visual inspection (with and without a mirror) to note any changes in contour or texture and manual inspection in standing and reclining positions to note any unusual lumps or thicknesses.

- **Clinical breast examinations** (CBE), are conducted by the woman's healthcare provider and should be performed every year starting at age 20. The exam consists of observing the breasts for signs such as dimpling, feeling the breast and underarm for abnormal signs or swollen lymph nodes, and squeezing the nipples for signs of discharge.[143]
- **Mammography**, a low-dose radiograph of the breast tissue, can detect smaller breast lesions that cannot

---

Breast Self-Examination

Breast self-examination should be done once a month so you become familiar with the usual appearance and feel of your breasts. Familiarity makes it easier to notice any changes in the breast from month to month. Early discovery of a change from what is "normal" is the main idea behind BSE. The outlook is much better if you detect cancer in an early stage.

If you menstruate, the best time to do BSE is 2 or 3 days after your period ends, when your breasts are least likely to be tender or swollen. If you no longer menstruate, pick a day such as the first day of the month, to remind yourself it is time to do BSE.

Here is one way to do BSE:

1. Stand before a mirror. Inspect both breasts for anything unusual, such as any discharge from the nipples or puckering, dimpling, or scaling of the skin.

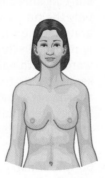

The next two steps are designed to emphasize any change in the shape or contour of your breasts. As you do them, you should be able to feel your chest muscles tighten.

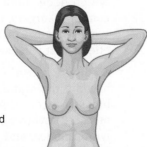

2. Watching closely in the mirror, clasp your hands behind your head and press your hands forward.

3. Next, press your hands firmly on your hips and bow slightly toward your mirror as you pull your shoulders and elbows forward.

Some women do the next part of the exam in the shower because fingers glide over soapy skin, making it easy to concentrate on the texture underneath.

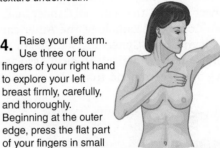

4. Raise your left arm. Use three or four fingers of your right hand to explore your left breast firmly, carefully, and thoroughly. Beginning at the outer edge, press the flat part of your fingers in small circles, moving the circles slowly around the breast. Gradually work toward the nipple. Be sure to cover the entire breast. Pay special attention to the area between the breast and the underarm, including the underarm itself. Feel for any unusual lump or mass under the skin.

5. Gently squeeze the nipple and look for discharge. (If you have any discharge during the month—whether or not it is during BSE—see your doctor.) Repeat steps 4 and 5 on your right breast.

6. Steps 4 and 5 should be repeated lying down. Lie flat on your back with your left arm over your head and a pillow or folded towel under your left shoulder. This position flattens the breast and makes it easier to examine. Use the same circular motion described earlier. Repeat the exam on your right breast.

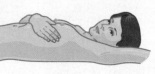

Figure 10.23   Breast self-exam.

be felt through BSE or CBE. This technology has the potential to detect breast cancer at the earliest stages of development. Mammography involves compressing the breast between two flat disks. The radiographs are taken of each breast lying flat and another of the breasts from above (see **Figure 10.24**). Although mammograms can detect some breast cancers before they can be felt, other tumors may be felt through BSE or CBE that could not be detected by the mammogram. Therefore, it is critical to conduct a BSE, have a CBE, and have a regular mammogram.[143–145]

The question remains regarding how often a woman should have a mammogram. A major controversy emerged in 2009 when the U.S. Preventive Services Task Force recommended a change in screening frequency.[146] They stated, based upon examination of the data, that the frequency of mammogram screenings could be done every 2 years starting at the age of 50. However, those recommendations are currently being updated and it is not entirely clear whether there will be substantive changes.

This caused a major controversy among many different cancer organizations regarding the appropriate action women should take. Major cancer organizations (the American Cancer Society, the National Cancer Institute, the American College of Radiology, the American College of Obstetricians and Gynecologists, Susan G. Komen for the Cure, and the American Medical Association) firmly believe and recommend that mammogram

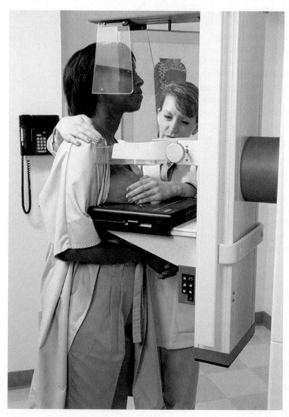

Figure 10.24 Mammogram.
© Keith Brofsky/Getty Images

screening should be done every 1 to 2 years starting at age 40. While scientific opinions differ, the bottom line is that every woman should talk with her healthcare provider about her risks and how often she should have a mammogram. In the meantime, the National Institutes of Health's National Cancer Institute has current recommendations that can be appropriately and safely followed until the issues are resolved.[147]

Magnetic resonance imaging (MRI) has been in use for a number of years but until recently has not been used for breast cancer screening. The scans appear to be especially useful in pre- and perimenopausal women, especially those who have dense breast tissue. For women who are at increased risk for breast cancer, MRI scans appear to be better at detecting tumors at an earlier stage. However, sometimes the test can show abnormalities when none exist. Therefore, this screening test is still being studied.[148]

Treatment and Reconstruction Although a breast tumor may be suspected with an examination or a mammogram, the ultimate diagnosis is made by a biopsy. The **biopsy** removes a sample of the suspected tissue, which is then examined for abnormal cell growth.

Surgery is the primary treatment for breast cancer, although it may be combined with radiation therapy or hormone therapy. There are several types of breast cancer surgery.

- **Lumpectomy**: A lumpectomy is often used for early-stage localized tumors when it is possible to remove only the tumor and some surrounding tissue. A separate incision may be made to remove the axillary lymph node (lymph nodes in the armpit area). In women with early cancer, a lumpectomy with subsequent radiation therapy has become the primary alternative to modified radical mastectomy. Lumpectomies are usually limited to those breast tumors that are well defined and less than 1–2 inches in total diameter.

- **Simple mastectomy**: This treatment involves the complete removal of the breast, but not the lymph nodes under the arm or the chest wall muscles.

- **Radical mastectomy**: This is the removal of the entire affected breast, the underlying chest muscles, and the lymph nodes under the arm. Although once a very common surgery, this procedure is used less often today because of the disfigurement and the side effects that it causes.

- **Modified radical mastectomy**: This procedure has become the standard surgical procedure for most breast cancers that require removal of the entire breast. It involves removing the breast, some of the lymph nodes, and the lining of the chest muscles. This procedure has survival rates comparable to those with a radical mastectomy, but it is more conducive to breast reconstruction and results in greater mobility and reduced swelling.[148]

■ **Adjuvant therapies**: There are treatments that enhance surgical effectiveness, including chemotherapy, hormone therapy, and radiation therapy. Chemotherapy and hormone therapy may be used to treat localized tumors as well as to control metastatic conditions. Hormone therapy may block the effects of certain hormones that promote the growth of some breast cancers. Tamoxifen and raloxifene, known as selective estrogen reduction modulators (SERMs), are the most common anti-estrogen drugs used to reduce the risk of breast cancer in high-risk women. Side effects include hot flashes and night sweats and, sometimes, irregular menstrual periods. There are some serious but rare side effects: endometrial cancer and blood clots.[149]

■ Targeted therapy is also used. In this type of therapy, special substances known as monoclonal antibodies or tyrosine kinase inhibitors, such as Herceptin, attack specific cancer cells without killing normal cells. In addition, even more advanced therapies are currently being tested.[150]

After a mastectomy, a woman faces the decision of whether to undergo breast reconstruction. Reconstruction of breast tissue may be an important part of breast cancer recovery for some women. The degree of difficulty associated with reconstruction varies with the extent of the proposed surgery. In addition, emotional support and social support are important components of recovery. Support groups may provide valuable information and assistance with physical and psychological breast cancer recovery issues.[151,152]

Gynecological Conditions

A variety of malignant and benign conditions can develop in a woman's upper and/or lower reproductive tract. This section reviews major benign and malignant conditions of the cervix, uterus, and ovaries. It also discusses the risk factors, screening, and treatment of these conditions.

Benign Cervical Changes

Polyps are small, benign growths that develop in the endocervical canal, often after the onset of menstruation. Polyps usually produce mild symptoms such as abnormal vaginal bleeding or discharge. Although they are rarely cancerous, the growth should be examined. Treatment of a cervical polyp consists of removing the polyp and examining the tissue.

Cervical dysplasia, which involves abnormal changes in the cells of the cervix, is usually a benign condition.

GENDER DIMENSIONS: Health Differences Between Men and Women

Sex/Gender Differences in Breast Cancer

Breast cancer is well known and feared among women. Unfortunately, because it is far less common, breast cancer is not usually thought of as a threat to men's health, often with disastrous consequences. Data from the American Cancer Society states that in 2015, an estimated 2350 new cases will be detected and approximately 440 men will die from breast cancer.[203]

Men and women both have breast tissue. Both sexes also have male and female hormones, such as testosterone and estrogen, just in different amounts. The major difference in females and males is the amount of breast tissue and the hormonal influence on it. Females have more breast tissue than men and make far more female hormones than men do. These female hormones cause the breasts to develop and grow. In men, male hormones, made largely in the testicles, inhibit breast growth spurred by female hormones. Yet breast tissue, in both males and females, can become cancerous.

Several risk factors are associated with breast cancer in men:

■ Radiation exposure in the chest area, as in radiation treatment for a disease

■ Diseases that produce high levels of estrogen (female hormone) in the body, such as cirrhosis of the liver or Kleinfelter's syndrome (a genetic disorder in which men have more than one X chromosome, e.g., XXY)

■ Female relatives who have alternations of the *BRCA1* or *BRCA2* gene

■ Obesity, because fat cells produce estrogen

Known mutations in breast cancer susceptibility genes—*BRCA1*, *BRCA2*, and *CHEK2*—pose a heightened breast cancer risk in women. *BRCA1* and *BRCA2* are also associated with breast cancer in men, and *CHEK2* may also prove a risk. *BRCA2* is the genetic mutation that appears most commonly in men and accounts for an estimated 5–10% risk. *BRCA1* is less common and seems to appear more often in men of Jewish heritage.[204,205]

In general:

■ Men are less likely to be diagnosed early.

■ Poorer and younger Black men had higher death rates from breast cancer compared with younger White men.

■ Both Black and White older men had less chemotherapy compared with women.[206,207]

This is a disease that deserves attention in both sexes. Yet for many reasons, men are more reluctant to acknowledge or be tested for the disease. Fortunately, men are becoming more aware and making efforts to educate both men and women about the disease in men. Websites are more prevalent and men are becoming more comfortable discussing it. However, much work remains to be done to promote public awareness of breast cancer in men.

It is considered precancerous, however, because severe, untreated **dysplasia** can result in invasive cervical cancer. Low-grade or mild dysplasia usually occurs in women around the ages of 25 to 35 and can often be detected with a Pap smear. High-grade or moderate-to-severe dysplasia refers to the presence of a large number of precancerous cells covering the surface of the cervix. Also referred to as **carcinoma-in-situ**, severe dysplasia is more likely to become cancerous, but it can be successfully cured if detected early. Treatment varies depending on the severity of the dysplasia.[153]

Cervical Cancer

Cervical cancer is a type of uterine cancer afflicting the lower part of the uterus, which is referred to as the cervical canal. Most cancers of the cervix originate in the cells lining the surface of the cervix. Cervical cancer is classified into five stages, 0 to 4:

- **Stage 0:** In its localized first stage, or carcinoma-in-situ, cervical cancer involves only the cervix's innermost lining.

- **Stage I:** This cancer remains only in the cervix. There are two stages of this level: Stage IA1 and IB2. In Stage IB2, the cancer is advanced slightly farther than in IA1.

- **Stage II:** This cancer has spread beyond the cervix, but not to the pelvic wall. Stage II cancer is defined as either Stage IIA or Stage IIB. In Stage IIB, the cancer has spread to the tissue around the uterus.

- **Stage III:** This cancer has spread to the pelvic wall and the vagina and may affect the kidneys. Again, it is presented in two stages: Stage IIIA and Stage IIIB.

- **Stage IV:** This cancer has spread past the pelvic wall and may be found in the bladder or the rectum. It has two substages: Stage IVA and Stage IVB. In Stage IVB the cancer has spread to other body parts—liver, lungs, or distant lymph nodes.[154]

It's Your Health

The cervix is technically part of the uterus, but because characteristics and risk factors for uterine and cervical cancer are distinctive, they are discussed separately.

Risk Factors   Cervical cancer is primarily caused by persistent infection with certain high-risk strains of human papillomavirus (HPV). Some strains of HPV can cause genital warts, while others can, in some cases, lead to cervical cancer. HPV is a sexually transmitted infection that most sexually active women contract during their twenties. In fact, according to the CDC, it is estimated that 79 million people are presently infected with HPV, and some 14 million new persons are infected each year.[155]

Most women who become infected with HPV will clear the virus on their own through the body's natural immune system. A few women will not clear the virus, however, and will develop a long-term, persistent infection. These women are at a higher risk for developing cervical cancer.[156]

Other factors that may contribute to the development of cervical cancer include lower immune system suppression, often from taking immunosuppressant drugs; having HIV/AIDS; having multiple sexual partners; having other sexually transmitted diseases; smoking cigarettes; having a mother who took the drug diethylstilbestrol (DES); and having a family history of cervical cancer. Women can now be treated for HPV when they get their Pap smear.[156]

Invasive cervical cancer rarely occurs in women who have regular gynecological examinations. When it does occur, however, symptoms may include bleeding between menstrual periods, spotting after intercourse, and increased vaginal discharge. By the time the symptoms of cervical cancer appear, a tumor is usually quite large and may have already invaded nearby tissue.

Screening and Diagnosis   Cervical cancer is one of the few cancers that is effectively preventable through regular screening. The Pap test, also known as the **Pap smear**, provides a method of screening for cellular changes before cancer develops and detecting cancer at an early stage.

A newer screening method, the HPV test, looks for the DNA of cancer-causing types of HPV. The HPV test was first approved by the U.S. Food and Drug Administration (FDA) for follow-up evaluation in women whose Pap results are uncertain—typically referred to as ASC-US (atypical squamous cells of undetermined significance).

The U.S. Preventive Services Task Force released Cervical Cancer Screening Guidelines in 2012.[157,158] Having a positive HPV test does not mean that a woman will get cervical cancer. It just means that she should be followed more closely by her healthcare provider. If a Pap smear is abnormal, regardless of the results of the HPV test, the clinician will want to perform a colposcopy, a procedure to more closely examine the cervix, vagina, and vulva, and possibly a biopsy to view the cervical cells more closely. If the Pap test results are inconclusive, the HPV test can help the clinician clarify a woman's risk of cervical cancer. A negative HPV test means a woman is not at risk of developing cervical cancer in the next few years. Even when results are negative, women should continue to visit their healthcare provider for an annual exam.

Treatment   Treatment following an abnormal Pap smear depends on the results of the cervical biopsy. Inflammation of the cervix, known as **cervicitis**, may be associated with a vaginal infection or discharge and requires only local treatment with a specific vaginal cream or suppositories. Treatment for dysplasia depends on the severity and usually consists of cryosurgery, cone biopsy, or laser cone biopsy.

Cryosurgery destroys tissue by a freezing process. It is most often used to treat mild or moderate dysplasia. As a procedure, cryosurgery has the advantage of producing little or no discomfort. It also presents few risks for complications such as bleeding, further infection, or infertility from scarring. A watery vaginal discharge is common for about 2 weeks after cryosurgery. It is generally recommended that a woman avoid intercourse, douching, or tampons during the recovery period.

A cone biopsy, or **conization**, is considered to be both a diagnostic and therapeutic procedure, because it provides tissue for an accurate diagnosis and removes the abnormal tissue. Cone biopsy procedures are less common today than they were several years ago because of the widespread use of colposcopy. **Colposcopy** is usually performed in the physician's office using a **colposcope**, a special microscope that permits close examination of the cervix and vagina as well as biopsy.

Treatment of cervical cancer depends on the tumor's stage when diagnosed. Carcinoma-in-situ may be treated with cone biopsy in a woman who wishes to have children. Surgery to remove abnormal tissues in or near the cervix will remove the tumor but leave the uterus and the ovaries intact. Definitive treatment of carcinoma-in-situ, however, may require a hysterectomy (surgical removal of the uterus) to ensure complete removal of the cancerous cells. Lymph nodes, as well as fallopian tubes and ovaries, may also need to be removed. Depending on the stage of the cancer, radiation therapy or chemotherapy may be used as adjuvant therapy. Even after hysterectomy, a small percentage of women experience cancer in the vagina, so lifelong gynecological follow-up is very important.[159]

Benign Uterine Conditions

Fibroids are benign tumors composed of muscular and fibrous tissue in the uterus (see **Figure 10.25**). Fibroids have different names depending on the type of fibroid: fibromyomas, leiomyomas, or myomas. The cause of uterine fibroids is not entirely understood. Hormones, estrogen and progesterone, other bodily chemicals such as insulin growth factor, and perhaps other genes may contribute to their development.[160] Risk factors for uterine fibroids also vary. Heredity and race appear to play a role. Fibroids are more common in Black women than any other race.[161] Clinical studies are also investigating whether obesity affects their development and whether oral contraceptives may be a deterrent.

Fibroids often begin developing in women between the ages of 25 and 35. They are the primary cause of an abnormally enlarged uterus and one of the most common reasons for hysterectomy. Although single fibroid tumors occur, multiple tumors are more common.

Symptoms depend on the size and location of the tumors and may include the following:

- Irregular vaginal bleeding
- Vaginal discharge
- Pain in the lower back
- Pain during sexual intercourse
- Frequent urination

Fibroids may grow under the influence of estrogen produced during pregnancy, from oral contraceptives, or from HT. They often shrink and disappear with menopause. These tumors are usually detected during routine pelvic examinations because they create an enlarged and irregular uterus.

Hormone-based treatments can temporarily reduce the size of the fibroid and relieve symptoms. A gonadotrophin-releasing hormone (GnRH) agonist may be used to block the production of hormones, particularly estrogen, by the ovary. The most commonly used GnRH agonist in the United States is Lupron, which is given by an injection either once a month or every 3 months. Fibroids usually regrow, however once treatment stops.[162,163]

Surgery may be indicated for fibroids if they cause severe pain or bleeding. Surgery involves removing either the fibroid alone, **myomectomy**, or the entire uterus, hysterectomy. A hysteroscopic resection may be used for certain types of fibroids. In this procedure, a fiber-optic scope is inserted through the vagina and curettage is used to remove the fibroid.

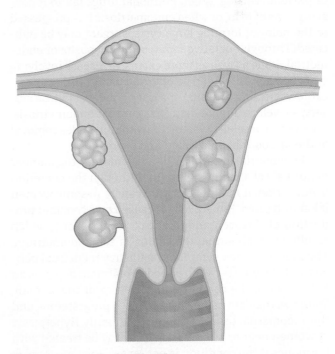

Figure 10.25   Uterine fibroids.

Nonsurgical procedures are another option to remove fibroids. In uterine artery embolization, a surgeon injects small particles of plastic or gelatin sponge through a catheter placed in the uterine artery. The particles block the blood supply to the fibroid, resulting in the death of the fibroid tissue. The fibroid shrinks and symptoms are usually relieved without the need for surgery. Focused ultrasound surgery is a surgery that uses an MRI scanner to locate the fibroids and then uses high-frequency and high-energy sound waves to destroy the fibroids.[163]

Endometriosis **Endometriosis** is another benign condition of the uterus. In this condition, tissue that looks and acts like endometrial tissue begins to grow outside the uterine lining. This progressive condition is most common in women aged 30 to 40 years. Because endometrial tissue responds to hormonal influences during the menstrual cycle, women who have this disorder often feel pain just before or during menstruation. Endometriosis also may cause abdominal upset during menstruation and abnormal vaginal bleeding. Many women, however, have advanced lesions without any symptoms.[164]

For those with minimal or no symptoms or those women who do not want to have any or more children, regular gynecological checkups (every 6 to 12 months), exercise/relaxation efforts, and the use of anti-inflammatory medications such as ibuprofen (Advil) or naproxen (Aleve) may be sufficient to manage any symptoms of discomfort.

For others, options include pain medications, hormonal medications, or surgery. Hormones can prevent ovulation and associated discomfort. However, hormonal therapy does not reverse damage that has already occurred or prevent scarring. When hormonal drugs fail to relieve symptoms of pain, or when endometriosis has progressed to the point of forming large cysts, surgery may be indicated. Through operative **laparoscopy**, deposits of endometrial tissue as well as more extensive disease involving cysts and adhesions can be removed using either electrocautery (burning of tissue) or a laser. The most radical surgery, as well as a more definitive cure for endometriosis, involves a complete hysterectomy that includes removal of the uterus, fallopian tubes, and ovaries.[165]

Endometrial hyperplasia is an increase in the number of normal cells lining the uterus. Although the condition is not cancer, it may develop into cancer in some women if left untreated. Hyperplasia is caused by a constant production of estrogen and a lack of progesterone, which results in an abnormal thickening of the endometrium. The most common symptoms are heavy menstrual periods and bleeding between periods. Treatment depends on the extent of the condition and the age of the woman. Young women are usually treated with progesterone and the endometrial tissue is checked frequently. Hyperplasia in women near or after menopause may be treated with hormones if the condition is not severe. Hysterectomy is the usual treatment for severe cases.[166]

Malignant Uterine Tumors

Uterine cancer typically begins in the tissue lining of the uterus, the **endometrium**. Endometrial cancer is most common in women ages 55 and older. Carcinoma-in-situ is found only on the surface layer of the endometrium. As the cancer progresses to Stage I, it spreads to the muscle wall of the uterus. Stage II cancer spreads to the cervix and, possibly, tissue supporting the cervix. By Stage III, cancer has spread to the vagina, pelvic lymph nodes, and other membranes or organs in the pelvic cavity. The final stage of this cancer involves the bladder, rectum, and possibly the abdominal lymph nodes.[167]

Risk Factors   Endometrial cancer accounts for most uterine cancers. The greatest risk for endometrial cancer is being older than 45 years of age. It is estimated that over 54,000 new cases of uterine cancer will be diagnosed in 2015. Risk factors of uterine cancer appear to involve excess stimulation of the endometrial cell proliferation by estrogen in the absence of progesterone. Obesity increases endometrial cancer risk perhaps owing to estrogen production in fat cells. Other risk factors include high blood pressure, diabetes, early menarche (before 12 years of age), late menopause (after age 55), and never being pregnant. Failure to ovulate and a history of infertility also increase risk and may be associated with estrogen imbalance. Other risk factors include postmenopausal long-term, high-dose estrogen replacement therapy.

Family history of endometrial cancer and personal history of breast, ovarian, or colon cancer increase a woman's risk as well. Finally, women using tamoxifen treatment for breast cancer are also at higher risk. Further research is needed to ascertain the mechanism and roles of these risk factors for endometrial cancer.[168]

Screening and Diagnosis   Because endometrial cancer affects the inside of the uterus, the tumor initially cannot be seen or felt during a pelvic examination. Thus, a pelvic exam and Pap smear are only partially effective in the diagnosis of endometrial cancer and therefore the disease is not usually detected until the symptoms appear. The most common symptoms of endometrial cancer include pain in the pelvic area, difficult or painful urination, pain during intercourse, and change in bowel patterns.

The American Cancer Society recommends that women at increased risk for endometrial cancer (those with a history of infertility or obesity) have an endometrial biopsy at menopause. Women on unopposed estrogen replacement therapy should have such biopsies repeated on a regular basis. A **transvaginal ultrasound** has also proven useful as a screening tool for endometrial cancer.

Diagnosis of endometrial cancer is made by biopsy, ultrasound, dilatation and curettage (D&C), or **hysteroscopy**. These procedures permit the evaluation of the tissue and cell lining in the uterine cavity.[169]

Treatment   Treatment of endometrial cancer depends on several factors, including the stage of the disease. Because uterine cancer may spread rapidly, treatment of early-stage disease involves removal of the uterus as well as the fallopian tubes and ovaries. A combination of surgery and radiotherapy is effective in the treatment of localized disease. Regional spread of the cancer outside the uterus is treatable by radiation. Advanced, metastatic endometrial cancer is generally treated by the administration of progesterone, which usually results in long-term survival, but not cure. Treatment for later-stage disease includes removal of not only the uterus, fallopian tubes, and ovaries but also the cervix, part of the vagina, and lymph nodes.[169]

Benign Ovarian Growths

Cysts are fluid-filled growths that are extremely common. Ovarian cysts are usually benign and rarely cause discomfort or pain. If symptoms do occur, they may include pain or pressure in the pelvic cavity, irregular periods, and pain during intercourse.

Different types of cysts exist depending on the tissue and the makeup of the cyst. The most common type results from the follicle that surrounds the mature egg. If the follicle does not rupture to release the egg during ovulation, it becomes a cyst. Many of these cysts go away without treatment in a few months.

Several treatments are available. Birth control pills are a common treatment for women who have recurrent cysts. If the cyst does not resolve, then surgery may be required. Laproscopy, which is only mildly invasive, is often used for small cysts. Laparotomy, which involves an abdominal incision, is preferred for larger cysts and tumors.[170]

Polycystic ovarian syndrome, a condition that affects women of reproductive age, causes the formation of numerous cysts in the ovaries. This disorder results from increased levels and, often, the imbalance of hormones, including estrogen and testosterone. Women with polycystic ovarian syndrome are often obese (which contributes to excess estrogen) and have many obesity-related risk factors: diabetes, high blood pressure, and high cholesterol levels. In addition, because of the effects of testosterone, some women may experience an excess of body and facial hair. The treatment for this condition may include losing weight; hormonal medications, such as birth control pills, to regularize the menstrual cycle; and antitestosterone medication. Sometimes, medications for diabetes are also used.[171]

Ovarian Cancer

Ovarian cancer, the fifth leading cause of cancer death in women, leads to more deaths than any other cancer of the female reproductive system. This cancer usually affects women around the time of menopause or later (ages 50 to 70). There are four stages considered in the diagnosis of ovarian cancer:

- **Stage I:** Cancer cells are limited to the ovaries or fallopian tubes.
- **Stage II:** Cancer cells have migrated from the ovaries to other parts of the pelvis (uterus, fallopian tubes, bladder, colon, or rectum).
- **Stage III:** Cancer cells have spread to the lymph nodes and to other areas within the abdominal cavity.
- **Stage IV:** Cancer cells have moved outside the abdomen and pelvis to other organ systems such as the lungs.[171]

Risk Factors   The risk factors for ovarian cancer:

- A family or personal history of cancer, especially breast, uterine, colon, or rectal
- Genetic mutations—BRCA1 or BRCA2 gene
- Age greater than 55 years
- Infertility or never been pregnant
- Possibly the use of hormone replacement therapy, especially estrogen

Other potential risk factors include obesity and certain fertility drugs. However, it is not yet clear whether they are strong predictive risk factors. Currently there are "risk-reducing" actions that are being taken such as using oral contraceptives, tubal ligation (having the fallopian tubes "tied"), hysterectomy, having one or more children before age 30, breastfeeding.[172,173]

Screening and Diagnosis   Ovarian cancer, often called the "silent cancer," usually remains asymptomatic until it is relatively advanced. Unfortunately, it cannot be detected by Pap smears. Early detection is best accomplished though regular pelvic examinations, transvaginal ultrasound, and a laboratory test for an ovarian tumor marker in the blood, called CA-125. Elevated levels of CA-125 are associated with ovarian cancer but also may indicate other conditions.

Early symptoms of ovarian cancer include pelvic pressure, abdominal swelling, gas pains, indigestion, and vague abdominal discomfort. These symptoms are rarely attributable to ovarian cancer because they are also symptoms of other common benign conditions. Diagnosis of ovarian cancer is confirmed through ultrasound and/or biopsy.[174]

Treatment   Definitive treatment for ovarian cancer consists of surgery, radiation, hormone therapy, and chemotherapy. Surgical treatment involves removal of the uterus, fallopian tubes, and ovaries. If a woman wishes to have children and has a slow-growing tumor, the doctor may remove only the affected ovary. Chemotherapy and radiation therapy are used after surgery to destroy remaining cancer cells and improve survival.[174]

Other Cancers of Special Concern to Women

Women are susceptible to cancer anywhere in their bodies. The following section discusses the risk factors, screening guidelines, and treatment for the following cancers: lung cancer, colorectal cancer, and skin cancer.

Lung Cancer

Lung cancer is the leading cause of cancer death among White, Black, Asian/Pacific Islander, and American Indian/Alaska Native women and second among Hispanic women (see **Figure 10.26**).[175]

Lung cancer is almost twice as deadly as breast cancer, although breast cancer is twice as common in women. There were 232,670 estimated new cases of breast cancer compared to 108,210 new cases of lung cancer in 2014. However, overall deaths from lung cancer were 72,330 compared to 40,000 from breast cancer.[176,177] Although overall deaths from lung cancer have declined since the 1990s, they have remained relatively stable since then. New lung cancer cases and deaths in women vary considerably by state. Some of the lowest rates of new cases in women are in western states such as Utah, Wyoming, Colorado, North Dakota, Hawaii, and California, whereas some of the highest are in northeastern states such as Delaware, Maine, Massachusetts, and Vermont. The state with the highest new incidence rate is West Virginia.[178,179]

Most cases of lung cancer start in the lining of the bronchus, but the disease can originate anywhere in the lungs. Lung cancer develops over many years, and it often spreads before it can be detected radiographically. Causes of lung cancer vary, but most cases share a common factor—persistent exposure to lung irritants, particularly those that are inhaled, such as cigarette smoke.[179]

Risk Factors Although exposure to radon, asbestos, radioactive materials, and some industrial compounds has been associated with lung cancer, cigarette smoking is clearly the most significant risk factor. Cigarette smoking is responsible for 90% of lung cancer cases and 80% of lung cancer deaths.[180,181] What we do not yet know is the role of electronic cigarettes in the development of lung cancer. Studies are under way. However, the American Cancer Society referred to a study done by the FDA that cancer-causing substances were found in about half of the e-cigarettes tested.[182] The bottom line is that we simply do not know the extent of the danger in such devices. Wisdom strongly suggests that they be avoided.

A diagnosis of cancer usually reflects the cumulative effect of many years of smoking. Lung cancer in women appears to be different from lung cancer in men. Women who develop lung cancer typically have better survival rates than do men, possibly because women

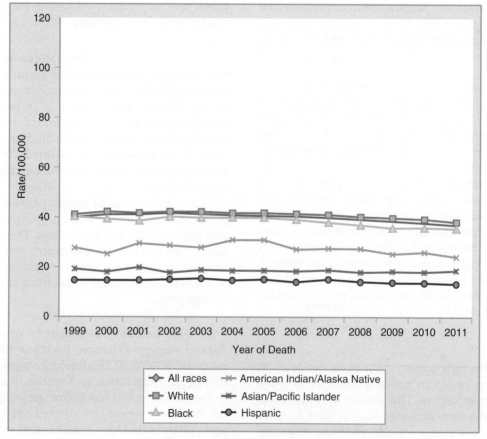

Figure 10.26   Lung and bronchus cancer death rates in women by racial/ethnic group, 1999–2011.

may metabolize chemicals in cigarettes differently than do men.[183]

Secondhand smoke is also a risk factor. An individual living with a smoker has a 20–30% greater risk of developing lung cancer. The CDC states that "exposure to secondhand smoke causes nearly 42,000 deaths each year among adults in the United States" from lung cancer and heart disease as a result of breathing secondhand smoke.[184] A family history of lung cancer may also increase a person's risk, although this increase may be associated with exposure to secondhand smoke from family members as opposed to a hereditary factor.

> *My mom died of lung cancer at the age of 50. She never smoked a day in her life. But my dad smoked, my uncle who lived with us smoked, all her friends smoked, and many of her coworkers smoked in her office before her workplace became smoke-free. It makes me so angry when I see people smoking. Don't they realize that they're not just killing themselves but they're also killing their family and friends?*
>
> **—32-year-old woman**

Workplace exposure to asbestos has been, especially in the past, a substantial risk for a specific type of lung cancer called mesothelioma. Today, with much more stringent workplace regulations, asbestos exposure is much less common. Most women have not been exposed to work-related asbestos commonly found in plants, mills, mines, and related workplaces. However, women may have been exposed via indirect means. This is especially true for women married to or living with men who work or have worked in such places. The exposure for women comes largely from the dust in the worker's clothing or workplace equipment brought home. Exposure to asbestos substantially increases a person's risk of developing lung cancer. Furthermore, workers exposed to asbestos and who smoke have a greatly increased risk of lung cancer.[185,186]

Other cancer-causing environmental agents exist such as radon, radioactive ores, minerals, and, potentially, air pollution.

Diagnosis Early detection of lung cancer is difficult because symptoms often do not appear until the disease has reached an advanced stage. A persistent cough may then present as the predominant symptom. Along with the cough, common symptoms of lung cancer include weight loss, bloody **sputum**, recurring bronchitis or pneumonia, chest pain, and/or voice changes. There are no specific screening techniques or guidelines for the early detection of lung cancer, but clinical studies are going forward to determine the best methods for early detection of the disease. Newer tests, such as low-dose helical CT scans and molecule markers in sputum, have the potential to detect early lung cancer. A person with symptoms may have a chest radiograph, sputum tests,

and fiber-optic examination of the bronchial passages for a more definitive diagnosis.[187] However, care must be taken in administering too many high-radiation tests because they, themselves, present a risk.

Treatment Lung cancer treatment usually includes one or more of the following: surgery, radiation, chemotherapy, and targeted therapy. Because most lung cancers are not diagnosed until they are in advanced stages, however, treatment options are often limited. In the early stages of lung cancer, surgery is generally employed. Treatment typically includes surgical removal of the affected regions. A **segmentectomy** removes a section of a lobe of the lung. A **lobectomy** removes a lobe of the lung. A **pneumonectomy** removes the entire lung. Depending on the stage of the lung cancer, different additional therapies may be added such as radiation, chemotherapy, and targeted therapy.[188]

Colorectal Cancer

Colorectal cancer is the third most common cancer in women and men. In 2014, the estimated number of colon cancer cases was 96,830 and 40,000 of rectal cancer.[189] This disease develops in a gradual, progressive manner and may present anywhere in the colon and rectal area (see **Figure 10.27**). Cancers affecting different areas of this anatomical region present with different symptoms. The stages of colorectal cancer are:

- **Stage 0** (carcinoma-in-situ): Cancer is found in the lining of the colon or rectum.
- **Stage I:** Cancer has moved from the lining of the colon to the muscles.
- **Stage II:** Cancer has spread through the muscle layers into the serosa (outer layers of the colon wall).
- **Stage III:** Cancer has spread through the muscle wall and into the lymph nodes.
- **Stage IV:** Cancer has spread, via the blood and lymph nodes, to other organ systems such as the ovaries, abdominal wall, liver, or lungs.[170]

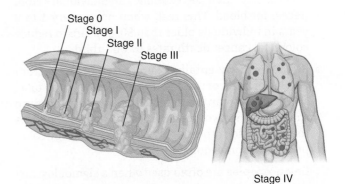

Stage 0
Stage I
Stage II
Stage III
Stage IV

Figure 10.27   Colon cancer stages.

By far, the most common colon cancer is **adenocarcinoma**, which begins in the glandular structure lining the colon. This is a slow-growing cancer and it may not manifest symptoms for years.[189]

Risk Factors   Increasing age is the primary risk factor for colorectal cancer. Ninety percent of people with colorectal cancer are older than 50 years of age. The risk of developing colon and rectal cancers is about twice as high for individuals with an immediate family member who has had colorectal cancer or certain conditions such as **familial adenomatous polyposis (FAP)**. FAP is characterized by the presence of hundreds of polyps in the colon and rectum.[189,190]

Likewise, a history of inflammatory bowel disease is associated with a high risk of developing colon cancer. An individual who has developed a polyp or carcinoma in the past is also at increased risk of developing a second carcinoma.

Dietary factors are important determinants of colon and rectal cancer risk. An increased incidence of these cancers is associated with diets that are high in fat and low in fiber and other components of fruits and vegetables. In particular, the most definitive dietary risk for colorectal cancer is a high-fat diet.[189]

Screening and Diagnosis   In its early stages, colorectal cancer usually presents no symptoms. Warning signs for advanced colorectal cancer include rectal bleeding, blood in the stool, a change in bowel habits, and cramping in the lower abdomen. Similar to other forms of cancer, early detection greatly improves the likelihood of recovery. Approaches to the detection of colorectal cancer include fecal occult blood test, sigmoidoscopy, colonoscopy, and double contrast barium enema.[190] In addition, clinical studies continue to investigate new and more efficient methods to screen for the disease.[191]

- **Digital rectal examination** is a simple part of a routine physical examination. However, it is relatively insensitive as a screening test because very few colorectal lesions develop within range of the examining finger.

- **Fecal occult blood test** examines an individual's stool (feces) for blood. This test, when done every 1 to 2 years in individuals older than 50, appears to reduce colorectal cancer death rates by one-third.

- **Sigmoidoscopy** entails examination of the rectum and lower parts of the colon with a thin, lighted tube. More tumors can be detected with this procedure than with the two previous tests. This test requires that the patient thoroughly cleanse her lower colon prior to the procedure.

- **Colonoscopies** are often used when a sigmoidoscopy detects a polyp or abnormality or a person is at high risk for colorectal cancer. Whereas signoidoscopies screen only the rectum and lower portion of the colon, a colonoscopy examines the entire colon. If a healthcare provider detects an abnormality, he or she can use the colonoscope to remove all or part of the polyp or inflamed tissue by passing tiny instruments through the scope. Medicines, lasers, and heat probes can be passed through the scope to stop bleeding.

- **Double contrast barium enema** requires that the individual have an enema with barium solution followed by X-rays. The pictures from these X-rays provide an outline of both the rectum and the colon. This procedure, although useful, may not discover small polyps.[192,193]

> *I am a 65-year-old woman who for years was terrified of getting a colorectal screening. I went for mammograms, monitored my blood pressure and cholesterol, and exercised regularly. But the thought of a colorectal exam seemed so uncomfortable and painful. When my daughter showed me the statistics, I realized that I needed to take care of myself. Now, both my husband and I have gone for screening and it's so good to know we're healthy.*
>
> **—65-year-old grandmother of two**

Treatment   Treatment depends on several factors: the stage of the cancer, whether this is a first-time discovery or recurrence, and the patient's health. In general, there are four standard treatment options: surgery, chemotherapy, radiation therapy, or targeted therapy.

- Surgery can be done in several ways.
    - An incision into the abdomen to remove the tumor
    - Removal of the diseased part of colon and then sewing the healthy parts of the colon back together
    - Removal of the diseased portion of the colon and, if unable to connect the healthy parts back together, then creating a *stoma* (an opening) to the outside of the abdomen. A bag is attached to the stoma to collect the fecal matter that is produced.

- Targeted therapy: radiofrequency ablation (a special probe using electrodes that can destroy cancer cells) or cryosurgery (a method that freezes the cancerous tissue).

- **Chemotherapy** employs anticancer medications that destroy the tumor.

- **Radiation therapy** uses powerful "high-energy" X-rays to destroy the cells.[194]

The death rates from colorectal cancer have declined during the past several decades. While rates are declining among most female racial and ethnic groups, the highest death rates are among African American women (see **Figure 10.28**).

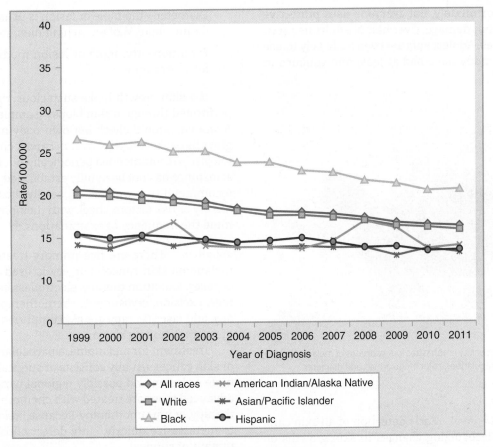

Figure 10.28   **Colorectal death rates among women by race/ethnicity, 1999–2011.**

Unfortunately, the decline is not even across the United States. Death rates are highest in the District of Columbia and the following states: Alabama, Alaska, Arkansas, Illinois, Kentucky, Nebraska, Nevada, New Jersey, and West Virginia.[195]

Skin Cancer

Cancer of the skin, the most common of all cancers, comes in a number of different forms.

- *Melanoma:* The **melanocyte** cells in the skin, which are responsible for making pigment (coloring), can form a cancer known as melanoma. Although it can occur on any skin area, it is usually found between the shoulders and hips. However, some sex differences are noted. Men tend to develop melanomas on the head, while women often develop them on their legs. This skin cancer is unusual in individuals with dark skin, but it can occur on the soles of their feet or palms of their hands. Occupational exposure to coal tar, pitch, creosote, arsenic compounds, or radium is also a risk factor.

- *Basal cell carcinoma:* This cancer is formed in the outer layer of the skin (epidermis). This is the most common cancer in individuals who are fair-skinned. The skin sites most vulnerable are those most exposed to the sun.

- *Squamous cell carcinoma:* This cancer is formed on the skin surface in the squamous cells. In individuals who have darker skin, this tends to be the most common skin cancer. The most common sites are the feet and legs—areas less commonly exposed to the sun.[196]

Risk Factors   A major risk factor is ultraviolet radiation from sunlight. Lifetime exposure, severe sunburn, and tanning each enhance the risk. People with lighter skin are especially vulnerable because darker skin appears to provide some protection from the negative effects of the sun's rays. In addition, an individual's family history of skin cancer can play a role.

The presence of benign growths, such as moles, is not generally dangerous. Although they are benign, certain types of moles, such as dysplastic nevi, can increase a person's risk. **Dysplastic nevi** is the term for irregular moles (nevi is the medical term for moles), and this condition often runs in families. Moles are considered irregular when they have an uneven border or color. A family history of melanoma is another important risk factor. Individuals with a first-degree relative who has had melanoma are eight times more likely to develop a melanoma themselves.[197]

Preventive measures for skin cancer include limiting or avoiding sun exposure during midday hours (10 a.m. to 4 p.m.), using sunblock with a sun protective factor (SPF) of 15 or greater, and avoiding tanning beds and sun lamps. Unfortunately, not everyone uses protective factors against sun damage. Over half of adults use sun-protective devices. Adolescents are even less likely to use protection and many have had at least one sunburn in the past year.[198]

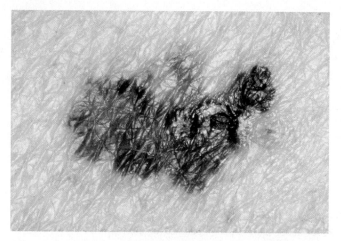

The American Cancer Society emphasizes four warnings of melanoma: asymmetry, border irregularities, color irregularities, and diameter.
Courtesy of National Cancer Institute

Screening and Diagnosis   Early detection of all skin cancers is critical. Recognizing changes in skin growths or the appearance of new growths is the best way to find skin cancer.

Screening is best accomplished by skin examination. Basal cell carcinomas often appear as flat, scaly red areas or a small, raised translucent area. Squamous cell carcinomas are growing lumps or flat reddish patches. Melanomas may develop within a mole or as a new mole-like growth. They are characterized by increasing size and changes in color. The Skin Cancer Foundation emphasizes five warning signs of melanoma (the ABCDE system).[199]

- Asymmetry—the shape of one-half of a lesion or mole is different from the other.

- Border irregularities—the edge may be uneven, ragged, or blotched.

- Color irregularities—different colors (tan, brown, black, red, blue, or sometimes white) may be present in the mole or lesion.

- Diameter—the mole or lesion is usually greater than 6 mm (about ¼ of an inch) in diameter.

- Evolution—the mole or lesion modifies its appearance over time.

If a skin growth looks suspicious, diagnosis will be performed through a skin biopsy (sample of the growth). A woman should check her own body monthly for new growths or skin changes. A skin cancer check by a dermatologist is recommended periodically, but the frequency of screenings has not been fully established. Dermatologists recommend that women, especially those with a family history or risk factors, check with their physician to determine the frequency of examinations.[200]

Treatment   There are five primary treatments for non-melanoma skin cancer. Surgery is used in the majority of cases. Radiation therapy, electrodessication and curettage, excision, cryosurgery, chemotherapy, biologic therapy, and laser therapy are also employed for early forms of nonmelanoma skin cancer.[201,202]

Treatment for melanoma, a particularly virulent form of skin cancer, usually consists of surgical removal of the mole or lesion and possibly regional lymph nodes. More advanced cases are treated with chemotherapy, radiation therapy, or immunotherapy. Because melanomas are able to metastasize quickly, early detection is a major determinant of survival.

INFORMED DECISION MAKING

Women can reduce their risk of cardiovascular disease and cancer in several ways. For most women, prevention and taking good care of their daily and long-term health are critical actions. The old adage "An ounce of prevention is worth a pound of cure" is still correct. It is much more effective to reduce your risk of suffering a life-threatening or disabling heart attack at 55 by never smoking, eating a prudent diet, and exercising—all behaviors that should begin in childhood. Although it is better to begin these lifesaving behaviors in childhood, changing as one ages can still reduce one's risk.

Prevention Through Lifestyle

Lifestyle is a critical part of maintaining a woman's health. Such efforts also help to minimize problems when a woman is affected by disease. Prevention and health enhancement include quitting smoking (or never starting), limiting alcohol intake, avoiding illegal and dangerous substances, practicing safe sex, being physically active, using sunblock and proper covering when in the sun, maintaining an appropriate weight, and eating a healthy diet. Enjoying life and maintaining a positive mental outlook are also important factors. These activities should be taught in childhood, adopted at the

I had so many sunburns as a child. My mom has had basal cells removed from her face and my grandfather had melanoma, so I know I'm at high risk for skin cancer. I get checked regularly by a dermatologist, but so far, the moles that she has removed from my back have been normal. I finally understand how important it is to protect myself from the sun.

—30-year-old fair-skinned woman

appropriate ages, and maintained throughout life. Each woman should work with her healthcare provider and have regular checkups and address any issues that might arise.

Prevention Through Health Screening

Cardiovascular disease prevention involves getting screened and knowing one's family history of heart disease and stroke. When a woman visits her doctor, she should be ready to discuss her health and health concerns and to present her lifestyle habits: smoking, alcohol, dietary status, sexual activity, and any other issues that might affect her health. Her blood pressure, height, and weight should be measured. In addition, she should have regular blood tests to check for heart disease and risk factors: blood cholesterol, triglycerides, and fasting blood glucose.

Mammography is the best way to detect breast cancer in its earliest and most treatable stage—an average of 1.7 years before a woman can feel a lump. Clinical breast exams and monthly breast self-examinations are recommended for women younger than age 40 and should supplement mammograms for women older than age 40. Any breast lumps, skin changes such as flaking or crusting, weeping eruptions around the nipple, discharge from the nipple, or dimpling or retraction of the skin should be evaluated by a physician.

Pap smears and HPV testing are screening methods that can greatly reduce invasive cervical cancer morbidity and mortality. Because cervical cancer is a slow-growing disease, screening programs starting at age 21 dramatically decrease the risk of developing advanced disease. In fact, when cervical cancer is detected at its earliest stage, the 5-year survival rate is more than 90%. Pelvic exams are also essential for women to detect any abnormal changes of the reproductive system.

Self-examination of one's skin enables a woman to detect early forms of skin cancer. Women should become familiar with their bodies to be able to recognize any of the warning signs of cancer.

I had a lump in my breast, and it had been there for some time. It didn't hurt. I guess that I was hoping it was nothing and would go away. I waited too long. This has been a rough year, but I am trying to tell other women not to make the same mistake. If you feel a lump, regardless of the size, have it checked right away.

—**42-year-old woman**

It's Your Health

Quitting Tobacco

The positive effects of quitting begin very soon after you stop using tobacco and continue long after you have quit.

Short-Term Benefits

- Your blood pressure, pulse, and body temperature, which were abnormally elevated by nicotine, return to normal. Persons taking blood pressure medication should continue doing so until told otherwise by their physician.

- Your body starts to heal itself. Carbon monoxide and oxygen levels in your blood return to normal.

- Your chance of having a heart attack goes down.

- Nerve endings start to regrow. Your ability to taste and smell improves.

- Your breathing passages (bronchial tubes) relax, lung capacity goes up, and your breathing becomes easier.

- Your circulation improves.

- Your lungs become stronger, making it easier to walk.

- In your lungs, the cilia (hair-like structures on the lining) begin to regrow, increasing the ability of your lungs to handle mucus, to clean themselves, and to reduce infection.

- Coughing, sinus congestion, fatigue, and shortness of breath decrease. Your overall energy level increases.

Long-Term Benefits

- As a former smoker, your chance of dying from lung cancer is less than it would be if you continued to smoke. Your chance of getting cancer of the throat, bladder, kidney, or pancreas also decreases.

Source: National Cancer Institute, U.S. National Institutes of Health. Available at: http://www.cancer.gov/cancertopics/factsheet/Tobacco/quitting-benefits

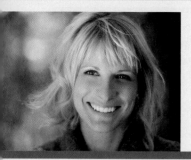
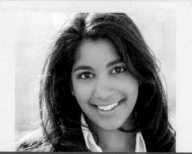
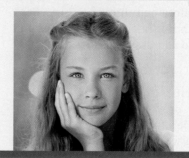
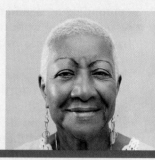

CASE STUDY

Imagine that you are an English teacher in a high school in a very diverse community in an American city. The community residents have emigrated from many different countries and have come to the United States to achieve a better life. Many of the residents have limited incomes and work in low-level jobs. In addition, they often have difficulty with the English language. Yet, many firmly believe that their children should advance and, thus, they make certain that the children attend school.

One thing that you, the teacher, have noticed is that the knowledge of health promotion and disease prevention is limited. You have decided that you may be able to help them, and possibly their families, by providing some health education opportunities both in the classroom and in special after-school meetings.

You decide to develop a health education plan that can be tested initially with a small group of students and then expanded as you see what works. Because you are a female teacher, you decide that you will focus initially on female students in the ninth and tenth grades. Having discussed the project with some of the students, you decide, based on their recommendations, to focus on cardiovascular and cancer risk factors: smoking, overweight, and exercise in an after-school program.

If you were the teacher, how would you proceed?

Questions

1. How would you design the after-school program: lectures, discussions, presentations by local advocates, and ... ?

2. How would you market the program to the ninth- and tenth-grade girls?

3. What materials would you design to engage them in learning about the health risks?

4. Would you serve snacks?

Please develop an action plan for a 6-month period of time. Make certain to state your goal and objectives, the plan for implementing the action, and how you will evaluate the results of the plan.

■ Summary

Together, cardiovascular disease and cancer represent the greatest risks to women's health. The underpinnings of disease causality and progression have been shown to be a complex interrelationship among an individual's family history, environment, lifestyle, and comorbid conditions. Though family history is not the only risk factor, women with genetic predispositions to cardiovascular disease and certain types of cancers are at an increased risk for developing disease. Recognizing that these diseases affect women of all ages should be an incentive for women to begin making lifestyle changes in diet, physical activity, tobacco use, and health screening as early as possible.

Jacqueline Dunbar-Jacob, PhD, RN, FAAN

Jacqueline Dunbar-Jacob is distinguished service professor and dean of the School of Nursing at the University of Pittsburgh and professor of psychology, epidemiology, and occupational therapy. She has been the dean of the School of Nursing since 2001.

Dunbar-Jacob received her Bachelor of Science degree in nursing from Florida State University, her Master of Science in psychiatric nursing with a postmaster certificate in child psychiatric nursing at the University of California, San Francisco, and her PhD in counseling psychology, focusing on health psychology, at Stanford University. She is both a registered nurse and a licensed psychologist.

She has worked as a staff nurse, unit manager, and nursing director and has taught nursing at both undergraduate and graduate levels.

Dunbar-Jacob has been actively funded by the NIH for the past 25 years for studies on patient adherence, including a PO1 designed to examine factors relevant to the translation of interventions to clinical settings. She has served as a behavioral scientist in key multicenter clinical trials and as an NIH data and safety monitoring board member for three multicenter trials. She has written over 130 papers and chapters, primarily focusing on patient adherence. She has received research awards from the University of Pittsburgh, Pennsylvania Nightingala, and Sigma Theta Tau International Honor Society.

Dunbar-Jacob has been the president and fellow of the Society for Behavioral Medicine and the Academy of Behavioral Medicine Research, as well as president of the Friends of the National Institute for Nursing Research and a fellow of the American Academy of Nursing, the American Psychological Association, and the American Heart Association. She is a former Robert Wood Johnson Executive Nurse Fellow. In 2015, she was named as one of the 30 most influential nursing deans.

Nanette K. Wenger, MD, MACC, MACP, FAHA (1930–)

Nanette K. Wenger is professor of medicine in the Division of Cardiology at the Emory University School of Medicine. She is a consultant to the Emory Heart and Vascular Center.

Coronary heart disease in women is one of Wenger's major clinical and research interests. She chaired the U.S. National Heart, Lung, and Blood Institute Conference on Cardiovascular Health and Disease in Women. Wenger has expertise in cardiac rehabilitation. She chaired the World Health Organization Expert Committee on Rehabilitation after Cardiovascular Disease, and co-chaired the Guideline Panel on Cardiac Rehabilitation for the U.S. Agency for Health Care Policy and Research. Wenger has had a longstanding interest in geriatric cardiology, is a past president of the Society of Geriatric Cardiology, and was editor-in-chief of the *American Journal of Geriatric Cardiology* for more than 15 years.

Wenger received the Outstanding Professional Achievement Award from Hunter College (1993) and the Physician of the Year Award of the American Heart Association (1998). In 1999, Wenger received the Distinguished Achievement Award from the Scientific Councils of the American Heart Association and its Women in Cardiology Mentoring Award. She was chosen by Atlanta Women in Law and Medicine for a Shining Star Award, recognizing her distinguished career in cardiology and women's health issues.

In 2000, Wenger was presented the James D. Bruce Memorial Award of the American College of Physicians for distinguished contributions in preventive medicine. In 2002 she received the Distinguished Fellow Award of the Society of Geriatric Cardiology. In 2003, she was included in the National Library of Medicine Exhibition Changing the Face of Medicine: A History of American Women Physicians. Wenger received the Gold Heart Award, the highest award of the American Heart Association (2004).

At the Emory University 2004 commencement, Wenger received the Emory Williams Distinguished Teaching Award of the University and the Evangeline Papageorge Alumni Teaching Award of the Emory University School of Medicine. Wenger was selected to deliver the 2004 Laennec Lecture of the American Heart Association. In 2006, Wenger received the Hatter Award, international recognition for the advancement of cardiovascular science. The Georgia Chapter of the American College of Cardiology presented Wenger its Lifetime Achievement Award in 2009. She was selected Georgia Woman of the Year for 2010. In 2011, Wenger was selected to deliver the James B. Herrick lecture by the American Heart Association for her outstanding achievement in clinical cardiology. She was elected a member of Emory's 175 history makers during Emory's first 175 years.

In 2012, Wenger received the Charles R. Hatcher, Jr., MD, Award for Excellence in Public Health from Emory University and was honored in 2013 by the establishment of the J. Willis Hurst, R. Bruce Logue, and Nanette K. Wenger Cardiovascular Society for Emory Cardiology Trainee Alumni. In 2013, she received the Inaugural Distinguished Mentor Award of the American College of Cardiology and the Arnall Patz Lifetime Achievement Award of the Emory University School of Medicine Medical Alumni Association. The American Society of Preventive Cardiology honored Wenger by naming an annual Nanette K. Wenger Distinguished Lecture focusing on cardiovascular prevention in women (2014).

In 2015, she was awarded the Inaugural Bernadine Healy Leadership in Women's CV Disease Award, American College of Cardiology.

Wenger has participated as an author of several American College of Cardiology/American Heart Association Clinical Practice Guidelines. She is past chair, board of directors, of the Society for Women's Health Research. Wenger serves on the editorial boards of numerous professional journals and is a sought-after lecturer for issues related to heart disease in women, heart disease in the elderly, cardiac rehabilitation, coronary prevention, and contemporary cardiac care. She is listed in *Best Doctors in America*.

Wenger has authored or coauthored over 1500 scientific and review articles and book chapters.

Profiles of Remarkable Women

Vivian W. Pinn, MD

Vivian W. Pinn was the first full-time director of the Office of Research on Women's Health (ORWH) at the National Institutes of Health (NIH), an appointment she held from 1991 until her retirement in August 2011, and was also NIH associate director for research on women's health since 1994. Pinn came to NIH from Howard University College of Medicine in Washington, DC, where she had been professor and chair of the Department of Pathology since 1982. She has been invited to present the ORWH's programs and initiatives to many national and international organizations with an interest in improving women's health and the health of minorities. The ORWH was established by Congress to ensure the inclusion of women (and minorities) in clinical research funded by the NIH; Pinn led NIH efforts to implement and monitor these inclusion policies. Another of her efforts was to raise the perception of the scientific community about the importance of sex differences in research and health care. Until her retirement, Pinn helped establish and cochaired with the director of NIH the NIH Working Group on Women in Biomedical Careers, which developed and implemented programs and policies to improve the advancement of women in biomedical careers. Since her retirement, Pinn has been named as a senior scientist emerita at the NIH Fogarty International Center.

Pinn earned her BA from Wellesley College in Massachusetts and received her MD from the University of Virginia School of Medicine in 1967, where she was the only woman and only minority in her class. She completed her postgraduate training in pathology at the Massachusetts General Hospital, during which time she also served as teaching fellow at Harvard Medical School. She was associate professor of pathology and assistant dean of student affairs at Tufts University School of Medicine before leaving to join the faculty at Howard, when she became the third woman and first African American woman in the United States to chair an academic department of pathology. She is a member of long standing in many professional and scientific organizations in which she has held many positions of leadership, including being the second woman president of the National Medical Association in 1989. Pinn has more than 200 publications in scientific journals and chapters related to renal diseases, minorities in medicine, women's health research and related career issues, in addition to other posters and abstracts.

Pinn serves as an IOM (National Academy of Medicine) representative on the Committee on Women in Science, Engineering, and Medicine of the National Research Council of the National Academies. She has received numerous honors, awards, and recognitions and has been granted 13 Honorary Degrees of Laws and Science since 1992. She is a fellow of the American Academy of Arts and Sciences and was elected to the Institute of Medicine (now the National Academy of Medicine) in 1995. Among her honors is the 1993 Alumni Achievement Award from Wellesley College, where she formerly served on the Wellesley College Board of Trustees. She also received the second annual Distinguished Alumna Award from the University of Virginia, was honored by the UVA medical school as one of their Alumni Luminaries, and was invited to serve as the 2005 speaker for the University of Virginia commencement, the first African American woman to be so honored. The UVA School of Medicine further honored her in the fall of 2010 by establishing one of its four advisory colleges for medical students in her name, the "Vivian Pinn College of UVA." In May 2011 she was presented with the distinguished Tufts University School of Medicine Dean's Medal, conferred only rarely to individuals whose service to the school and career in medicine have enhanced the university's national standing. Tufts University also established the Vivian W. Pinn Office of Student Affairs in her honor, and her former students and the medical school also honored her by the establishment of a scholarship fund in her name to assist disadvantaged students. Pinn has since been appointed to the Board of Advisors of Tufts University School of Medicine.

Pinn was elected as an honorary fellow of the New York Academy of Medicine and received the (NY) Academy Medal for Distinguished Contributions in Health Policy. She was also elected as the first ever honorary member of the North American Menopause Society in 2011. A special tribute by Senator Olympia Snowe, "The Retirement of Dr. Vivian Pinn," was published in the Congressional Record in November 2011 commending her contributions during her tenure at the NIH. The Association of American Medical Colleges awarded her a Special Recognition Award for exceptional leadership in promoting the health of women and minorities over a 40-year career. She was awarded the first Bernadine Healy Award for Visionary Leadership in Women's Health by the Women's Health Congress in 2012. Pinn was elected as chairperson of the NMA Past Presidents Council at the 2012 Annual NMA Convention and a Member of the Inaugural Class of the W. Montague Cobb/NMA Health Institute Senior Fellows. The national organization of The Links, Incorporated, awarded her its prestigious Co-Founder's Award for her contributions to the nation in health and human services at its 2012 Annual Assembly. And the National Organization for Women presented her the third annual Victoria J. Mastrobuono Women's Health Award at its 2012 national conference. In 2013, she received the Founder Award from National Medical Fellowships and the Foremother Award from the National Research Center for Women and Families. Pinn was also a 2014 Honoree of the Howard University College of Medicine as a Magnificent Professor and was featured on the DC Lottery 2014 Black History Month Poster, "African Americans in Medicine," which celebrated pioneers in medicine and was distributed to public libraries, schools, and the general public in the Washington, DC, area. Her oral history is included in the National Library of Medicine's exhibit on women physicians: "Changing the Face of Medicine," the University of Virginia's project, "Explorations in Black Leadership" conducted by Julian Bond, and in the HistoryMakers collection, which is now housed in the Library of Congress.

■ Topics for Discussion

1. What factors influence women of different ages and cultures to adopt healthier lifestyles and engage in preventive action to reduce their risks of cardiovascular disease and cancer? Discuss factors for different age groups beginning with the teen years.

2. How can women increase their awareness of cardiovascular and cancer threats? Discuss for different cultures and age groups beginning with the teen years.

3. What can public health agencies and community organizations do to increase women's awareness of cardiovascular and cancer risk factors?

4. Substantial differences exist in the incidence and prevalence of cancer and cardiovascular diseases across racial and ethnic groups. Discuss which factors influence these differences and why.

5. How can academic institutions take a more active role in disease prevention for young women?

■ Key Terms

Acute coronary syndrome

Adenocarcinoma

Adjuvant therapies

Aneurysm

Angina pectoris

Aorta

Aortic valve

Arrhythmia

Arteries

Arterioles

Arteriosclerosis

Atherosclerosis

Atrial fibrillation

Balloon angioplasty

Benign tumor

Bicuspid valve

Biopsy

Blood

Breast self-examination

C-reactive protein

Cancer

Capillaries

Carcinogenesis

Carcinogens

Carcinoma

Carcinoma-in-situ

Cardiovascular disease

Cardiovascular system

Cerebrovascular accident

Cervical dysplasia

Cervicitis

Chemotherapy

Clinical breast examination

Colonoscopy

Colposcope

Colposcopy

Congenital heart disease

Congestive heart failure (CHF)

Conization

Coronary artery bypass graft (CABG) surgery

Cryosurgery

Cysts

Diastolic

Digital rectal examination

Double contrast barium enema

Dysplasia

Dysplastic nevi

Electrocardiograph (ECG)

Embolism

Embolus

Endometriosis

Endometrium

Environmental tobacco smoke (ETS)

Erythrocytes

Familial adenomatous polyposis (FAP)

Fecal occult blood test

Fibroadenoma

Fibroids

Heart attack

Hemoglobin

Hemorrhagic stroke

Homocysteine

Hyperplasia

Hypertension

Hysteroscopy

Inferior vena cava

Ischemic stroke

Laparoscopy

Left atrium

Left ventricle

Leukocytes

Lipoprotein

Lobectomy

Lumpectomy

Magnetic resonance imaging (MRI)

Malignant neoplasm

Malignant tumor

Mammography

Melanocyte

Metabolic syndrome

Metastasis

Mitral valve

Modified radical mastectomy

Myocardial infarction

Myomectomy

Neoplasm

Pap smear

Patent ductus arteriosus

Peripheral artery disease (PAD)

Plaques

Platelets

Pneumonectomy

Polycystic ovarian syndrome

Polyps

Pulmonary arteries

Pulmonary stenosis

Pulmonary veins

Radiation therapy

Radical mastectomy

Red blood cells

Rheumatic heart disease

Right atrium

Right ventricle

Segmentectomy

Septum

Sigmoidoscopy

Simple mastectomy

Sphygmomanometer

Sputum

Statins

Stent

Sternum

Stroke

Superior vena cava

Systolic

Thrombocytes

Thrombus

Transvaginal ultrasound

Tricuspid valve

Triglycerides

Tumor

Vasocontrictors

Ventricular fibrillation

Venules

Very-low-density lipoprotein

White blood cells

■ References

1. Centers for Disease Control and Prevention (CDC). *Heart disease facts.* Available at: http://www.cdc.gov/heartdisease/facts.htm

2. CDC. *Women and heart disease fact sheet.* Available at: http://www.cdc.gov/dhdsp/data_statistics/fact_sheets/fs_women_heart.htm

3. CDC. *Health, United States, 2013.* Table 26: Death rates for diseases of the heart by sex, race, Hispanic origin and age. Available at: http://www.cdc.gov/nchs/data/hus/hus13.pdf

4. Million Hearts. *About heart disease and stroke.* Available at: http://millionhearts.hhs.gov/abouthds/cost-consequences.html

5. Ibid.

6. Women's Heart Foundation. *Women and heart disease facts.* Available at: http://www.womensheart.org/content/heartdisease/heart_disease_facts.asp

7. American Heart Association. *Women have a higher risk of stroke.* Available at: http://www.strokeassociation.org/STROKEORG/AboutStroke/UnderstandingRisk/Women-Have-a-Higher-Risk-of-Stroke—Text-Version_UCM_460399_Article.jsp

8. CDC. *Health, United States, 2013.* Table 27: Death rates for cerebrovascular disease by sex, race, Hispanic origin, and age, p. 110. Available at: http://www.cdc.gov/nchs/data/hus/hus13.pdf

9. CDC. *Health, United States, 2013.* Table 27: Death rates for cerebrovascular disease by sex, race, Hispanic origin, and age, pp. 111–112. http://www.cdc.gov/nchs/data/hus/hus13.pdf

10. Mozaffarian, D., et al. (2015). Heart disease and stroke statistics—2015 update. *Circulation* 131: e29–322. Available at: https://circ.ahajournals.org/content/early/2014/12/18/CIR.0000000000000152

11. World Heart Federation. *Cardiovascular disease in women.* Available at: http://www.world-heart-federation.org/fileadmin/user_upload/documents/Fact_sheets/2012/CVD_women.pdf

12. ProCon.org. *Obesity pros and cons.* Available at: http://obesity.procon.org/view.resource.php?resourceID=004371

13. Sreeramareddy, C. T., Pradhan, P. M. S., Mir I. A., et al. (2014). *Smoking and smokeless tobacco use in nine South and Southeast Asian countries: Prevalence estimates and social determinants from demographic and health surveys, population health metrics.* Published online August 28, 2014. DOI: 10.1186/s12963-014-0022-0

14. American Lung Association. *Lung cancer fact sheet.* Available at: http://www.lung.org/lung-disease/lung-cancer/resources/facts-figures/lung-cancer-fact-sheet.html

15. CDC. *Health, United States, 2014.* Table 53: Current cigarette smoking among adults aged 18 ad over by sex, race, and age: United States, selected years 1990–2013. Available at: http://www.cdc.gov/nchs/data/hus/hus14.pdf

16. American Heart Association (AHA). (2015). *How the healthy heart works.* Available at: http://www.heart.org/HEARTORG/Conditions/CongenitalHeartDefects/AboutCongenitalHeartDefects/How-the-Healthy-Heart-Works_UCM_307016_Article.jsp

17. AHA. (2015). *Anatomy of the heart and lungs.* Available at: http://watchlearnlive.heart.org/CVML_Player.php?moduleSelect=bldflo

18. National Heart, Lung, and Blood Institute (NHLBI). (2015). *What is an electrocardiogram?* Available at: http://www.nhlbi.nih.gov /health/health-topics/topics/ekg

19. NHLBI. (2015). *Types of blood tests.* Available at: http://www.nhlbi .nih.gov/health/health-topics/topics/bdt/types

20. NHLBI. (2015). *What is Atrial Fibrillation?* Available at: http://www .nhlbi.nih.gov/health/health-topics/topics/af

21. NHLBI. *What is coronary heart disease?* Available at: http://www .nhlbi.nih.gov/health/health-topics/topics/cad

22. NHLBI. *How is coronary heart disease treated?* Available at: http:// www.nhlbi.nih.gov/health/health-topics/topics/cad/treatment

23. AHA. *Acute coronary syndrome.* Available at: http://www.heart .org/HEARTORG/Conditions/HeartAttack/AboutHeartAttacks /Acute-Coronary-Syndrome_UCM_428752_Article.jsp

24. AHA. *Heart attack symptoms in women.* Available at: http:// www.heart.org/HEARTORG/Conditions/HeartAttack/Warning SignsofaHeartAttack/Heart-Attack-Symptoms-in-Women _UCM_436448_Article.jsp

25. Cleveland Clinic. *Heart failure in women.* Available at: http:// my.clevelandclinic.org/services/heart/disorders/heart-failure -what-is/heart-failure-women

26. Medline Plus. *Congenital heart disease.* Available at: http://www .nlm.nih.gov/medlineplus/ency/article/001114.htm

27. CDC. *Congenital heart defects (CHDs): Data and statistics.* Available at: http://www.cdc.gov/ncbddd/heartdefects/data.html

28. NHLBI. *Ten leading causes of infant mortality.* Available at: http:// www.nhlbi.nih.gov/about/documents/factbook/2012/chapter4

29. AHA. *Congenital cardiovascular defects, statistical fact sheet, 2014 update.* Available at: http://www.sciencedaily.com /releases/2010/11/101122172131.htm

30. Medscape. *Pathology of rheumatic heart disease.* Available at: http://emedicine.medscape.com/article/1962779-overview

31. AHA. *Angina pectoris (stable angina).* Available at: http://www .heart.org/HEARTORG/Conditions/HeartAttack/Symptoms DiagnosisofHeartAttack/Angina-Pectoris-Stable-Angina _UCM_437515_Article.jsp

32. AHA. (2015). *About peripheral artery disease (PAD).* Available at: http://www.heart.org/HEARTORG/Conditions/More /PeripheralArteryDisease/About-Peripheral-Artery-Disease -PAD_UCM_301301_Article.jsp

33. PubMed Heath. (2015). *Metabolic syndrome.* Available at: http:// www.ncbi.nlm.nih.gov/pubmedhealth/PMHT0024493/

34. Kaur, J. (2014). *A comprehensive review on metabolic syndrome, cardiology research and practice.* Available at: http://www.hindawi .com/journals/crp/2014/943162/

35. Fruge, A. D., Byrd, S. H., Fountain, B. J., et al. (2014). Race and gender disparities in nutrient intake are not related to metabolic syndrome in 20–59 year old US adults. *Metabolic Syndrome Related Disorders* 12(8): 430–436.

36. Beltran-Sanchez, H., Harhay, M. O., Harhay, M., et al. (2013). Prevalence and trends of metabolic syndrome in the adult US population, 1999–2010. *Journal of the American College of Cardiology* 62(8): 697–703. Available at: http://content.onlinejacc.org/article .aspx?articleid=1709463

37. MedlinePlus. *Stroke.* Available at: http://www.nlm.nih.gov /medlineplus/ency/article/000726.htm

38. NHLBI. *What is a stroke?* Available at: http://www.nhlbi.nih.gov /health/health-topics/topics/stroke

39. Stroke Awareness Foundation. *What is the standard treatment for stroke?* Available at: http://strokeinfo.org/signsandsymptoms /stroke-facts/treatment-for-stroke

40. Healthline. *Symptoms of stroke in women.* Available at: http://www .healthline.com/health-slideshow/stroke-symptoms-women#8

41. NHLBI. *How is stroke treated?* Available at: http://www.nhlbi.nih .gov/health/health-topics/topics/stroke/treatment

42. National Institute of Neurological Disorders and Stroke. *Poststroke rehabilitation fact sheet.* Available at: http://www.ninds.nih .gov/disorders/stroke/poststrokerehab.htm

43. AHA. *Cognitive challenges after stroke.* Available at: http://www .strokeassociation.org/STROKEORG/LifeAfterStroke/Regaining Independence/EmotionalBehavioralChallenges/Cognitive -Challenges-After-Stroke_UCM_309904_Article.jsp

44. Women's Health. *I Had a Mini-Stroke at 24.* Available at: http:// www.womenshealthmag.com/health/mini-stroke

45. CDC. (2013). *Health, United States, 2013.* Table 27: Death rates for cerebrovascular diseases by sex, race, Hispanic origin, and age, United States selected years 1950–2010. Available at: http:// www.cdc.gov/nchs/data/hus/hus13.pdf

46. CDC. *Stroke facts.* Available at: http://www.cdc.gov/stroke/facts .htm

47. CDC. Current cigarette smoking among adults—United States, 2005–2012. *Morbidity and Mortality Weekly Report* 63(02): 29–34. Available at: http://www.cdc.gov/tobacco/data_statistics /fact_sheets/adult_data/cig_smoking/

48. CDC. *Smoking during pregnancy.* Available at: http://www.cdc.gov /tobacco/basic_information/health_effects/pregnancy/

49. City, M. D. *What happens when you quit smoking?* Available at: http://www.healthline.com/health-slideshow/quit -smoking-timeline#1

50. CDC. *Health Effects of Secondhand Smoke.* Available at: http://www.cdc.gov/tobacco/data_statistics/fact_sheets /secondhand_smoke/health_effects/

51. Chen, I.-L., & Husten, C. G. (2014). Introduction to tobacco control supplement. *Tobacco Control* 23(5): ii–1. DOI: 10.1136/ tobaccocontrol-2013-051504

52. Callahan-Lyon, P. (2014). Electronic cigarettes: Human health effects. *Tobacco Control* 23(5): ii36. DOI: 10.1136/ tobaccocontrol-2013-051470

53. Crotty Alexander, L. E., et al. (2014). Electronic cigarette vapor (ECV) exposure decreases *Staphylococcus aureus* susceptibility to macrophage and neutrophil killing. American Thoracic Society International Conference, San Diego. May 18, 2014.

54. Grana, R., Benowitz, N., & Glantz, S. A. (May 13, 2014). E-cigarettes: A scientific review. *Circulation* 129: 1972. DOI: 10.1161/ circulationaha.114.007667

55. Kosmider, L., et al. (2014). Carbonyl compounds in electronic cigarette vapors—effects of nicotine solvent and battery output voltage. *Nicotine & Tobacco Research.* Published online May 15, 2014. DOI: 10.1093/ntr/ntu078

56. NHLBI. (2015). *What is High Blood Pressure?* Available at: http:// www.nhlbi.nih.gov/health/health-topics/topics/hbp

57. Practical Clinical Skills. *Blood pressure measurement.* Available at: http://www.practicalclinicalskills.com/blood-pressure -measurement.aspx

58. AHA. *Cholesterol conditions.* Available at: http://www.heart.org /HEARTORG/Conditions/Cholesterol/Cholesterol_UCM_001089 _SubHomePage.jsp

59. NHLBI. (2015). *What is Cholesterol?* Available at: http://www.nhlbi.nih.gov/health/health-topics/topics/hbc/

60. Eckel, R. H. (2014). LDL cholesterol as a predictor of mortality, and beyond. *Circulation* 30: 528–529. Available at: http://circ.ahajournals.org/content/130/7/528.short

61. Jug, B., Papazian, J., & Budoff, M. J. (2013). Association of lipoprotein subfractions and coronary artery calcium in patient at intermediate cardiovascular risk. *American Journal of Cardiology* 15(1): 111, 213–218.

62. Acharjee, S., Boden, W. E., Hartigan, P. M., et al. (2013). Low levels of high-density lipoprotein cholesterol and increased risk of cardiovascular events in stable ischemic heart disease patients: A post-hoc analysis from the COURAGE trial. *Journal of the American College of Cardiology* 62(20): 1826–1833. Available at: http://www.ncbi.nlm.nih.gov/pubmed/23973693

63. Medscape. (2014). *Low HDL cholesterol (hypoalphalipoproteinemia).* Available at: http://emedicine.medscape.com/article/127943-overview

64. Medscape. (2014). *High HDL cholesterol (hyperalphalipoproteinemia).* Available at: http://emedicine.medscape.com/article/121187-overview#a0199

65. National Cholesterol Education Program. (2001). Executive Summary of the Third Report of the National Cholesterol Education Program (NCEP) Expert Panel on Detection, Evaluation, and Treatment of High Blood Cholesterol in Adults (Adult Treatment Panel III). *Journal of the American Medical Association* 285(19): 2486–2497.

66. CDC. *Health, United States, 2013.* Table 66: Cholesterol among adults aged 20 and over by selected characteristics, pp 217–219. Available at: http://www.cdc.gov/nchs/data/hus/hus13.pdf

67. MedlinePlus. *C-reactive protein.* Available at: http://www.nlm.nih.gov/medlineplus/ency/article/003356.htm

68. Ndrepepa, G., Braun, S., Fusaro, M., et al. (2013). C-reactive protein and prognosis in women and men with coronary artery disease after percutaneous coronary intervention. *Cardiovascular Revascularization Medicine* 14(5): 264–269. Available at: http://www.ncbi.nlm.nih.gov/pubmed/23969223

69. Life Extension. *Homocysteine reduction.* Available at: http://www.lef.org/protocols/heart-circulatory/homocysteine-reduction/Page-01

70. AHA. *Cardiovascular disease and diabetes.* Available at: http://www.heart.org/HEARTORG/Conditions/Diabetes/WhyDiabetesMatters/Cardiovascular-Disease-Diabetes_UCM_313865_Article.jsp

71. Levine, J. (2011). Poverty and obesity in the U.S. *Diabetes* 60(11): 2667–2668. http://diabetes.diabetesjournals.org/content/60/11/2667.full

72. American Diabetes Association. (2015). *Gestational diabetes.* Available at: http://www.diabetes.org/diabetes-basics/gestational/

73. AHA. *Obesity information.* Available at: http://www.heart.org/HEARTORG/GettingHealthy/WeightManagement/Obesity/Obesity-Information_UCM_307908_Article.jsp

74. CDC. (2015). *Overweight and obesity.* Available at: http://www.cdc.gov/obesity/index.html

75. Niswas, A., Oh, P. I., Faulkner, G. E., et al. (2015). Sedentary time and its association with risk for disease incidence, mortality, and hospitalization in adults. *Annals of Internal Medicine* 162: 123–132.

76. CDC. *Health, United States, 2013.* Table 68: Participation in leisure-time aerobic and muscle-strengthening activities that meet the federal 2008 Physical Activities Guidelines for Americans among adults aged 18 and over by selected characteristics. Available at: http://www.cdc.gov/nchs/data/hus/hus13.pdf

77. Harvard School of Public Health. *Physical activity guidelines: How much exercise do you need?* Available at: http://www.hsph.harvard.edu/nutritionsource/2013/11/20/physical-activity-guidelines-how-much-exercise-do-you-need/

78. Sun, C., Burger, D. P., Ponsonby, A. L., et al. (2013). Effects of early-life environment and epigenetics on cardiovascular disease risk in children: Highlight the role of twin studies. *Pediatric Research* 73: 523–530. Available at: http://www.nature.com/pr/journal/v73/n4-2/full/pr20136a.html

79. Briana, D. D., & Malamitsi-Pucher, A. (2008). Intrauterine growth restriction and adult disease: The role of adipocytokines. *European Journal of Endocrinology* 160: 337–347. Available at: http://www.eje-online.org/content/160/3/337

80. AHA. *Menopause and heart disease.* Available at: http://www.heart.org/HEARTORG/Conditions/More/MyHeartandStrokeNews/Menopause-and-Heart-Disease_UCM_448432_Article.jsp

81. Suk, D. J., et al. (2008). Lipoprotein(a), hormone replacement therapy, and risk of future cardiovascular events. *Journal of the American College of Cardiology* 52(2): 124–131.

82. Committee on Gynecologic Practice. (2013). Committee opinion: Hormone therapy and heart disease. *American College of Obstetricians and Gynecologists* 565: 1–4. Available at: http://www.acog.org/Resources-And-Publications/Committee-Opinions/Committee-on-Gynecologic-Practice/Hormone-Therapy-and-Heart-Disease

83. Lidegaard, O., Lokkegaard, E., Jensen, A., et al. (2012). Thrombotic stroke and myocardial infarction with hormonal contraception. *New England Journal of Medicine* 366: 2257–2266. Available at: http://www.nejm.org/doi/full/10.1056/NEJMoa1111840?query=featured_home&

84. Bellin, J. P., & McCarthy, C. R. (2013). Cardiovascular risk and combined oral contraceptives: Clinical decisions in settings of uncertainty. *American Journal of Obstetricians and Gynecologists* 208: 39–41. Available at: http://www.ajog.org/article/S0002-9378(12)00128-7/fulltext

85. Alias, G., Gabellari, I. C., De Lorenzo, C., et al. (2009). Oral contraceptives in migraine. *Expert Review of Neurotherapeutics* 9(3): 381–393. Available at: http://www.medscape.com/viewarticle/589439

86. Constano, S., Di Castelnuovo, A., Donati, M. B., et al. (2010). Cardiovascular and overall mortality risk in relation to alcohol consumption in patients with cardiovascular disease. *Circulation* 1(21): 1951–1959. Available at: http://circ.ahajournals.org/content/121/17/1951.full

87. AHA. *Cocaine, other drugs and heart disease.* Available at: http://www.heart.org/HEARTORG/Conditions/Cocaine-Marijuana-and-Other-Drugs_UCM_428537_Article.jsp

88. Samad, Z., Boyle, S., Ersboll, M., et al. (2014). Sex differences in platelet reactivity and cardiovascular and psychological response to mental stress in patients with stable ischemic disease. *Journal of the American College of Cardiology* 64(16): 1669–1678.

89. Go, A. S., Mozaffarian, D., Roger, V. L., et al. (2014). AHA statistical update. *Circulation* 1(29): e28–e292. Available at: http://circ.ahajournals.org/content/129/3/e28.figures-only

90. AHA. *Statistical fact sheet: Women and cardiovascular disease, 2014 update.* Available at: http://circ.ahajournals.org/content/129/3/e28.figures-only

91. Moser, D. K., Kimble, L. P., Alberts, M. J., et al. (2006). Reducing delay in seeking treatment by patients with acute coronary

syndrome and stroke. *Circulation* 114: 168–182. Available at: http://circ.ahajournals.org/content/114/2/168.full

92. AHA. *Time of arrival at hospital impacts time to treatment and survival of heart attack patients.* Available at: http://blog.heart.org/time-of-arrival-at-hospital-impacts-time-to-treatment-and-survival-of-heart-attack-patients/

93. CDC. *Women and heart disease fact sheet.* Available at: http://www.cdc.gov/dhdsp/data_statistics/fact_sheets/fs_women_heart.htm

94. CDC. *Health, United States, 2013.* Table 70: Obesity among children and adolescents ages 2–19 years. Available at: http://www.cdc.gov/nchs/data/hus/hus13.pdf

95. CDC. *Health, United States, 2013.* Table 68: Participation in leisure-time aerobic and muscle strengthening activities that meet federal 2008 Physical Activity Guidelines. Available at: http://www.cdc.gov/nchs/data/hus/hus13.pdf

96. Johns Hopkins Medicine. *What is cancer?* Available at: http://pathology.jhu.edu/pc/BasicTypes1.php

97. National Cancer Institute (NCI). *Metastatic cancer.* Available at: http://www.cancer.gov/cancertopics/factsheet/Sites-Types/metastatic

98. NCI. *Cancer prevention overview: Carcinogenesis.* Available at: http://pathology.jhu.edu/pc/BasicTypes1.php

99. Boston University. *Behind the vapor.* Available at: http://www.bu.edu/research/articles/behind-the-vapor/

100. World Health Organization (WHO). *Backgrounder on WHO report on regulation of e-cigarettes and similar products.* Available at: http://www.who.int/nmh/events/2014/backgrounder-e-cigarettes/en/

101. American Cancer Society (ACS). *Known and probable carcinogens.* Available at: http://www.cancer.org/cancer/cancercauses/othercarcinogens/generalinformationaboutcarcinogens/known-and-probable-human-carcinogens

102. Fruits and Vegetables MORE Matters. *What are phytochemicals?* Available at: http://www.fruitsandveggiesmorematters.org/what-are-phytochemicals

103. Phytochemicals. *What are phytochemicals?* Available at: http://www.phytochemicals.info/

104. ACS. *Known and probable human carcinogens.* Available at: http://www.cancer.org/cancer/cancercauses/othercarcinogens/generalinformationaboutcarcinogens/known-and-probable-human-carcinogens

105. ACS. *Estimated number of new cancer cases and deaths by sex, US, 2014.* Available at: http://www.cancer.org/acs/groups/content/@research/documents/document/acspc-041780.pdf

106. Siegel, R. (January 5, 2015). Facts and figures report: 1.5 million cancer deaths avoided in 2 decades, cancer statistics. Published early online in *CA: A Cancer Journal for Clinicians.* Atlanta, GA: American Cancer Society. Available at: http://www.cancer.org/cancer/news/news/facts-figures-report-cancer-deaths-avoided-in-2-decades

107. CDC. *Smoking and tobacco use.* Available at: http://www.cdc.gov/tobacco/data_statistics/fact_sheets/adult_data/cig_smoking/

108. Jampel, S. *What a pack of cigarettes costs now state by state, August 2014.* Available at: http://www.theawl.com/2013/07/what-a-pack-of-cigarettes-costs-now-state-by-state

109. ACS. (2014). *Cancer facts and figures,* p. 4. Available at: http://www.cancer.org/acs/groups/content/@research/documents/webcontent/acspc-042151.pdf

110. CDC. (2015). *Current cigarette smoking among adults in the United States.* Available at: http://www.cdc.gov/tobacco/data_statistics/fact_sheets/adult_data/cig_smoking/

111. Kulwin, N. (2014). *What a pack of cigarettes costs, state by state.* Available at: http://www.theawl.com/2014/08/how-much-a-pack-of-cigarettes-costs-state-by-statehttp://www.theawl.com/2014/08/how-much-a-pack-of-cigarettes-costs-state-by-state

112. ACS. *Colorectal cancer facts and figures, 2014–2016,* p 3. Available at: http://www.cancer.org/acs/groups/content/documents/document/acspc-042280.pdf

113. NCI. *Surveillance, epidemiology, and end results program.* Available at: http://seer.cancer.gov/statfacts/html/corp.html

114. NCI. *Endometrial cancer treatment, general information about endometrial cancer.* Available at: http://www.cancer.gov/cancertopics/pdq/treatment/endometrial/HealthProfessional/page1

115. ACS. *What is ovarian cancer?* Available at: http://www.cancer.org/cancer/ovariancancer/detailedguide/ovarian-cancer-what-is-ovarian-cancer

116. CDC. *Ovarian cancer death rates by race and ethnicity, 1999–2011.* Available at: http://www.cdc.gov/cancer/ovarian/statistics/race.htm

117. NCI. *Surveillance, epidemiology, and end results program, cervix uteri cancer.* Available at: http://seer.cancer.gov/statfacts/html/cervix.html

118. NCI. *Surveillance, epidemiology, and end results program, SEER stat fact sheets, pancreas cancer.* Available at: http://seer.cancer.gov/statfacts/html/pancreas.html

119. NCI. *A snapshot of pancreatic cancer.* Available at: http://www.cancer.gov/research/progress/snapshots/pancreatic

120. NCI. *Skin cancer.* Available at: http://www.cancer.gov/cancertopics/types/skin

121. ACS. (2014). *Cancer facts and figures,* p 20. Available at: http://www.cancer.org/research/cancerfactsstatistics/cancerfactsfigures2014/

122. CDC. *Skin cancer, indoor tanning is not safe.* Available at: http://www.cdc.gov/cancer/skin/basic_info/indoor_tanning.htm

123. Skin Cancer Foundation. *Skin cancer facts.* Available at: http://www.skincancer.org/skin-cancer-information/skin-cancer-facts#men/women

124. NCI. *State cancer profiles.* Available at: http://statecancerprofiles.cancer.gov/data-topics/mortality.html

125. Kingsley, C., & Bandolin, S. (2011). Cultural and socioeconomic factors affecting cancer screening, early detection and care in the Latino population. *Ethnomed.* Available at: https://ethnomed.org/clinical/cancer/cultural-and-socioeconomic-factors-affecting-cancer-screening-early-detection-and-care-in-the-latino-population

126. Marlow, L. A., Waller, J., & Wardle. J. (January 12, 2015). Barriers to cervical cancer screening among ethnic minority women: a qualitative study. *Journal of Family Planning and Reproductive Health Care* [E-pub ahead of print]. Available at: http://www.ncbi.nlm.nih.gov/pubmed/25583124

127. Ramirez, A. S. (2014). Fatalism and cancer risk knowledge among a sample of highly acculturated Latinas. *Journal of Cancer Education* 29(1): 50–55.

128. Pampel, F. C., Krueger, P. M., & Denney, J. T. (2010). Socioeconomic disparities in health behaviors. *Annual Review of Sociology* 36: 349–370. Available at: http://www.ncbi.nlm.nih.gov/pmc/articles/PMC3169799/

129. ACS. *Economic impact of cancer.* Available at: http://www.cancer.org/cancer/cancerbasics/economic-impact-of-cancer

130. WHO. (2014). *Cancer fact sheet.* Available at: http://www.who.int/mediacentre/factsheets/fs297/en/

131. WHO, International Agency for Research on Cancer. (February 3, 2014). *Global battle against cancer won't be won with treatment alone: Effective prevention measures urgently needed to prevent cancer crisis.* [Press Release Number 224]. Available at: http://www.iarc.fr/en/media-centre/pr/2014/pdfs/pr224_E.pdf

132. Susan G. Komen. *The who, what, where, when and sometimes, why: Benign breast conditions.* Available at: http://ww5.komen.org/BreastCancer/BenignConditions.html

133. Breastcancer.org. *Stages of breast cancer.* Available at: http://www.breastcancer.org/symptoms/diagnosis/staging

134. Center for Restorative Breast Surgery. *Heredity and breast cancer—the BRCA gene.* Available at: http://www.breastcenter.com/breast-reconstruction-procedures/brca-reconstruction/?utm_source=googleppc&utm_medium=cpc&utm_term=brca%252Bjewish%252Bwomen&utm_content=ad2&utm_campaign=genetic&gclid=CMPdvcjboMMCFdgjvQodCFQA2g

135. Susan G. Komen. *The who, what, where, when, and sometimes why: Race and ethnicity.* Available at: http://ww5.komen.org/BreastCancer/RaceampEthnicity.html

136. Cancer.net. *Race and breast cancer.* Available at: http://www.cancer.net/research-and-advocacy/health-disparities-and-cancer/race-and-breast-cancer

137. Kaplowitz, P. B. (2015). Precious puberty. *Medscape.* Available at: http://emedicine.medscape.com/article/924002-overview

138. Healthy Women. *Estrogen overview.* Available at: http://www.healthywomen.org/condition/estrogen

139. Healthy Women. *Progesterone overview.* Available at: http://www.healthywomen.org/condition/progesterone

140. National Institute on Aging. *Hormones and menopause.* Available at: http://www.nia.nih.gov/health/publication/hormones-and-menopause

141. eMed Expert. *Birth control pills advantages and disadvantages.* Available at: http://www.emedexpert.com/compare/birth-control-advantages.shtml

142. NCI. *Oral contraceptives and cancer.* Available at: http://www.cancer.gov/about-cancer/causes-prevention/risk/hormones/oral-contraceptives-fact-sheet

143. Cleveland Clinic. *Treatments and procedures, clinical breast examination.* Available at: http://my.clevelandclinic.org/health/treatments_and_procedures/hic_clinical_breast-examination

144. NCI. *Mammograms.* Available at: http://www.cancer.gov/cancertopics/factsheet/detection/mammograms

145. ACS. *American Cancer Society recommendations for early breast cancer detection in women without breast symptoms.* Available at: http://www.cancer.org/cancer/breastcancer/moreinformation/breastcancerearlydetection/breast-cancer-early-detection-acs-recs

146. U.S. Preventive Services Task Force. *Breast cancer: Screening, recommendation summary.* Available at: http://www.uspreventiveservicestaskforce.org/Page/Topic/recommendation-summary/breast-cancer-screening

147. NCI. *Breast cancer.* Available at: http://www.cancer.gov/types/breast; Breast cancer screening. Available at: http://www.cancer.gov/types/breast/patient/breast-screening-pdq

148. NCI. *Surgery choices for women with DCIS or breast cancer.* Available at: http://www.cancer.gov/types/breast/surgery-choices/surgerychoices.pdf

149. ACS. *Medicines to reduce breast cancer risk.* Available at: http://www.cancer.org/cancer/breastcancer/moreinformation/medicinestoreducebreastcancer/medicines-to-reduce-breast-cancer-risk-toc

150. ACS. *Targeted therapy for breast cancer.* Available at: http://www.cancer.org/cancer/breastcancer/detailedguide/breast-cancer-treating-targeted-therapy

151. Nilsson, M. I., Peterson, L. M., Wennman-Larsen, A., et al. (2013). Adjustment and social support at work early after breast cancer surgery and its association with sickness absence. *Psychooncology* 22(12): 2755–2762.

152. Susan G. Komen. *How to go on after all you've been through.* Available at: http://ww5.komen.org/LifeAfterTreatment.html

153. Johns Hopkins Medicine, The Sidney Kimmel Comprehensive Cancer Center. *Cervical dysplasia treatment.* Available at: http://www.hopkinsmedicine.org/kimmel_cancer_center/centers/cervical_dysplasia/treatment.html

154. NCI. *Stages of cervical cancer.* Available at: http://www.cancer.gov/cancertopics/pdq/treatment/cervical/Patient/page2

155. CDC. *Incidence, prevalence and cost of sexually transmitted infections in the United States.* Available at: http://www.cdc.gov/std/stats/sti-estimates-fact-sheet-feb-2013.pdf

156. Satterwhite, C. L., Torrone, E., Meites, E., et al. (2013). Sexually transmitted infections among U.S. women and men: Prevalence and incidence estimates, 2008. *Sexually Transmitted Diseases* 40: 187–193.

157. U.S. Preventive Services Task Force. *Cervical cancer screening recommendations.* Available at: http://www.uspreventiveservicestaskforce.org/uspstf/uspscerv.htm

158. U.S. Preventive Services Task Force. *Guidelines on cervical cancer screening.* Available at: http://www.acog.org/~/media/Districts/District%20II/PDFs/USPSTF_Cervical_Ca_Screening_Guidelines.pdf

159. NCI. *Cervical cancer treatment, treatment options by stage.* Available at: http://www.cancer.gov/cancertopics/pdq/treatment/cervical/Patient/page5

160. Womenshealth.gov. *Uterine fibroids fact sheet.* Available at: http://www.womenshealth.gov/publications/our-publications/fact-sheet/uterine-fibroids.html

161. National Institute of Child Health and Human Development. *How many people are affected by uterine fibroids?* Available at: http://www.nichd.nih.gov/health/topics/uterine/conditioninfo/pages/people-affected.aspx

162. Mayo Clinic. *Uterine fibroids, treatments and drugs.* Available at: http://www.mayoclinic.org/diseases-conditions/uterine-fibroids/basics/treatment/con-20037901

163. Office of Women's Health. *Uterine fibroids fact sheet.* Available at: https://www.womenshealth.gov/publications/our-publications/fact-sheet/uterine-fibroids.html

164. Endometriosis Association. *What is endometriosis?* Available at: http://www.endometriosisassn.org/endo.html

165. Womenshealth.gov. *Endometriosis.* Available at: http://www.womenshealth.gov/publications/our-publications/fact-sheet/endometriosis.html

166. American College of Obstetricians and Gynecologists. *Endometrial hyperplasia.* Available at: http://www.acog.org/Patients/FAQs/Endometrial-Hyperplasia

167. Florida Hospital. *Uterine cancer (endometrial cancer), stages of uterine cancer.* Available at: https://www.floridahospital.com/uterine-cancer/stages

168. ACS. *What is endometrial cancer?* Available at: http://www.cancer.org/cancer/endometrialcancer/detailedguide/endometrial-uterine-cancer-what-is-endometrial-cancer

169. ACS. *Endometrial (uterine) cancer.* Available at: http://www.cancer.org/cancer/endometrialcancer/detailedguide/endometrial-uterine-cancer-diagnosis

170. Office of Women's Health. *Ovarian cysts.* Available at: http://www.womenshealth.gov/publications/our-publications/fact-sheet/ovarian-cysts.html

171. WebMD. *Ovarian cysts and tumors.* Available at: http://www.webmd.com/women/guide/ovarian-cysts?page=3

172. NCI. *Ovarian epithelial cancer.* Available at: http://www.cancer.gov/cancertopics/pdq/treatment/ovarianepithelial/Patient/page1

173. Memorial Sloan Kettering Cancer Center. *Ovarian cancer risk factors.* Available at: http://www.mskcc.org/cancer-care/adult/ovarian/risk-factors

174. NCI. *Ovarian epithelial cancer treatment, treatment option overview.* Available at: http://www.cancer.gov/cancertopics/pdq/treatment/ovarianepithelial/Patient/page4

175. CDC. *Cancer among women.* Available at: http://www.cdc.gov/cancer/dcpc/data/women.htm

176. ACS. (2014). *Cancer facts and figures,* p 4. Available at: http://www.cancer.org/acs/groups/content/@research/documents/webcontent/acspc-042151.pdf

177. Ibid, p 7.

178. Ibid, p 15.

179. CDC. *What are the risk factors for lung cancer?* Available at: http://www.cdc.gov/cancer/lung/basic_info/risk_factors.htm

180. ACS. *Lung cancer (non-small cell).* Available at: http://www.cancer.org/acs/groups/cid/documents/webcontent/003115-pdf.pdf

181. CDC. *What are the risk factors for lung cancer?* Available at: http://www.cdc.gov/cancer/lung/basic_info/risk_factors.htm

182. ACS. *What about electronic cigarettes? Are they safe?* Available at: http://www.cancer.org/cancer/cancercauses/tobaccocancer/questionsaboutsmokingtobaccoandhealth/questions-about-smoking-tobacco-and-health-e-cigarettes

183. American Lung Association. *Lung cancer fact sheet.* Available at: http://www.lung.org/lung-disease/lung-cancer/resources/facts-figures/lung-cancer-fact-sheet.html

184. U.S. Department of Health and Human Services. (2014). *The health consequences of smoking—50 years of progress. A Report of the Surgeon General.* Atlanta, GA: U.S. Department of Health and Human Services, Centers for Disease Control and Prevention, National Center for Chronic Disease Prevention and Health Promotion, Office on Smoking and Health. Available at: http://www.cdc.gov/tobacco/data_statistics/fact_sheets/health_effects/tobacco_related_mortality/. Accessed February 6, 2014.

185. CDC, National Institute for Occupational Safety and Health (NIOSH). *Environmental tobacco smoke in the workplace: Lung cancer and other health effects.* Available at: http://www.cdc.gov/niosh/docs/91-108/

186. CDC, NIOSH. *Women's safety and health issues at work.* Available at: http://www.cdc.gov/niosh/topics/women/manufacturing.html

187. ACS. *Lung cancer prevention and early detection.* Available at: http://www.cancer.org/cancer/lungcancer-non-smallcell/moreinformation/lungcancerpreventionandearlydetection/lung-cancer-ped-toc

188. Cancer.net. *Lung cancer: Treatment and options.* Available at: http://www.cancer.net/cancer-types/lung-cancer/treatment-options

189. ACS. (2014). *Facts and figures: Colon and rectum,* p. 11. Available at: http://www.cancer.org/acs/groups/content/@research/documents/webcontent/acspc-042151.pdf

190. NCI. *Colon cancer treatment, stages of colon cancer.* Available at: http://www.cancer.gov/cancertopics/pdq/treatment/colon/Patient/page2

191. NCI. *The cancer genome atlas, colorectal adenocarcinoma.* Available at: http://cancergenome.nih.gov/cancersselected/colorectaladenocarcinoma

192. CDC. *Colorectal cancer, what are the risk factors?* Available at: http://www.cdc.gov/cancer/colorectal/basic_info/risk_factors.htm

193. CDC. *Colorectal cancer, what should I know about screening?* Available at: http://www.cdc.gov/cancer/colorectal/basic_info/screening/

194. ACS. *Treatment of colon cancer by stage.* Available at: http://www.cancer.org/cancer/colonandrectumcancer/detailedguide/colorectal-cancer-treating-by-stage-colon

195. ACS. (2014). *Facts and figures,* p 8. Available at: http://www.cancer.org/acs/groups/content/@research/documents/webcontent/acspc-042151.pdf

196. Skin Cancer Foundation. *Skin cancer facts.* Available at: http://www.skincancer.org/skin-cancer-information/skin-cancer-facts

197. CDC. *What are the risk factors for skin cancer?* Available at: http://www.cdc.gov/cancer/skin/basic_info/risk_factors.htm

198. CDC. *What can I do to reduce my risk of skin cancer?* Available at: http://www.cdc.gov/cancer/skin/basic_info/prevention.htm

199. Skin Cancer Foundation. *Do you know your ABCDEs?* Available at: http://www.skincancer.org/skin-cancer-information/melanoma/melanoma-warning-signs-and-images/do-you-know-your-abcdes

200. Cancer.net. *Cancer screening.* Available at: http://www.cancer.net/navigating-cancer-care/prevention-and-healthy-living/cancer-screening

201. NCI. *Skin cancer treatments.* Available at: http://www.cancer.gov/cancertopics/pdq/treatment/skin/Patient/page4

202. ACS. *How is melanoma skin cancer treated?* Available at: http://www.cancer.org/cancer/skincancer-melanoma/detailedguide/melanoma-skin-cancer-treating-general-info

203. ACS. *Breast cancer in men.* Available at: http://www.cancer.org/cancer/breastcancerinmen/

204. ACS. (2015). *What are the risk factors for breast cancer in men?* Available at: http://www.cancer.org/cancer/breastcancerinmen/detailedguide/breast-cancer-in-men-risk-factors

205. NCI. *Male breast cancer.* Available at: http://www.cancer.gov/types/breast/patient/male-breast-treatment-pdq

206. Sineshaw, H. M., Freedman, R. A., Ward, E. M., et al. (2015). Black/White disparities in receipt of treatment and survival among men with early-stage breast cancer. *Journal of Clinical Oncology* 33(211): 2337–2344.

207. Kiluk, J. V., Lee, M. C., Park, C.K., et al. (2011). Male breast cancer: Management and follow-up recommendations. *Breast Journal* 17(5): 503–509.

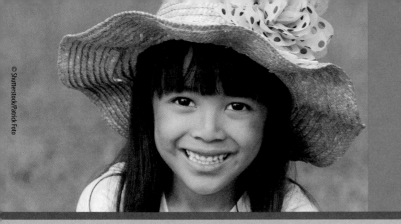

CHAPTER 11

Other Chronic Diseases and Conditions

Learning Objectives

On completion of this chapter, the student should be able to discuss:

1. Major chronic diseases and their effects on women.

2. Differences between racial and ethnic groups in the incidence rates of chronic diseases.

3. The individual and societal costs of various chronic diseases.

4. Risk factors, screening tests, and preventive and treatment measures for osteoporosis.

5. The process of bone resorption, bone formation, and osteoporosis development.

6. The two major forms of arthritis that disproportionately afflict women.

7. Risk factors and symptoms of arthritis and methods for pain management.

8. How diabetes affects individuals and society as a whole.

9. Special risks that pregnancy presents to the diabetic mother.

10. Diabetes management and responding in emergency situations.

11. Symptoms, risk factors, and treatment of fibromyalgia.

12. Autoimmune diseases that most commonly affect women.

13. Types of lupus and the clinical manifestations of the disease.

14. The basics of Hashimoto's disease, Graves' disease, and other thyroid disorders.

15. The development of Alzheimer's disease and the resulting symptoms.

16. Methods for diagnosing Alzheimer's disease and ways to manage living with the disease.

17. Ways that a woman can recognize symptoms of a disease so as to seek treatment and prevent future disease-related complications.

INTRODUCTION

Chronic diseases persist or progress over a long time. They develop slowly, do not resolve spontaneously, and are rarely cured completely. While infections cause a few chronic diseases, genetics and lifestyle factors, such as diet, physical activity, and environmental exposures, play the biggest role in how chronic diseases appear and develop. Many of these diseases manifest themselves in young women, creating health issues that these individuals must learn to live with for the rest of their lives.

Living with a chronic disease can become an encompassing process, especially when the disease causes frequent illness and necessitates many visits to physicians. Some women begin to consider the management of their illness to be a full-time job. Others try to live as they did before diagnosis, not wanting their condition to become central to their lives. Women's responses to chronic disease are as individual as the women themselves. In all cases, however, active support networks via family, friends, healthcare providers, disease support groups, or therapy can help ease the burden of disease management. Support can help these woman cope with the physical, emotional, and financial ramifications of living with a chronic disease.

Unhealthful diets, smoking, lack of exercise, continuous stress, and other risks contribute to the progression of many chronic diseases. These lifestyle risk factors contribute to high blood pressure, high cholesterol levels, diabetes, obesity, arthritis, and other conditions, which in turn can lead to conditions such as stroke, heart attack, some forms of cancer, chronic bronchitis, and emphysema. Other chronic conditions are the result of fluctuations in hormone levels, due to disorders in the endocrine system.

Chronic diseases are the leading cause of death in the United States and around the world. They are also the most costly and preventable of all health conditions. Data from the World Health Organization (WHO) indicate that chronic diseases caused about 38 million (68%) of the 56 million deaths in 2012.[1] The four main diseases are cardiovascular diseases, cancers, diabetes, and chronic lung diseases. The leading causes of chronic disease deaths in 2012 were cardiovascular diseases, cancers, respiratory diseases, and diabetes (46%, 22%, 10%, and 4% of chronic disease deaths, respectively).[1]

This chapter reviews osteoporosis, arthritis, diabetes, fibromyalgia, major autoimmune diseases, and Alzheimer's disease—chronic diseases that have dramatic effects on the health of women in the world today.

DIMENSIONS OF CHRONIC DISEASES

Epidemiological Overview

Understanding, preventing, and managing chronic conditions are important steps for maintaining satisfactory health. The prevalence of chronic conditions is difficult to ascertain because of differences and inconsistencies in diagnostic criteria and the lack of national reporting systems. Many chronic diseases affect women more often than they do men. For example:

- Of the 10.2 million U.S. adults estimated to have osteoporosis, 8.2 million are women and 2 million are men. An additional 27.3 million women and 16.1 million men have low bone mass.[2]

- Osteoarthritis and rheumatoid arthritis, two of the most common health problems in the United States, are far more prevalent in women than in men; 60% of all people with arthritis are women.[3]

- Diabetes affects 29 million people in the United States: 13.4 million women and 15.5 million men. This means that roughly 11% of adult U.S. women have diabetes.[4]

- Of the 50 million Americans living with autoimmune diseases, more than 75% are women. These diseases typically appear during a woman's childbearing years. **Table 11.1** shows the disproportionate female-to-male ratios in autoimmune diseases. Reproductive hormones appear to affect when (and how often) these diseases appear. For example, many autoimmune diseases improve during pregnancy and then reappear after delivery, appear after menopause, or get worse during pregnancy.[5]

It's Your Health

The Endocrine System

The endocrine system is made up of glands that produce and release hormones. Hormones affect body processes such as growth and development, metabolism, sexual function, reproduction, and mood. Each gland of the endocrine system releases specific hormones into the bloodstream. Parts of the endocrine system include:

- Adrenal glands: Two small glands, one located on top of each kidney. The adrenal glands produce sex hormones and cortisol. They also help to control blood sugar.

- Hypothalamus: A part of the lower middle brain that tells the pituitary gland when to release hormones.

- Ovaries: The female reproductive organs that release eggs and produce sex hormones.

- Islets of Langerhans (in the pancreas): Cells in the pancreas that control the release of the hormones insulin and glucagon, which help to maintain healthy blood sugar levels.

- Parathyroid: Four pea-sized glands on the thyroid gland in the neck. Parathyroid glands make parathyroid hormone, which helps the body keep the right balance of calcium and phosphorus. This is vital to bone development.

- Pineal gland: A gland found near the center of the brain that releases melatonin and may be linked to sleep patterns.

- Pituitary gland: A pea-sized gland found at the base of the brain. It is often called the "master control gland" because it affects growth as well as the functions of other glands in the body.

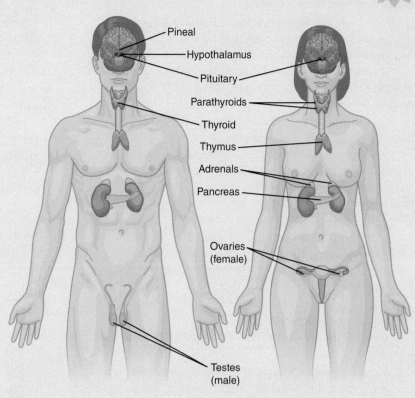

- Testes: The male reproductive glands that produce sperm and sex hormones.

- Thymus: A gland in the upper chest that helps develop the body's immune system early in life.

- Thyroid: A butterfly-shaped gland in the front of the neck that controls metabolism.

Even the slightest alteration in the functioning of one of the endocrine glands can lead to an endocrine disorder. Endocrine disorders include diseases such as diabetes, hypothyroidism, and hyperthyroidism, among many other conditions.

Table 11.1	Female-to-Male Ratios in Autoimmune Diseases
Hashimoto's thyroiditis	10:1
Lupus	9:1
Sjögren's syndrome	9:1
Graves' disease	7:1
Scleroderma	4:1
Rheumatoid arthritis	3:1
Multiple sclerosis	2:1

Source: Adapted from Fairweather, D., Frisancho-Kiss, S., & Rose, N. (2008). Sex differences in autoimmune disease from a pathological perspective. *American Journal of Pathology* 173(3): 600–609.

- Women are more likely than men to develop Alzheimer's disease, primarily because women live longer than men and the likelihood of developing Alzheimer's disease increases as a person ages. Women are also most likely to be the primary caregivers for their parents, spouses, and other family members with the disease.

Racial/Ethnic and Socioeconomic Dimensions

Rates and severity of chronic diseases vary among racial and ethnic groups, often in complex ways. Black women, for example, typically have a higher bone mineral density than White and Asian American women. This puts Black women at a lower absolute risk of developing osteoporosis. However, due to other factors, such as general health status and reduced access to health care, Black

It's Your Health

Global Burden of Chronic Diseases

Chronic diseases, also referred to as noncommunicable diseases or NCDs, are the leading cause of death globally. NCDs were responsible for 38 million (68%) of the world's 56 million deaths in 2012. Almost three-quarters of these deaths and the majority of premature deaths of people younger than age 70 (82%) occurred in low- and middle-income countries.

All age groups and all areas of the world are affected by NCDs. The globalization of unhealthy lifestyles, such as tobacco use, physical inactivity, unhealthy diet, and the harmful use of alcohol, has lead to an increase in NCDs. These behavioral risk factors lead to conditions such as hypertension, high cholesterol, and obesity, which in turn can lead to cardiovascular diseases or exacerbate conditions such as diabetes.

In 2013, the World Health Assembly adopted a comprehensive global monitoring framework with 25 indicators and nine voluntary global targets in order to accelerate national efforts for addressing NCDs by 2025. The global targets are as follows:

1. A 25% relative reduction in overall mortality from cardiovascular diseases, cancer, diabetes, or chronic respiratory disease. These four diseases are responsible for 82% of NCD deaths.

2. At least 10% relative reduction in the harmful use of alcohol as appropriate, within the national context. In 2012, an estimated 5.9% of all deaths worldwide were attributable to alcohol consumption; more than half of these deaths resulted from NCDs.

3. A 10% relative reduction in the prevalence of insufficient physical activity. Insufficient physical activity contributes to 3.2 million deaths each year.

4. A 30% relative reduction in the mean population intake of salt/sodium. Globally, 1.7 million annual deaths from cardiovascular causes have been attributed to high sodium intake.

5. A 30% relative reduction in prevalence of current tobacco use in persons aged 15 and older. Annually, 6 million people are estimated to die from tobacco use, with more than 600,000 deaths due to exposure to secondhand smoke.

6. A 25% relative reduction in the prevalence of high blood pressure. High blood pressure is estimated to have caused 9.4 million deaths in 2010. The global prevalence of hypertension in adults aged 18 and older was 22% in 2014.

7. Halt the rise in diabetes and obesity. In 2014, the global prevalence of diabetes was estimated to be 9%; 11% of men and 15% of women were obese. More than 42 million children under age 5 were overweight in 2013.

8. At least 50% of eligible people receive drug therapy and counseling to prevent heart attacks and strokes. CVD was the leading cause of NCD deaths in 2012 and was responsible for 46% of all NCD deaths.

9. An 80% availability of the affordable basic technologies and essential medicines required to treat major NCDs in both public and private facilities

Source: World Health Organization. (2014). *Global status report on noncommunicable diseases 2014*. Available at: http://www.who.int/global-coordination-mechanism/publications/global-status-report-ncds-2014-eng.pdf?ua=1

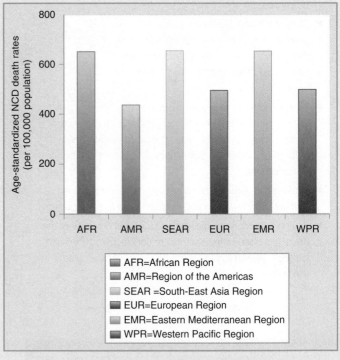

Data from World Health Organization (2014). Global status report on noncommunicable diseases 2014.

women are more likely to die if they have a serious osteoporosis-related injury. Racial differences are also evident with arthritis. Although Black women are about as likely as White women to have arthritis, they are more likely (10.1% versus 7.9%) to have more serious symptoms that limit their daily activities. Overall, Black people with doctor-diagnosed arthritis have a higher prevalence of severe pain attributable to arthritis compared with White people (34.0% versus 22.6%).[6] Diabetes is also more prevalent among non-White populations. As **Figure 11.1** shows, American Indians/Alaska Natives, followed by non-Hispanic Blacks, Hispanics, and then Asian Americans, have the highest prevalence rates of diabetes in the United States.[7]

Economic Dimensions

As of 2012, about half of all adults in the United States—117 million people—had one or more chronic

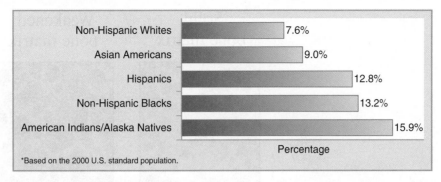

Figure 11.1   Age-adjusted percentage of people aged 20 years or older with diagnosed diabetes, by race/ethnicity: United States, 2010–2012.

Source: Centers for Disease Control and Prevention (CDC). (2014). *Diabetes Report Card 2014.* Atlanta, GA: CDC, U.S. Department of Health and Human Services.

health conditions.[8] In addition to harming individuals, chronic diseases have major effects on the economy. In 2010, 86% of all healthcare spending was for people with one or more chronic medical conditions.[9]

The costs associated with specific chronic diseases are huge. The total annual costs of diagnosed diabetes were estimated to be $245 billion in 2012—about $176 billion in direct medical expenses, and $69 billion in decreased productivity, including work loss, absenteeism, and disability.[10] Arthritis and related conditions create expenses of more than $128 billion a year.[11] Bone fractures caused by osteoporosis and low bone mass cost $19 billion per year in the United States.[12] The costs of caring for Alzheimer's patients in the United States—including health care, home care, and hospice—is estimated to be $226 billion in 2015.[13]

People with chronic diseases often struggle to pay for appropriate medical care. Men and women with diabetes have, for example, more than twice the average medical expenses of people without diabetes.[10] People with chronic diseases also experience costs in their personal relationships as the strain of dealing with chronic disease damages marriages, friendships, or other relationships. As the major primary caregivers, women often are forced to miss work in order to care for their loved ones and family members with chronic diseases. This can pose financial challenges for women, as they may have to endure reduced work hours, take family leave, or elect early retirement.

OSTEOPOROSIS

Osteoporosis is an age-related disease characterized by a reduction in bone mass and structural deterioration of bone tissue. Bone is living, growing tissue that changes throughout life. **Bone remodeling** is the process that removes older bone (resorption) and replaces it with new bone (formation) to maintain a healthy skeleton. Until a woman's mid-20s, new bone forms faster than resorption

occurs, until peak bone mass is reached—after age 30, bone resorption begins to exceed bone formation. The first few years after menopause are the most significant for bone loss. As bone is lost, the skeletal structure weakens, leading to an increased risk of fracture. Osteoporosis develops when bone resorption occurs too quickly or bone replacement occurs too slowly (**Figure 11.2**).

Osteoporosis is a major cause of bone fractures in postmenopausal women and a leading cause of frailty. It affects approximately 8 million women, with millions more at increased risk of developing osteoporosis due to low bone mass. This translates to one in two women older than age 50 having an osteoporosis-related fracture in her lifetime. **Table 11.2** outlines major risk factors for osteoporosis.

Osteoporosis is responsible for more than 2 million fractures per year.[12] One of every two women and one of every four men older than age 50 will suffer a fracture related to osteoporosis. Hip fractures are especially serious and can present long-term problems when they occur. Hip fractures account for 350,000 hospital admissions each year and 60,000 nursing home admissions.[14] Women suffer three-quarters of all hip fractures.

Risk Factors

Smoking is detrimental to bone health, as it can cause early menopause and increase the rate of bone loss. The effects of smoking on bone health have been difficult to analyze in more detail because possible confounding factors, such as lifestyle differences between smokers and nonsmokers, may also play a role. Smokers are often thinner, drink more alcohol, are more likely to lead sedentary lifestyles, and tend to have earlier menopause than nonsmokers do—all of which are risk factors for poor bone health. Additionally, inadequate calcium intake and a lack of regular weight-bearing exercise increase the risk for developing osteoporosis.

Some medications used to treat other chronic conditions may also cause bone loss. For example, long-term

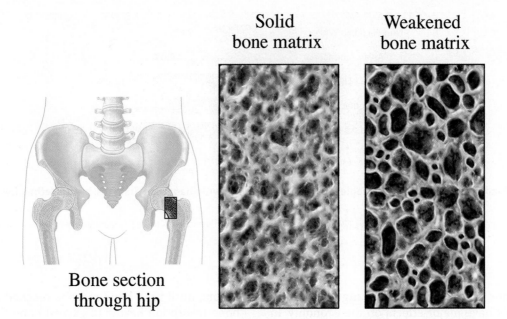

Solid bone matrix

Weakened bone matrix

Bone section through hip

Figure 11.2   A–B. Left to right, healthy bone vs. osteoporotic bone. "Osteoporosis" literally means "porous bone."
© Nucleus Medical Art/Visuals Unlimited/Getty Images

use of glucocorticoids (medicines prescribed for diseases including arthritis, asthma, Crohn's disease, and lupus) can lead to a loss of bone density and increase in fractures. Antiseizure drugs, gonadotropin-releasing hormone (GnRH) analogs, excessive use of aluminum-containing antacids, certain cancer treatments, and excessive thyroid hormone also may cause bone loss. The health benefits of these medications may be worth the

risk of possible bone loss, however. Women using these medications should discuss their options for osteoporosis prevention and best treatment regimens with their healthcare providers.

Medical conditions, including diseases of the thyroid gland such as hyperthyroidism and hypothyroidism, may lead to bone loss. Amenorrhea (lack of menstrual periods) or diseases that lead to amenorrhea, such as anorexia nervosa, cause estrogen deficiencies, which in turn lead to accelerated bone loss (see Table 11.2).

Signs and Symptoms

Osteoporosis is often called a "silent disease" because neither pain nor specific symptoms are associated with this condition. Only one out of four women who has osteoporosis is aware of the condition.[15] Some women notice a loss of height as the vertebrae weaken, collapse, and consequently fracture. When the bones in the spine fracture, a woman loses a small amount of height. The spine also begins to curve as multiple fractures occur.

Screening and Diagnosis

One red flag that signals a woman might have osteoporosis is a bone fracture that results from minimal trauma. To test for osteoporosis, a bone mass measurement (also referred to as a bone mineral density test) must be taken.

Methods for measuring bone mineral density are painless, noninvasive, and safe. Traditional tests measure bone density in the areas most susceptible to fractures caused by osteoporosis: the spine, the hip, and the wrist. Newer machines measure density in the finger, the patella (or kneecap), the tibia (or shinbone), and the heel.

Table 11.2   Risk Factors for Osteoporosis
Modifiable Risk Factors
■ Diet low in calcium and vitamin D
■ Sedentary lifestyle
■ Cigarette smoking
■ Estrogen deficiency
■ Low weight and body mass index
■ Certain medications, such as glucocorticoids, some anticonvulsants, and thyroid hormones
■ Abnormal absence of menstrual periods (amenorrhea)
■ Anorexia nervosa or bulimia
Nonmodifiable Risk Factors
■ Being female
■ Increased age/postmenopausal status
■ Small frame and thin-boned
■ White or Asian race
■ Family history of osteoporosis or fractures
Having one or more of these risk factors increases the risk of developing osteoporosis. The more risk factors a woman has, the greater her risk.

My mother just found out that she has osteoporosis. I have watched my grandmother shrink with it. The doctor says that my mother can do some things to prevent further bone loss. The message for me is to prevent it from happening. I am now much more interested in diet and exercise.

—26-year-old woman

Women who should be tested include:

- All women age 65 or older

- All postmenopausal women younger than age 65 who have one or more additional risk factors for osteoporosis besides menopause

- Women age 50 and older with fractures

- Women with a condition or taking a medication associated with low bone mass or bone loss

- Women who are considering therapy for osteoporosis or who want to monitor the effectiveness of certain osteoporosis treatments

Prevention and Treatment

In the absence of a cure, prevention and management are the best strategies available for women with osteoporosis and for women at all stages of life. Lifestyle and personal behaviors are the key osteoporosis prevention strategies. A woman should not start smoking, and she should quit if she already smokes. An inadequate supply of calcium over a woman's lifetime is a major risk factor for developing osteoporosis. Calcium plays an important role in achieving peak bone mass, maintaining bone mass before menopause, and preventing bone loss in the postmenopausal years.

Vitamin D is necessary for intestinal absorption of calcium. Calcium and vitamin D reduce the risk of fracture of the spine, hip, and other sites. The typical diet of U.S. women contains less than 600 milligrams of calcium per day, about half the recommended amount for women. Dietary calcium is preferable; however, supplements can help a woman meet the recommended dose of 1000–1200 milligrams per day. (See Chapter 9.) The skin manufactures vitamin D after exposure to sunlight; vitamin D–fortified milk, cereal, egg yolks, saltwater fish, and liver can also provide vitamin D through the diet. Those people who cannot obtain enough vitamin D naturally should include 200–600 IU (International Units) in their diets per day.

Regular weight-bearing and muscle-strengthening exercises are important for osteoporosis prevention and overall health. These exercises improve agility, strength, and balance, thus reducing a woman's risk of falls and decreasing her risk of fractures. Weight-bearing exercises (exercises in which bones and muscles work against gravity) include walking, hiking, jogging, stair climbing,

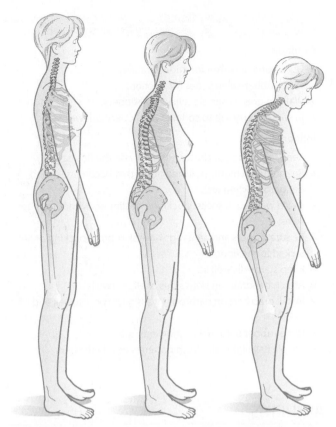

Osteoporosis in the vertebrae can cause women to lose height and cause a curving of the spine.

dancing, and tennis. Muscle-strengthening exercise, such as weight-lifting, improves muscle mass and bone strength. Treatment involves managing osteoporosis-associated fractures, universal prevention measures, and medical treatment of the underlying disease. Current osteoporosis recommendations indicate that women 50 and older who have had osteoporotic vertebral or hip fractures and those with a bone mineral density diagnosis of osteoporosis should receive treatment. In women with a bone mineral density above the osteoporosis range, treatment may be indicated depending on the number and severity of other risk factors.[16] The Food and Drug Administration (FDA) has approved several classes of medications that can help reduce or prevent the progress of osteoporosis; women with osteoporosis or who are at risk for developing osteoporosis should speak with their healthcare providers about these treatments.

Preventing fall-related fractures is a special concern for women with osteoporosis. Many factors can cause falls, including impaired vision or balance, certain chronic diseases, and certain medications. A woman with osteoporosis should be aware of any factors that may affect her balance or gait, and she should discuss these changes with her healthcare provider. Making some simple adjustments to one's living area and behaviors can also greatly lower risk of falls (**Table 11.3**).

Table 11.3 Tips for Fall Prevention
Outdoors
▪ Use a cane or walker for added stability.
▪ Wear rubber-soled shoes for traction.
▪ Walk on grass when sidewalks are slippery.
▪ In winter, carry salt to sprinkle on slippery sidewalks.
Indoors
▪ Keep rooms free of clutter, especially on the floors.
▪ Be careful on highly polished floors that become slick and dangerous when wet.
▪ Avoid walking in socks, stockings, or slippers without rubber soles.
▪ Be sure carpets and area rugs have skid-proof backing or are tacked to the floor.
▪ Keep stairwells well lit.
▪ Attach handrails on both sides of all stairwells.
▪ Install grab bars on bathroom walls near tub, shower, and toilet.
▪ Use a rubber bath mat in shower or tub.
▪ Keep a flashlight with fresh batteries beside the bed.

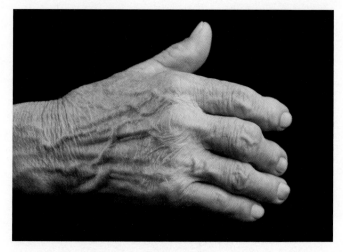

Arthritis can be physically debilitating as well as painful.
© Catalin Petolea/Dreamstime.com

ARTHRITIS

The term arthritis, which means "inflamed joints," includes more than 100 diseases and conditions that affect joints, the surrounding tissues, and other connective tissues. **Arthritis** affects about 50 million adults in the United States, making it the most common cause of disability in the country. Common forms of arthritis are osteoarthritis, rheumatoid arthritis, and gout. The underlying cause of arthritis can result from injury, wear and tear on the joints, an autoimmune response, or a bacterial or viral infection. No matter the cause, however, similar processes occur in the joints as the disease develops. Healthy joints are usually protected by cartilage, a flexible connective tissue, and synovial fluid, a viscous, protective fluid. Cartilage and synovial fluid cushion joints from impacts and allow them to move smoothly. If something damages or wears down the cartilage and synovial fluid, the bones may rub together, and stiffness, rigidity, and pain during movement may result. Eventually a scar between the bones may develop, resulting in joint deformity.

Arthritis and other rheumatic conditions (conditions affecting the joints and muscles) are among the most common chronic conditions and the leading causes of disability in the United States. Arthritis affects more than one out of five adults, most of whom are women, and limits the activity of more than 20 million Americans. The prevalence of arthritis will continue to increase as the population ages. Although aging is a risk factor, nearly two-thirds of people with arthritis are younger than 65 years of age. By 2030, 67 million Americans 18 years or older will have doctor-diagnosed arthritis.[17]

Osteoarthritis

Osteoarthritis, also called degenerative joint disease, is the most common form of arthritis, affecting more than 27 million people. A milder form of arthritis than rheumatoid arthritis, it is seen in all age groups but is most common among older adults. Osteoarthritis is more common in women than in men, especially after age 50.[18]

In osteoarthritis, the surface layer of cartilage erodes, causing bones under the cartilage to rub together. This friction causes joint pain, swelling, and loss of movement of the joints. This disease most often affects the knees, but it also affects the hips, hands, neck, lower back, and other joints. Hip and knee osteoarthritis are the leading causes of arthritis disability and the primary reasons for joint replacement surgery.

Rheumatoid Arthritis

Rheumatoid arthritis is a chronic inflammatory disease with increasing prevalence among older adults. It currently affects 1.5 million people in the United States, and is two to three times more common in women than in men.[19]

Rheumatoid arthritis is an autoimmune disease, meaning that the person's immune system attacks the body's own cells. The exact causes for this immune response are still unknown. In this condition, the immune system attacks the cells inside the synovial fluid and cartilage in the joint, causing inflammation, pain, and swelling. Eventually, the synovial fluid and cartilage may be mostly destroyed (**Figure 11.3**), which can lead to severe disability. In addition to attacking the joint lining, the immune system may also attack other tissues. If a faulty immune response affects other organs, such as the lung and the heart, a person may be more likely to die from respiratory and infectious diseases. Rheumatoid arthritis generally occurs in a symmetrical pattern, meaning that it will involve both the left and right hands, not just one of them. The disease varies significantly between

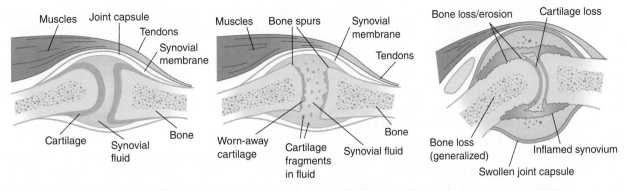

Figure 11.3   Left to right: healthy joint, joint affected by osteoarthritis, and joint affected by rheumatoid arthritis.

individuals: Some people have flare-ups followed by periods of remission, whereas others have severe disease that is continuously active. Rheumatoid arthritis can also go away and not return.

> *I am twenty-three, and I have arthritis. Sometimes I am frightened that I will end up with gnarled hands like my grandmother. I hope that new treatments will prevent my disease progression.*
>
> **—23-year-old student**

Gout

Gout is a painful and potentially disabling form of arthritis that was first described more than 2000 years ago by the Greek physician Hippocrates. Unlike other forms of arthritis, which are typically persistent, symptoms of gout can appear, typically for a few days or a few weeks, and then disappear for long periods. However, when symptoms are present, they can be quite painful and debilitating.

Gout is caused by an excess of uric acid in the body. This excess can result from an increased production of uric acid due to a metabolic disorder or the inability of the kidneys to adequately clear uric acid. Consumption of certain foods (such as shellfish) and an excess of alcoholic beverages may increase uric acid levels and precipitate gout attacks, but studies are not conclusive on these associations. Some medications and transplant drugs can also increase uric acid levels. With time, elevated levels of uric acid in the blood may be deposited around joints, especially in the feet and toes. Eventually, the uric acid may form needle-like crystals in joints, leading to acute painful gout attacks. Uric acid may also collect under the skin, where it is known as tophus, or in the urinary tract as kidney stones.

About 8.3 million people in the United States have gout.[19] While gout and its complications occur more commonly in men, gout is also common among women who have experienced menopause and people with kidney disease. Gout is strongly associated with obesity, hypertension, hyperlipidemia, and diabetes. Some families have a genetic predisposition to gout. African Americans and people with poor kidney function are more likely to have gout attacks.

Diagnosing gout can be difficult because infections or other kinds of arthritis can mimic a gout attack. Given that its treatment is specific to gout, proper diagnosis is essential. The definitive diagnosis of gout depends on finding uric acid crystals in the joint fluid during an acute attack. However, uric acid levels in the blood alone are often misleading and may provide "false positive" (indicating gout when it is not present) or "false negative" (missing gout when it exists) results.

Treatments can now control most cases of gout; however, because of their potential side effects, individual patients often work with their healthcare providers to find a treatment that is best for them. Colchicine has been a standard treatment for acute gout since the 1800s. However, while colchicine is effective, it can cause nausea, vomiting, diarrhea, and other side effects. Because of these side effects, nonsteroidal anti-inflammatory drugs (NSAIDs) have become the treatment of choice for most acute attacks of gout. NSAIDs may also have significant toxicity, but if used over a short term, they are generally well tolerated. However, some people are unable to take NSAIDs because of other medical factors such as ulcer disease, poor kidney function, or use of blood thinners. Elderly patients often cannot tolerate NSAIDs because of their multiple side effects. Corticosteroid-type medications are also used to treat gout attacks and can be given as pills or by injection. Decisions about appropriate treatments must be tailored to the individual and depend on his or her kidney function and other medical factors. With correct treatment, gout can be well controlled in almost all cases.

Risk Factors

Arthritis is the leading chronic condition among women and a major cause of activity limitation.[20] Risk for arthritis increases with age, with nearly half of the elderly population being affected by some form of arthritis. Some people are genetically predisposed to arthritis, placing them at higher risk for developing the disease. Other risk factors are modifiable, although altering these factors does not guarantee prevention. Obesity, which increases the risk of many types of arthritis, is one such factor. Among persons who are obese, 33.8% of women reported doctor-diagnosed arthritis.[21] Joint injuries from sports, infectious diseases such as Lyme disease, and occupations that require repetitive joint use and knee bending are other factors that increase a person's risk of arthritis. Because women are more likely than men to have rheumatoid arthritis, researchers have been studying the role of hormones in the development of the disease, though investigations conducted to date have produced contradictory results. **Table 11.4** summarizes the major risk factors associated with arthritis.

Arthritis is not uniformly distributed across the United States. The reasons for the inequitable distribution are unclear but are the subject of ongoing research. As **Figure 11.4** shows, arthritis is most common in the Midwest and the South, but arthritis affects at least one in six adults in every state.

Symptoms

Symptoms of arthritis depend on the specific disease affecting the joints. Osteoarthritis evolves slowly. Early in the disease, joints may ache after physical work or exercise. Small bony knobs may appear on the joints of the fingers, causing the fingers to become enlarged, gnarled, achy, stiff, and numb. Osteoarthritis in the knees or hips may make it difficult for a person to walk or bend. Rheumatoid arthritis is typically the most painful, disabling

form of arthritis. Symptoms, which include pain, stiffness, and swelling of multiple joints, do not always respond to treatment. As a result of these symptoms, people with arthritis typically lead inactive or less active lives, placing them at greater risk for other diseases, including heart disease, hypertension, diabetes, colon cancer, obesity, depression, and anxiety.

Diagnosis

No single test can diagnose arthritis. Instead, healthcare providers use a variety of tools, such as a medical history, family history, and physical exams to check the joints, reflexes, and muscle strength. Radiographs can determine the amount of damage done to a joint by showing cartilage loss, bone damage, and bone spurs. In the early stages of arthritis, before damage is evident, radiographs are not useful; however, they are helpful in later stages for monitoring the progression of the disease. Blood tests to determine the cause of the symptoms, a test for rheumatoid factor (an antibody present in most rheumatoid arthritis patients), and a joint aspiration (drawing fluid from the joint for examination) may also be used for diagnosing arthritis.

Prevention and Treatment

Maintaining an appropriate weight is an important preventive measure. For people who are overweight or obese, losing weight through healthful eating and regular exercise also can help reduce the effects of osteoarthritis. Taking precautions during exercise can also reduce the chance of joint injury. Women should participate in warm-up and cool-down periods when performing any type of exercise or sports-related activities. They should also incorporate strength-training exercises into their routines. Other methods for preventing joint injury and damage to ligaments and cartilage, which in turn can prevent osteoarthritis, include avoiding contact sports and repetitive joint motion; wearing braces, pads, and proper shoes; and exercising on appropriate surfaces. Regular exercise decreases impairment by increasing muscle and joint function. Research has shown that weakness in a woman's quadriceps muscles is a risk factor for osteoarthritis of the knee, and that exercise can significantly benefit knee osteoarthritis pathology.[22]

Another cause of arthritis is **Lyme disease**, a disease caused by the bacterium *Borrelia burgdorferi*. These bacteria are transmitted to humans by the bite of infected deer ticks. About 30,000 cases of Lyme disease are reported each year; however, studies suggest that the number of people diagnosed with Lyme disease each year in the United States is around 300,000.[23] After several months of being infected, more than half of people who are not treated with antibiotics experience recurrent attacks of painful and swollen joints. About 10 to 20% of these people develop chronic arthritis.[24] Strategies to prevent Lyme disease include using insect repellants, wearing long-sleeved shirts and pants when walking in wooded

---

Table 11.4   Risk Factors for Arthritis

Modifiable Risk Factors

- Overweight and obesity: Overweight and obesity can contribute to both the appearance and development of knee osteoarthritis.
- Joint injuries: Damage to a joint increases the likelihood that osteoarthritis will develop in that joint.
- Infection: Bacteria and viruses can infect joints and cause the development of some kinds of arthritis.
- Occupation: Jobs involving repetitive knee bending can lead to osteoarthritis of the knee.

Nonmodifiable Risk Factors

- Age: The risk of developing most types of arthritis increases with age.
- Gender: About 60% of arthritis cases develop in women.
- Genetics: Some genes are associated with rheumatoid arthritis and other types of arthritis.

Source: Modified from Centers for Disease Control and Prevention (CDC). (2014). Available at: http://www.cdc.gov/arthritis/basics/risk_factors.htm

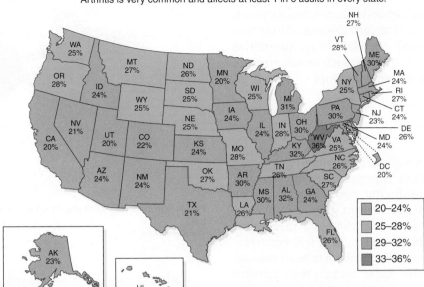

Arthritis is very common and affects at least 1 in 6 adults in every state.

Age-adjusted population prevalence of arthritis among adults ages ≥18 years, 2013 BRFSS.

Figure 11.4 **Percentage of adults with arthritis, 2013.**

Source: Reproduced from Centers for Disease Control and Prevention. (2013). *Arthritis prevalence estimates by state, Behavioral Risk Factor Surveillance System 2013.* Available at: http://www.cdc.gov/arthritis/data_statistics/state-data-current.htm

areas, and checking one's body for ticks immediately upon return.

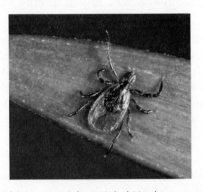

Infected deer ticks can transmit bacteria by biting humans, causing Lyme disease, which has many possible adverse outcomes, including arthritis.
Courtesy of Jim Gathany/CDC

The goals of treating arthritis are to decrease pain, improve joint care by slowing down or stopping joint damage, and improve a person's sense of well-being and ability to function. Exercise is one of the best treatments for arthritis. Physical activity supports healthy and strong muscles, preserves joint mobility, and maintains flexibility. It is important to exercise when pain is least severe and to recognize when rest is necessary. Resting the body reduces active joint inflammation and pain and prevents pain from overexercising. Canes, splints, or braces can temporarily take pressure off joints or provide extra support. Controlling body weight through a healthful diet also helps reduce stress on weight-bearing joints and limit further injury.

Many people with osteoarthritis or rheumatoid arthritis use medications to reduce pain and inflammation, as well as to prevent joint damage, including:

- NSAIDs, either in prescription or over-the-counter form, can reduce pain, swelling, and inflammation.

- Topical pain-relieving creams, rubs, and sprays, such as those containing capsaicin, can be applied directly to the skin to relieve pain.

- Corticosteroids (anti-inflammatory hormones) can provide short-term relief of pain, stiffness, and swelling and can reduce the risk of joint swelling.

- Hyaluronic acid, a medication for joint injection, can relieve pain associated with osteoarthritis of the knee.

- For rheumatoid arthritis, disease-modifying anti-rheumatic drugs (DMARDs) may produce significant improvement. DMARDs can alter the course of rheumatoid arthritis and prevent joint and cartilage destruction. These medications, however, can cause serious side effects and are not appropriate for everyone.

- Biologic response modifiers (BRMs) inhibit proteins called cytokines that contribute to inflammation and joint damage in rheumatoid arthritis. BRMs must be injected under the skin or given as an infusion into a vein.

- Immunosuppressants appear to be very effective in restraining the active immune system, the causal factor behind rheumatoid arthritis. These medications can cause side effects, however, and their effectiveness appears to diminish over time.

Surgery can also be a treatment option for arthritis. Surgery can resurface and reposition bones, replace joints, remove loose pieces of bone or cartilage, reconstruct tendons, or remove inflamed synovial tissue. Alternative methods of treatment for arthritis, such as acupuncture and yoga, can also help relieve symptoms.

DIABETES

Diabetes is a disease characterized by abnormal glucose production or metabolism. A person with diabetes has either a deficiency of insulin (the hormone produced by the pancreas and needed to convert glucose to energy) or a decreased ability to use insulin. As a result, glucose builds up in the bloodstream, and, without treatment, will damage organs and contribute to heart disease. Cells without glucose also starve without their primary source of energy, leading to fatigue, irritability, and other symptoms. Diabetes has become an extremely harmful and pervasive epidemic; it is now the seventh leading cause of death in the United States. Additionally, every year, millions of people experience diabetes-related complications, including blindness, nerve damage, lower-limb amputations, kidney failure, heart disease, and stroke.[4]

There are three major kinds of diabetes: type 1, type 2, and gestational diabetes. Type 1 diabetes is often classified as an autoimmune disease, though genetic and environmental factors can also influence its development. In this type of diabetes, the body's immune system attacks the cells that produce insulin, the hormone that regulates blood glucose. Type 1 diabetes often first appears in childhood or adolescence, and it accounts for about 5% of total cases of diabetes. About 90 to 95% of people with diabetes have type 2 diabetes. In this form of diabetes, cells develop insulin resistance, meaning that cells need increasing doses of insulin in order to absorb and use glucose. **Gestational diabetes** occurs when women become intolerant to glucose during pregnancy. After pregnancy, gestational diabetes usually goes away but may return during later pregnancies or as type 2 diabetes. Women who have had gestational diabetes are at an increased risk of developing type 2 diabetes within the next 5 to 10 years.

Most people with type 1 diabetes develop the disease early in life, while type 2 diabetes generally occurs later in life; however, the rise in childhood obesity is leading to a dramatic surge in the incidence of type 2 diabetes among children and adolescents.

In 2012, 29.1 million people, or 9.3% of the U.S. population, had diabetes.[4] More than 8 million of those 29.1 million were undiagnosed. **Figure 11.5** shows the number of people diagnosed with diabetes over the past 30 years. According to the most recent analysis by the Centers for Disease Control and Prevention (CDC):

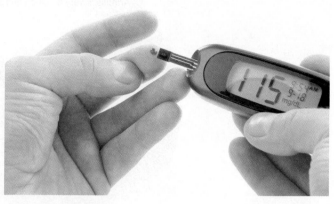

People with diabetes should check their blood sugar levels on a regular basis.
© Dmitry Lobanov/Shutterstock

- Almost one-half of people with diabetes are female. About 11.2% of women age 20 or older have diabetes.

- Women of color are the hardest hit by type 2 and gestational diabetes.

- The prevalence of diabetes is highest in American Indians/Alaska Natives (15.9%), followed by non-Hispanic Blacks (13.2%), Hispanics (12.8%), Asian Americans (9.0%), and then non-Hispanic Whites (7.6%).

- The risk of diabetic ketoacidosis (DKA), often called diabetic coma, is 50% higher among women than men.

- Heart disease is the leading cause of diabetes-related death; at least 65% of people with diabetes die from some form of heart disease or stroke. Adults with diabetes have heart disease rates and risk for stroke rates that are about two to four times higher than adults without diabetes.[25]

My grandmother had diabetes, but she was not always good about taking care of herself. She always loved taking us out for ice cream when I was a girl, and I worry that these habits may have contributed to her stroke. I also worry about myself and my father—a strong sweet tooth runs in our family—but I don't want either of us to suffer like my grandmother did.

—24-year-old woman

Researchers have also identified *prediabetes*, a condition in which a person has abnormally high blood glucose levels but does not have diabetes. An estimated 86 million adults in the United States—about 37% of all U.S. adults aged 20 or older—had prediabetes in 2012.[4] Prediabetes often progresses to type 2 diabetes, but weight loss and regular exercise can prevent or delay this progression.

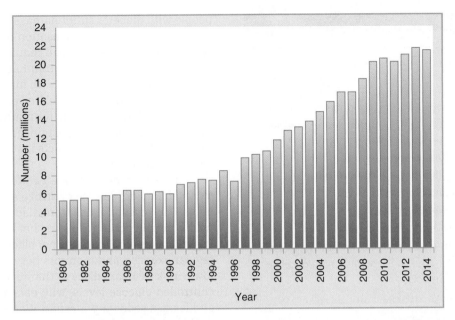

Figure 11.5 Number of persons with diagnosed diabetes, United States. The number of people with diabetes in the United States has more than tripled over the past 30 years. Because this figure shows only diagnosed cases, the true number of cases is even higher than this estimate.

Sources: Data from Centers for Disease Control and Prevention. (2015). *Diabetes public health resource*. Available at: http://www.cdc.gov/diabetes/statistics/prev/national/figpersons.htm; CDC, National Center for Health Statistics, Division of Health Interview Statistics. *National Health Interview Survey*; Statistical analysis by CDC, National Center for Chronic Disease Prevention and Health Promotion, Division of Diabetes Translation.

> *I was diagnosed with diabetes at the age of five. I still remember being in the hospital and how scared I was. My father died young from diabetes complications. I am determined to learn as much as I can to take care of myself.*
>
> **—32-year-old woman**

Risk Factors

Risk factors for diabetes include having a first-degree relative (mother, father, or sibling) with diabetes, and, for type 2 diabetes, being overweight, having hypertension, or having abnormal high-density lipoprotein (HDL) or triglyceride levels. African Americans, Hispanics, and American Indians/Alaska Natives are at increased risk for developing type 2 diabetes (see Figure 11.1). American Indians have the highest rate of diabetes in the United States.[4] **It's Your Health** provides a checklist of factors to ascertain personal risk for diabetes.

Symptoms and Complications

Symptoms of type 1 diabetes usually develop over a short period of time. Symptoms include increased thirst and urination, constant hunger, weight loss, blurred vision, and extreme fatigue. A person with type 1 diabetes needs insulin on a regular basis to survive. Without insulin, a person can lapse into a coma and will eventually die. Symptoms of type 2 diabetes develop gradually. Although they are not as noticeable as symptoms of type 1 disease,

type 2 symptoms are similar and include frequent urination, unusual thirst, weight loss, blurred vision, feelings of fatigue or illness, frequent infections, and slow healing of sores.

The most alarming part of diabetes is the severity of the complications associated with the disease (**Table 11.5**). Diabetes is the leading cause of new cases of blindness in adults 20 to 74 years of age: Each year, an estimated 12,000 to 24,000 people become blind because of diabetic eye disease. Early detection and treatment can prevent

Table 11.5   Complications of Diabetes
■ Heart disease: including peripheral vascular disease, coronary heart disease, and cardiac failure
■ Stroke
■ High blood pressure
■ Retinopathy (broken blood vessels in retina)/blindness
■ End-stage renal disease (kidney failure)
■ Damage of the nervous system
■ Lower-extremity amputations
■ Periodontal disease
■ Congenital malformations/spontaneous abortions
■ Neonatal mortality
■ Macrosomia (large-birth-weight babies)
■ Diabetic ketoacidosis (coma)
■ Susceptibility to infections and illness, such as pneumonia

It's Your Health

Am I at Risk for Diabetes?

- I am 45 or older.
- I am overweight.
- I have a parent, brother, or sister with diabetes.
- My family background is Alaska Native, American Indian, African American, Hispanic/Latino American, Asian American, or Pacific Islander.
- I have had gestational diabetes, or I gave birth to at least one baby weighing more than 9 pounds.
- My blood pressure is 140/90 mm Hg or higher, or I have been told that I have high blood pressure.
- My cholesterol levels are not normal. My HDL cholesterol ("good" cholesterol) is below 35 mg/dL or my triglyceride level is above 250 mg/dL.
- I am fairly inactive. I exercise fewer than three times per week.
- I have polycystic ovary syndrome (women only).
- On previous testing, I had impaired glucose tolerance (IGT) or impaired fasting glucose (IFG).
- I have other clinical conditions associated with insulin resistance (acanthosis nigricans).
- I have a history of cardiovascular disease.

The more items you checked, the higher your risk.

Anyone 45 years old or older should consider getting tested for diabetes. If you are 45 or older and overweight, getting tested is strongly recommended. If you are younger than 45, are overweight, and have one or more of the risk factors above, you should consider testing. Ask your doctor for a fasting blood glucose test or an oral glucose tolerance test. Your doctor will tell you if you have normal blood glucose, prediabetes, or diabetes.

Source: Centers for Disease Control and Prevention (CDC). (Page last updated 2015). *Women at High Risk for Diabetes: Physical Activity, Healthy Eating, and Weight Loss.* Available at: http://www.cdc.gov/diabetes/pubs /pdf/womenHighRiskDiabetes.pdf

people with diabetes suffer damage to their nervous system, including impaired sensation or pain in the feet. If severe, the nerve damage can require lower-limb amputation. More than 60% of nontraumatic lower-limb amputations occur among people with diabetes.[4] Amputations are also caused by infection related to nonhealing diabetic foot ulcers. New treatments for nonhealing diabetic foot ulcers include genetically engineered replacement dermis, growth hormone products, and better wound management programs.

Adults with diabetes are two to four times as likely to develop heart disease or stroke as those without diabetes. The additional risk from diabetes is related to how well a person cares for his or her condition. A woman with diabetes who manages her blood glucose levels, gets regular exercise, and monitors her diet will have a much lower risk of heart disease than a woman with poorly controlled glucose levels, who eats an unhealthful diet and leads a sedentary lifestyle. Women with poorly controlled diabetes also are at risk of diabetic ketoacidosis (DKA), a serious condition in which acid levels increase in the blood. Diabetes is known to affect brain function and increase the risk for cognitive decline, dementia, depression, and stroke. These complications frequently occur together, leading to poor quality of life and compounding the need for medical care. Diabetes, often associated with high blood pressure, may contribute to cognitive decline in elderly diabetics as well as to increased frequency and severity of cerebral vascular events.[26,27]

Pregnancy presents special risks to diabetic women. Women are more likely to have healthy pregnancies if their diabetes is well controlled before they become pregnant and throughout the pregnancy. The risk of serious congenital malformations and macrosomia (large birth weight) in babies born to mothers with diabetes is greater than in the general population. Due to the increased incidence of babies with high birth weight, women with diabetes are three to four times more likely to have a cesarean delivery than are women without diabetes. In addition, stillbirths among women with diabetes are five times greater than for women who do not have diabetes.[28]

Diagnosis

The routine test for diagnosing diabetes is a fasting plasma glucose test. A doctor may choose to perform an oral glucose tolerance test, which involves a fasting blood sample followed by numerous blood samples after glucose syrup is ingested. The "gold standard" for diagnosing diabetes is an elevated blood sugar level after an overnight fast (not eating anything after midnight). A value above 126 mg/dL on at least two occasions typically means a person has diabetes. People without diabetes have fasting sugar levels that generally run between 70 and 110 mg/dL. A fasting glucose level of 100 to 125 mg/dL indicates prediabetes, as well as a higher chance of developing type 2 diabetes in the future.[29]

90% of these cases of blindness. Diabetes is also the leading cause of end-stage renal disease (ESRD) or kidney failure, accounting for about 44% of new cases. At least half of the new cases of diabetes-related kidney failure could be prevented each year. Severe complications of diabetes, however, should not be considered an unavoidable part of diabetes. With proper care and management, most diabetes complications can be prevented.

Because the high glucose levels of unregulated diabetes can literally thicken the blood, people with diabetes often develop complications relating to poor circulation. As a result, many people have trouble healing from injuries, especially in their extremities. About 60 to 70% of

Prevention and Treatment

Managing type 1 diabetes requires a regimen of multiple daily insulin injections, a carefully calculated diet, planned physical activity, and home blood glucose testing several times a day. Treatment of type 2 diabetes is also based on diet control, exercise, and blood glucose testing, and for some people may entail oral medications or insulin. Daily management is important to prevent blood sugar levels from going too high or too low. A person with diabetes should eat a healthful diet and monitor the amount of carbohydrates (starches and sugars) that he or she eats. Because simple carbohydrates, such as sugars and refined grains, can quickly raise blood glucose levels, their consumption should be limited. If blood sugar levels rise too high, as in **hyperglycemia**, a person may become very ill. Early signs of hyperglycemia include high blood sugar, high levels of sugar in the urine, frequent urination, and increased thirst. Hyperglycemia should be treated as an emergency situation and emergency services (such as 911) should be called immediately. The opposite problem, **hypoglycemia** (low blood sugar levels), may occur if a person with diabetes takes too much insulin. Hypoglycemia can cause a person to become nervous, shaky, or confused, or even to pass out. Consumption of food or drink with sugar in it can counteract low blood sugar.

FIBROMYALGIA

Fibromyalgia is a disease characterized by pain. People with fibromyalgia experience widespread pain throughout their bodies for most, if not all, of their waking lives. This pain lowers quality of life and reduces peoples' ability to function. Other symptoms associated with fibromyalgia include fatigue, depression, trouble sleeping, headaches, tingling or numbness in the limbs, and irritable bowel syndrome. The causes of fibromyalgia are largely unknown. One theory is that people with fibromyalgia have a low pain threshold, meaning that the brain overinterprets stimuli as pain. Some evidence indicates that fibromyalgia may develop after certain viral infections; from sudden trauma to the brain, as an autoimmune response; or through a combination of physical and emotional stressors.

About 5 million people in the United States, or about 2% of the population, have fibromyalgia.[30] Accurate estimates are difficult, however, because the condition often goes undiagnosed. This may be because the symptoms are nonspecific or because providers believe that the condition is "all in the head" of the sufferer (it was not until 1990 that the medical community recognized fibromyalgia as a genuine, diagnosable condition). Diagnosis of fibromyalgia is made if a person feels pain in response to a firm touch in 11 out of 18 defined points on the head, legs, chest, and arms, and if other conditions are ruled out.

Fibromyalgia is about seven times more common in women than it is in men. It is most likely to appear during or after middle age, though it also appears among young adults. Other risk factors include obesity, repetitive injuries, and having rheumatoid arthritis, lupus, or family history of fibromyalgia.[30]

Although fibromyalgia is rarely deadly, it can be an extremely debilitating condition. On average, working adults with fibromyalgia miss three times the number of days from work due to illness as people without fibromyalgia. On average, people with fibromyalgia also incur about $3500 a year in medical bills.[30]

Treatment for fibromyalgia focuses on managing and learning to live with symptoms. Medications, such as acetaminophen (Tylenol), antidepressants, and anti-seizure drugs, may help some people with fibromyalgia. However, the effects of these medications are modest, usually reducing pain by 30 to 50% in about one-half of patients.[31] Regular physical exercise appears to reduce pain and insomnia and improve quality of life; exercise also provides the same benefits to people with fibromyalgia as it does to people without the condition. Cognitive-behavioral therapy (CBT), in which the patient works with a psychologist to develop and maintain healthful thoughts and behaviors, helps to reduce symptoms and helps people cope with them. A multimodal approach to treatment that includes medication, exercise, and CBT appears to provide the most overall benefits.

AUTOIMMUNE DISEASES

Autoimmune diseases are those diseases in which the immune system attacks normal components of the body. More than 80 serious, chronic illnesses are collectively referred to as autoimmune diseases, and these diseases involve the nervous, gastrointestinal, and endocrine systems, as well as skin and other connective tissue, eyes, blood, and blood vessels. Autoimmune diseases are about three times more common in women than they are in men, and they most frequently first manifest during the childbearing years.[32] Autoimmune diseases include multiple sclerosis, type 1 diabetes, scleroderma, rheumatoid arthritis, thyroid disorders, Sjögren's syndrome, and systemic lupus erythematosus (SLE). Rheumatoid arthritis, type 1 diabetes, SLE, and thyroid disease are the most common autoimmune diseases. Together, autoimmune diseases represent the fourth-largest cause of disability among women in the United States.[32]

Lupus

Lupus is an autoimmune disease that is still not fully understood. In patients with lupus, the immune system forms antibodies that target healthy tissues and organs. Lupus can be a mild, moderate, or severe disease. Although lupus may affect men and women of any age, it is primarily a disease that affects women during their childbearing years. Lupus affects women 10 to 15 times more often than it does men, and it affects African American women 2 to 3 times more often than it does White women.[33]

Lupus presents in three forms. Discoid lupus, also known as cutaneous lupus, only affects the skin and causes a rash that usually appears on the face and upper body. Only about 10% of people with discoid lupus will progress to the systemic form of lupus, which can involve any organ or system of the body. Systemic lupus erythematosus (SLE) is the most common and more severe form of the disease; it is characterized by unpredictable periods of disease activity and periods of symptom-free remission. SLE can affect many parts of the body, including joints, skin, kidneys, lungs, heart, blood vessels, nervous system, blood, and brain. Drug-induced lupus is a reaction to some prescription medicines. The symptoms of this type of lupus are similar to SLE but do not affect the kidneys or central nervous system. Drug-induced lupus usually disappears when the medication is discontinued.

Risk Factors

The cause of lupus is unknown, although genetic, hormonal, and environmental factors appear to play a role.

Lupus is known to occur within families, although no specific gene for it has been found. Environmental factors, including infections, exposure to sunlight, stress, and certain medications, play a role in triggering flare-ups of the disease. Because the cause of lupus is unknown, it has been difficult to determine its risk factors.

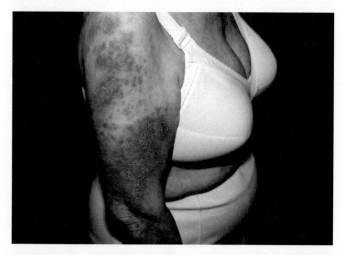

A rash is a common symptom of lupus.
© Custom Medical Stock Photo/Alamy Stock Photo

Symptoms

Lupus has been called "the great imitator" because of its varied symptoms, which often mimic other, less serious illnesses. Lupus is characterized by periods of remission when no symptoms are present. The two most common symptoms are painful, swollen joints and a skin rash. In addition to being nonspecific, symptoms of lupus vary from person to person because lupus can affect any organ or organ system. Although lupus can affect any part of the body, most people experience symptoms in only a few organs.

The origins of lupus remain a mystery and have been the subject of considerable speculation and research. Cigarette smoking is one type of environmental exposure hypothesized to be linked to the development of SLE, as are exposures to infectious agents, silica, and ultraviolet light; hormonal and dietary factors such as vitamin D deficiency are also believed to be connected to development of the disease.[34] However, the root causes of lupus likely involve more than these factors.

Diagnosis

The clinical diagnosis of systemic lupus involves noting potential symptoms, such as skin rash, joint pain, chest pain, seizures, and photosensitivity, and reviewing a person's history of medications. A complete blood count and urinalysis may provide evidence of the involvement of the kidneys and blood vessels. The antinuclear antibody (ANA) test may be used to rule out a diagnosis of lupus, as it is positive in virtually all people with lupus and is the best diagnostic tool available for lupus. Antinuclear antibody is not a definitive test, however, because other illnesses, certain medications, or other factors can produce a "false positive" for ANA in a person without lupus.

Treatment and Prevention

Lupus is characterized by periods of symptoms called "flare-ups." The symptoms are unpredictable and inconsistent when they present.

Women with lupus can take preventive measures to help prevent flare-ups. People who are photosensitive should avoid sun exposure and regularly use sunscreen to prevent rashes. Exercise is important to prevent muscle weakness and fatigue, while support groups, counseling, meditation, and other techniques can help to reduce stress. Treatment usually involves nonsteroidal anti-inflammatory drugs (NSAIDs) to ease muscle and joint pain. Corticosteroids are used on a short-term basis to treat skin rashes. Some people find antimalarial agents, such as Plaquenil or Aralen, are helpful for skin and joint symptoms as well as oral ulcers. Immunosuppressant drugs may be used in serious cases of lupus, when major organs are losing their ability to function. These drugs suppress, or turn down, the immune system to limit the damage done to the organ(s) and reduce inflammation. Serious side effects may occur with their use, including nausea, vomiting, hair loss, bladder problems, decreased fertility, and increased risk of cancer and infection.

THYROID DISEASE

The thyroid is a small gland, shaped like a butterfly, located in the middle of the lower neck. Its primary function is to control the body's metabolism—the rate at which cells perform duties essential to living. To control body metabolism, the thyroid produces two hormones, T_4 and T_3, that regulate cell energy.

A properly functioning thyroid will maintain the right amount of hormones needed to keep the body's metabolism functioning at a steady state. The pituitary gland, located in the center of the skull below the brain, monitors and controls the quantity of thyroid hormones in the bloodstream. When the pituitary gland senses either a lack of thyroid hormones or a high level of thyroid hormones, it will adjust its own thyroid-stimulating hormone (TSH) and send messages to the thyroid to regulate hormone production.

Thyroiditis is an inflammation of the thyroid gland (**Figure 11.6**). When the thyroid produces too much hormone, the body uses energy faster than it should; this condition is called hyperthyroidism. When the thyroid doesn't produce enough hormone, the body uses energy more slowly than it should; this condition is called hypothyroidism. An estimated 20 million Americans have overactive or underactive thyroid glands, and more than half of them go undiagnosed. Women are five to eight times more likely than men to have thyroid problems.[35]

Hypothyroidism results from an underactive thyroid. Hypothyroidism can be caused by a lack of iodine in the diet. Another common cause is a condition known as Hashimoto's thyroiditis, or Hashimoto's disease. This autoimmune condition occurs when the immune system reacts against the thyroid gland. About 4.6% of the U.S. population has hypothyroidism; women are more likely than men to develop hypothyroidism and the disease is more common among people age 60 and older.[36] Because people with hypothyroidism lack enough thyroid hormones to properly run their metabolisms, they often have symptoms associated with having low energy. (See **Table 11.6** for a full list of symptoms.)

Hyperthyroidism occurs when the body produces too much thyroid hormone. Because the excess of thyroid hormone increases the body's metabolism by as much as 60 to 100%, people with hyperthyroidism often feel symptoms associated with being overstimulated.[36] Graves' disease, an autoimmune disorder in which the immune system stimulates the thyroid, causes about 80% of hyperthyroid cases. Like hypothyroidism, hyperthyroidism is more common in women than in men. People with hyperthyroidism may develop moderate to severe eye problems, which may cause bulging of the eyes, blurring of vision, or damage to the eyes. (See Table 11.6 for a full list of symptoms.)

Risk Factors

Both Hashimoto's disease and Graves' disease are inherited conditions. Women over 20 years old are at an increased risk for these conditions, though the disorders

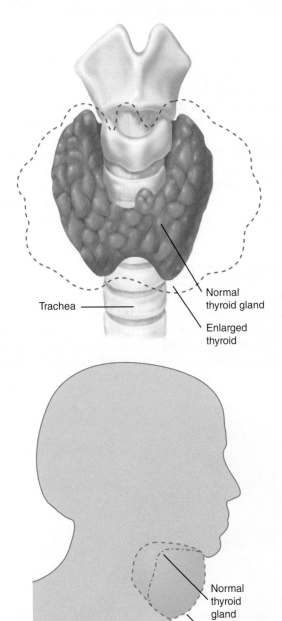

Trachea —

Normal thyroid gland

Enlarged thyroid

Normal thyroid gland

Enlarged thyroid

Figure 11.6 Thyroiditis.

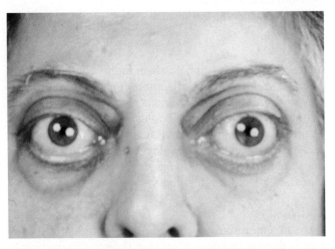

There are many symptoms of Graves' disease, including increased appetite, weight loss, nervousness, insomnia, and bulging appearance of the eyes.
© Chet Childs/Custom Medical Stock Photo

Table 11.6	Symptoms of Hypothyroidism and Hyperthyroidism

Many people have no symptoms.

Hypothyroidism

- Fatigue
- Sensitivity to cold
- Constipation
- Dry skin
- Difficulty concentrating
- Unexplained weight gain or difficulty losing weight
- Puffy face
- Hoarseness or difficulty swallowing
- Muscle weakness, cramping, and achiness
- Elevated blood cholesterol level
- Muscle aches, tenderness, and stiffness
- Pain, stiffness, or swelling in the joints
- Heavier or irregular menstrual periods
- Coarse, dry, or thinning hair (hair loss)
- Slowed heart rate
- Depression
- Irritability
- Impaired memory
- Decreased libido

Hyperthyroidism

- Sudden weight loss
- Rapid heartbeat (tachycardia), irregular heartbeat (arrhythmia), or heart palpitations
- Change in appetite
- Feeling nervous or irritable
- Tremor or shakiness
- Sweating more than normal
- Lighter or missed menstrual periods
- Increased sensitivity to heat
- Frequent bowel movements and possibly diarrhea
- Muscle weakness
- Difficulty sleeping
- Fine, brittle, and thinning hair
- Problems with fertility
- Vision changes and eye irritation

Screening and Diagnosis

Thyroid disease can be difficult to diagnose because its symptoms are easily confused with other conditions. A comprehensive history and physical examination are integral to a diagnosis of thyroiditis. An examination typically includes weight, blood pressure, pulse rate, cardiac rhythm, and examination of the thyroid, neuromuscular system, eyes, skin, and the cardiovascular and lymphatic systems.

Laboratory testing is also important. The thyroid-stimulating hormone (TSH) test is generally used as a screening test because it can often identify thyroid disorders before the onset of symptoms. Blood tests measuring levels of thyroxine (T_4) can confirm the presence of thyroid disease.

If thyroid disease is caught early, treatment can control the disorder before symptoms become severe.

Treatment

Treatment for Hashimoto's disease is based on determining the correct amount of thyroid hormone (thyroxine) needed to stimulate the thyroid gland. Gradually increasing doses of thyroxine are given until a person's blood levels become normal. Annual checkups are necessary to confirm that the prescribed dose is still appropriate. During pregnancy, doses of thyroxine usually increase; as a person ages, doses usually decrease. Overtreatment of hypothyroidism with thyroid hormone can result in bone loss. Graves' disease is treated with antithyroid drugs to prevent the thyroid gland from manufacturing thyroid hormone.

ALZHEIMER'S DISEASE

Alzheimer's disease is an irreversible, progressive brain disorder that affects thinking, memory, and behavior. The changes result from the death of brain cells and the breakdown of the connections between them. The progression of Alzheimer's disease and the resulting cognitive decline

may occur at any age and do affect men. Other risk factors associated with thyroid disorders include a family history of thyroid disease, previous thyroid concerns (such as enlargement, goiter, or nodules), or a transient thyroid condition during pregnancy. Having one of these risk factors increases the risk of developing a thyroid disorder but does not inevitably lead to one. Likewise, people without known risk factors can still develop thyroid disorders.

Symptoms

Table 11.6 summarizes clinical manifestations of Hashimoto's disease and Graves' disease. However, many people have no symptoms, and symptoms rarely occur all at once.

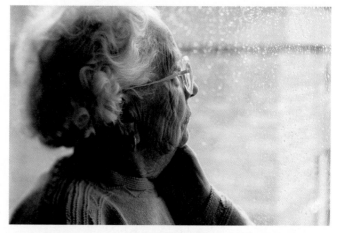

Alzheimer's disease is a devastating disease that results in memory loss, behavior and personality changes, and a decline in cognitive abilities.
© Photodisc

vary from person to person. People with this disease usually live anywhere from 3 to 20 years after first showing symptoms. Alzheimer's disease is the most common cause of **dementia**, accounting for an estimated 60 to 80% of cases of dementia. Approximately 5.3 million Americans had Alzheimer's in 2015.[13] This number will grow as the population ages. The risk of developing Alzheimer's disease increases with age; however, the disease and symptoms of dementia are not a part of normal aging.

Alzheimer's disease affects many areas of mental function, including memory, language, behavior, and thought processes. These changes are linked with distinct changes in the brain, most notably the development of amyloid plaques and neurofibrillary tangles. Plaques are dense deposits of protein and cellular material that form outside and around the brain's neurons. Researchers are not certain whether the plaques cause the disease or are simply a by-product of the disease process. Tangles are insoluble twisted fibers that build up inside neurons. A form of a protein called tau is the main component of the tangles. In healthy neurons, tau proteins help stabilize a cell's structure. In brains affected by Alzheimer's disease, the tau protein is chemically altered and cannot hold the structure together; the resulting collapse is responsible for malfunctions in communication. These brain changes may begin 20 or more years before symptoms actually appear.

There are two forms of Alzheimer's disease. Late-onset Alzheimer's disease is the most common form, usually occurring in people over the age of 60. This form of the disease progresses slower and has less of a genetic link than early-onset Alzheimer's disease. Early-onset Alzheimer's is less common but more severe than the late onset form of the disease. Early-onset Alzheimer's disease can appear in a person's 40s or 50s and progress rapidly within a few years.

Risk Factors

The causes of Alzheimer's disease are not fully known. Multiple factors, including age, genetic background, and possibly lifestyle, influence its development and progression. Some studies have implicated severe or repeated head injuries, lower education levels, and environmental agents as risk factors; however, more research is needed to determine the exact relationship among these risk factors and the development of Alzheimer's.

The risk of developing Alzheimer's increases with age. One out of every 10 persons 65 years or older is a victim of Alzheimer's disease, although early-onset victims may be in their 40s or 50s. Approximately 20% of Americans between the ages of 75 and 84, and almost one-half of those 85 years or older, suffer from Alzheimer's disease.[11]

Genetics play a strong role in the development of early-onset Alzheimer's disease. As many as 50% of early-onset cases are caused by defects in three genes located on three different chromosomes. Even if only one of these mutations is inherited from a parent, a person will inevitably develop a form of early-onset Alzheimer's.

Genetics play a role in late-onset disease as well; however, a person can inherit the gene associated with late-onset Alzheimer's and not get the disease. Similarly, people with late-onset Alzheimer's may not have any genetic factor. Certain forms of the apolipoprotein E (APOE) gene can also influence the development of late-onset disease. Scientists are now intensively searching for other genes that may be linked to Alzheimer's.

Newer evidence suggests that the health of the brain is closely linked to the overall health of the heart and blood vessels. Factors that increase the risk of cardiovascular disease, such as smoking, obesity, diabetes, hypertension, and high cholesterol, also appear to increase the risk of dementia. This association also provides a key to potential protective factors. Physical activity and a heart-healthy diet appear to be associated with a reduced risk of developing Alzheimer's.[13]

Symptoms

Alzheimer's disease disrupts three key processes in the nerve cells of the brain: communication, metabolism, and repair. This disruption causes many nerve cells to stop functioning, lose connections with other nerve cells, and die. The disease advances by stages, from early, mild forgetfulness to severe loss of mental function (i.e., dementia). Symptoms usually first appear after age 65.

The disease first destroys neurons in parts of the brain that control memory; as a result, a person's ability to do easy and familiar tasks begins to decline. The most common initial symptom is the inability to remember new information. People in the initial stages of disease often think less clearly and start forgetting the names of familiar people and common objects. Later in the disease, they may forget how to do simple tasks, such as brushing their teeth. The cerebral cortex, particularly the area responsible for language and reasoning, is affected next, disrupting a person's language skills and ability to make judgments. Personality changes also may occur. Emotional outbursts and disturbing behavior, such as wandering and agitation, become more frequent as the disease runs its course. Eventually, many other areas of the brain are involved. All brain regions atrophy, and the person becomes bedridden, incontinent, totally helpless, unresponsive to the outside world, and susceptible to a variety of illnesses and infections. People with Alzheimer's disease often die from pneumonia.

Diagnosis

In the absence of a conclusive diagnostic test, healthcare providers rely on symptoms, medical and family history, and physical and neurological examinations to diagnose Alzheimer's disease. Although these tests allow healthcare providers looking for Alzheimer's disease to diagnose it with high accuracy, many people with Alzheimer's disease are never diagnosed. The only way to conclusively identify the disease is through autopsy, by examining the characteristic plaques and tangles in the brain.

It is important to rule out other illnesses or medications that can cause dementia. Severe depression in the elderly, which can often be treated successfully, is frequently accompanied by memory loss and therefore may be confused with Alzheimer's. However, depression and Alzheimer's disease do coexist in many patients.

Researchers are studying brain-imaging techniques to better detect biological changes or signs of dysfunction in the brain. The earlier an accurate diagnosis of disease can be made, the better the chance of managing symptoms and helping patients and their families plan for future care while the patient is still able to take part in the decision-making process.

> *My grandfather has Alzheimer's disease. My mother tries to take care of him but it is very difficult. Sometimes my sisters and I feel angry that she does not have time for us even when we understand that he needs her attention.*
>
> **—20-year-old woman**

Treatment

There is no cure for Alzheimer's disease. The FDA has approved several medications that temporarily improve symptoms of Alzheimer's; however, the effectiveness of these medications varies from person to person. In addition, none of these treatments slows or stops the underlying degeneration of brain cells, and thus the progression of Alzheimer's. In the absence of effective medication, treatment for Alzheimer's disease focuses on managing symptoms and making lifestyle changes to help the patients and their caregivers cope with the progression of the disease. Therapies include the management of problematic behaviors, home or "environmental" modifications, music and reminiscence therapy (using photos and other items to elicit memories), exercise, cognitive activity (such as gardening, puzzles, or cooking), and the use of appropriate communication techniques.

Physical activity, good nutrition, and social interaction are important for keeping Alzheimer's patients as functional as possible. Maintaining a calm, safe, structured environment also helps patients feel better and remain independent longer. Drugs can help soothe agitation, anxiety, depression, and sleeplessness and may help boost participation in daily activities.

The care of a person who has Alzheimer's disease is challenging on many fronts. Care can be emotionally devastating, physically demanding, and a financial burden. Caregivers are subject to high levels of chronic stress, and caregiver burnout is a major factor in the inability to continue caring for a person with Alzheimer's at home. Support and education for caregivers and family members are crucial to the best care of people with Alzheimer's.

INFORMED DECISION MAKING

Lifestyle changes are often the first step in preventing the development of chronic conditions or in slowing their progression. A healthy diet, regular exercise, and avoidance of harmful substances are standard methods for health promotion. Other important approaches toward disease prevention include being knowledgeable about chronic diseases and their symptoms and visiting one's healthcare provider regularly. A woman who knows her body may be able to recognize changes or problems readily and prevent or slow progression of disease before symptoms begin or complications arise.

For osteoporosis prevention purposes, a woman usually only needs to have a bone mineral density test two or three times during her lifetime. Preventive measures such as medication may be an appropriate option for women with decreasing bone density. A significant aspect of arthritis treatment involves learning ways to ease pain and perform daily activities. A diagnosis of arthritis should encourage women to become more active in their own health care and learn better ways to manage their diseases. Some diseases can cause significant damage if left undiagnosed and therefore untreated. Uncontrolled diabetes, for example, can lead to serious illness and possibly death. With appropriate treatment and by managing their condition, however, women with diabetes can live complete and satisfying lives.

A disease such as Alzheimer's presents different issues. Early diagnosis appears to have little effect on treatment or management of the disease. It does, however, afford both the patient and family members time to arrange for who will make future healthcare, financial, long-term care, and any other decisions necessary for the patient. Many issues need to be considered with Alzheimer's disease because as the disease progresses, a person will no longer be able to make rational decisions or care for himself or herself. A woman who is considering becoming a caregiver for a person with this disease needs to understand the time and commitment involved before making such a decision. Early diagnosis assists people in this preparation.

The Internet can help patients and their families learn more about chronic diseases and cope with their effects. It provides individuals with information about symptoms, diagnosis, and treatment and offers a connection to support groups and individuals who understand first-hand what it is like to live with a chronic disease. As with all information sources, there are risks related to information received on the Internet, including claims for supposed "miracle cures" for certain disorders, and information that is misleading or inaccurate. As with all other topics, women should make every effort to go to trusted sources to get information about chronic diseases.

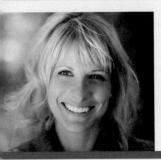 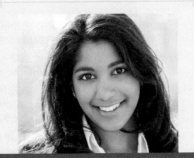 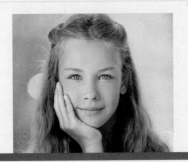 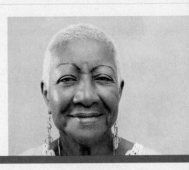

CASE STUDY

Sally is a 60-year-old woman who is experiencing some pain in her knee. She is moderately overweight and smokes half a pack of cigarettes per day. Her mother had severe arthritis that began when she turned 70. She is concerned that she may be showing signs of arthritis.

Questions

1. What are some preventive measures Sally can take to slow down joint damage and reduce the effects of arthritis?

2. Since she had her children 30 years ago, both of which were 10-pound babies, Sally has had high blood pressure and low HDL levels. Are there any other diseases for which she also may be at high risk?

■ Summary

Chronic diseases are major causes of death and disability in the United States. Because these diseases usually lack definitive cures, medical focus falls on preventing the diseases when possible and managing them through medication and behaviors when they develop. Knowledge, healthful behaviors, and lifestyle modifications are the best measures by which a woman can reduce her chances of developing chronic conditions. In the cases of chronic diseases with genetic components, women can better understand their risks by learning about their family history. Health screenings can alert a woman to an increased risk of disease, allowing her to make decisions on lifestyle changes and treatment options. Although prevention is the first step, chronic diseases can affect a woman who has followed a healthy lifestyle and has adhered to screening guidelines for various conditions. The next step is to

Profiles of Remarkable Women

Mary Tyler Moore (1936–)

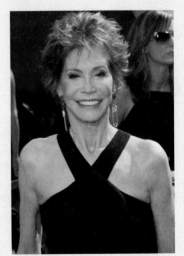
© s_bukley/Shutterstock

Mary Tyler Moore began her career as a dancer and actress in TV commercials. After a series of unsuccessful TV series and specials, she landed a role on *The Dick Van Dyke Show* in the early 1960s. From that point, Moore's career took off. *The Mary Tyler Moore Show* ran from 1970 to 1977 and was followed by *Mary* (1978), *The Mary Tyler Moore Hour* (1979), and *Mary* (1985–1986). Moore won five Emmy awards for her roles on *The Dick Van Dyke Show* and *The Mary Tyler Moore Show*. Her career has continued with roles in movies and on Broadway.

Moore has overcome many hardships in her personal life. Her son committed suicide at the age of 24; soon thereafter, she divorced her husband. She later checked herself into the Betty Ford Clinic with alcohol abuse problems.

Since early adulthood, Moore also has had diabetes. As the International Chairwoman of the Juvenile Diabetes Foundation (JDF), Moore has advocated for diabetes education, awareness, and increased funding for diabetes research. She has been featured in a series of public service announcements for the JDF. In June 1999, Moore led 100 child delegates in the first Juvenile Diabetes Foundation Children's Congress before the Senate Committee on Appropriations, Subcommittee in Labor, Health and Human Services, and Education. She and the children, as well as other advocates, called on lawmakers to increase funding for diabetes research to help speed up the discovery of a cure. Moore has continued to lead the Children's Congress to Capitol Hill every other year, making the event one of the largest media and grassroots efforts held in support of finding a cure for juvenile diabetes, raising national awareness, and representing personal advocacy.

Over the course of her disease, Moore has experienced several flare-ups of diabetic retinopathy, which until recently have been kept under control with laser surgery. She is now nearly blind as a result of her disease. She has also recently suffered heart and kidney problems.

understand how to control or treat a condition, through lifestyle modifications and appropriate treatment.

■ Topics for Discussion

1. What type of ethical issues may arise with testing for genetic predisposition for various chronic diseases?

2. Have you, a close friend, or a family member ever been diagnosed with a chronic disease? How has that diagnosis changed your or his or her life?

3. How can lifestyle changes affect chronic disease management?

4. What differences exist between chronic diseases that occur early in life versus those that manifest later in life?

5. In what ways does early diagnosis help a woman and her family to cope with her disease?

■ Key Terms

Arthritis

Bone remodeling

Dementia

Diabetes

Fibromyalgia

Gestational diabetes

Hyperglycemia

Hyperthyroidism

Hypoglycemia

Hypothyroidism

Lupus

Lyme disease

Osteoarthritis

Rheumatoid arthritis

Thyroiditis

■ References

1. World Health Organization. (2015). *Global Health Observatory (GHO) data.* Available at: http://www.who.int/gho/ncd/en/

2. National Osteoporosis Foundation. (2014). *54 million Americans affected by osteoporosis and low bone mass.* Available at: http://nof.org/news/2948

3. Centers for Disease Control and Prevention (CDC). (2015). *Arthritis: Risk factors.* Available at: http://www.cdc.gov/arthritis/basics/risk_factors.htm

4. CDC. (2014). *National diabetes statistics report: Estimates of diabetes and its burden in the United States.* Atlanta, GA: U.S. Department of Health and Human Services. Available at: http://www.cdc.gov/diabetes/pubs/statsreport14/national-diabetes-report-web.pdf

5. National Institutes of Health (NIH). (2005). *Progress in auto-immune disease research: Report to Congress.* Available at: http://www.niaid.nih.gov/dait/pdf/ADCC_Final.pdf

6. CDC. (2005). Racial/ethnic differences in the prevalence and impact of doctor-diagnosed arthritis—United States, 2002. *Morbidity and Mortality Weekly Report* 54(5): 119–123.

7. CDC. (2014). *Diabetes Report Card 2014.* Atlanta, GA: CDC, U.S. Department of Health and Human Services.

8. Ward, B. W., Schiller, J. S., & Goodman R. A. (2014). Multiple chronic conditions among U.S. adults: A 2012 update. *Preventing Chronic Disease* 11: 130389. DOI: http://dx.doi.org/10.5888/pcd11.130389

9. Gerteis, J., Izrael, D., Deitz, D., et al. (2014). *Multiple chronic conditions chartbook.* AHRQ Publications No. Q14-0038. Rockville, MD: Agency for Healthcare Research and Quality.

10. American Diabetes Association. (2013). *The cost of diabetes.* Available at: http://www.diabetes.org/advocate/resources/cost-of-diabetes.html

11. CDC. (2007). National and state medical expenditures and lost earnings attributable to arthritis and other rheumatic conditions. *Morbidity and Mortality Weekly Report* 56(1): 4–7.

12. Burge, R., Dawson-Hughes, B., Solomon, D. H., et al. (2007). Incidence and economic burden of osteoporosis-related fractures in the United States, 2005–2025. *Journal of Bone and Mineral Research* 22(3): 465–475.

13. Alzheimer's Association. (2015). *2015 Alzheimer's disease facts and figures.* Available at: https://www.alz.org/facts/downloads/facts_figures_2015.pdf

14. American Academy of Orthopaedic Surgeons. (2008). *Burden of musculoskeletal diseases in the United States: Prevalence, societal and economic cost.* Rosemont, IL: American Academy of Orthopaedic Surgeons.

15. Delaney, M. F. (2006). Strategies for the prevention and treatment of osteoporosis during early menopause. *American Journal of Obstetrics and Gynecology* 194(2 Suppl.): S12–S23.

16. National Osteoporosis Foundation. (2014). *Clinician's guide to prevention and treatment of osteoporosis.* Available at: http://nof.org/files/nof/public/content/file/2791/upload/919.pdf

17. CDC. (2015). *Arthritis: Addressing the nation's most common cause of disability at a glance 2015.* Available at: http://www.cdc.gov/chronicdisease/resources/publications/aag/arthritis.htm

18. Buckwalter, J. A., Saltzman, C., & Brown, T. (2004). The impact of osteoarthritis. *Clinical Orthopaedics Related Research* 427(Suppl.): S6–S15.

19. Zhu, Y., Pandya, B. J., Choi, H. K. (2011). Prevalence of gout and hyperuricemia in the US general population: The National Health and Nutrition Examination Survey 2007–2008. *Arthritis and Rheumatism.* 63(10): 3136–3141.

20. Lawrence, R. C., Felson, D. T., Helmick, C. G., et al. (2008). Estimates of the prevalence of arthritis and other rheumatic conditions in the United States: Part II. *Arthritis and Rheumatism* 58(1): 26–35.

21. CDC. (2010). Prevalence of doctor-diagnosed arthritis and arthritis-attributable activity limitation—United States, 2007–2009. *Morbidity and Mortality Weekly Report* 59(39): 1261–1265.

22. Miyaguchi, M., Kobayashi, A., Kadoya, Y., et al. (2003). Biochemical change in joint fluid after isometric quadriceps exercise for patients with osteoarthritis of the knee. *Osteoarthritis and Cartilage* 11: 252–259.

23. CDC. *How many people get Lyme disease?* Available at: http://www.cdc.gov/lyme/stats/humancases.html

24. NIH. (2005). *Lyme disease: The facts, the challenge.* National Institute of Allergy and Infectious Diseases and National Institute of Arthritis and Musculoskeletal and Skin Diseases. NIH

Publication #05-7045. Bethesda, MD: National Institute of Allergy and Infectious Diseases.

25. American Heart Association. (2012). *Cardiovascular disease and diabetes*. Available at: http://www.heart.org/HEARTORG /Conditions/Diabetes/WhyDiabetesMatters/Cardiovascular -Disease-Diabetes_UCM_313865_Article.jsp/

26. Bauduceau, B., Bourdel-Marchasson, I., Brocker, P., et al. (2005). The brain of the elderly diabetic patient. *Diabetes Metabolism* 2: 92–97.

27. Kumari, M., & Marmot, M. (2005). Diabetes and cognitive function in a middle-aged cohort: Findings from the Whitehall II study. *Neurology* 65(10): 1597–1603.

28. Perrson, M., Norman, M., & Hanson, U. (2009). Obstetric and perinatal outcomes in type 1 diabetic pregnancies. *Diabetes Care* 32(11): 2005–2009.

29. National Institutes of Health, National Institute of Diabetes and Digestive and Kidney Diseases. (2014). *Diagnosis of diabetes and prediabetes*. Available at: http://www.niddk.nih.gov/health -information/health-topics/Diabetes/diagnosis-diabetes -prediabetes/Pages/index.aspx#3

30. CDC. (2015). *Fibromyalgia*. Available at: http://www.cdc.gov /arthritis/basics/fibromyalgia.htm

31. Arnold, L. (2009). Strategies for managing fibromyalgia. *American Journal of Medicine* 122(12 Suppl.): S31–S43.

32. American Autoimmune Related Diseases Association. (n.d.). *Autoimmune disease in women*. Available at: http://www.aarda .org/autoimmune-information/autoimmune-disease-in-women/

33. Lupus Foundation of America. (2015). *What is lupus?* Available at: http://www.lupus.org/answers/entry/what-is-lupus

34. Lupus Foundation of America. (2015). *What causes lupus?* Available at: http://www.lupus.org/answers/entry/what-causes-lupus

35. American Thyroid Association. (2014). *Prevalence and impact of thyroid disease*. Available at: http://www.thyroid.org/media-main /about-hypothyroidism/

36. Golden, S. H., Robinson, K. A., Saldanha, I., et al. (2009). Prevalence and incidence of endocrine and metabolic disorders in the United States: A comprehensive review. *Journal of Clinical Endocrinology & Metabolism* 94(6): 1853–1878.

CHAPTER 12

Mental Health

Learning Objectives

On completion of this chapter, the student should be able to discuss:

1. Basic definitions of mental health, and why mental health is important.

2. How biological, social, and environmental factors contribute to and affect mental health.

3. Epidemiological, economic, legal, and political dimensions of mental health.

4. Basic types of mental illness, including mood, anxiety, and eating disorders, as well as schizophrenia, dissociative disorders, and personality disorders.

5. Mental illnesses that disproportionately affect women, as well as biological and cultural factors that influence how mental illnesses affect women.

6. The stress response, how stress affects mental and physical health, and healthy methods of coping with stress.

7. Risk factors for suicide in the United States and developing world, and methods of preventing suicide.

8. Strategies for improving and developing mental health.

9. When to consider seeking treatment for mental illness.

10. Different methods of treating mental disorders, including pharmaceutical treatments and counseling.

INTRODUCTION

Mental health is at least as important as physical health for a happy, meaningful life. Poor mental health can interfere with maintaining relationships, having a sense of satisfaction in one's self and one's work, and functioning in day-to-day life. Mental illnesses can dull or block even our basic interests in food, sleep, and sexual contact.

So how should a topic as important, yet as nebulous, as "mental health" be defined? One definition of mental health is "how we think, feel, and act as we cope with life."[1] By this definition, good mental health could be considered a state of well-being that allows a person to be productive, have fulfilling relationships, adapt to changes, and cope with difficult circumstances; poor mental health could be considered a mental or emotional state that interferes with these abilities. Mental illnesses, or mental disorders, on the other hand, can be defined as distinct, diagnosable illnesses, typically marked by changes or abnormalities in mood, thinking, or behavior (or a combination of the three) that affect mental health.[2]

Making more specific definitions without going into extensive detail is difficult. *The Diagnostic and Statistical Manual of Mental Disorders, Fifth edition* (DSM-V), the manual the American Psychological Association uses to classify mental disorders, uses more than 140 words to define "mental disorder" and uses nearly 1000 pages to define and describe every recognized mental illness.

Defining terms like "mental health," "mental disorders," and "mental illness" is also difficult because the distinction between mental and physical health is largely artificial. The brain governs our ability to think, feel, and respond—everything we think of as "mental health." But the brain, like any other organ, requires nutrients and oxygen. It can be damaged or otherwise affected by nutritional deficiencies, thyroid problems, tumors, or physical trauma. Mental health also influences physical health. Depression, for example, makes people less likely to exercise, more likely to engage in substance abuse, and less able to take good care of themselves, greatly increasing their risk for heart disease and other conditions. The environment also affects a person's mental health. An otherwise healthy person will eventually develop scurvy if you restrict his or her vitamin C intake; similarly if you prevent a person from getting enough oxygen, he or she will have a panic attack, even if that person is otherwise a brave, disciplined person in good mental health.

Social context also influences how cultures conceptualize mental health. The DSM previously, but no longer, classified homosexuality as a mental illness. Today, suicide is considered the ultimate symptom of mental illness; but in feudal Japan, this act was sometimes expected of an honorable person. Freud said the mark of a mentally healthy individual was the ability to love and to work, but even this definition carries certain social judgments about what is important for a good life.

Finally, mental health is difficult to define because it is a matter of degree. People normally considered "mentally healthy" may engage in behaviors that, if taken further, are associated with mental illness. A woman may be considered mentally healthy, and even sensible, for washing her hands several times a day during cold or flu season. If that same woman washes her hands 30 or 40 times a day and her hand washing interferes with her ability to work, she could be diagnosed with obsessive-compulsive disorder (OCD). Drawing a line between mental health and someone with a mental illness requires a judgment call that may vary from person to person, just as people have different definitions about at what point water turns from "hot" to "cold," even if everyone agrees that boiling water is hot and ice is cold.

Mental illness is extremely common. The National Institute of Mental Health (NIMH) estimates that one in five American adults (19.5%) have experienced at least one mental disorder in the past year.[3] Just as a person's physical health varies throughout his or her lifetime, so too does his or her mental health. Many people with mental illnesses are otherwise normal people who love and are loved and who contribute to society. People with mental illnesses can be politicians, artists, bus drivers, accountants, doctors, or any other profession. They may seek treatment and recover fully, or they may cope with their disorder as best they can by themselves. In some cases, the perspectives people gain from dealing with mental illness may be of great value to society; some historians have argued that Abraham Lincoln and Winston Churchill were better leaders because of their depressive tendencies.

Half of all Americans experience mental illness in their lifetimes, but most of these people will not seek professional treatment.[2] Many factors contribute to this lack of care. Sometimes good mental health care is not available or affordable, or people do not know where they can find it. The stigma associated with mental illness—many people are afraid to seek help because they are afraid of being thought of as "crazy"—prevents people from seeking needed care. Even as science continues to make enormous strides in mapping the brain and understanding cognitive function, the basic problem of improving access to mental health care remains one of the major health challenges of the next 20 years.

FACTORS AFFECTING MENTAL HEALTH

Biological, environmental, and social factors all influence mental health. At the biological level, a person's genes, physical health, and possibly hormone levels may determine her susceptibility to certain kinds of mental illness. Many aspects of a person's physical and social environment, from sources of real or perceived danger; to relationships with friends, family, and colleagues; to societal expectations based on a person's gender, race, relative wealth, or other factors, also have numerous effects on mental health.

Biological Factors

Biological factors affecting mental health include genetic predisposition to a disease, head or brain injuries, or prenatal exposure to illegal drugs or alcohol.

There are clearly genetic components to some mental illnesses. Many people with a mental illness have family members who have also dealt with the same condition. Studies following separated identical twins find that if one twin has bipolar disorder, the other twin has about a 59% chance of developing the disease—clearly greater than the proportion of bipolar disorder in the general population.[2] In this case, both of these twins may be genetically vulnerable to developing bipolar disease, but some aspect of a person's social or physical environment may ultimately trigger the onset of bipolar disorder (or help prevent bipolar disorder from occurring).

Reproductive hormones can sometimes play a part in women's mental health. Although hormonal changes do not normally cause mental illness, shifts in hormone levels may affect the severity of depression during premenstrual syndrome, postpartum depression, and postpartum psychosis. Brain structure and function, as well as neurotransmitter levels, also have been studied to identify gender-related differences and differences between people with and without mental illness.

Social and Psychosocial Factors

Social and psychosocial factors change throughout a woman's lifetime and influence the way a woman views herself and how she interacts with others. Any of these factors can affect a woman's mental health. Women with low incomes; low levels of education; and who work in difficult, stressful, and low-status jobs are disproportionately vulnerable to mental illness. This vulnerability may be due to both the undervalued or nonvalued roles that these women fill and the financial difficulties that accompany such roles. Women who live in poverty, for example, are more likely than other women to experience disruptive events, such as being evicted from one's home, facing overt discrimination, or being the victim of a crime. They are also less likely to have access to mental health services or other resources that can aid in recovery from a mental illness that does develop. Women who are trying to fill multiple roles as career women, mothers, and caretakers often feel overwhelmed, which may lead to low self-esteem, increased stress, and, in some cases, depression.

Societal expectations and the way parents treat their children also influence mental health. In the United States, for example, parents may consciously or subconsciously encourage girls to be delicate, nurturing, nonaggressive, and sensitive to the feelings of others and teach boys to be assertive, aggressive, and dominant. This may lead women and girls to turn their aggression inward, toward themselves, rather than directing it at others, thus increasing the likelihood of depression and other mental illnesses.

As children reach puberty, gender differences, both physically and culturally, become more apparent. A girl's success often comes from popularity and attractiveness, whereas a boy's success is often based on athleticism and academic achievement. Factors such as these lead many girls to base their self-esteem on their physical appearance and body weight. These pressures, along with the physical and hormonal and social changes that accompany adolescence, make the teenage years an especially difficult period.

Girls continue to receive less attention than boys in academic settings. Girls generally achieve better grades than do boys, but despite this academic success, girls experience more internal costs—worry, anxiety, and depression. As the authors of one study note, "Although girls may

GENDER DIMENSIONS: Health Differences Between Men and Women

Gender Differences in Mental Illness

Strong gender differences exist both in the prevalence of specific mental disorders and in the way the diseases manifest themselves. Some of these differences are:

- Women have twice the rate of clinical depression as men.
- Women have four times the incidence of seasonal affective disorder.
- Women experience more of the depressed phase of bipolar disorder and have more rapid cycling between mania and depression.
- Women are nine times more likely to suffer from anorexia nervosa and bulimia nervosa.

- Twice as many women suffer from panic disorder.
- Women are more likely to have phobias and experience more intense symptoms.
- Borderline personality disorder and histrionic personality disorder are diagnosed more often in women.
- Men are more than three times as likely to be diagnosed with antisocial personality disorders than women.
- More women attempt suicide, although more men die from their attempts.

have the edge over boys in terms of their performance in school, this edge is lost when it comes to the experience of internal distress."[4] Another study showed that women tend to attribute their successes to luck and their failures to lack of ability, whereas men tend to attribute their successes to ability and their failures to bad luck.[5]

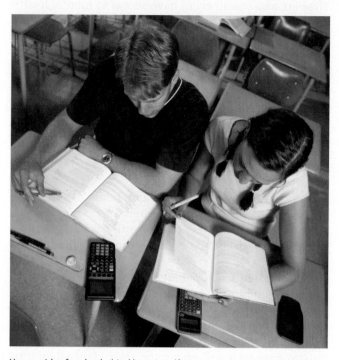

Young girls often lag behind boys in self-esteem and they are more likely to experience depression.
© AbleStock

During and after adolescence, girls must create an identity for themselves, deal with their sexuality, make educational and career choices, and become independent. For adolescents, risk factors for mental disorders include lack of parental support, sexual abuse, low self-esteem, and weak relationships with friends or family. Some teens may not exhibit obvious signs of emotional distress while expressing their lack of mental wellness through substance abuse, disordered eating, behavior problems, and sexual promiscuity.

Teenage girls are more likely than teenage boys to experience depression. Female high school students are more likely to have anxiety disorders, eating disorders, and adjustment disorder than their male counterparts, who have higher rates of disruptive behavior disorders, attention deficit disorder, autism, and learning disabilities.

Early adulthood brings many decisions, including those concerning career choices, long-term relationships, and childbearing. Reproductive events at this time in a woman's life, such as pregnancy, childcare, infertility, or the decision not to have children, may create both personal stress and relationship tension. Women

also experience increased independence at this time in their lives, as well as increased financial obligations and responsibilities at work and at home. All of these factors can affect a woman's mental health.

Many women begin to experiment with recreational drug use during adolescence and early adulthood. Among women with mental health disorders, substance abuse is a common occurrence. Women with mood disorders, anxiety disorders, or other mental illness are about twice as likely as women without a mental illness to abuse alcohol or other drugs.[6] Substance abuse may occur when these women attempt to self-medicate to cope with a mental illness, if a mental illness affects a woman's reasoning skills, or for any of the other myriad reasons that substance abuse occurs in mentally healthy women. The prolonged use of illicit drugs can put people at higher risk for developing mental illness and can make existing illnesses worse, causing people to self-medicate with drugs more intensely or more frequently. This pattern creates a vicious cycle in the relationship between drug use and mental illness.

Women who have substance abuse problems are also at a greater risk than other women for depression, attempted suicide, eating disorders, and other forms of mental illness. Women with eating disorders may abuse cocaine, heroin, or methamphetamines as appetite suppressants to lose weight. Concurrent treatment that addresses both the mental illness and the substance abuse problem is especially important for successfully treating women dealing with both of these problems. Unfortunately, the current healthcare system in the United States is often designed to treat each of these issues separately: physicians or psychiatrists who treat mental illness are often unable or unwilling to successfully treat a substance abuse problem, and providers or

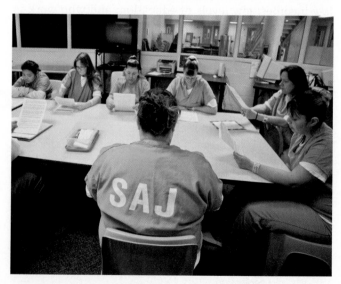

Six out of 10 female inmates in federal prisons are mentally ill; more than 7 in 10 female inmates in state prisons and jails are mentally ill.
© absolut/Shutterstock

treatment centers that can help with substance abuse problems are often unprepared to deal with problems brought on by mental illness.[6]

As women reach midlife, many continue to deal with career issues and financial burdens while struggling to balance their many roles of mother, wife, daughter, friend, sibling, employer, employee, and self. Women also may be dealing with stress from caring for growing children and aging parents. The support and joy that good relationships offer a woman are often important counterbalances to the stress of managing her everyday life. As she nears late adulthood, a woman may be fortunate enough to feel satisfied with her accomplishments and be financially secure. Women who struggle with retirement issues, physical health, unaccomplished areas of their lives, ill parents, or adult children with difficulties, however, may feel overwhelmed by stressors not fully within their control.

Depression and **dementia** resulting from Alzheimer's disease are serious mental health issues that affect the elderly. A majority of people with Alzheimer's disease are women, in part because women constitute a larger percentage of the elderly population than men. Depression is widely underdiagnosed and undertreated in the elderly population. One in every 14 Americans age 65 or older currently has a diagnosable depressive illness.[7]

Poor physical health, limited independence, loss of privacy and freedom, and loss of one's partner or friends all contribute to stress and poor mental health in older women. Cognitive impairments in the elderly often result from some form of dementia but may also result from severe depression. In many cases, depression occurs alongside chronic medical conditions such as heart disease, diabetes, cancer, and dementia. Because of the common occurrence of depression in the elderly, many healthcare providers, as well as patients and caregivers, falsely believe that symptoms of depression are a normal part of aging or a normal consequence of chronic disease. Depression in older women can lead to disorientation, loss of short-term memory, verbal difficulty, and inappropriate reasoning skills. Personality changes also may result from dementia or depression or from a decrease in overall physical health.[7]

Discrimination—being singled out by others based on sexuality, gender, ethnicity, age, or other physical characteristics, including the presence of a mental disorder—is another risk factor for mental illness that women of all age groups experience. Discrimination can affect any aspect of a woman's life, including her work, marriage, and social status. Both mental and physical abuse put women at high risk for developing depression, posttraumatic stress disorder, or obsessive-compulsive disorder. Mental illness is more likely to occur if a person has experienced childhood abuse or trauma. This factor may partly account for women's increased incidence of certain mental illnesses, because women are at a higher risk for rape, abuse, and sexual harassment.

Other reasons that women suffer from mental illness may relate to their individual personality traits. Women who are prone to pessimistic thinking, have low self-esteem, feel they have little control over life events, and worry excessively are at higher risk for depressive and anxiety disorders. Many women also have a heightened sense of sympathy and empathy, which leaves them more vulnerable to suffering from depression after tragic events, even if they were not directly affected by the events themselves.

Stress

Stress is the body's response to any demand or change.[8] All animals have developed some kind of stress responses to help them cope with unexpected circumstances. For most of human history, sources of stress might include the arrival of a sudden storm, contact with a rival tribe, or running into a dangerous animal. In the modern world, common sources of stress range from daily events such as a traffic jam or work or school deadline to major life events, such as a wedding, new job, or the loss of a family member.

The stress response emerged to improve the body's short-term ability to respond to physical danger. The body releases hormones, primarily adrenaline and cortisol, which increase heart rate and blood pressure. Blood is diverted from the digestive, reproductive, and immune systems to the muscles and brain, temporarily speeding reflexes and increasing muscle strength, preparing a person to either flee or attack.[8]

For most women living in the 21st century, exposure to physical danger is a relatively rare event. Even so, acute (short-term) stress is not always harmful. Acute stress can make a situation feel exciting or motivate a person to succeed. However, repeated exposure to stress over time, or a stress response that lasts too long, can cause serious mental, emotional, and physical harm (see **It's Your Health**).

Unfortunately, today's women face many potential sources of long-term stress. College students often face heavy course (and often work) loads as well as pressure to succeed and choose a career. For working women, a weakened economy, along with continuing high rates of unemployment, has increased financial insecurity and made it harder to earn a living wage. More women, especially those with young children, are becoming members of the paid workforce, even as they continue to do more housework and spend more time caring for dependent family members than men. Domestic chores, childcare, and running errands can sap women of their energy and cause stress that affects both their home life and their work life. And women of all ages face stress from events such as the sudden end of a relationship, financial difficulties, the loss of a job or family member, or an injury or illness.

It's Your Health

Chronic Stress and Health

The same stress response that temporarily increases physical performance, over time, can cause serious harm to the body. Repeated exposure to stress over days or weeks makes a person more prone to viral infections, such as the common cold or flu. Reduced blood flow to the digestive system and other areas may cause other symptoms such as heartburn, digestive problems, headaches, irritability, anxiety, and insomnia.[8] These symptoms can reduce performance at school or at work and make a person's home life more difficult and less enjoyable. Over time, cumulative effects of stress responses on blood pressure, heart rate, and blood glucose levels raise the risk for chronic conditions such as heart disease, stroke, type 2 diabetes, and depression. In addition to these direct physical effects, chronic stress has other, more insidious effects on physical and mental health. People under stress are more likely to fall back on harmful habitual behaviors, such as unhealthy eating, sedentary recreational habits such as binge television watching, or alcohol, tobacco, or recreational drug use.[9]

Although there are no ways to eliminate stress, there are healthy ways of coping with it. In some cases, planning, such as setting aside enough time for a project to avoid a last-minute rush, or avoiding recreational activities that add to one's stress level, can prevent some stressful situations entirely. For sources of stress that are unavoidable or unforeseeable, positive methods of coping include:

- Regular physical exercise (ideally at least 30 minutes per day on 5 or more days per week, but any exercise has benefits)

- Getting at least 8 hours of sleep per night

- Scheduling time for relaxation or other enjoyable activities

- Meditation, yoga, or mindfulness practice

- Having supportive, positive interactions with friends and family

- Avoiding tobacco, recreational drug use, or excessive alcohol

PERSPECTIVES ON MENTAL HEALTH

Epidemiological Data

Almost one out of five American adults—about 44 million people—experience a diagnosable mental illness in a given year.[3]

About 10 million, or 1 out of 25, American adults will suffer from a severe mental illness that seriously disrupts their day-to-day activities. Among adults ages 15 to 44, mental illnesses cause more death and injury than cancer.[3]

Men and women are equally likely to suffer from mental illness, but the frequencies of specific mental disorders vary by gender. Men and women may also experience the same disorders in different ways, including the average age that disorders appear, frequency of psychotic symptoms, course of disease progression, social adjustment, and long-term outcome.[10] Variations in mental illnesses may be partially a result of distinct brain structures and the presence of different hormone levels (as well as different responses to hormones) in the body. The development of brain hemispheres differs by gender; men and women use their brains in different ways when decoding words, deciphering emotion, and performing other basic tasks. Other gender differences in mental illness may be due to how men and women cope with problems, view themselves, and express emotions. The **Gender Dimensions** box lists gender differences in common mental health disorders.

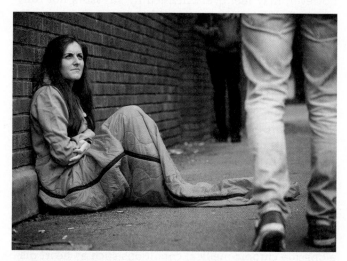

Mentally ill homeless people present a host of legal and ethical dilemmas for society.
© SpeedKingz/Shutterstock

Economic Dimensions

In addition to their harmful effects on individual health, mental illnesses carry a great economic cost—according to one estimate, more than $193 billion per year in the United States alone.[11] This estimate does not include the billions of dollars spent on medical care such as medications, clinic visits, and hospital visits; nor does it include the time and resources spent by families and caregivers of people with mental illnesses or the cost of social problems such as increased crime and threats to public safety.

Treating mental illness is often a costly undertaking. Prescription drugs can be very expensive, especially for people who do not have health insurance or who are **underinsured**. Because individual responses to medications vary and medications sometimes have serious side effects, time and medical care must often be spent on determining, often by trial and error, the correct medication and dosage for a person's individual needs. Inpatient and outpatient mental healthcare services are also expensive and require commitments of time and resources for patients and facilities providing care. Because people with serious mental illnesses sometimes have difficulty holding down jobs for long periods of time, they are at increased risk for being both uninsured and economically vulnerable.

Legal Dimensions

Most people with mental illness are law-abiding citizens. With access to proper treatment, people with mental illness are not more likely than the general population to commit crimes. However, if women are unable or unwilling to receive treatment, or if their illnesses are not treated properly, a correlation between mental illness and crime does exist, especially among individuals with psychotic and mood disorders. Many people are not identified as suffering from a mental illness during the legal and criminal process. More than half of prison and jail inmates suffer from at least one mental illness, most often mania, depression, and psychotic disorders. Female inmates are more likely to have some form of mental illness than male inmates: 73% of women in state prisons, 61% of women in federal prisons, and 75% of women in jails had a significant mental illness. Less than one-third of prisoners who had a mental health problem had received treatment since they were incarcerated.[10] These numbers likely reflect both a link between untreated mental illnesses and crime as well as increased rates of mental illness that result from the trauma related to committing a crime, going to trial, and adjusting to a life in prison.

Mentally ill homeless people also create legal and ethical dilemmas for society. During the 1980s, thousands of mentally ill people became homeless after cuts in federal and state funding to inpatient mental facilities and outpatient mental health clinics. These funding cuts forced facilities to release thousands of patients who were not capable of caring for themselves and also removed a source of mental health care for thousands of others who were caring for themselves but who were economically vulnerable. For this and other reasons, homeless people with mental illnesses have a high incidence of arrests and encounters with the law for threatening behavior, substance abuse, or other disorderly conduct. They also face numerous health problems that develop from unhealthy living conditions. The connection between the inability of many mentally ill people to access appropriate care and the incidence of criminal behavior underscores the continued need for social programs that improve the quality of life for the mentally ill in the United States.

Political Dimensions

The National Institute of Mental Health (NIMH) is the largest research organization in the world dedicated to improving mental health. Part of the National Institutes of Health, which itself is part of the federal government, the NIMH researches new ways to understand the mind, brain, and behavior; examine, treat, and prevent mental disorders; and promote and maintain good mental health. The Substance Abuse and Mental Health Services Administration (SAMHSA), another agency of the federal government, is responsible for preventing death and preventing, treating, and rehabilitating disability caused by mental illness and substance abuse. Whereas the NIMH deals primarily in research that furthers scientific understanding, SAMHSA focuses on aid and research that more directly helps people who suffer from poor mental health or substance abuse.

Federal, state, and local policies and laws have enormous, far-reaching effects on mental health. The connections between these causes and effects are not always obvious, however. An overseas conflict that sends U.S. armed forces into combat could also increase rates of post-traumatic stress disorder (PTSD) as those troops react to injuries and their experiences on the battlefield. Changes in the way police departments deal with and prosecute cases of rape and sexual assault could help reduce mental health issues associated with these traumatic events. A program offering low-interest loans to small businesses could reduce rates of depression if it lifts large numbers of people out of poverty and thus reduces the stresses and risk factors associated with living below the poverty line.

Laws and policies affect the affordability of mental health care. For years, people who had health insurance often found that the plans charged more for mental health services than for other services or that the plans did not cover mental health services at all. This discrepancy often resulted in people being unable to afford mental health care and contributed to the false idea that mental health services are either unimportant or a luxury. Legislation now requires health insurance plans that offer mental health services to give those services the same coverage they offer for other physical health services; however, this law only affects insurance plans that offered mental health coverage to begin with.

CLINICAL DIMENSIONS OF MENTAL ILLNESS

Mood Disorders

Mood disorders (also known as **affective disorders**) are mental disorders characterized by extreme disturbances of mood, the dominant emotion (or emotional tendency) a person feels at any given moment. Biological, genetic, psychological, and environmental factors can all contribute to a mood disorder or influence how a given disorder progresses. Depression and dysthymia are associated with persistent sadness, whereas bipolar disorder is associated with rapid mood changes or sustained elevations in mood.

Depression

Depression is a medical illness affecting the mind as well as the body. Usually triggered by stressful life events, depression is characterized by persistent, inescapable feelings of sadness or apathy. These emotions are often accompanied by feelings of inadequacy and hopelessness, physical exhaustion, and other symptoms (**Table 12.1**). Symptoms of depression are so intense that they usually disrupt a person's basic activities, including eating, sleeping, maintaining relationships, and taking pleasure in life.[12] People with depression often feel undesirable and inadequate. They anticipate rejection and dissatisfaction from their interactions and experiences, and they blame themselves when their negative expectations are fulfilled. People with depression often know their feelings are unhealthy and unproductive and want desperately to feel better but are unable to do so. This inability to "snap out of it" makes them feel even more weak and inadequate.[12] Feelings of hopelessness and worthlessness also make people with depression unlikely to seek professional help. Fewer than one-third of people with depression seek help from a mental health professional.[13]

Depression often coexists with other physical and mental illnesses. Among the elderly, for example, depression is often mistaken for, or present with, Alzheimer's disease. Medical conditions, such as thyroid disease, multiple sclerosis, and cancer, also increase a person's risk of getting depression. Depression also may arise as a response to a serious illness, a consequence of substance abuse, or a side effect of certain medications. In addition, depression frequently accompanies chronic diseases, such as coronary heart disease, diabetes, stroke, cancer, and HIV/AIDS, that disrupt a person's life, require hospitalization or major life changes, and force a person with one of these conditions to face his or her own mortality. Estimates of the number of women currently or recently experiencing a depressive episode vary from about 6% to about 10%.[13,14] However, more than 1 in 5 women will experience at least one depressive episode during their lives.[13]

Hormonal shifts during reproductive-related events may also affect a woman's chances of developing a mood disorder. For some women predisposed toward depression, hormones may trigger depression-like symptoms.

A severe form of depression during PMS, called premenstrual dysphoric disorder (PMDD), affects 3 to 7% of menstruating women.[15]

Postpartum depression is a type of depression that affects 10 to 15% of all new mothers.[13] This condition is different from the "baby blues," or postpartum blues, which occurs in the first 10 days after delivery and is quite common and typically mild. Postpartum depression typically begins 3 to 6 weeks after delivery and is much more severe (**Table 12.2**), although less severe than **postpartum psychosis**. Postpartum depression is more common in women with a history of depression, marital issues, lack of social support, or negative life experiences. Although it often goes unnoticed and untreated, postpartum depression can greatly affect the mother and child as well as damage the relationship between the parents. For women who are already at risk, menopause can be another hormone-related event that can trigger depression.

> *My grandmother suffered from severe depression. My mother also had it, and now I've got it too. I've been in counseling for six years and on antidepressants for three years. I feel I've finally gained control of my life, but I'm scared for my children. I don't want my daughter to have to suffer like all of the other generations in my family have suffered.*
>
> **—33-year-old woman**

Levels of the neurotransmitter **serotonin** are lower in people with major depression. Medications that boost levels of serotonin, called selective serotonin reuptake inhibitors (SSRIs), can often relieve symptoms of depression. One study found that men's brains make 52% more serotonin than do women's brains, possibly explaining why depression can manifest differently in men and women.[16]

Genetics also play a major role in depression. Someone with a family history of depression is significantly more likely to develop depression than someone with no family history of the disease. Studies have shown that children with one depressed parent are two to three times more likely to experience depression by age 18 than are children without depressed parents. The risk doubles if both parents suffer from depression.[17]

Table 12.1   Symptoms of Depression
Persistent sad mood
Constant feelings of sadness
Excessive crying
Low energy
Feelings of worthlessness or hopelessness
Difficulty concentrating or making decisions
Loss of interest in pleasurable activities
Sleep disturbances
Appetite and weight changes
Thoughts of death or suicide
Physical symptoms that do not respond to treatment

Table 12.2   Symptoms of Postpartum Depression
Anxiety
Feelings of hopelessness and guilt
Panic attacks
Insomnia
Lack of interest in the baby
Thoughts of suicide
Thoughts of hurting self or baby

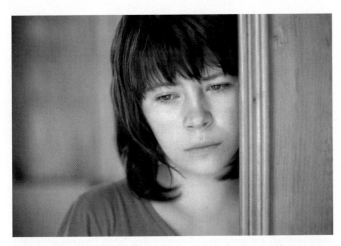

Depression is characterized by persistent, intense feelings of sadness, inadequacy, and hopelessness.
© luxorphoto/Shutterstock

Seasonal shifts in daylight hours, which affect a person's circadian rhythm or sleep–wake cycle, can cause a particular form of depression called **seasonal affective disorder (SAD)**. Seasonal affective disorder often affects women in their reproductive years, producing symptoms such as increased appetite, lethargy, and carbohydrate cravings. Researchers believe the cause of SAD may be related to melatonin disturbances. Therapeutic doses of bright light in the morning can help to relieve this condition.

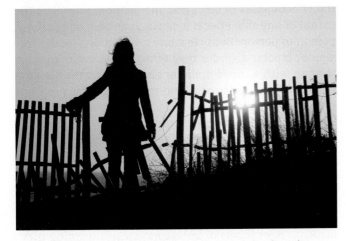

Therapeutic doses of bright light in the morning can help relieve depression caused by seasonal affective disorder (SAD).
© Francisco Caravana/Shutterstock

Depression is the most common mood disorder among women and is about twice as common in women as it is in men. Adolescent females have especially high rates of depression. Before puberty, boys are more likely than girls of the same age to be diagnosed with depression or depressive symptoms. After puberty, however, girls are far more likely to be diagnosed with depression.[13] Between the ages of 30 and 44—typically the years of childbearing and childrearing—rates of depression are three times greater for women than they are for men. Elderly women,

especially women who are widowed, are in poor physical health, or have lost some or all of their independence, are also at risk for developing depression. Medical illness and the effects of multiple medications in the elderly make diagnosing depression especially difficult.

Rates of depression vary significantly by race/ethnicity and socioeconomic characteristics. People of color are significantly more likely to be depressed than White people. Education, employment status, and poverty are also predictors for depression. People without a high school diploma are two and a half times more likely to be depressed than people who have gone to college; people who are unemployed or unable to work are three to five times more likely to be depressed than people who work, and people living in poverty are about twice as likely to be depressed as people who are not poor.[13] People living in poverty are more likely than people who are not poor to be affected by traumatic events such as the loss of a job, a financial crisis, or being the victim of violent crime; they are also less likely to have the kinds of support, from access to mental health care, to a savings account, that can prevent difficult life events from becoming catastrophic ones.

Researchers are examining whether higher rates of depression in women truly represent a greater incidence of depression or whether the rates reflect gender-based differences in the acknowledgment of mental illness or ability to recognize symptoms. Rates of depression in men may be underestimated because women are more likely than men to discuss feelings associated with being depressed, to admit to feeling depressed, and to seek help. Men are also more likely to direct negative feelings outward rather than inward, toward the self, which may make them both less vulnerable to depression and more likely to engage in self-destructive behaviors, such as substance abuse and violent behavior directed at others. In Amish culture, where women's roles as mothers and

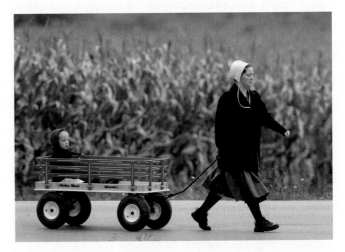

In most parts of the United States, rates of depression are much greater in women than in men. In Amish society, rates of depression are equal by gender. Social and cultural factors are the likely cause for the difference.
© Amy Sancetta/AP Photos

homemakers are more highly valued than in U.S. society as a whole and where society frowns on self-destructive "macho" behaviors and alcohol consumption, rates of depression are equal for men and women.[18] Depression may also be more common in women because women are more likely to be affected by physical abuse, sexual harassment, and rape. Acts of violence such as these directly cause mental and physical trauma and also foster low self-esteem, a sense of helplessness, social isolation, and ultimately depression. Being a caregiver for young children, aging parents, or ill family members—roles often filled by women—also has been noted as a risk factor for depression.

Dysthymia

Dysthymia is a milder but persistent form of depression. Even though dysthymia's symptoms are less severe than other forms of depression, dysthymia is still a serious, debilitating disease. It is diagnosed when symptoms last at least 2 years in adults or 1 year in adolescents and children. People with dysthymia exhibit a depressed mood and at least two other symptoms of depression, such as poor appetite, overeating, sleep difficulties, or low self-esteem. Dysthymia often begins in childhood or adolescence, but it can occur at any age. When dysthymia develops at a young age, the depressed state can become integrated within the woman's personality, affecting her self-esteem and motivation, as well as her ability to live a satisfying life and function normally. Dysthymia affects about 1.7% of the adult population (about 3.9 million adults) in any given year.[14]

Bipolar Disorder

Bipolar disorder, sometimes also referred to as **manic-depressive disorder**, is characterized by shifts in emotion, not by a single mood. A person with bipolar disorder experiences episodes of both mania ("highs") and depression ("lows"). During manic episodes a person with bipolar disorder typically has an excess of energy, activity, and restlessness. During a manic episode a person could feel wonderful and euphoric or overly stimulated and easily irritated. Other symptoms of a manic phase include racing thoughts, extreme distractibility, overconfidence, and an increased sex drive. People experiencing depressive episodes typically have deep, persistent feelings of sadness, anxiety, hopelessness, or guilt; they might also have low energy, a reduced sense of pleasure, a lowered sex drive, and thoughts of suicide. Between manic and depressive episodes, a person with bipolar disorder could have extended periods of being within the normal range of moods. People with bipolar disorder are at great risk for abusing alcohol and other drugs and engaging in other self-destructive behaviors.

About 0.4% of the adult population (900,000 people) will be affected by bipolar disorder in any given year.[14] Bipolar disorder typically first appears during a person's 20s.[19] Gender differences influence the manifestation of the disease, however, with women typically having more depressed episodes and more rapid cycling between depression and mania than do men.

Treatment

Although there is no "quick fix" that can easily cure a mood disorder, treatment for a mood disorder can provide great benefits and allow a person to live a satisfying, functional, and healthy life. Between 70 and 80% of people who experience one episode of depression will experience depression again at some point in their lives;[14] bipolar disorder typically requires ongoing treatment for a person to stay within a stable mood range. For both depression and bipolar disorder, the earlier a person seeks treatment, the better chance that person will have of making a recovery and of preventing further episodes.

Mood disorders can be treated with medications, psychosocial treatment (some form of "talk therapy"), or both of these forms used together. A combined approach usually works better than either form used alone.[13] Medications are a powerful, yet imperfect tool to treat people with mood disorders. Medications can gradually bring a person with depression or bipolar disorder back into a normal range of moods, but they may take days or even weeks to have any noticeable effects. Individuals with a mood disorder should work with their psychiatrists to find the medication and dosage that work best for them: the effectiveness of any given medication, as well as the extent of any side effects it causes, can vary widely from person to person. Because some medications for depression or bipolar disorder may affect fetal development, a woman with a mood disorder should talk with her psychiatrist about her medication routine if she is pregnant or wishes to conceive.

Antidepressant medications attempt to restore a depressed person's levels of **neurotransmitters**, particularly serotonin, norepinephrine, and dopamine, to a normal level. There are several types of antidepressant medications. The two newest, most commonly used types are called selective serotonin reuptake inhibitors (SSRIs) and serotonin and norepinephrine reuptake inhibitors (SNRIs). Older forms of antidepressants, including tricyclics or monoamine oxidase inhibitors (MAOIs), are more likely to have side effects, though these medications may be best for some individuals. Possible side effects of antidepressant medications include headaches, nausea, insomnia, constipation, and reduced sexual desire and function.

Bipolar disorder is usually treated with one or more of several kinds of medications known as "mood stabilizers." Mood-stabilizing drugs include lithium and several classes of anticonvulsant drugs. These drugs help to keep a person's mood within a consistent, central range. To be effective, these drugs should be taken on a regular basis. Sometimes a person with bipolar disorder can "feel" a mood shift approaching; if a person notices this and talks with his or her psychiatrist, a temporary change in his or her treatment plan can often prevent an episode from occurring.[19]

Psychosocial treatment for depression may focus on treating a single episode or may be maintained on a continuous basis, depending on the individual's needs and desires. Cognitive behavioral therapy (CBT) and interpersonal therapy (IPT) are the two most popular forms of psychotherapy used to treat depression. Cognitive behavioral therapy teaches a depressed person to recognize patterns of thinking and behaving that contribute to depression and helps that person find new thoughts and behaviors that support recovery, whereas IPT helps people to understand and improve their own personal relationships and interactions with other people. Psychotherapy is often the best treatment option for people with mild to moderate depression; for people with major depression, psychotherapy can be combined with antidepressant medications.[20]

For people with bipolar disorder, psychosocial treatment includes:

- Cognitive behavioral therapy, which helps patients to recognize and change harmful thought patterns and behaviors associated with the disorder

- Psychoeducation, which teaches patients (and sometimes relatives or loved ones) about the effects, treatment, and management of bipolar disorder

- Family therapy, which examines family interactions to improve harmful relationships or patterns of interaction that contribute to or result from the patient's symptoms

- Interpersonal and social rhythm therapy, which helps patients improve their personal interactions and establish regular daily routines[19]

Anxiety Disorders

Anxiety is an adaptive mental function that helps us live safe, productive lives. At healthy levels, anxiety can motivate a person to study for a test, look both ways before crossing the street, double-check that the front door is locked, or refrain from stealing or committing some other crime. **Anxiety disorders** occur when anxiety grows to unhealthy levels or when anxiety appears in situations in which no risks exist. People with anxiety disorders often know that the worries, fears, or behaviors caused by the disorders are unhelpful and unrealistic, but this knowledge does not eliminate the symptoms (**Table 12.3**). Anxiety disorders include generalized anxiety disorder (GAD), social phobias (also known as social anxiety disorder), specific phobias, panic disorder, obsessive-compulsive disorder (OCD), and posttraumatic stress disorder.

About 6% of American adults (about 13 million people) have, or have had, an anxiety disorder within the past year. Of the major anxiety disorders, generalized anxiety

Table 12.3   Symptoms of Anxiety Disorder
Feelings of terror and dread
Feelings of apprehension and uncertainty
Nervousness
Irritability
Rapid heartbeat
Chest pain
Fainting
Difficulty breathing
Sweating
Belief that feelings are signs of a heart attack

disorder and phobias are the most common.[13] Women are two to three times more likely than men to suffer from anxiety disorders. People with an anxiety disorder are disproportionately likely to experience some form of depression or another anxiety disorder or engage in substance abuse in efforts to self-medicate. Anxiety disorders usually appear earlier than other mental illnesses: Three-fourths of people with an anxiety disorder experience their first symptoms before they turn 21.[21]

Generalized Anxiety Disorder

Generalized anxiety disorder (GAD) is characterized by chronic and exaggerated worry and tension that lasts for at least 6 months. People with GAD may worry about disasters befalling themselves or their loved ones, or about routine events of everyday life. This constant worrying eventually affects the body in many ways, producing symptoms such as an inability to relax, nausea, muscle tension or pain, trembling, or having to go to the bathroom frequently. The worrying can also interfere with concentration and memory. The severity of GAD varies from person to person: It can be relatively mild, or the anxiety can be intense and disabling enough to prevent a person from carrying out daily activities, holding a job, or interacting with others. About 1.8% of adults (4.1 million people) have experienced generalized anxiety disorder within the past year.[14]

Phobias

Phobias are intense fears of something that poses little or no threat. People can develop phobias about specific animals, objects, places, or social interactions. Phobias may involve heights, closed spaces, flying, spiders, elevators, the sight of blood, or other things or situations. A phobia involves more than a moderate level of fear—a person can be afraid of any of the previously mentioned things without having a phobia. Phobias involve powerful, overwhelming fear that occurs not only when the object of the phobia appears but also often when it is merely even thought about. Phobias can be especially disabling if the object of the phobia is common or difficult to avoid in a person's daily life.

The most common specific phobia is social phobia, or social anxiety disorder, which involves a powerful, lasting fear of interacting with other people. People with this mental disorder become very self-conscious in social settings, often imagining that they are being watched or judged, or that they are doing something embarrassing. A social phobia may create anxiety surrounding all human interactions, or it may be limited to specific situations, such as eating or drinking in public or speaking in front of a group. Anxiety can last for days or weeks before a social event and can continue afterward. Specific, non-social phobias and social phobias affect about 1.6% and 1.0% of the adult U.S. population, respectively.[14]

Panic Disorder

Panic disorder is characterized by periods of intense fear accompanied by physical and emotional distress that may last anywhere from 5 to 20 minutes.[21] These periods are called panic attacks. Panic disorder currently affects about 2 million U.S. adults (about 1% of the adult population) and is twice as common in women as in men.[14] Panic attacks typically strike without warning. They often cause physical symptoms such as a pounding heart, sweating, faintness, dizziness, chest pain, and nausea; they also cause emotional symptoms such as a feeling of impending doom or of losing control. In many cases the intensity of the symptoms, as well as their unexplainable nature, makes the panic attacks themselves a major source of anxiety.

Panic attacks typically appear for the first time during a person's 20s.[21] A panic attack may occur during transition periods, times of considerable stress or crises, and often sends the individual to the emergency room. Some women have an isolated attack without ever developing the disorder; nevertheless, repeated panic attacks are a definitive sign of panic disorder. Panic attacks can be extremely disabling if they occur on a regular basis.

Obsessive-Compulsive Disorder

Obsessive-compulsive disorder (OCD) is an anxiety disorder in which a person develops intense, persistent fears, worries, or superstitions (obsessions) and uses specific rituals (compulsions), often repeated over and over again on a daily basis, for relief. One of the classic obsessions in OCD is an overwhelming fear of germs; a woman with this obsession might wash her hands dozens of times a day or be afraid to touch a doorknob or any item that someone else has touched. Other obsessions include fear of social embarrassment, thoughts about having harmed a loved one, worries about having forgotten something or left something out of place, and intrusive sexual thoughts. The ritual adopted to find relief varies from person to person, but some common themes emerge. Rituals often involve repeatedly checking, counting, or touching things in a specific pattern or order. The rituals are distracting and time-consuming and do not actually bring pleasure; at most, they just provide short-lived relief from symptoms.[21]

About 700,000 adults (0.3% of the population) in the United States have OCD, which affects men and women in equal numbers. Obsessive-compulsive disorder usually appears in the first 20 to 30 years of a person's life, often appearing in childhood. It also runs in families, suggesting that genetics can predispose a person to the disorder.[14]

Posttraumatic Stress Disorder

Posttraumatic stress disorder (PTSD), also referred to as posttraumatic stress injury, is a debilitating disorder that occurs after an exposure to a terrifying event involving violent harm or the threat of violent harm. PTSD can result from situations such as armed combat, a car accident, sexual assault, mugging, or natural disaster. A person can develop PTSD if he or she was threatened directly or if he or she witnessed a threat to a friend or family member. People with PTSD may be easily startled or may be constantly anxious and hypervigilant. Situations that remind them of the traumatic event can trigger "flashbacks" in which they relive part or all of their experience. Flashbacks can also occur in dreams or for no apparent reason while the person is awake. People with PTSD can also become emotionally numb, unable to maintain personal relationships or take pleasure from daily life. People with PTSD may become violent or aggressive; alternatively they may become depressed or turn to substance abuse for relief.

PTSD was originally identified in male Vietnam veterans, but PTSD is a major public health concern for women as well. Women are more than twice as likely as men to develop PTSD after exposure to a traumatic event, in part because they are more likely to blame themselves. Women are also more likely than men to be victims of sexual assault, a major trigger event for PTSD. Women are more likely to experience PTSD if they have more than one traumatic experience, had or have a mental disorder before the trauma, or do not have good social support.[22] At the same time, women may be able to recover from PTSD more easily than men because they are more likely to be comfortable talking about their feelings and difficult personal issues. At least 1.7 million U.S. adults (0.7% of the population) have PTSD,[21] but this number may be an underestimate.

Over the past decade, millions of women have been subject to traumatic events that have made them more vulnerable to PTSD. Hundreds of thousands of women and have lost their jobs, homes, or financial security as a result of the lagging recovery of the last decade's global economic crisis. Women veterans have had to adjust to coping with daily life after returning from the wars in Iraq and Afghanistan—about one out of seven military personnel who have experienced combat in Iraq is a woman.[22]

Sexual assault, as well as combat, remains a major source of PTSD for women. Despite some progress over the past 5 years, close to 20,000 sexual assaults, most of them among women, occur in the U.S. military every year; barely one in four of those assaults is actually reported.[23]

Treatment

Like many other mental illnesses, anxiety disorders can be treated with medications, psychotherapy, or a combination of the two, depending on individual needs and preferences. Without treatment, people with anxiety disorders may find themselves making serious life decisions based on their likelihood of encountering a phobic or anxiety-producing object or situation. Treatment can provide great benefits for people living with anxiety disorders, but time, effort, and a qualified therapist that matches an individual's needs are necessary to see improvements; people sometimes believe that they cannot be treated, or that the treatment does not work for them, when more time or an adjustment to the treatment is all that is needed. Commonly prescribed medications for anxiety disorders include antidepressants, antianxiety medications, and beta-blockers, a type of drug originally developed to treat heart conditions. Cognitive behavioral therapy can help people with anxiety disorders learn to recognize and change thoughts and behaviors associated with the disorder. Another form of therapy used for anxiety disorders is called exposure/response therapy. Exposure/response therapy aims to desensitize sufferers to their fears by supporting them in staying calm while gradually confronting more and more anxiety-producing situations. Certain forms of group therapy can also help people with anxiety disorders, especially people with PTSD or social phobia. If a person with an anxiety disorder is experiencing another form of mental illness or has a substance-abuse problem, these issues also need to be treated.

Eating Disorders

Eating disorders are serious mental illnesses characterized by dysfunctional eating patterns. But an eating disorder is much more than an unhealthy eating habit or a desire "not to eat." Like other mental illnesses, eating disorders have biological and environmental causes, distinct symptoms, and harmful consequences for the body.[24] Eating disorders are treatable, but success requires the person to acknowledge the seriousness of the issue and seek professional medical help.

The most common eating disorders are anorexia, bulimia, and binge eating disorder (BED). Eating disorders are relatively rare: on average, 0.3% of adults will develop anorexia, 0.9% will develop bulimia, and 1.6% will develop binge-eating disorder, respectively.[25] However, men and women with eating disorders represent a population at high risk: People with eating disorders are also likely to have other mental illnesses, including depression, anxiety disorders, and substance-abuse problems, as well as an increased risk of medical complications, early death, and suicide.[25]

Eating disorders evolve for many reasons. Disordered behavior often begins with dieting; however, before dieting, other factors have already affected a person's mindset. Some women may have a biological vulnerability to eating disorders. Levels of neurotransmitters and hormones that affect one's mood, appetite, and eating behavior may be altered in some women with eating disorders. For example, the hormone serotonin, which creates feelings of satiety after eating, may be present at lower levels in women with bulimia. Therefore, these individuals tend to not feel as satisfied after eating and may binge as a result. Poor self-image, depression, anxiety, loneliness, and unhealthy family and personal relationships may contribute to the development of an eating disorder. The stresses associated with adolescent and adult life can also precipitate anorexia or bulimia.[26]

Our culture, with its unrelenting idealization of thinness, "the perfect body," and its presentation of weight loss as an accomplishment, is also partly to blame. Consider

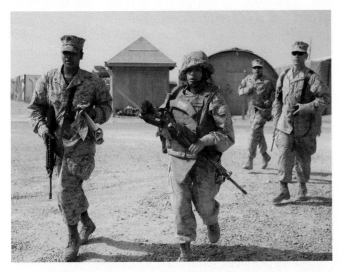

Rates of posttraumatic stress disorder among women have increased as more women have joined the U.S. military.
Courtesy of Gunnery Sgt. Katesha Washington/U.S. Marines

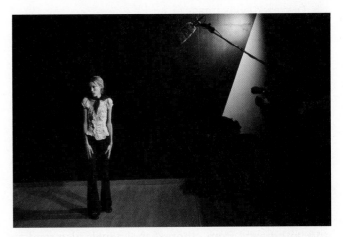

Anorexia creates numerous problems for physical and mental health.
© Villard/Sipa/AP Images

the rise in pro-eating-disorder websites that share information among those with eating disorders on how to better meet their disordered goals of weight loss and behavior control. Women (and men) use personal blogs and webpages such as Pinterest to share photographs, stories, and techniques in an effort to create a sense of support and community among people of like thinking. Many health professionals, however, believe these websites encourage harmful eating habits and have mounted campaigns with Internet service providers to have the sites removed.

Eating disorders have harmful consequences for the mind and the body. People with eating disorders are more likely to suffer from other mental illnesses; they can also develop health complications, including dental problems, kidney failure, and heart conditions.[27]

The female athlete triad is a particularly harmful interrelationship among disordered eating, **amenorrhea** (the absence of a regular menstrual cycle in a woman of reproductive age), and **osteoporosis**. The triad usually begins with disordered eating. Poor nutrition and intense athletic training cause weight loss and a decrease in or shutdown of estrogen production. These stresses on the body lead to a cessation of the menstrual cycle. The final condition in the triad, osteoporosis, may follow if estrogen levels remain low and the woman's diet is lacking in calcium and vitamin D. Although the triad can occur in any athlete, those at greatest risk are endurance athletes such as distance swimmers and runners and athletes in sports where slim appearance is highly valued, such as gymnasts and figure skaters.

Anorexia Nervosa

Anorexia nervosa is characterized by deprivation of food and a body weight of at least 15% below the normal weight for a person's height and age. The *DSM-V* classifies anorexia as an eating disorder associated with the following factors:

- Refusal to maintain an adequate weight
- Intense fear of gaining weight
- Distorted body image
- In women, three consecutive missed periods without pregnancy

Physical symptoms of anorexia nervosa include a significant loss of weight, a refusal to eat, amenorrhea, and a denial of unusual eating behaviors or weight change. As an anorexic person's metabolism slows to adjust to the lack of nourishment, other symptoms appear, including muscle weakness, constipation, brittle hair and nails, lethargy, and a lowering of the body temperature, which causes a constant feeling of coldness and slowness. Psychological symptoms include a distorted or confused body image, a sense of being incompetent, depression, and withdrawal from others.[26] Individuals also tend to become socially withdrawn as the disorder progresses.

The most notable belief shared by women with anorexia is that weight, shape, or being thin is the predominant reference for establishing personal value or self-worth.[27] Other identified psychological features of the illness include:

- A frustration over becoming overweight
- A fear of losing control over eating
- A loss of judgment relative to the requirement of food as a basic need for the body
- An unrealistic sense of body image

> *I look in the mirror and see myself as grotesquely fat—a real blimp. My legs and arms are really fat and I can't stand what I see. I know that others say I am too thin, but I can see myself and I have to deal with this my way.*
>
> **—100-pound anorexic girl**

Women with anorexia often display obsessive-compulsive behaviors, such as obsessing about becoming fat and, consequently, compulsively exercising or practicing odd eating rituals to avoid weight gain. Other compulsive activities may include constant weighing, looking in the mirror, and taking body measurements. Women with anorexia also are obsessed with food and eating and will often cook, prepare, and purchase food for others. They will eat in secret and reject food in public.

Anorexia nervosa usually strikes in early to late adolescence. The typical anorexic woman is highly critical of herself, has poor self-esteem, and believes that she is quite inadequate in most areas of personal and social functioning. She often feels powerless and unable to control many areas of her life, so she establishes power over her food intake and weight. Because of her perfectionist tendencies, the woman with anorexia may believe that the ultimate sign of control is a "perfect" body. Symptoms of depression with large mood swings are commonly seen in individuals with the disorder. The increased risk for heart and kidney failure, suicide, and other serious consequences makes people with anorexia about 10 times more likely to die early than people without this condition.[24]

Bulimia Nervosa

Bulimia nervosa is an eating disorder characterized by cyclic binge eating (**bingeing**) followed by purging (behaviors such as inducing vomiting to remove the food before it can be digested).

The *DSM-V* associates four distinguishing characteristics of bulimia:

- Recurrent episodes of binge eating (at least two episodes per week for at least 3 months)
- A feeling of lack of control over eating behavior during the binge

- Regular engagement in purges
- Persistent overconcern with body shape and weight

Bulimia is a progressive disorder that usually begins with extreme hunger as a result of long periods of food deprivation from fasting or dieting. This hunger is followed by attempts at eating while still trying to control weight. Women with this eating disorder often maintain normal body weight but are extremely dissatisfied with their bodies. Some bulimics have reported that in their preadolescent years, they gained feelings of control and power through this self-denial. The situation progresses to out-of-control binges/purges because the artificial elimination methods have relieved the feeling of being "stuffed," and the bulimic believes it is a good way to lose weight.

Binges often occur when bulimics feel that they have passed a self-imposed limit on acceptable food intake. Consequently, they feel defeated and generally gorge until they are interrupted or the food runs out, often eating 2000 to 3000 calories in a single sitting. The binge foods of choice are usually high-calorie, easily ingested "junk" food that requires little preparation and can be obtained while keeping the behavior secret from others. Bulimics may use several modes of purging, including induced vomiting, diuretics, laxatives, fasts, enemas, diet pills, chewing for hours and then spitting out the food, and excessive exercise. The number of different methods of purging is a stronger index of the severity of the woman's condition than is the frequency of use of any one type.

The binge–purge cycle may occur anywhere from once or twice weekly to several times daily. The cycle often begins in response to a strong emotion, either positive or negative. These emotions can come from a food craving, stress, sleeplessness, anxiety, joy, excitement, physical or emotional pain, helplessness, hopelessness, loneliness, or sadness. After the binge, some women say they initially feel relaxed and soothed, but these feelings turn to shame, guilt, and self-hatred. The women then feel the need to purge to relieve the fear of weight gain and to regain a sense of control and purity. After the purge, bulimics may feel relieved that they have controlled their weight but guilty and negative about succumbing to the cycle again. These feelings of guilt invariably lead the bulimic to perpetuate the behavior.

People with bulimia are often independent high achievers and of normal weight. Bulimia has traditionally afflicted adolescent and young adult females from middle-class backgrounds, but it affects other groups of women and men as well. Bulimics are often perfectionist, obsessive-compulsive, depressed, intense, insecure, sensitive to rejection, anxious to please, and dependent on others. They may be socially isolated as a result of their all-consuming preoccupation with food and weight and their struggle to hide their eating behavior. The majority of women who suffer from bulimia are aware that their eating habits are abnormal but may believe that they have the ultimate weight control secret of being able to "have

their cake and eat it, too." Other factors that may contribute to the development of bulimia include family problems, maladaptive behavior, self-identity conflicts, history of sexual abuse, and cultural overemphasis on physical appearance. In addition to the psychological problems, bulimia nervosa can cause a variety of physical problems, including hypoglycemia, a slowed metabolism, spontaneous regurgitation, erosion of tooth enamel or tooth loss, bleeding and sores in the mouth and esophagus, and mineral deficiencies. **Table 12.4** compares the symptoms of anorexia nervosa with those of bulimia nervosa.

Binge Eating Disorder

Binge eating disorder (BED) is characterized by compulsive overeating without attempting to purge. Defining factors of BED include recurrent episodes of binge eating 2 days per week or more for at least 6 months, as well as an overall sense of loss of control over the binges.

Women with BED also have a preoccupation with food and weight, as well as a distorted body image.

Most people who suffer from BED are obese and have a long history of weight fluctuations. Women who suffer from BED are at high risk for medical problems associated with obesity as well as depression and anxiety due to guilt and feelings of self-disgust. Many people with BED have histories of major family dysfunction and childhood abuse.

Table 12.4 Symptoms of Eating Disorders
Symptoms of Anorexia Nervosa
Loss of at least 15% of body weight
Intense fear of weight gain
Distorted body image (feeling fat even when too thin)
Absence of three consecutive menstrual periods (amenorrhea)
Insistence on keeping weight below a healthy minimum
Symptoms of Bulimia Nervosa
Repeated (usually secretive) episodes of bingeing and vomiting
Feeling out of control during a binge
Purging after a binge (vomiting, use of laxatives or diuretics, excessive exercise)
Frequent dieting
Extreme concern with body weight and shape

My friends confronted me about my anorexia in my senior year of high school. By that point it had gotten so bad that even I had to admit it—I got lost on the way to school because I couldn't think straight. It was really tough for the first year, and was still difficult after that, but now I'm really okay with it. In fact, I'm eating a healthier diet than I ever was before, even though I don't think about food nearly as much.

—**22-year-old woman**

Treatment

People with eating disorders are usually intensely secretive about them. However, observant friends and family members often have an idea when an eating disorder is occurring. Many people try to ignore their suspicions so as to protect the privacy of their friend or family member or out of a wish not to interfere. Women with bulimia and BED are often able to identify the disorder themselves. In contrast, women with anorexia are often in denial about their condition and usually are brought to treatment by concerned family members. Many women enter therapy to treat an eating disorder only after being persuaded to do so by friends or family members. It thus becomes extremely important for people to confront the women in their lives when they suspect disordered eating and to provide them with support in finding the appropriate help. As with all health interventions, being sensitive, caring, and understanding of the central and painful role the disorder may play in a person's life is essential when discussing an eating disorder.

Several approaches are used to treat eating disorders, including motivating the patient, enlisting family support, behavior modification therapy, drug therapy, nutrition counseling, and psychotherapy. Hospitalization may be required for patients with life-threatening complications or extreme psychological problems. If the patient's life is not in danger, treatment may be provided on an outpatient basis and may last for a year or longer.

Treatment is often a lengthy and difficult process, with many women suffering from relapses. Stopping the pattern of dysfunctional eating is essential for successfully treating an eating disorder, but this is only the start. Healthful eating habits must be learned and established to replace the harmful behaviors. Additionally, people with eating disorders also need professional help to develop a realistic body image, develop positive self-esteem, and resolve the underlying issues that may have contributed to the eating disorder.

Other Disorders

Personality Disorders

Personality disorders are characterized by distorted and inflexible thoughts and behaviors that make it impossible for a person to live a productive life or establish fulfilling relationships. These types of disorders have created controversy in the field of psychiatry because it is often difficult to decide when the personality of a person becomes clinically deviant. A diagnosis of a personality disorder requires observing long-term patterns of distorted thoughts and behaviors that seriously interfere with a person's life. Several personality disorders exist (**Table 12.5**), with histrionic and borderline personality disorders being the most common in women.

People with histrionic personality disorder are deeply emotional, have low self-control, and feel a strong need for

Table 12.5   Types and Symptoms of Personality Disorders
Antisocial: disrespectful of others; often in trouble with authorities
Avoidant: extremely inhibited socially; low self-esteem; intense fear of rejection
Borderline: poor self-image; unstable relationships; mood swings; impulsive behavior; extreme fear of being abandoned; self-destructive behaviors such as drug abuse, casual sex, and binge eating
Dependent: submissive; feelings of worthlessness; allows others to make important decisions; common in women who have suffered domestic abuse
Histrionic: seeks attention; acts overly emotional to attract desired attention; constantly seeks approval; is demanding and needy in relationships
Narcissistic: needs constant admiration and attention; has low self-esteem and an exaggerated sense of her own importance; constantly worried what others think of her
Obsessive-compulsive: obsessive about certain areas of life, including work; perfectionist tendencies; controlling personality
Paranoid: extremely distrustful; suspicious of others; extremely jealous, unforgiving, and quick to anger
Passive-aggressive: passively resists taking on responsibilities; consistently fails to live up to demands placed on her; often is irritable and complaining, resulting in problems in relationships
Schizoid: cannot form close relationships; has a very limited range of emotions; may lead to schizophrenia
Schizotypal: cannot form close relationships; eccentric in behavior; experiences distorted thinking and strange speech and behavior patterns; suffers from extreme social anxiety; often suspicious of others

attention. People with this mental disorder feel uncomfortable and unappreciated unless they are constantly the center of attention. Because people with this disorder are very sensitive, they can be easily hurt by real or imagined slights. People with histrionic disorder often have a difficult time maintaining stable jobs, living arrangements, and relationships. Additionally, their suggestibility, and need for attention and approval, can lead people with histrionic disorder to engage in risky sexual behaviors.[28]

Borderline personality disorder (BPD) is also characterized by instability in moods, relationships, identity, and behavior. People with BPD may develop intense feelings of anxiety, anger, or depression that appear and disappear within several hours. The intensity of these feelings makes people with BPD more likely to hurt themselves, engage in substance abuse, and commit suicide. The same intense, changing emotional pattern also makes it very difficult for people with BPD to build and maintain stable relationships. A combination of environmental and genetic factors likely play a part in whether a person develops histrionic personality disorder or BPD.[28]

Many people with personality disorders never enter treatment. Those who do usually seek help for depression or anxiety. Treatment often involves long-term psychotherapy, cognitive behavioral therapy, and/or family or group therapy. Medications may be given with psychotherapy to relieve symptoms of depression or anxiety.

Schizophrenia

Psychosis is a severe mental disorder characterized by loss of contact with reality and severe personality changes. Although mood disorders primarily affect how a person feels, psychosis disorders primarily affect how a person thinks and perceives the world. **Schizophrenia**, a type of psychosis, is a severe, chronic, and disabling type of psychosis disorder. Many subtypes of schizophrenia exist, each of which has specific symptoms and a certain degree of disease severity. Although the word "schizophrenia" comes from the Greek word for "split," it does not mean that a schizophrenic person has a "split" personality or multiple personalities. Instead, this meaning describes the splitting of coherent thoughts in those who suffer from the illness.

My brother had schizophrenia. He started hearing voices when he was in his twenties. He was married, in graduate school, and he just fell apart. I took care of him, but my family was too embarrassed to deal with him. He hated the way the medication made him feel and he hated how he was when he was off the drugs, so he took his own life. I was so angry with him for doing that, at myself for not being able to prevent it, and at my family for not helping him. But now I feel that I need to do something—to educate people about mental illness, to advocate for research to get better treatment, and to help erase the stigma that goes along with mental disorders.

—26-year-old woman

Schizophrenia affects about 2.4 million U.S. adults (about 1% of the adult population).[14] Women and men are equally likely to develop schizophrenia, but there are gender differences in the development of the disease. Men are more likely to be affected between the ages of 16 and 25, while women are more likely to develop schizophrenia between the ages of 25 and 30. Women typically start with a milder form of the disease, experiencing more mood symptoms than psychoses. A significant proportion of women with schizophrenia experience an increase in symptoms during pregnancy and the postpartum period.

Living with schizophrenia can be terrifying. People with schizophrenia experience hallucinations (usually voices and other sounds, but also smells and sights that are not there) and delusions (beliefs that are not true, such as that people are reading the person's mind, planning to harm or trap the person, or controlling the person's thoughts). To the person experiencing them, these hallucinations and delusions appear utterly real.[2] These and other symptoms can appear suddenly or gradually over a period of years. Other symptoms of schizophrenia include disordered thinking, difficulty interacting with others, and difficulty thinking clearly. Some women with schizophrenia may experience symptoms for years or decades at a time, whereas others may experience random episodes of symptoms throughout life.

Treatments for schizophrenia are improving and can provide some relief, but most people with schizophrenia experience symptoms throughout their lives.[29] Fewer than half of people with schizophrenia get adequate treatment. New medications that cause fewer side effects have been developed over the last decade. A newly developed class of drugs, called atypical antipsychotics, are more effective than older types of drugs but have much more severe side effects. Psychotherapy and support groups also may help some patients. Schizophrenia is a difficult disease; only 1 in 5 people recovers completely and 1 in 10 eventually takes his or her own life.[29]

Dissociative Disorders

Dissociative disorders develop as an unconscious way to protect oneself from emotional traumas by detaching from a part of one's identity, thoughts, memory, behavior, or personality.

The DSM-V describes three types of dissociative identity disorders:

- Dissociative amnesia, in which a person has difficulty remembering important information about one's past or self, often resulting in memory gaps that typically last between a few minutes to a few days. (Contrary to depictions in popular culture, a person is much more likely to forget about a recent traumatic event or time period than to forget his or her name or identity.)

- Depersonalization disorder can involve persistent feelings of depersonalization, where a person loses either his or her sense of attachment to the world or to events, almost as if that person is watching a movie of his or her life. Alternatively, this disorder can involve derealization—the feeling that people or other aspects of the world are fake or unreal.

- Dissociative identity disorder (formerly known as "multiple personality disorder") in which a person unconsciously creates and acts out multiple identities in addition to his or her "own" personality. This disorder most often results from sexual or other forms of abuse that occur at a very young age.

Temporary symptoms that mimic some of the symptoms of dissociative identity disorders are a fairly common response to trauma. Short-term detachment or memory loss, for example, may occur after a car accident, sexual assault, or fight. Symptoms in dissociative identity disorders are more persistent, lasting for weeks or months, and occur in about 2.5% of the population.[30]

SUICIDE

The taking of one's own life is the most drastic consequence of mental illness. There are almost always warning signs that a person is at risk of suicide. More than 90% of people who kill themselves have depression, another diagnosable mental illness, or a substance abuse disorder. Adverse life events like a death in the family, a relationship breakup, or financial ruin, along with other risk factors, also may make a person more likely to take his or her own life. However, suicide is not a normal or acceptable response to stress. Many people have briefly considered suicide at some point in their lives when they were depressed or experienced something very bad; however, most people do not act on these thoughts, and are thus not considered suicidal. Risk factors for someone committing suicide include the following:

- Adverse life events along with other factors such as depression
- Prior suicide attempt
- Family history of mental disorder or substance abuse
- Family history of suicide
- Family violence, including physical or sexual abuse
- Firearms in the home
- Incarceration
- Exposure to suicidal behavior of others, including family members, peers, and even the media

Suicide rates differ sharply by gender. Males account for about 80% of all suicides, but this is in part due to the way men and women choose to end their lives—women are actually more likely than men to have suicidal thoughts. Men are more likely than women to kill themselves impulsively or to use firearms to commit the act; women are more likely than men to use poison or other methods in an attempt to kill themselves. For adults of all ages, suicide is the 10th leading cause of death in the United States—the 9th leading cause of death for males, and the 16th leading cause of death for females. For men and women younger than the age of 44, who are less likely than older adults to die of chronic diseases, suicide is consistently among the top five causes of death.[31]

For many people, an attempt at suicide is both a "cry for help" and a very real health risk. Having a previous suicide attempt is a risk factor for a future suicide attempt. In addition, a person may face serious, lasting health consequences from the original attempt. At the same time, however, most suicidal thoughts (as well as the pain, mental illness, or emotional trauma that causes those thoughts)

are only temporary. Providing a suicidal person with immediate, compassionate, and effective treatment can help a person cope long enough to get through a suicidal impulse; later, additional treatment can help a person deal with the underlying root causes of suicidal thoughts. Similarly, many cases of suicide can be prevented by limiting access to effective ways for a person to kill him- or herself. Suicide barriers or nets have prevented many people from killing themselves by jumping off of tall bridges. Many studies have also found that suicides are much less likely to occur in houses without firearms.

Friends and family members of people with known depression or risk factor(s) for suicide should pay close attention to their loved ones. If someone you know demonstrates suicidal behaviors or discusses suicidal wishes, seek professional psychiatric, social work, or medical help immediately. Treatments for a suicide attempt or suicidal thoughts depend on the underlying root cause but often involve learning new coping skills, recognizing the underlying factors causing thoughts of self-harm, and receiving appropriate treatment for existing mental and substance abuse disorders.

Globally, more than 800,000 people commit suicide each year, accounting for about 1% of global deaths.[32] Women living in low- and middle-income countries face the same risk factors for suicide as do women living in upper-income countries, but they are also more likely to face additional challenges at the societal level. Facing discrimination or persecution, whether due to one's gender, sexual identity, racial or ethnic group, or other factors, greatly increases a person's risk for suicide, as does living in poverty, without access to education or mental health care, or under unstable living conditions (such as being a refugee).[32] Together, these factors have a devastating impact: women in low- and middle-income countries make up about three-fourths of all global suicides. The World Health Organization is working to reduce suicide around the world by establishing programs and working with national governments to fight these root causes.[32]

INFORMED DECISION MAKING

Just as good physical health is more than the absence of disease, good mental health is more than the absence of mental illness. Being able to engage in rational thought and decision making; feeling a variety of emotions without being controlled by those emotions; being able to maintain stable, fulfilling relationships; and being able to cope with difficult circumstances are all signs of a healthy mind.

Maintaining good mental health requires taking care of oneself. Some women tend to put other people's needs before their own. Doing this on a consistent basis can be extremely stressful and increases the likelihood of mental illness. Finding appropriate coping mechanisms can help women deal with stressful situations and difficult circumstances. Some good coping mechanisms include taking time to relax and having a trusted friend, family member, or mentor to talk to. Other basic healthy behaviors, like getting a good night's sleep, eating a nutritious diet, and integrating physical activity into one's daily routine, benefit the mind as well as the body. Regular exercise yields benefits for people suffering from depression and anxiety disorders in particular. See **It's Your Health** for a list of healthful activities that can relieve stress and promote good mental health.

People have different vulnerabilities to mental disorders based on their genetic inheritance, physical condition, social situation, and life experiences, but mental health is a concern for everyone. No one is immune to mental disorders. Even if you are fortunate enough to never experience one, it is almost certain that you will know and care for someone who has had one, has one now, or will have one.

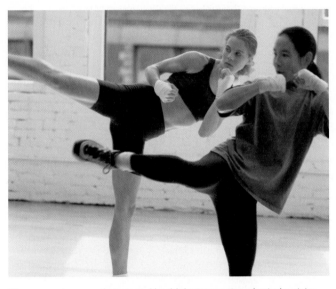

Women can improve their mental health by integrating physical activity into their day.
© Photodisc

Seek professional help if you notice a pattern of disturbing thoughts, find yourself unable to cope with life's daily challenges, or feel anxious or unhappy most of the time. Seeking help is not always easy. Many people who could benefit from mental health services decide not to seek care out of fear that they will be labeled "crazy" or "unstable." Other people believe either that "things will get better on their own" or that treatment would be useless. Millions of Americans already benefit from (or would benefit from) some form of mental health treatment. Although some mental disorders may go away on their own, others do not, and treatment can often dramatically shorten the course of a disorder. **Self-Assessment 12.1** can help determine whether you or someone you care about needs to seek help.

Psychiatrists, clinical psychologists, and social workers are all trained, certified practitioners who have been trained to help people with mental illnesses. Many colleges and universities have professional mental health services available, or at least can give referrals to nearby services. A good match between a patient and provider that includes mutual trust is key. To help decide whether a provider is right for you, feel free to ask a mental health provider questions about his or her training, number of years in practice, experience treating someone with a similar problem, fees, types of insurance accepted, and methods of therapy.

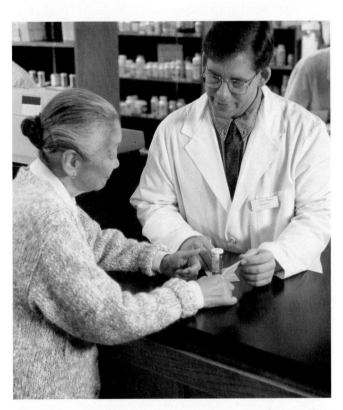

When used properly, medications can be an enormous benefit to people coping with a mental illness.
© Keith Brofsky/Photodisc/Thinkstock

Prescribed medications can help many people deal with the symptoms or underlying causes of many mental illnesses. However, although medications can be of great benefit, they should not be thought of as a "magic bullet" that can instantly fix or eliminate mental illness. Medications usually take days or weeks to have any effects. Medications may require professional help and personal observation to determine the correct choice of medication and dosage; they also may cause unpleasant or dangerous side effects. For dealing with a persistent issue, a combination of therapy with medication often works better at treating mental illness than either medication or therapy alone.

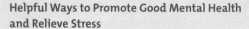

It's Your Health

Helpful Ways to Promote Good Mental Health and Relieve Stress

Here is a list of common activities that can provide relief from stress, anxiety, and depression, as well as promote good mental health.

- Watching a funny movie or video, telling and listening to jokes, or other activities that bring laughter
- Exercise (30 minutes or more per day is best, but any amount of exercise brings benefits)
- Meditation, prayer, or visualization (imagining yourself on a calm beach, in a quiet meadow, or in some other peaceful, relaxing situation)
- Spending time with trusted friends, family, or pets
- When a problem arises, thinking about potential ways you can solve the problem (or take steps toward solving it)
- Listing things for which you feel grateful
- Napping or simply lying down, closing one's eyes, and relaxing
- Creative endeavors (writing, drawing or painting, dancing, singing, etc.)

There are four basic forms of psychotherapy:

- Traditional psychotherapy, which deals with psycho-social aspects of depression and is often referred to as "talk therapy"
- Psychodynamic psychotherapy, which deals with experiences from childhood to resolve rooted problems
- Cognitive behavioral therapy, which works to identify and correct patterns of thinking and behaviors
- Interpersonal psychotherapy, which focuses on present problems and helps with improving relationships, communication skills, and coping skills

Self Assessment 12.1

Determining One's Need to Seek Professional Help

Experiencing any of the following symptoms for several weeks may be an indication to seek professional help.

- Feelings of sadness, hopelessness, or worthlessness
- Loss of energy and drive
- Behavioral changes, such as restlessness, irritability, or self-destructive behavior
- Physical symptoms, such as headache, nausea, backache, or unexplained pain without another medical explanation
- Prolonged worry or anxiety without any identifiable cause or reason
- Sudden episodes of intense and overwhelming fear for no apparent reason
- Irrational and uncontrollable fear or panic when exposed to a particular object or situation
- Frequent thoughts or talk about death or suicide

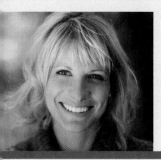
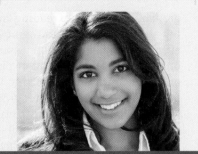
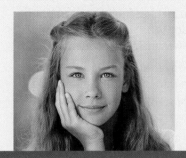
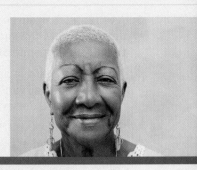

■ Summary

Mental health is a complicated concept to define. Like physical health, it varies from person to person and can even change within a person over time. Mental health includes a person's ability to find peace in life, feel emotions without being controlled by them, build and maintain stable relationships, and cope with difficult circumstances. Biological, social, psychological, and environmental factors all influence mental health.

Mental illnesses affect the way people feel, think, perceive reality, and interact with the world. Three major categories of mental illnesses include mood disorders, anxiety disorders, and eating disorders. Mood disorders, such as depression, dysthymia, and bipolar disorder, interfere with a person's ability to feel and control their emotions. Anxiety disorders, including GAD, phobias, panic disorder, OCD, and PTSD, occur when anxiety grows to unhealthy levels, or appears in situations where no danger exists. Eating disorders, such as anorexia, bulimia, and BED, are characterized by dysfunctional eating patterns. Other major mental illnesses include schizophrenia, dissociative disorders, and personality disorders. Most people with mental illnesses are functional members of society. Even so, untreated mental illnesses cause a variety of harmful effects, the most harmful and dramatic of which is suicide. Treatment may involve psychotherapy, medications, or a combination of both. Mental health should involve not just avoiding and treating specific types of mental illness but also practicing behaviors that reduce stress and promote good mental health.

■ Topics for Discussion

1. Freud defined mental health as "the ability to love and to work." What do you think of this definition? Can you create a better one?

2. If you were president of the United States, what laws would you change to promote better mental health?

3. Why does stigma around mental illness exist? What can be done to reduce this stigma?

4. What are some of the advantages and disadvantages of prescribing medication for a mental disorder?

Profiles of Remarkable Women

Dorothea Lynde Dix (1804–1887)

Dorothea Lynde Dix was a nurse and humanitarian who was instrumental in the reform of treatment of the mentally ill in the 19th century. Dix became interested in this issue when she visited a Massachusetts prison that housed mentally ill people. She saw naked prisoners who were kept chained, in filthy quarters, with visible signs of harsh treatment and abuse. Dix spent the next 2 years researching the situation and then reported her findings to the Massachusetts legislature. Responding to her plea for humane care for the mentally ill, Massachusetts took action and moved the mentally ill people to an asylum. Dix sought change all over the United States through legislative reform, and her work prompted the establishment of 32 mental health hospitals across the United States. Dix also made an international impact, recommending reforms for prisons in Italy, France, Russia, Scotland, and Turkey.

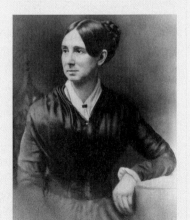

© Universal Images Group Limited/Alamy Images

5. A young woman suspects that her friend has an eating disorder. What can she do? What if her friend denies the disorder in spite of overwhelming evidence?

6. A young woman suspects that her grandfather is depressed. What can she do? What if her grandfather tells her he doesn't know what "being depressed" means?

7. What are steps that you can take (as a class or as individuals) to promote good mental health?

CASE STUDY

You have had the same roommate since the start of freshman year, so by halfway through your sophomore year, you feel you know Julia pretty well: she's generally quiet but calm, kind, and a really good listener. Julia studies hard but also loves to go dancing and see a local comedy group perform improv sketches. Every morning, Julia takes antidepressant medications. She tells you she's been on them since she was 16.

Three months into your second semester living together, Julia has been acting differently. She doesn't smile as much, seems more nervous, sometimes even grouchy. She stays up reading late into the night, saying she can't sleep, and then oversleeps, sometimes even missing her morning classes. Last Friday you tried ordering her favorite kind of pizza and she only ate one slice. She didn't want to go with you that evening to watch the improv theater group either. In addition, Julia hasn't been bothering to brush her hair—she just pushes it back into a ponytail—and has been wearing the same sweatpants for days. You come back one afternoon from class and find her curled up in bed, crying. When you ask her, "What's wrong?" she says, "Nothing… life… everything… don't worry about it."

(Julia's story has been drawn from the experiences of multiple women coping with depression. Her name and other identifying information have been changed to preserve anonymity.)

Questions

1. Based on the information provided, Julia is showing symptoms of what mental illness?

2. As Julia's roommate, what could you say or do (now or in the near future) that might be helpful?

3. What are some things you should avoid doing in order to not make this situation worse?

Profiles of Remarkable Women

Joanne Rowling (1965–)

Joanne "J. K." Rowling is the author of the *Harry Potter* series of novels, the best-selling book series in history. More than 400 million copies of the seven-part *Harry Potter* books have been sold, and the movies based on the series have grossed almost $6 billion worldwide. Rowling's journey from a poor, single, working mother to a billionaire and world-famous author has become a well-known rags-to-riches story. What is less well known, however, is that Rowling suffered from severe depression for a 3-year period during her mid-20s.

Rowling first became depressed shortly after the breakdown of her first marriage in 1993. This time was an especially traumatic one for her: Rowling was left without a job after her marriage ended, and she struggled to support herself and her 1-year-old daughter. Rowling's own mother had also died the year before.

Rowling described her time with depression as the worst part of her life. "We're talking suicidal thoughts here, we're not talking 'I'm a little bit miserable,'" Rowling said in a 2008 interview. Rowling's concern for her daughter eventually convinced her to seek counseling. With time and help, Rowling eventually overcame her depression. During this period, Rowling also completed the manuscript for *Harry Potter and the Sorcerer's Stone*.

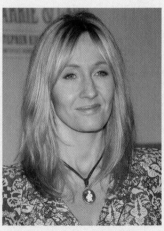

© Everett Collection Inc/Alamy Images

Rowling's time with depression had at least one silver lining: Rowling was able to incorporate her experiences with depression into the *Harry Potter* series. Dementors, evil wraith-like creatures in the books, induce a state much like permanent depression after consuming the souls of their victims. One character describes Dementors as "drain[ing] peace, hope, and happiness out of the air around them . . . Get too near a Dementor and every good feeling, every happy memory will be sucked out of you. . . . You will be left with nothing but the worst experiences of your life."

Rowling continues to speak about her time with depression and recommends that anyone experiencing the disease not blame themselves and seek help instead. "The funny thing is, I have never been remotely ashamed of having been depressed," Rowling said in a 2010 interview.

■ Key Terms

Amenorrhea

Anxiety disorder

Binge eating disorder (BED)

Bingeing

Bipolar disorder (manic-depressive disorder)

Dementia

Depression

Dissociative disorder

Dysthymia

Generalized anxiety disorder (GAD)

Mood disorder (affective disorder)

Neurotransmitter

Obsessive-compulsive disorder (OCD)

Osteoporosis

Panic disorder

Personality disorder

Phobia

Postpartum psychosis

Posttraumatic stress disorder (PTSD)

Psychosis

Seasonal affective disorder (SAD)

Schizophrenia

Serotonin

Underinsured

■ References

1. Kellogg, R. (2008). Quoted in *What is mental health?* [Press release]. Available at: http://www1.dshs.wa.gov/mediareleases/2008/pr08057.shtml

2. U.S. Department of Health and Human Services. (1999). *Mental health: A report of the Surgeon General.* Available at: http://www.surgeongeneral.gov/library/mentalhealth/home.html

3. Substance Abuse and Mental Health Services Administration (SAMHSA). (2013). *Results from the 2012 National Survey on Drug Use and Health: Mental health findings.* Rockville, MD: Substance Abuse and Mental Health Services Administration.

4. Pomerantz, E., Rydell Altermatt, E., & Saxon, J. (2002). Making the grade but feeling distressed: Gender differences in academic performance and internal distress. *Journal of Educational Psychology* 94(2): 396–404.

5. Stewart, W. F., Ricci, J. A., Chee, E., et al. (2003). Cost of lost productive work time among U.S. workers with depression. *Journal of the American Medical Association* 289(23): 3135–3144.

6. National Institute on Drug Abuse. (2010). *Comorbidity: Addiction and other mental illnesses.* Available at: http://www.drugabuse.gov/sites/default/files/rrcomorbidity.pdf

7. Almeida, O. (2012). Approaches to decrease the prevalence of depression in later life. *Current Opinion in Psychiatry* 25(6): 451–456.

8. National Institute of Mental Health (NIMH). (2015). *Fact sheet on stress.* Available at: http://www.nimh.nih.gov/health/publications/stress/index.shtml

9. Lipschitz, J., Paiva, A., Redding, C., et al. (2013). Co-occurrence and coaction of stress management with other health risk behaviors. *Journal of Health Psychology* 20: 1002–1012.

10. James, D., & Glaze, L. (2006). *Mental health problems of prison and jail inmates.* Bureau of Justice Statistics. Available at: http://www.bjs.gov/content/pub/pdf/mhppji.pdf

11. Kessler, R. C., Heeringa, S., Lakoma, M. D., et al. (2008). Individual-level and societal-level effects of mental disorders on earnings in the United States: Results from the National Comorbidity Survey Replication. *American Journal of Psychiatry* 165(6): 703–711.

12. NIMH. (2008). *Depression.* Available at: http://www.nimh.nih.gov/health/publications/depression/complete-index.shtml

13. Centers for Disease Control and Prevention (CDC). (2010). Current depression among adults—United States, 2006 and 2008. *Morbidity and Mortality Weekly Report* 59(38): 1229–1235.

14. Karg, R., Bose, J., Batts, K., et al. (2014). Past year mental disorders among adults in the United States: Results from the 2008–2012 Mental Health Surveillance Study. Available at: http://www.samhsa.gov/data/sites/default/files/NSDUH-DR-N2MentalDis-2014-1/Web/NSDUH-DR-N2MentalDis-2014.htm

15. Halbreich, U., Borenstein, J., Pearlstein, T., et al. (2003). The prevalence, impairment, impact, and burden of premenstrual dysphoric disorder (PMS/PMDD). *Psychoneuroendocrinology* 28(3): 1–23.

16. Nishizawa, S., Benkelfat, C., Young, S. N., et al. (1997). Differences between males and females in rates of serotonin synthesis in the human brain. *Proceedings of the National Academy of Science* 94(10): 5308–5313.

17. Rasic, D., Hajek, T., Alda, M., & Uher, R. (2014). Risk of mental illness in offspring of parents with schizophrenia, bipolar disorder, and major depressive disorder: A meta-analysis of family high-risk studies. *Schizophrenia Bulletin* 40(1): 28–38.

18. O'Connor, R. (1997). *Undoing depression.* New York, NY: Little, Brown.

19. NIMH. (2015). *Bipolar disorder.* Available at: http://www.nimh.nih.gov/health/publications/bipolar-disorder/complete-index.shtml

20. Scott, J. (2006). Depression should be managed like a chronic disease. *British Medical Journal* 332: 985–986.

21. NIMH. (2015). *Anxiety disorders.* U.S. Department of Health and Human Services. Available at: http://www.nimh.nih.gov/health/publications/anxiety-disorders/summary.shtml

22. National Center for Posttraumatic Stress Disorder. (2014). *Women, trauma and PTSD.* U.S. Department of Veteran's Affairs. Available at: http://www.ptsd.va.gov/public/PTSD-overview/women/women-trauma-and-ptsd.asp

23. Department of Defense. (2014). *Department of defense annual report on sexual assault in the military: Fiscal year 2013.* Available at: http://sapr.mil/public/docs/reports/FY13_DoD_SAPRO_Annual_Report_on_Sexual_Assault.pdf

24. NIMH. (2015). *Eating disorders.* Available at: http://www.nimh.nih.gov/health/topics/eating-disorders/index.shtml

25. Swanson, S. (2011). Prevalence and correlates of eating disorders in adolescents. *Archives of General Psychiatry* 68(7): 714.

26. Vitiello, B., & Lederhendler, I. (2000). Research on eating disorders: Current status and future prospects. *Biological Psychiatry* 47(9): 777–786.

27. Blank, S., Zadik, Z., Katz, I., et al. (2002). The emergence and treatment of anorexia and bulimia nervosa. A comprehensive and practical model. *International Journal of Adolescent Medicine and Health* 14(4): 257–260.

28. American Psychiatric Association. (2013). *Diagnostic and statistical manual of mental disorders* (5th ed.). Washington, DC: American Psychiatric Association.

29. NIMH. (2015). *Schizophrenia*. Available at: http://www.nimh.nih.gov/health/publications/schizophrenia/complete-index.shtml

30. Devillé, C., Moeglin, C., & Sentissi, O. (2014). Dissociative disorders: Between neurosis and psychosis. *Case Reports in Psychiatry* 2014: 1–6.

31. Xu, J., Kochanek, K., Murphy, S., et al. (2014). *Mortality in the United States, 2012.* NCHS Data Brief 168. Hyattsville, MD: National Center for Health Statistics.

32. World Health Organization. (2014). *Preventing suicide: A global imperative.* Available at: http://www.who.int/mental_health/suicide-prevention/world_report_2014/en/

4

PART FOUR

Interpersonal and Social Dimensions of Women's Health

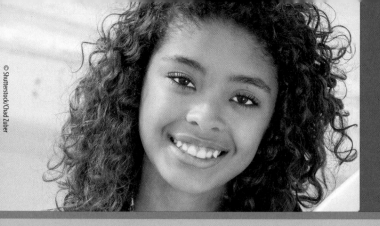
© Shutterstock/Chad Zuber

CHAPTER 13

Substance Abuse

Learning Objectives

On completion of this chapter, the student should be able to discuss:

1. Basic definitions of drugs, drug abuse, tolerance, and other concepts related to drug use and addiction.

2. Biological, cultural, and legal factors that influence how and why women use drugs.

3. Health consequences of smoking, including those particular to women, as well as consequences of secondhand and third-hand smoke.

4. Legal, economic, and cultural factors that influence smoking rates in women, both in the United States and around the world.

5. Reasons why quitting tobacco is difficult, and basic strategies for quitting smoking.

6. Epidemiological trends and various perspectives on alcohol use and abuse.

7. The physiological effects of alcohol on the body.

8. Alcoholism, the symptoms of alcoholism, and approaches to understanding and treating alcoholism.

9. The most common illicit drugs, their effects on the body, and their associated health risks.

10. Links between drug use and mental illness.

11. The development of drug dependency, tolerance, and basic approaches to drug abuse treatment.

12. Effective strategies for recognizing a drug problem and seeking help.

INTRODUCTION

A **drug** is any substance other than food taken to affect body processes. The development of medical drugs has been one of modern society's greatest advances. Drugs prevent or cure diseases, alleviate pain, treat a variety of conditions, and perform many other functions. **Recreational drugs**—or drugs taken for pleasure—such as alcohol and caffeine, can provide relief or enjoyment when used in moderation, and their use has become an important part of many cultures. However, drugs can also cause serious harm or death.

DRUG USE AND ABUSE

Drug abuse is the overuse or misuse use of any drug. Any drug has the potential for abuse, including tobacco, alcohol, medications purchased **over-the-counter (OTC)** or with a prescription, and illicit drugs (illegal drugs or legal drugs used for nonintended purposes). Substance abuse and problems related to substance abuse are among society's most pervasive health and social concerns. Tobacco use is the greatest preventable cause of death, disability, and disease in the United States; every year, it kills more than 480,000 people through cardiovascular disease, cancer, and other conditions.[1] Chronic alcohol use can cause permanent damage to the brain, heart, liver, and other organs, and it increases the risk for many cancers. In addition, drunk driving is a factor in one-third of all automobile accidents.[2] Illicit drugs directly cause about 38,000 deaths per year, and they contribute to deaths from accidents, homicides, and other causes. Individuals who abuse illicit drugs may experience addiction, cardiac illness and death, neurological damage, mental illness, fetal and infant morbidity and mortality, infection with HIV and hepatitis, and other consequences. On a societal level, illicit drug use contributes to accidents and violent crime and causes billions of dollars in medical expenses and lost productivity. Even drugs designed and tested for medical use can cause great harm. Every year, millions of people abuse or misuse drugs purchased over-the-counter or via prescription, sometimes intentionally and sometimes accidentally.

Although many people draw a clear distinction between drugs that are legal and those that are not, the line between these two categories is not always clear. Many drugs that are illegal today, such as LSD or most narcotics, were originally developed for legitimate medical purposes. In addition, the legal status of some drugs has changed with time and may vary by country or state. In the 1920s and 1930s, for example, alcohol was illegal and marijuana was legal. Today, the reverse is true. In the early 1900s, opium, morphine, and cocaine were openly advertised and sold as "remedies" in the form of tonics, syrups, and elixirs. Coca-Cola contained cocaine until 1906, when the cocaine was replaced by caffeine. Today, marijuana use is tolerated in the Netherlands and in small amounts in most of Europe. In the United States, marijuana inhabits a legal gray area in many states. Federal law, which applies to the entire country, prohibits the sale or possession of marijuana. Over the past decade, however, 4 states and the District of Columbia have legalized marijuana, and 21 states now allow some form of marijuana use with a doctor's approval. Although the federal government technically has the ability to override these state laws and arrest people who buy, sell, or use marijuana in these states, it has so far refrained from doing so.

In addition, some drugs, such as alcohol, are legal for some people to use, but not for others. The age at which a person can legally purchase and use alcohol varies throughout Europe and much of the Americas, from as young as 14 in Germany (with the presence and permission of a parent or guardian) to 21 for most of the United States. Many predominately Muslim countries have laws that either outlaw alcohol or severely restrict how it can be bought and sold. There are also age restrictions ranging from 18 to 21 on tobacco purchased throughout the United States and most of Europe.

Legal drugs in the United States include alcohol, nicotine, caffeine, OTC drugs, and drugs obtained with a medical prescription. Prescribed medications are legal drugs that can be obtained only through the authorization of a licensed physician or dentist. Besides marijuana, drugs that are illegal include cocaine, methamphetamines, and heroin. Despite a government-led "war on drugs," which has been ongoing since the Nixon administration, drug availability continues to grow. Nearly one-half of Americans older than the age of 12 have tried at least one illegal drug.[3]

The use of a drug for a purpose for which it was not originally intended is called **drug misuse**. Drug misuse, whether accidental or deliberate, includes using a prescribed or OTC drug in a manner different from its intended purpose, typically in terms of dose, timing, or

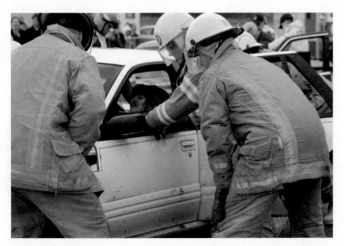

Every year, alcohol is responsible for one-third of all automobile accidents.
© Murray Wilson/Fotolia.com

by a person for whom it was not originally intended. Frequently misused OTC drugs include sleep aids, antihistamines, and cough suppressants containing dextromethorphan (DXM). Deliberate drug use inconsistent with or in excess of accepted medical practice constitutes drug abuse. The most frequently abused prescribed medications include opioid-based pain relievers, prescribed pain medicines used for anxiety and sleep disorders, and medications for attention-deficit hyperactivity disorders.

The dangers of misusing or abusing a particular drug are often associated with the drug's ability to cause addiction. Addiction has roots in physical dependence, where the body adjusts to having a drug in its system and goes through observable negative changes when the drug is removed. Many legal drugs—including alcohol, tobacco, and prescription painkiller medications—can cause physical dependence. Besides physical dependence, drugs can create a psychological dependence, called habituation. A combination of physical and psychological dependence can greatly increase a person's risk for addiction. Addictions can vary in their intensity. Some forms of addiction may feel akin to a strongly ingrained habit. Other forms of addiction may drive a person to direct all of his or her energies to compulsive drug-seeking behavior, even as those drugs increasingly provide less pleasure or relief.

Drugs typically enter the body through one of three ways:

- *Orally*—swallowing a drug in capsule, tablet, or liquid form is the most common way of consuming a drug. Drugs taken orally do not reach the bloodstream as quickly as those taken by other means.

- *Through the lungs*—sniffing a powder, such as cocaine; inhaling gases, aerosol sprays, or fumes from solvents or other compounds that evaporate quickly; or smoking tobacco or another substance.

- *By injection*—drugs may be injected subcutaneously (under the skin), intramuscularly (into the muscle tissue), or intravenously (directly into a vein) through the use of a syringe. An intravenous injection immediately introduces the drugs into the bloodstream. Intramuscular and subcutaneous injections are slower in action.

In addition to the dosage and the route of administration, several factors influence the intensity and the duration of a drug's effects:

- Physical conditions such as a cold, pregnancy, or menstruation may make the body more vulnerable to the effects of a drug.

- Genetic differences among individuals may account for varying drug responses. Some people appear to be more sensitive than others to specific classes of drugs or to drugs in general. Mindset or social setting can also influence a drug's effects. Someone who snorts cocaine to enhance sexual pleasure may feel more

stimulated simply because that is what she expects to happen or may experience different feelings if she or he takes a drug at a noisy, crowded party rather than in a secluded room.

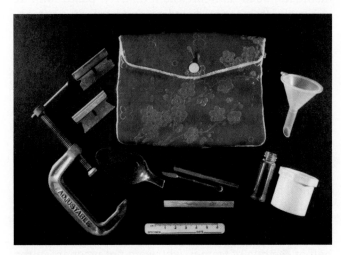

There are several ways that drugs can enter the body.
Courtesy of Orange County Police Department, Florida

Tolerance is the body's ability to withstand the effects of a drug. Continued use of many drugs increases tolerance so that increasingly large doses may become necessary to produce the same effects. Larger doses also increase the risk of toxicity—the level at which a drug becomes poisonous to the body. Toxicity-related damage may be temporary, permanent, mild, or even deadly, depending on the drug, dose, and individual.

Many people with substance abuse problems abuse more than one drug at once; the average user who enters treatment is on five different drugs. The more drugs used, the greater the chance of side effects, complications, and possible life-threatening situations.

Sociocultural Dimensions

Several sociocultural factors increase the likelihood of drug abuse in women, including:[3,4]

- Significant life stresses, such as divorce, loneliness, and dissatisfaction with a career

- Traumatic events, such as the loss of a home, a financial crisis, or being the victim of a violent crime

- Sexual abuse and physical abuse, beginning before the age of 11 and occurring repeatedly

- Mental illnesses, such as anxiety, depression, or personality disorder

Society's double standard for women prevails in drug use. Women face greater stigma for drug abuse than men, sometimes because of their potential position as mothers, sometimes because perceived irresponsibility is forgiven more easily in men than in women, and sometimes for other reasons. These social sanctions against addiction can make it harder for women to seek help or may make their friends and families less willing to recognize the addiction and intervene. Females also have a higher rate of substance abuse co-occurring with other psychiatric disorders, such as depression, anxiety, posttraumatic stress disorder, eating disorders, and borderline personality disorder. Connections between mental illness and drug abuse are not always clear. Some women with mental illness may use drugs in an attempt to self-medicate their symptoms, whereas in other cases, women may develop mental illnesses as a result of the consequences of drug abuse. In some cases, both mental illness and drug abuse may result from the same trauma or event.

Pregnant drug users are at increased risk for miscarriage, ectopic pregnancy, stillbirth, low weight gain, anemia, hypertension, low-birth-weight babies, and other medical problems. HIV infection, a possible consequence of intravenous drug use, is another risk among pregnant drug users. Approximately 4.4% of pregnant women between the ages of 15 and 44 use illicit drugs, less than half of the rate of women who were not pregnant in the same age group (10.9%). However, rates of drug use vary considerably among pregnant women of different age groups: 16.2% of pregnant women between the ages of 15 and 26 reported currently using illegal drugs, nearly 9 times the rate (1.9%) of pregnant women between the ages of 26 and 44.[3]

Legal Dimensions

Legal dimensions of drugs and women's health go far beyond the legal status of various drugs. Chief among these is how criminalizing drug use disproportionately affects people of color. While White, Black, and Hispanic Americans use drugs at roughly equal rates, Black and Hispanic Americans are much more likely to be arrested for using or selling drugs. Whereas African Americans constitute 14% of marijuana users in general, they account for nearly one-third of all marijuana arrests. Hispanic and African American drug offenders have a greater chance (40% and 20% greater, respectively) of being sentenced to prison than White drug offenders. African Americans also receive longer prison terms for drug offenses than Whites, serving nearly as much time in prison for a drug offense as Whites do for a violent offense.[5] Various factors contribute to these racial disparities. Greater Black and Hispanic drug-related arrests may be due in part to law enforcement agencies being more likely to focus on making arrests in low-income urban areas, where a disproportionate number of Black and Hispanic people live. Harsher sentences for Blacks and Hispanics arrested for drug possession may be due both to bias (whether conscious or unconscious) on the part of judges and to White arrestees being more likely to live in areas overseen by more judges. Whatever their origins, however, racial drug-related disparities have had numerous harmful consequences for the people who are arrested, their families, and their communities.

Although men are still more likely than women to be sentenced to prison, the number of women in prison has increased at nearly double the rate for men over the past 35 years. There are now nearly seven times as many women in state and federal prisons as there were in 1980; in particular, the number of women incarcerated for drug offenses has risen by more than 900% since that year. African American and Hispanic women represent a disproportionate share of this increase. Minority women are also less likely than White women to receive effective drug treatment. Once arrested, many addicts are incarcerated, where their addiction is either left untreated or worsens due to the widespread underground availability of drugs in many prisons.

Other legal considerations affecting women are associated with drug use during pregnancy. Several states now treat substance abuse among pregnant women as a criminal offense. This approach shifts the focus to punishment and away from the urgent need to provide appropriate drug treatment programs. These states may require healthcare professionals to report prenatal drug exposure; others have amended their child welfare laws to include prenatal substance abuse, using this as evidence of child abuse to end or diminish parental rights. Only a few states view drug use by pregnant women as a sign of the need for treatment. Punitive reproductive health policies have an especially negative effect on low-income women and women of color. Most pregnant women charged with crimes for drug abuse are women of color, and drug testing of newborns is implemented almost exclusively by public hospitals that predominantly serve low-income women. Such policies often discourage women from seeking needed prenatal care or drug treatment. The threat of criminal punishment fosters a climate of fear and mistrust between doctors and patients, potentially causing harm to the health of both women and their future children.

Economic Dimensions

The use and abuse of illicit drugs has a tremendous impact on American society and causes about $200 billion per year in economic damages.[6] Alcohol and tobacco also cost hundreds of billions of additional dollars every year in medical expenses, accidents, lost productivity at the workplace, and other factors.

Societal costs of drug abuse include:

- Treatment of physical damage, disease, and other complications resulting from inappropriate drug use
- Burden of drug-related crime
- Creation and maintenance of treatment facilities
- Loss of individual productivity
- Care for children of drug-dependent parents
- The policing of illicit drug availability

Each year, the federal government spends about $25.5 billion for drug control.[6] This money is used to reduce, prevent, and deal with the consequences of illicit drug use. Under President Obama, the Office of National Drug Control Policy (ONDCP) has shifted its approach to acknowledge drug control as a public health concern as well as a matter for law enforcement. The Obama administration has worked to reduce federal criminal penalties for the use of certain drugs. In addition, the ONDCP has focused on the following major areas:[6]

- Preventing illicit drug use and addiction

- Expanding access to treatment for Americans struggling with addiction

- Reforming the criminal justice system to break the cycle of drug use, crime, and incarceration while protecting public safety

- Supporting recovery from addiction by reducing the stigma associated with drug use and substance abuse disorders

Economic dimensions also affect who uses specific illicit drugs. Use of certain drugs, such as crack cocaine, which tend to be relatively affordable on a per-dose basis, are more common among poorer people than among affluent people. In addition, whereas drugs are most often exchanged for money, women living in poverty are more likely than other groups to exchange drugs for sex. Exchanging drugs for sex puts women at heightened risk for acquiring sexually transmitted infections and for becoming a target for sexual violence.

Tobacco use also has serious economic costs. Today, the price of a pack of cigarettes averages around $6 to $7, with state and city taxes sometimes bringing the cost up to more than $10 per pack. State, federal, and local taxes often make up half or more of the price of cigarettes sold in stores. State taxes on a package of cigarettes range from $4.35 in New York to $0.17 in Missouri, with some cities or counties imposing additional taxes.[7] As a result, a pack-a-day smoker may spend anywhere from $2000 to $4000 annually to fund her habit. In addition to collecting government revenue, cigarette taxes can act as a deterrent to smoking, both by discouraging nonsmokers from starting and by encouraging smokers to smoke less. The World Health Organization estimates that every 10% price increase would reduce smoking by about 4% in the United States, with greater effects on price among young smokers and smokers in the developing world.[8]

Some street vendors sell "black-market" cigarettes for below-market prices, pocketing the money that would otherwise go to taxes. Untaxed cigarettes are available on Indian reservations, in some foreign countries, and on the Internet for as little as $2.50 per pack. Organized crime and large-scale smugglers are now participating in the underground cigarette market. In addition to the cost of purchasing cigarettes, smokers may have to pay higher premiums for their health insurance coverage. Some companies have even implemented policies against hiring smokers in states where it is legal to do so.

TOBACCO

The consequences of smoking are devastating to women's health. Tobacco kills more people every year than alcohol, car accidents, all illicit drugs, HIV, murders, and suicides combined.[1] Half of all Americans who smoke will die from a smoking-related disease; millions of lifelong smokers who do not die from smoking will develop debilitating lung problems or other conditions. The costs of smoking-related illness in the United States are more than $300 billion every year, including $170 billion for direct medical care and $156 billion in lost productivity.[9]

Tobacco also affects people who do not use it directly. Environmental exposure to smoke exhaled from a cigarette (secondhand smoke) as well as leftover chemicals that accumulate in a room where someone has smoked (third-hand smoke) also increase the risk for lung cancer, asthma, and other conditions.[1] Although tobacco use has fallen substantially over the past 20 years, these reductions have slowed in recent years, and smoking rates remain high among vulnerable groups such as the poor or people with low education levels (**Figure 13.1**). Clearly, tobacco remains a major issue for public health and women's health.

Epidemiological Trends and Issues

Native Americans first cultivated and smoked tobacco in North America thousands of years ago. Tobacco became popular in Europe in the 16th century, when Spanish explorers brought it to their colonies and Europe from

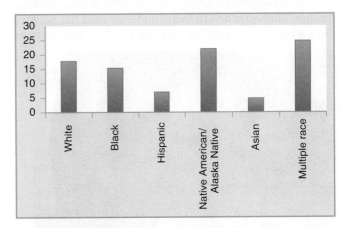

Figure 13.1   **Percentage of U.S. women who currently smoke, by race and ethnicity.**

Source: Centers for Disease Control and Prevention. (2014). *Current cigarette smoking among adults: United States, 2005–2013.* Available at: http://www.cdc.gov/mmwr/preview/mmwrhtml/mm6347a4.htm

the New World. Tobacco became an accepted component of early colonial life, though its use was largely limited to men. Through the next century, tobacco was also snuffed (inhaled), dipped, and chewed.

Cigarette smoking gradually increased in popularity throughout the 19th century. During this time, a few doctors noted that tobacco use was connected with certain diseases, but this information was not widely reported or believed. Most people believed that tobacco use either posed no harm or actually improved health. Over the course of the 1800s, a series of technological additions to cigarettes enhanced the ease of inhalation and modified their flavor and aroma.

The 1920s were a critical period of change for women, characterized by new social and cultural patterns, a newly won ability to vote, and a push for greater rights and emancipation. In an extremely effective series of advertising campaigns, the tobacco industry took advantage of this women's rights movement. Cigarette companies marketed smoking as a symbol of rebellion, romance, and emancipation for women—women could now smoke cigarettes alongside men as well as vote. Women began to smoke openly in public settings, and female cigarette smoking prevalence rates rose from 2% in 1930 to 34% in 1965.[10]

Just over one in seven women (15.3%) currently smoke in the United States.[11] Although this number represents tremendous progress—current smoking rates are less than half of what they were 50 years ago—this decline has not affected all groups of women equally.[11] Large disparities exist based on race, ethnicity, and other factors (**Table 13.1**).

Among adult women in the United States, smoking rates are the highest among people of Native American descent (22%). This is 50% above the national average and five times the smoking rate of Asian Americans, the racial group least likely to smoke. After Native Americans, the ethnic and racial groups most likely to smoke are people of mixed race, Whites, African Americans, and Hispanics. Women who are living under or near the poverty line, who do not have a college degree, or who identify as

Table 13.1	Percentage of U.S. Women Who Smoke, by Age, Education, Region, and Other Factors
Characteristic	**Percentage of Women**
Age (Years)	
18–24	15.4
25–44	17.1
45–64	18.1
≥ 65	7.5
Education*	
Some high school or less	18.0
GED diploma	39.7
High school graduate	17.6
Associate degree	17.7
Some college	19.5
Undergraduate degree	7.9
Graduate degree	5.5
Region	
Northeast	15.8
Midwest	17.4
South	16.2
West	11.5
Sexual Orientation	
Straight	15.0
Lesbian, bisexual, gay, or transgendered	26.7
Poverty Status	
At or above poverty level	13.8
Below poverty level	25.8

*Among adults aged ≥ 25 years

Source: Centers for Disease Control and Prevention. (2014). *Current cigarette smoking among adults: United States, 2005–2013.* Available at: http://www.cdc.gov/mmwr/preview/mmwrhtml/mm6347a4.htm

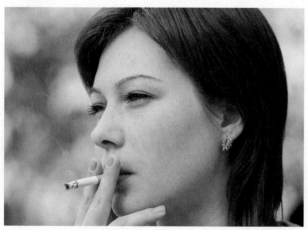

Smoking habits that start during teenage years often become lifelong addictions.
© DenisNata/Shutterstock

lesbian, gay, bisexual, or transgender are all more likely to smoke.[11]

Even though tobacco use is illegal for people under the age of 18, many teenagers and adolescents have tried tobacco. Four in 10 (40%) of all female high school students have tried smoking. About one in seven (15%) female high school students reported smoking in the past month, a rate slightly less than the smoking rate among male high school students (16%).[12] Women (and men) who have tried tobacco as teenagers are much more likely to become lifelong smokers. White high school students are most likely to smoke, followed by Hispanic and Black high

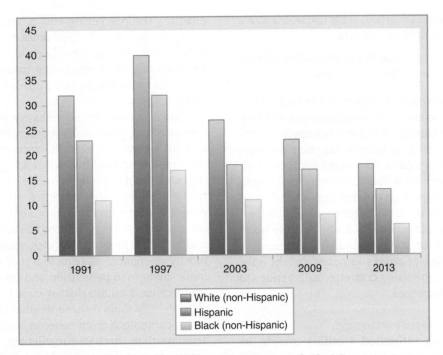

Figure 13.2   **Percentage of female high school students who smoke, by race and ethnicity, 1991–2013.**

Data from Centers for Disease Control and Prevention. (2010). Youth Risk Behavior Surveillance, United States, 2009. *MMWR*. Available at http://www.cdc.gov/mmwr/pdf/ss/ss5905.pdf

school students, though rates for all three groups have fallen over the past 20 years (**Figure 13.2**).

Water pipes, also known as hookahs, have become popular among some adolescents, college students, and young professionals. An old custom among some cultures in the Middle East, hookahs can now be found in fashionable clubs, restaurants, and cafes in many cities. Hookah smoking appears to be just as harmful as cigarette smoking.[13] In fact, it may be even more dangerous because the hookah is used over a longer period of time than smoking a cigarette (about 40 to 45 minutes compared to 5 to 10 minutes). This longer period of inhalation and exposure may lead a smoker to inhale as much smoke as consuming 10 or more cigarettes during a single hookah session.[13]

Electronic Cigarettes

Electronic cigarettes, also referred to as "vapes" or "e-cigarettes," are an alternative to cigarettes that have gained popularity over the past 5 years. These products are typically cigar or cigarette-shaped devices that produce a nicotine-containing vapor that may be inhaled, or "vaped," in place of smoke. Electronic cigarettes are a new, untested frontier in public health. Proponents argue that electronic cigarettes can provide nicotine, like nicotine gum or patches, and allow a person to indulge in a habit similar to smoking, while avoiding the cancer-causing elements of tobacco.

Other experts urge greater caution. These experts argue that electronic cigarettes, by being perceived as "harmless," may lure new users who have never tried cigarettes or persuade smokers to switch to vaping instead of quitting. Experts skeptical of electronic cigarettes also point out that nicotine, and possibly other components of the inhaled vapor, are still harmful, even if they are less harmful than tobacco smoke.

While the topic remains under continuing study, the evidence that exists so far indicates that electronic cigarettes are a more effective lure than they are a tool for quitting. A 2014 study found that more than 263,000 middle and high school students who had not smoked had tried electronic cigarettes—an increase of more than 300% in just 2 years.[14] These same students were also more likely than others to say they would be likely to smoke in the future.

Legal Dimensions of Tobacco Use

Federal and state governments share responsibility for controlling how tobacco products are bought and sold. In 2009, the U.S. Food and Drug Administration (FDA) gained the authority to regulate tobacco products and began issuing rules about how tobacco products could be sold, distributed, and marketed. Most of these changes were made to prevent people younger than 18 from purchasing or receiving tobacco products. These FDA requirements included:

- Banning the sale of tobacco products to people younger than 18

- Prohibiting the distribution of free cigarettes or the sale of packages containing fewer than 20 cigarettes

- Limiting the sale of cigarettes in vending machines to select locations where only adults are present

- Prohibiting tobacco company names from appearing as a sponsor of athletic, musical, or cultural events

- Requiring that audio advertisements use words alone rather than music or sound effects
- Banning the sale or distribution of promotional items with tobacco company brands or logos

State governments may tax cigarettes or place additional restrictions on when or where smoking is allowed. All 50 states and the District of Columbia impose a cigarette excise tax; the national average for state cigarette excise taxes is $1.63 per pack. City taxes can occasionally add to these taxes: New York City taxes each package $1.50, for a combined state-local tax rate of $5.85 per package.[7] These taxes have become a valuable revenue source for many state budgets. Many of these taxes were enacted to pay for state medical bills associated with smoking. However, as other sources of income have declined, many states are using cigarette tax revenues to pay for nonmedical expenses.

Smoking and Women Worldwide

Around the world, an estimated 1 billion people, or one-seventh of the total population, are smokers.[15] The World Health Organization (WHO) estimates that tobacco use kills almost 6 million people each year, with about 5 million dying as a direct result of tobacco use and about 600,000 dying from exposure to secondhand smoke.

As smoking rates have fallen in the United States, Western Europe, Australia, and New Zealand, tobacco companies have aggressively expanded their markets in the developing world. Four out of five of the world's smokers now live in low- and middle-income nations. In these countries, where there is typically less government regulation of tobacco sales and marketing, as well as less public knowledge about the health dangers of smoking, tobacco companies have used tactics such as widespread advertising, cigarette giveaways, and promotions at bars and nightclubs to encourage smoking. In addition, tobacco companies have used their financial and political power to block or prevent developing countries from enacting the marketing and promotion bans and price increases that have helped reduce smoking in the developed world. Women have been affected by these efforts as direct targets of marketing campaigns and indirectly as victims of second- and third-hand smoke in heavily smoking populations.

Tobacco companies are savvy in the ways they lure new smokers, particularly women. Many tobacco companies have cleverly linked the emancipation of women in the developing world with smoking, similar to methods that were used in Western countries in the early 20th century. According to the Institute for Global Tobacco Control, governments in developing countries may be less aware of the harmful effects of tobacco use on women and children and are often preoccupied with other health issues; they mostly see tobacco as a problem confined to men. If no dramatic changes in prevention and cessation occur, tobacco could cause 1 billion deaths over the course of the 21st century.[15] To reduce these deaths, WHO works to counteract campaigns from tobacco companies, obtain more accurate data through surveillance, and encourage governments to implement tighter tobacco-control laws and help people who want to stop smoking quit successfully.

Health Consequences for Women Who Smoke

Tobacco use kills roughly 50% of the people who use it. Cigarette smoke causes numerous health problems, primarily for the lungs, but also for almost every system in the body. Health risks to smokers vary depending on the amount smoked, the depth of cigarette inhalation, the tar and nicotine content of cigarettes, and the duration of smoking. Inhalation patterns and puffing behavior affect the degree of exposure to carbon monoxide and other toxic compounds. In addition to causing 90% of all lung cancer deaths and 30% of all cancer deaths, recent research has revealed that smoking is responsible for more deaths than previously thought, including deaths from hypertension and kidney failure.[1]

The health consequences of smoking also depend largely on when a person starts smoking, and when, if ever, he or she quits. On average, a woman who smokes will lose 14.5 years of her life from smoking. Symptoms of smoking-related illness usually take years to develop, although irritation symptoms such as watery eyes, nasal irritation, squinting, and coughing develop fairly soon after a woman starts (**Figure 13.3**). In addition, smoking causes premature signs of aging, including wrinkles, blotchy skin, and discolored teeth.

Cigarette smoking increases the risk of coronary heart disease, the number-one cause of death among both men and women in the United States. Smoking doubles a woman's risk of myocardial infarction (heart attack) and doubles to quadruples her risk of sudden cardiac death. Young and middle-age women who smoke have substantially higher rates of both fatal and nonfatal stroke than nonsmokers. Each year, more than 8800 deaths from stroke and 40,000 deaths from coronary heart disease are attributed to smoking in women (**Figure 13.4**).[16] Smoking is

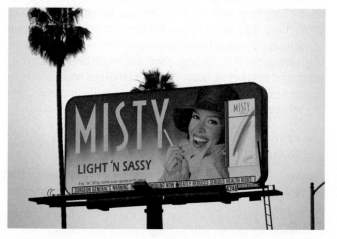

Tobacco companies are savvy in the ways they lure new smokers, particularly women.
© Michael Newman/PhotoEdit, Inc.

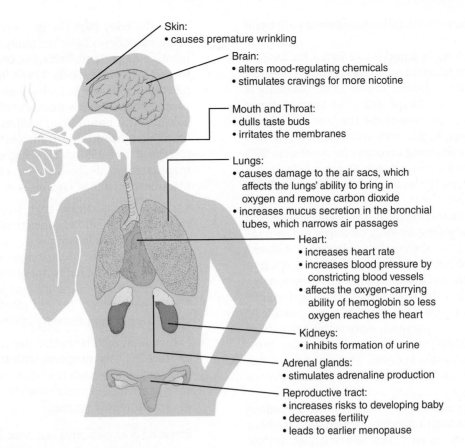

Figure 13.3 **Physiological effects of cigarette smoking.**

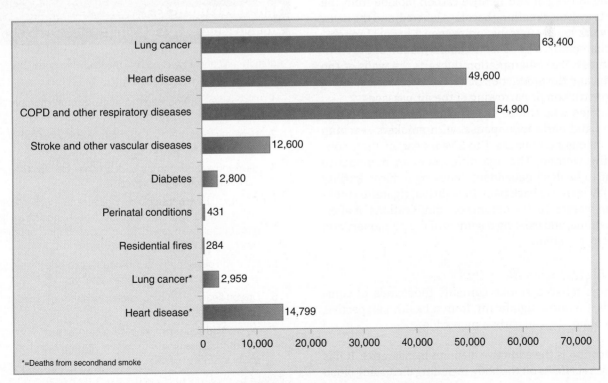

Figure 13.4 **Estimated annual deaths related to cigarette smoking among women and girls.**

Source: Centers for Disease Control and Prevention. (2014). *The health consequences of smoking—50 years of progress: A report of the Surgeon General.* Available at: http://www.surgeongeneral.gov/library/reports/50-years-of-progress/

also a major risk factor for arteriosclerosis and peripheral vascular disease.

Cigarette smoking is a major risk factor for cancers throughout the body. Cancer accounts for about one-third of all smoking-related deaths (Figure 13.4).[1] Smoking is associated with an increased risk of at least 15 types of cancer, including cancers of the lung, larynx, breast, pharynx, mouth, esophagus, kidney, pancreas, cervix, and bladder in women. Smoking accounts for more than 80% of lung cancer deaths. Lung cancer, an especially deadly form of cancer, is now the leading cause of cancer-related death among women.

In addition to increasing the risk for heart disease and cancer, cigarette smoking severely damages the respiratory system. **Chronic obstructive pulmonary disease (COPD)** is characterized by permanent airflow obstruction and extended periods of disability and restricted activity. Cigarette smoking is the major risk factor for developing COPD, with 80 to 90% of COPD deaths attributable to smoking. Over the past few years, more women than men have died from COPD (more than 70,000 females compared to 64,000 males).[15] Females who smoke also are nearly 13 times more likely to die from COPD than are female nonsmokers.

COPD encompasses many conditions, including emphysema and chronic bronchitis, which usually occur together. With **emphysema**, the limitation of airflow results from gradual, irreversible disease changes in the lung tissue after years of assault. The air sacs in the lungs are destroyed, which compromises the ability of the lungs to bring in oxygen and remove carbon dioxide from the body. As a result, breathing becomes labored, and the heart must work harder to transport oxygen. **Chronic bronchitis** is characterized by constant inflammation of the bronchial tubes. The inflammation thickens the walls of the bronchi, and the production of mucus increases, resulting in a constriction or narrowing of the air passages.

Women who smoke face an increased risk of osteoporosis and early menopause, with smokers reaching spontaneous menopause 1 to 2 years earlier than nonsmoking women. The age differences in menopause appear to be dose-dependent. Smoking reduces fertility and may increase back pain. In addition, cigarette smoking can worsen the symptoms or complications of allergies, asthma, and existing disorders of the pulmonary and circulatory system.

How Cigarettes Affect the Body

Although tobacco smoke contains thousands of compounds, the most significant, from a health perspective, are nicotine, tar, and carbon monoxide.

- **Nicotine** is the addictive element in cigarettes. It has several effects on the body, including increasing blood pressure, increasing heart rate, and negating hunger. Nicotine stimulates the pleasure centers of the brain, causing physical addiction. Although nicotine can harm the body over the long term, it also provides some short-term benefits: Many smokers state that nicotine helps them relax, concentrate, or complete some tasks more easily. These benefits, along with nicotine's addictive potential, help explain why many people continue to smoke despite knowing tobacco's harmful nature. Two studies published in 2007 found that the nicotine available in cigarettes steadily increased from 1997 to 2005, suggesting that cigarette manufacturers deliberately increased the amount of nicotine available in cigarettes.[17]

- **Tar** is a thick, sticky, dark fluid produced when tobacco is burned. Tar consists of hundreds of compounds, many of which are **carcinogenic** (capable of promoting growth of cancerous cells) in their own right. Through inhalation, tar settles and accumulates throughout the oral cavity and pulmonary system. The combination of tar and smoke further compromises the cardiopulmonary system.

- Carbon monoxide is another deadly by-product of cigarettes. This gas interferes with the blood's ability to carry oxygen, impairs normal functioning of the nervous system, and contributes to degradation of the cardiopulmonary system.

Smoking is an addictive behavior, with nicotine being the primary addictive pharmacological component. **Self-Assessment 13.1** provides an opportunity to assess whether

Self-Assessment 13.1
Are You Addicted to Cigarettes?

Carefully read and answer each of the following questions honestly.

1. Do you feel like you "need" to smoke a certain number of cigarettes per day? yes no

2. Have you made previous attempts to quit tobacco but been unable to do so? yes no

3. Have you ever tried to cut back on cigarettes and then gone back to previous levels? yes no

4. When you have not smoked a cigarette for a while, do you feel any withdrawal symptoms, such as an urge for a cigarette, irritability, anxiety, difficulty concentrating, or drowsiness? yes no

5. Have you developed any smoking-related side effects, such as a morning cough or a hoarse voice? yes no

6. Do you find yourself preoccupied with thoughts about smoking or cigarettes? yes no

7. Do you find yourself making life decisions (such as which friends to spend time with or where to live) based on your ability to smoke? yes no

If you answered "yes" to any of these questions, you may be addicted to tobacco. Consider quitting cigarettes, seeking help from your healthcare provider if necessary.

you or someone you know is addicted to cigarette smoking. Smoking cessation results in withdrawal, a period of unpleasant symptoms and an intense psychological and physiological demand for nicotine. Symptoms of withdrawal usually include the following:

- Cigarette craving
- Irritability
- Restlessness
- Anxiety
- Difficulty in concentrating
- Headache
- Drowsiness
- Depression (deep, overwhelming feelings of apathy, sadness, or anger)
- Varied gastrointestinal disturbances such as diarrhea and constipation

The physical and psychological withdrawal symptoms that occur with cigarette smoking cessation vary in their duration and intensity. For heavy smokers, withdrawal symptoms may occur within 2 hours of the last cigarette. The peak period of physiological symptoms from smoking cessation is usually 24 to 48 hours into abstinence, but many smokers report "cravings" for cigarettes for years.

Why Women Smoke

Women often begin cigarette smoking in adolescence in the context of social interactions with peers. Adolescents are more likely to be smokers if their parents, older siblings, or peers smoke. Many smokers report that their primary reason for smoking is to give them something to do in social situations and/or to "fill time." The social situations in which smoking occurs, as well as the physical effects of nicotine, strongly affect smoking dependence in women. (See **It's Your Health**.)

Many women hesitate to quit smoking over a fear of unwanted weight gain. Even many pregnant women who smoke indicate that their reason for doing so is to avoid weight gain. Smokers do tend to weigh less than nonsmokers. Some evidence indicates that nicotine elevates the body's basal metabolic rate (BMR). The average person gains between 4 and 10 pounds upon quitting smoking, but exercise combined with a smoking cessation program can decrease this weight gain and increase rates of abstinence from smoking.

Women's concerns about weight gain and the maintenance of their smoking behavior reflect their willingness to risk long-term detrimental—and potentially catastrophic—consequences in exchange for dealing with body image and weight-control issues. Teenage girls, in particular, often believe that smoking helps them control their weight, and this belief dissuades many from quitting

It's Your Health

Strategies to Quit Cigarettes Gradually

Wait 15 minutes after the initial urge for a cigarette. This delay gives a feeling of control, and sometimes the urge will go away or become manageable.

Distract yourself when you want to smoke by drinking water, making a phone call, chewing gum, taking a short walk, or brushing your teeth.

Avoid being around people who smoke or places where the smoking habit has thrived—a favorite chair, lingering after a meal, a coffee break.

Establish nonsmoking hours and gradually extend them.

Buy cigarettes only by the pack. Never buy the same brand twice in a row.

Ask that other smokers do not light up around you. Have friends and family help you fight the urge to smoke again.

Make it harder to get your cigarettes. Keep them in a locked drawer or with a friend.

Declare former smoking areas to be nonsmoking areas, such as the car, house, and office.

Keep a daily record to document and reinforce progress with quitting. Write down reasons why you want to quit.

Call 1-800-QUIT-NOW to connect with a local quit hotline.

Be willing to try again. Many people are able to quit after several attempts.

Consider nicotine replacement therapy (NRT) or other medications to help reduce the physical addiction of cigarettes.

this behavior. Health professionals, educators, mothers, and other female role models must strike a balance between recognizing that girls have concerns about their weight, while trying to refocus them on healthy behaviors, self-esteem, and safer coping strategies.

Smoking and Pregnancy

In addition to harming a woman directly, smoking also causes harm to a developing fetus. Smoking during pregnancy is responsible for 17 to 30% of low-birth-weight babies, 14% of preterm deliveries, and 5% of newborn deaths.[1] Pregnant women who smoke more are at additional risk. Nicotine and carbon monoxide are considered the two most important components in cigarettes that constitute major hazards to the fetus:

- Nicotine reduces fetal breathing movements and uterine blood flow and increases fetal heart rate.
- Carbon monoxide reduces the amount of oxygen available to the fetus by as much as 25%.

The prevalence of smoking during pregnancy has declined steadily over the past 20 years, with about 10% of pregnant women currently smoking during the last 3 months of pregnancy. About 45% of smoking women who become pregnant quit during pregnancy; half the women who quit during this time relapse within 6 months of delivery.[18]

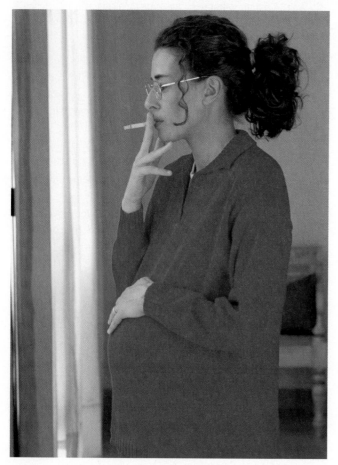

Smoking presents many risks to a woman and her unborn child.
© Pixal/Superstock

Secondhand and Third-hand Smoking

Smokers are not the only ones affected by cigarette smoke. **Secondhand smoke**, or environmental tobacco smoke (ETS), is air that is contaminated with chemicals from cigarette smoke. Nonsmokers who breathe second-hand smoke are at increased risk of developing asthma, lung cancer, heart disease, and other conditions; for smokers who spend much of their time with other smokers, secondhand smoke provides an additional source of exposure to carcinogens and dangerous chemicals. Secondhand smoke kills more than 40,000 adults each year in the United States—about 34,000 from heart disease and about 3000 from lung cancer.[1]

Infants and young children, whose lungs are more sensitive than the lungs of adults, are especially vulnerable to secondhand smoke. Secondhand smoke increases a child's risk of low birth weight; sudden infant death syndrome (SIDS); acute lower respiratory tract infections, such as bronchitis and pneumonia; induction and exacerbation of asthma; chronic respiratory symptoms; and middle-ear infections.

The greatest source of exposure to secondhand smoke for children, infants, and most adults is the home. For adults living in households where no one smokes, the workplace is the greatest source of exposure to ETS. The separation of smokers and nonsmokers within the same airspace reduces, but does not eliminate, exposure to ETS. Twenty-four states and the District of Columbia prohibit smoking in restaurants, bars, and government buildings, and seven states prohibit smoking in restaurants; the remaining states have weaker laws that allow smoking in at least some public locations. Many states have also legally mandated that most workplaces follow a nonsmoking policy.[1]

Third-hand smoke—the leftover nicotine and other chemicals that accumulate on walls, furniture, clothing, and other surfaces in areas where smoking has occurred—also creates health risks. These chemicals may last on surfaces for weeks or months. Although not as dangerous as secondhand smoke, third-hand smoke does increase the risk for asthma, lung cancer, and other conditions, with children and infants being more susceptible to its effects. More research is needed to fully understand the risks of third-hand smoke.[19]

Quitting Smoking

Quitting smoking is often the most significant personal behavior that a person can undertake to improve her or his health. Some health benefits of quitting begin shortly after the last cigarette. After a few weeks, a person's lungs and circulatory system improve; coughing and shortness of breath usually decline within a few months. The risk for cardiovascular disease and cancer also drops over time. A year after quitting, a person's risk of coronary heart disease falls by 50%. A person's risk of mouth, throat, and lung cancers also usually falls by 50% within 5 to 10 years. A person will experience greater benefits the earlier she or he quits, but quitting at any time significantly improves health.

Quitting smoking is not an easy process. Some people are able to quit on their first attempt, others are able to quit after several efforts, and some people are never able to quit. Typically, only about 8 to 10% of smokers who attempt to quit on their own are successful on any given attempt. This does not mean that quitting is impossible for anyone, simply that the act of quitting is typically a long-term process, characterized by gradual progress with many starts and stops along the way. Biologically, the most difficult period is usually the first 3 months, when a person's physical and psychological addiction to tobacco is the strongest. After that period, some people have an easy time staying away from smoking, while others continue to feel cigarette cravings for years. A second critical period is a relapse, or return to smoking. By itself, a single cigarette smoked during a quit attempt means little. Psychologically, however, the feelings of weakness and hopelessness a relapse can cause can often derail a quit attempt entirely. If you or someone you know is attempting to quit, it may help to compare a relapse to forgetting to brush one's teeth—a simple mistake and not something to repeat, but not something that should derail a quit attempt.

Some people decide to quit by going "cold turkey," or making a sudden, decisive break from cigarettes. Another approach involves gradually reducing the amount of nicotine the body receives. A person can do this either by reducing the number of cigarettes he or she smokes or by switching from smoking to an alternate form of nicotine, such as nicotine replacement therapy (NRT), to reduce withdrawal symptoms.

Nicotine replacement therapy allows a person to take a controlled, gradually decreasing source of nicotine without the additional harmful effects of tobacco. It is available as a patch, gum, lozenge, spray, or inhaler. Although these forms all provide the same drug, they differ in the speed at which it is delivered. The nicotine patch provides a slow, steady dose of nicotine that lasts for hours. Kept in the mouth, nicotine gum and lozenges may take about 30 minutes to take effect. Nicotine sprays (sprayed into the nose like some allergy medicines) and inhalers provide a strong, short-duration dose of nicotine that is felt within a few minutes. Studies have found that NRT improves a person's chances of quitting by 50 to 70% for the first 3 to 6 months.[20] However, the long-term effectiveness of NRT—whether it helps people quit tobacco for good—is less certain.

The FDA has also approved two medications to help people quit smoking: bupropion (Zyban) and varenicline (Chantix). Both of these medications appear to reduce cravings for tobacco and to block the pleasurable effects nicotine has within the brain. After taking these medications for a few weeks, a person who does smoke a cigarette may feel little or no enjoyment from the experience. Both of these medications are about as effective as NRT in helping people to quit; like NRT, there are still questions regarding their long-term efficacy.[20] A small percentage of people who take varenicline may experience disturbing psychological symptoms, ranging from changes in mood, to altered dreams, to thoughts of violence or suicide. Women who experience any of these symptoms should contact their healthcare provider immediately.

Another way to quit smoking is to enlist the help of other people. Counseling can help smokers identify their motivations for smoking and "triggers" that make them more likely to smoke. Support groups, conducted either online or in person, can help a person meet with and get sympathy, advice, and help from other people trying to quit. A person's own friends and family can be a valuable source of assistance by providing sympathy and gently but persistently encouraging them to continue their efforts to quit.

ALCOHOL

Ethyl **alcohol**, the type of alcohol found in alcoholic beverages, is a colorless liquid obtained by fermentation of a sugar-containing material. Pure alcohol is not drinkable on its own; most alcoholic beverages are at least 50% water and other ingredients. The amount of alcohol in a specific drink varies, from beer (typically 4–6% alcohol), to wine (about 10% alcohol), to distilled spirits (about 40% alcohol). Roughly the same amount of alcohol is present in a 12-ounce bottle or can of beer, 5 ounces of table wine (10% alcohol), and a 1.25-ounce "shot" of distilled spirits (40% alcohol)—each of these servings is often referred to as "one drink." For most people, drinking moderate amounts of alcohol (no more than one drink per day for women and no more than two drinks per day for men) is unlikely to cause any health problems and may even slightly lower the risk of heart disease. However, when a person drinks larger amounts of alcohol on a regular basis or engages in irresponsible drinking behaviors, death, serious injury, or other consequences can result.

Blood Alcohol Concentration

Blood alcohol concentration (BAC) is a physiological indicator that clinicians and law enforcement officials use to measure the content of alcohol in the body and determine whether a person is legally "drunk." Blood alcohol concentration represents the percentage of alcohol in the blood. A BAC of 0.10 indicates the presence of approximately one part of alcohol per 1000 parts of blood. As **Table 13.2** shows, a BAC of 0.10 or greater results in significant compromise of mental and psychomotor capabilities. Driving with a BAC of 0.08 or higher is illegal in all 50 states. The

Table 13.2	**Blood Alcohol Concentrations**
BAC	**Effects**
0.02–0.04	No overt effects; feelings of muscle relaxation and slight mood elevation
0.05–0.06	Relaxation and warmth; slight decrease in reaction time and slight decrease in fine muscle coordination
0.07–0.10	Balance, speech, vision, and hearing slightly impaired; euphoric feelings; increased loss of motor coordination
0.11–0.12	Difficulty with coordination and balance; distinct impairment of mental facilities and judgment
0.14–0.15	Major impairment of mental and physical control; slurred speech, blurred vision, and lack of motor skill
0.20	Loss of motor control; substantial mental disorientation
0.30	Severe intoxication with minimum conscious control of mind and body

Greater levels lead to unconsciousness, coma, and death from respiratory failure.

Source: Substance Abuse and Mental Health Services Administration.

punishment for violating this limit, as well as the number and kinds of other laws related to driving while intoxicated, varies from state to state.

Many factors affect BAC and an individual's response to alcohol. For example, BAC increases faster when alcohol is consumed at a faster rate and without food. Stronger drinks, smaller body size, older age, or being of Asian or Native American descent can also lead to increased BAC levels when drinking. In addition to higher BACs, some people of Native American or Asian descent experience effects such as nausea, headaches, and flushing of the skin when they drink.

With regular alcohol consumption, additional alcohol is required to achieve the same desired psychological effect, even though motor coordination and judgment are impaired at the same level. After years of heavy drinking, damage to the liver can sometimes cause "reverse tolerance." Reverse tolerance occurs when a person lacks enough liver enzymes to break down alcohol at normal rate; if this happens, a person can quickly become intoxicated after drinking only a small amount of alcohol.

Epidemiological Trends and Issues

Alcohol has been a constant component of American life since the colonial period. Attempts to control, restrict, or abolish alcohol in the United States have all met with failure. In 1919, the 18th Amendment to the Constitution was ratified in an attempt to stop the rapid growth of alcohol addiction. This amendment prohibited the manufacture, sale, and transportation of alcohol, ushering in the Prohibition era. During this time, illegal sales of "bootlegged" beverages and alcoholic prescription "medications" prevailed as people sought ways around the ban. Prohibition was officially repealed in 1933 by the 21st Amendment.

During the 19th and early 20th centuries, most people believed that alcoholics were morally weak. Today, there is a greater awareness of the complex nature of alcoholism. Public admissions of alcoholism by well-known women such as Drew Barrymore, Lindsay Lohan, and Nicole Richie have reinforced the fact that alcoholism is a personal and pervasive health problem that affects women from all walks of life.

In general, compared to men, women are less likely to drink, drink less, and are less likely to become alcohol dependent. About 48% of women aged 12 or older (compared to 57% of men) have had an alcoholic beverage within the past month. Women are most likely to drink between the ages of 18 and 25. More than half (57%) of women in this age group have had a drink within the past month, and almost one-third (31%) reported binge drinking. Current alcohol use is most common among Whites (58% of people 12 and older), followed by persons of two races (48%), Blacks (44%), Hispanics (43%), and people of Native American (37%) and Asian descent (34%).[3]

Cultural factors influence the prevalence of alcoholism. Heavy drinking is less common in many cultures where drinking is a part of family rituals or ceremonies or where there is great disapproval of public drunkenness. Gender-based social norms often contribute to alcohol consumption patterns. For example, in some cultures, men are drinkers while women generally abstain.

Social Dimensions

Many cultural factors affect women's drinking behavior. Society's double standard for women often prevails where alcoholism is concerned. Folklore and popular media may portray male drinkers as comical or lovable but a drunken woman as weak or immoral. Additionally, greater social sanctions applied to alcoholism make some women less willing to seek help and others less willing to recognize that they need help. Because alcoholic women violate the stereotype of feminine behavior, they often distress their families and friends and even the health professionals who might support them. For both women and men, depression is associated with excess alcohol consumption. In some cases alcohol may be a symptom of depression; in others, alcohol use may be a consequence of it.

Victimization is also associated with alcohol-related problems. Women who are sexually abused in childhood or physically abused as adults are more likely to experience alcohol-related problems later in life. The relationship between victimization and alcohol may be confounded by the fact that victimization often leads to depression, which is in turn associated with alcohol use.

Although the literature includes few studies on alcohol and drug use among lesbians, some evidence indicates that lesbians consume more alcohol and are more likely than heterosexual women to use alcohol with other drugs.[21] Lesbian women may be at greater risk of alcohol problems because of the social disapproval directed at their sexual orientation.

Societal Costs of Alcohol Use and Alcoholism

With more than 126 million Americans reporting current use of alcohol and 17 million calling themselves heavy drinkers, the economic, social, and personal costs of alcohol-related crimes, accidents, illnesses, and deaths are profound.[3] One estimate of cost of alcohol abuse and alcoholism in the United States is $224 billion per year, or about $750 per person.[22] This estimate includes healthcare costs of people who use or are affected by alcohol, lost productivity, law enforcement and criminal justice expenses, and motor vehicle accidents caused by drunk driving. Most of these costs come from binge or heavy drinking.

The costs to society from alcohol cannot be measured just in terms of dollars. More than 75,000 deaths in the United States are attributed to alcohol every year; just under one-third (21,000) of these deaths are women. About half of alcohol-related deaths are a result of chronic conditions, while the other half are a result of falls, homicides, motor vehicle accidents, suicides, and other acute conditions.[23] Chronic alcohol use contributes to several often-fatal illnesses, most notably liver disease, cancer, and cardiovascular disease, but it also contributes to infertility, immunity problems, and damage to the brain, stomach, colon, kidneys, and pancreas. Drunk driving, or driving under the influence of alcohol, affects not only the people who drink, but their passengers and other drivers. Alcohol is a factor in one in three automobile-related fatalities, causing an estimated 11,000 deaths a year.[24] Whereas men make up the majority (80%) of drunk drivers, both sexes drink and drive, and both sexes are injured or killed as a result of drunk driving.

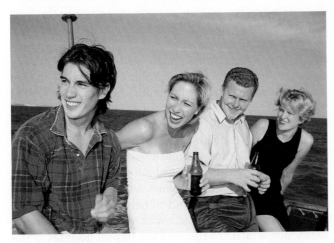

Alcohol is an accepted and often traditional part of many social events.
© Ingram Publishing/Index Stock Imagery, Inc.

Legal Issues of Alcohol Use and Alcoholism

There are many legal issues related to drinking. Although the 21st Amendment made alcohol legal after Prohibition, both states and the federal government have since enacted laws that limit alcohol use. Nationally, alcohol is legally restricted to people 21 and older; most other countries have legal drinking ages of 18 or 19.

In addition to setting age limits on alcohol use, states have enacted laws governing drinking and driving, drunk and disorderly behavior, purchase of alcohol for a minor, and driving with an open container of alcohol. Most of the penalties associated with alcohol abuse or misuse involve misdemeanor charges or fines, but some—for example, drunk driving violations—entail mandatory jail time in many states.

Effects of Alcohol

Alcohol is a central nervous system depressant that, when consumed in small quantities, has a mild, relaxing effect. Consumption of larger quantities results in compromised sensory motor coordination, judgment, emotional control, and reasoning capabilities. Once ingested, alcohol circulates throughout the body, affecting nearly every bodily function (**Figure 13.5**). Alcohol usually takes about 15 minutes to reach the bloodstream, and the peak effect occurs in 1 hour. Once in the bloodstream, alcohol quickly reaches the liver, heart, and brain.

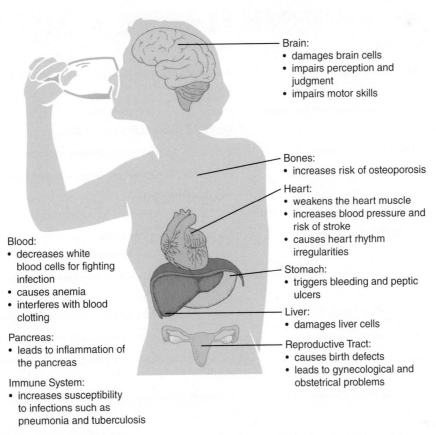

Figure 13.5   Physiological effects of alcohol.

The liver metabolizes alcohol and removes it from the body. This exposure makes the liver the organ most vulnerable to alcohol. Heavy drinking may eventually lead to alcoholic hepatitis, which is characterized by inflammation and destruction of liver cells, and **cirrhosis**, which produces progressive scarring of liver tissue. More than 90% of heavy drinkers develop fatty liver, a type of liver disease; 20% will develop liver cirrhosis.[25] Compared with men, women develop alcohol-induced liver disease over a shorter period of time and after consuming less alcohol.[26]

Chronic heavy alcohol consumption is also associated with cardiovascular damage. Consuming one or two alcoholic drinks per day may slightly lower the chances of developing coronary heart disease; however, heavier drinking greatly increases this risk. Chronic heavy alcohol use also increases the risk for cancers of the liver, mouth, throat, colon, and breast.

To an observer, the most noticeable effects of alcohol are on the brain and behavior. Alcohol alters the activity of brain neurons, impairing sensory, motor, and cognitive function. Even moderate amounts of alcohol result in reduced perception, judgment, and psychomotor skills. Alcohol's anesthetic effect may cause diminished perception of pain and temperature, possibly leading to serious injury or exposure to extreme temperatures. Although drinking may decrease judgment, increase interest, and reduce inhibitions related to sex, it also impairs a man's ability to achieve or maintain an erection and a woman's ability to achieve orgasm. Additional drinking progressively reduces behavioral activity, which may lead to sleep, general anesthesia, coma, and even death.

Alcohol is particularly dangerous when combined with other drugs, such as depressants and antianxiety medications. Of the 100 most frequently prescribed drugs, more than half contain at least one ingredient that interacts adversely with alcohol. Combining alcohol with drugs may heighten the effect of either drug or produce additional harmful effects (**Table 13.3**). Acetaminophen (brand name Tylenol) can be especially toxic to the liver when taken with many drinks, and in rare cases can lead to acute hepatic failure.

Heavy alcohol consumption typically leads to several nutritional problems for the chronic user. Because alcohol dulls the senses of taste and smell, heavy drinkers often skip meals and develop nutritional deficiencies. Alcohol consumption also has been associated with osteoporosis due to its ability to block the absorption of calcium. Chronic consumption disrupts normal digestive processes, resulting in gastritis (inflammation of the stomach lining), stomach ulcers, and intestinal lesions, which interfere with the metabolism of vitamins and minerals. In addition, alcoholism has been associated with thiamine (vitamin B1) deficiency, which can increase the risk for diseases of the nervous, digestive, muscular, and cardiovascular systems.

Table 13.3 Alcohol and Drug Interactions		
Type of Drug	**Examples**	**Possible Effects**
Analgesics (narcotic)	codeine, Demerol, Percodan	Increased CNS depression possibly leading to respiratory arrest and death
Analgesics (nonnarcotic)	aspirin, acetaminophen, ibuprofen	Gastric irritation and bleeding Increased susceptibility to liver damage
Antidepressants	Tofranil, tricyclics (Elavil)	Increased CNS depression, decreased alertness
Antianxiety drugs	Valium, Librium, Xanax, Ativan	Increased CNS depression, decreased alertness
Antihistamines	Actifed, Dimetapp, cold medications (prescribed and over-the-counter)	Increased drowsiness
Antibiotics	penicillin, erythromycin	Nausea, vomiting, headache Some antibiotics are rendered less effective
CNS stimulants	caffeine, Dexedrine, Ritalin, Adderall	Somewhat counter depressant effect of alcohol but do not influence level of intoxication
Diuretics	Lasix, Diuril, Hydromox	Reduction in blood pressure with possible lightheadedness
Psychotropics	Tindal, Mellaril, Thorazine	Increased CNS depression possibly leading to respiratory arrest
Sedatives	Dalmane, Nembutal, Quaalude	Increased CNS depression possibly leading to respiratory arrest and death
Tranquilizers	Valium, Miltown, Librium	Increased CNS depression, decreased alertness and judgment

CNS = Central nervous system.

Physiologically, women usually have less body water than men of similar body weight and produce less alcohol dehydrogenase, the enzyme responsible for ethanol metabolism. As a result, women absorb about 30% more alcohol than men do into the bloodstream before it can be metabolized in the liver.[26] In women, alcohol reaches the brain and other organs more quickly than it does in men, resulting in more rapid intoxication as well as more organ-specific ethanol toxicity. For a woman of average size, one drink has roughly the same effect as two drinks have on the average-sized man. Women alcoholics also are more likely to suffer liver damage than men.

Hormone levels affect alcohol metabolism. Studies have found that both the menstrual cycle and the use of oral contraceptives influence blood alcohol levels. The rate of alcohol metabolism and peak BAC attained with a certain amount of alcohol may vary depending on estrogen levels. Moderate alcohol consumption may increase the risk of breast cancer in postmenopausal women taking hormone replacement therapy.[27] These variances may help explain why some women have difficulty predicting their response to alcohol and their feelings of loss of control over their responses.

Alcohol can also affect reproductive health and cross the placental barrier. Alcohol's effects on the developing fetus vary depending on the degree and timing of exposure, genetic differences in maternal metabolism of alcohol, maternal nutritional status, and possible interaction with other drug compounds. Women who are alcoholics or who drink heavily during pregnancy are more likely to miscarry. A direct effect of alcohol in pregnant women is fetal alcohol syndrome (FAS), which causes physical and mental abnormalities in infants born to mothers who drank alcohol during pregnancy. (See Chapter 6.) Fetal alcohol syndrome has the following characteristics:

- Small body size and weight
- Slower than normal development and failure to catch up
- Skeletal deformities
- Facial abnormalities
- Organ deformities
- Central nervous system handicaps[28]

Alcohol consumption may inhibit the release of oxytocin and prolactin, two hormones important for initiation and maintenance of lactation. It also may alter the composition of a woman's breast milk and inhibit milk production.[29]

Alcohol plays an indirect role in many unwanted pregnancies and sexually transmitted infections (STIs). Because of impaired judgment and reasoning from intoxication, a woman may forget or ignore contraception, make judgments she later regrets, or miss signs of danger. In addition to increasing the risk for unwanted pregnancies and STIs, alcohol is often a factor in acquaintance rape cases and incidents of pressured sex.

Alcoholism

An alcoholic is a person who is addicted to alcohol and whose consumption of alcohol interferes with major aspects of her or his life. Alcoholics have problems controlling the amount of alcohol they drink or when they drink it, suffer physical withdrawal symptoms when they stop or slow their drinking, and are unable to control their actions while drunk. Alcoholism is different and more severe than simply drinking at unhealthy levels: a woman who drinks two to three glasses of wine a night, but is otherwise functional, may have a drinking problem without being an alcoholic. Until the early to mid-20th century, dependence on alcohol was largely seen as a sign of weakness or moral failure. Since then, however, **alcoholism** has been recognized as a chronic disease with genetic, psychological, environmental, and behavioral components. Alcoholism has a generational cyclic effect. Children of alcoholics are more likely to suffer abuse, to have psychological or emotional problems, to become alcoholics, and to marry alcoholics. Approximately one in five U.S. adults has lived with an alcoholic relative while growing up.[30]

Chronic alcohol abuse usually manifests itself as one of the following patterns:

- Daily intake of large amounts of alcohol
- Regular heavy drinking on weekends
- Periods of sobriety between binges of daily heavy drinking that may last for weeks or months

Alcoholism most often appears between the ages of 20 and 40 but can present in childhood or early adolescence. Alcohol becomes a problem when an individual is no longer able to control when and how much drinking takes place.

Clinical diagnosis of alcoholism is based on the presence of at least three of the following symptoms, persisting for a month or more or occurring repeatedly over a longer period of time:

- Consistent consumption of large amounts of alcohol (five or more drinks per day)
- Persistent desire to quit drinking, or one or more unsuccessful attempts to cut down or quit alcohol
- Considerable time spent obtaining, using, or recovering from alcohol
- Continued drinking despite social, psychological, or physical harm
- Withdrawal symptoms, such as physical trembling, sweating, high blood pressure, delusions, and hallucinations, when alcohol intake is curbed
- The avoidance or relief of withdrawal symptoms by drinking

- Desire or need for a drink to start the day
- Denial of an alcohol problem
- Sleep problems
- Trying, but being unable to stay away from alcohol
- Depression and paranoia
- Failure to recall what happened during a drinking episode
- Dramatic mood swings
- Behaviors or activities while drinking that are regretted later
- The experience of the following symptoms after drinking: headaches, nausea, stomach pain, heartburn, gas, fatigue, weakness, muscle cramps, irregular or rapid heart rate

Risk Factors for Alcoholism

A family history of alcohol problems, early initiation of drinking, and victimization increase a woman's risk for alcohol abuse or alcoholism. Some people do appear to have a genetic predisposition to alcohol. Identical twins, for example, have closer rates of alcohol dependence, abuse, and heavy consumption than fraternal twins. There is also a significant association between alcoholism in people who were adopted and their biological parents, further reinforcing this hypothesis.[30] Yet a person's childhood environment also plays a part; women who were sexually, verbally, or physically abused also reported more alcohol-related problems.

Alcoholism is associated with personality disorders, depression, and other mental illnesses. This association may result if a person resorts to alcohol abuse to cope with the symptoms of a mental illness or if a person develops depression or another mental illness as a result of alcohol abuse. Alcoholism is also associated with antisocial behavior and low self-esteem.

Treating Alcoholism

The most difficult and significant step for an alcoholic is admitting to an alcohol problem. Often well-intended friends or family members, out of fear, embarrassment, loyalty, or hope, help shield the alcoholic from the truth. Confrontation—either personal or via an accident or drunk-driving conviction—that makes the individual acknowledge the alcohol problem is often a turning point in seeking assistance (**Self-Assessment 13.2**). Recovery from

Self-Assessment 13.2
National Council on Alcoholism Self-Test: Do You Have a Drinking Problem?

1. Do you occasionally drink heavily after a disappointment, a quarrel, or when your parents give you a hard time? yes no

2. Do you drink more heavily than usual as a response to stress or other problems in life? yes no

3. Have you noticed that you are able to handle more liquor than you did when you were first drinking? yes no

4. Did you ever wake up on "the morning after" a bout of heavy drinking and discover that you could not remember the evening before, even though your friends tell you that you did not pass out? yes no

5. When drinking with other people, do you try to have a few extra drinks that others don't notice? yes no

6. Are there occasions when you feel uncomfortable if alcohol is not available? yes no

7. Have you recently noticed that when you begin drinking you are in more of a hurry to get the first drink than you used to be? yes no

8. Do you sometimes feel guilty about your drinking? yes no

9. Are you irritated when your family or friends discuss your drinking? yes no

10. Have you noticed an increase in the frequency of your memory blackouts? yes no

11. Do you often find that you wish to continue drinking after your friends say that they have had enough? yes no

12. Do you usually have a reason for the occasions that you drink heavily? yes no

13. When you are sober, do you often regret things you did or said while drinking? yes no

14. Have you tried switching brands or following different plans for controlling your drinking? yes no

15. Have you often failed to keep the promises you have made to yourself about controlling or cutting down on your drinking? yes no

16. Have you ever tried to control your drinking by changing jobs or moving to a new location? yes no

17. Do you try to avoid family or close friends while you are drinking? yes no

18. Are you having an increasing number of financial and academic problems? yes no

19. Do more people seem to be treating you unfairly without good reason? yes no

20. Do you eat very little or irregularly when you are drinking? yes no

21. Do you sometimes have the shakes in the morning and find that it helps to have a little drink? yes no

22. Have you recently noticed that you cannot drink as much as you once did? yes no

23. Do you sometimes stay drunk for several days at a time? yes no

24. Do you sometimes feel very depressed and wonder whether life is worth living? yes no

25. Sometimes after periods of drinking, do you see or hear things that are not there? yes no

26. Do you get terribly frightened after you have been drinking heavily? yes no

Those who answer "yes" to two or three of these questions may wish to evaluate their drinking in these areas. "Yes" answers to several of these questions indicate the following stages of alcoholism:

Questions 1–8: Early stage—drinking is a regular part of your life.

Questions 9–21: Middle stage—you are having trouble controlling when, where, and how much you drink.

Questions 22–26: Beginning of the final stage—you can no longer control your desire to drink.

Source: National Council on Alcoholism and Drug Dependence, Inc. http://www.ncadd.org.

---

alcoholism is more likely when the person has a strong emotional support system, including concerned family, friends, and employers.

Alcoholism is a complex problem. Each case must be treated with sensitivity and recognition of its unique situation and contributing factors. Standard treatment programs focus on the relief of physiological dependence but do not eliminate the underlying disease. Individual personality, psychological factors, and sociocultural factors must be addressed to help the alcoholic regain control of her life. Treatment programs for alcoholism often follow three steps:

1. Managing acute intoxication episodes

2. Correcting chronic health problems associated with alcoholism

3. Changing long-term behavior

The most successful treatments combine different approaches and provide ongoing support as a person learns to live without alcohol. Many alcohol treatment facilities assist clients in overcoming their physical addiction to alcohol and helping them deal with their withdrawal symptoms (**Table 13.4**) through detoxification programs. Detoxification programs are generally available in medical or psychiatric hospitals.

Psychological addiction is usually addressed shortly after the detoxification process is completed. Programs such as Alcoholics Anonymous (AA), which is entirely run by volunteers who are also recovering alcoholics, provide help and support for people trying to maintain their abstinence from alcohol. Studies conducted by Alcoholics Anonymous show that the average length of sobriety for its members is more than 8 years; 50% of members have been sober for more than 5 years, 24% for between 1 and 5 years, and 26% for less than 1 year. Since the organization began in 1935, AA has supported more than 100,000 groups and has more than 2 million members in 150 countries.[31] Alcoholics Anonymous meetings can be found in towns and cities across the country on almost

Table 13.4 Alcohol Withdrawal Symptoms
Irritability
Agitation
Depression
Lack of concentration
Body tremors
Nausea and vomiting
Generalized weakness, achiness
Sweating
Fever
Dry mouth
Elevated blood pressure
Headache
Anxiety
Puffy, blotchy skin
Fitful sleep with nightmares
Brief hallucinations
Delirium tremens (DTs)

every day of the week. Alcoholics Anonymous maintains a relatively rigid approach based on entirely abstaining from alcohol. Although this method has its proponents, some advocates now argue that other approaches, such as moderate (but controlled) drinking, or the use of new medications that may reduce the body's desire for alcohol, may be more effective for some women.

Women alcoholics who enter treatment programs have special needs. Their treatment programs must be culturally sensitive and incorporate issues such as age, socioeconomic status, drug use, and sexual orientation into their format. Strategies that can help women address their alcohol problems include using culturally appropriate, nonstigmatized language; supportive case management; mentoring or buddy systems; childcare services; and multimedia campaigns that educate and welcome women.

ILLICIT DRUGS

Illicit drugs include drugs that are banned outright, such as heroin, cocaine, and marijuana, as well as legal drugs used for illegal purposes, such as prescription drugs used either by someone for whom they were not intended or for nonmedical purposes. About half of the 4 million visits to emergency departments that occur in the United States every year are some sort of overdose, accident, or injury related to drug use (**Figure 13.6**). In addition to causing harm directly, some drugs expose people to harm indirectly. Sharing needles to inject heroin or other drugs can transmit hepatitis B and C, and HIV, for example, while heavy alcohol use may make a person more vulnerable to sexual assault.

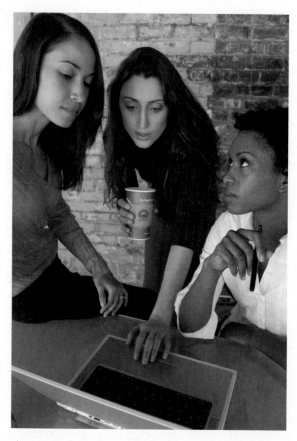

There is no particular stereotype of a drug-dependent woman.
© Photos.com

Epidemiological Trends and Issues

In 2013, 24.6 million Americans aged 12 or older (9.4% of the population) had used at least one illicit drug within the past month. This increase, from 7.9% of the population in 2003, is due to increased marijuana use; use of most other illicit drugs, such as cocaine or heroin, actually decreased during the same period.[3] Women are less likely to use illicit drugs, including marijuana, cocaine, crack, hallucinogens, and inhalants, than men.[3] Users of illicit drugs are more likely to be young, with rates highest for 18- to 25-year-olds (21.5%), but all age groups use

U.S. emergency department visits due to drug abuse or misuse, 2009*

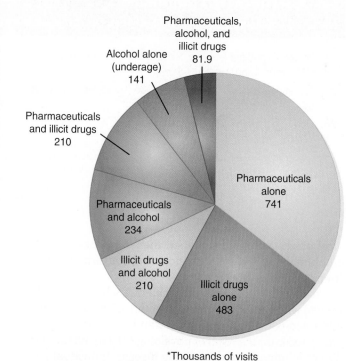

*Thousands of visits

Figure 13.6   **Annual emergency department visits due to drug abuse or misuse.**

Source: Data from Substance Abuse and Mental Health Services Administration. (2011). Drug abuse warning network, 2009: National estimates of drug-related emergency department visits. Available at: http://www.icpsr.umich.edu/icpsrweb/NACJD/studies/31921

illicit drugs. Marijuana, used by 19.8 million people (7.5% of Americans aged 12 or older), is by far the most commonly used illicit drug, followed by prescription drugs used for nonmedical purposes (6.6 million people, or 2.5% of Americans aged 12 or older) and cocaine (1.5 million users, or 0.6% of the population).[3]

Among older women, drug overuse and misuse are particular problems. Although they are generally not users of illicit drugs, older women may be likely to be consumers of high levels of medications. Women age 65 or older represent 12% of the general population, but they receive more than 25% of all written prescriptions.[3] Sedatives, hypnotics, antianxiety drugs, antihypertensive drugs, vitamins, analgesics, diuretics, laxatives, and tranquilizers are prescribed for elderly women two and a half times more often than they are for elderly men. Women are diagnosed with anxiety and depression disorders more often than men, and so are prescribed drugs more often to treat these disorders. Gender differences in weight, body composition, gastric emptying time, cerebral blood flow, and use of hormones in contraception and hormone therapy can influence the effects of these drugs.

Cannabis (Marijuana)

Cannabis, known as marijuana, "pot," or "weed," consists of a mixture of dried, crushed leaves and flower buds of the plant *Cannabis sativa*; this drug is usually smoked but is also sometimes cooked and eaten. Marijuana is by far the most-used illicit drug in the United States. More Americans use marijuana than the number of Americans abusing nonmedical prescription drugs, cocaine, heroin, inhalants, and hallucinogens combined. **Hashish** is an extract of cannabis that is 2 to 10 times as concentrated as marijuana that is sometimes used in its place. Tetrahydrocannabinol (THC) is the primary psychoactive ingredient in both drugs.

Marijuana use has increased dramatically over the past 15 years. From 2002 to 2012 alone, the number of people who have ever smoked marijuana in the United States grew by more than 50%.[3] This trend has been accompanied by a greater social acceptance of marijuana. Compared to 15 years ago, Americans today are less likely to believe that marijuana is a serious health threat, and a narrow minority now believes that marijuana should be legalized.[32]

When taken in low-to-moderate doses, marijuana may produce feelings of relaxation as well as a "high," or feeling of mild euphoria. Other immediate physical effects include an increased heart rate, bloodshot eyes, and dry mouth and throat. High doses diminish the ability to perceive and react and cause sensory distortion. Hashish users may experience hallucinations and LSD-like psychedelic reactions, and some people experience acute panic attacks.

Marijuana does not typically cause the same rapid deterioration of mind and body seen in users of drugs like heroin, methamphetamine, or cocaine. Studies show conflicting results regarding smoking marijuana and its relationship to cancer. However, medical evidence does indicate that marijuana, especially when used chronically, is a harmful drug. In the short term, marijuana impairs problem-solving ability and lowers coordination; over the long term, marijuana may increase the risk for heart disease and cause respiratory problems. On a personal level, chronic marijuana use is associated with reduced physical and mental health, a lower career status, and absenteeism in school and at work.[33]

In women, chronic use of marijuana appears to suppress ovulation and alter hormone levels. Frequent use of this drug during pregnancy may result in low-birth-weight infants and may be associated with impaired verbal, perceptual, and memory skills, as well as difficulties with decision making and sustained attention in children.[33]

Marijuana for medical use has been a subject of controversy for many years. The drug has been studied for its pain-relieving benefits; its potential for reducing spasms and spasticity produced by multiple sclerosis and partial spinal cord injury; its use for relieving chemotherapy-related nausea and vomiting; its ability to lower intraocular pressure to treat glaucoma; and its work as an appetite stimulant for wasting syndrome due to HIV infection, anorexia, and cancer. However, whereas medicinal marijuana does have legitimate potential, many claims about the value of medicinal marijuana have been clouded by bias, either by proponents or opponents of legalizing marijuana. Further research is needed to ascertain the full extent, if any, of many of the proposed health benefits of medicinal marijuana.

Prescription and Over-the-Counter Drugs

The most commonly abused class of drugs after alcohol, tobacco, and marijuana is prescription and OTC medicines, which include:

- Opioids prescribed for pain relief, such as Oxycontin, Vicodin, morphine, and codeine

- Central nervous system depressants, prescribed for anxiety and sleep disorders, such as Valium, Librium, and Xanax

- Stimulants, prescribed for attention-deficit hyperactivity disorder, such as Dexedrine, Adderall, and Ritalin

- OTC cough syrups and other OTC medicines[3]

Of all these medicines, prescription opioid pain relievers pose the biggest public health problem, with more than 2 million Americans currently abusing these medicines. Over the past 20 years, deaths from overdoses of these drugs have more than quadrupled. The rise in abuse of opioid pain relievers can be traced in part to their being prescribed more often than needed. Other factors that may have contributed to the rise in opioid pain reliever abuse include their potential for addiction and their perceived status as "non-harmful," legal drugs.[34]

Stimulants

Stimulants affect the central nervous system and increase heart rate, blood pressure, strength of heart contractions, blood glucose level, and overall muscle tension. Collectively, these effects place additional stress on the body. Some stimulants, such as nicotine and caffeine, are legal. Caffeine, one of the most widely used stimulants in the world, is found in many different sources. It has a variety of effects:

- Relief of drowsiness

- Help in the performance of repetitive tasks

- Improved mental capacity for work

- Increased basal metabolic rate

Caffeine can also cause anxiety, insomnia, irregular heartbeat, faster breathing, upset stomach and bowels, dizziness, and headaches in some women. Women who drink a lot of caffeine and then suddenly stop may experience headaches, irritability, and fatigue. Caffeine may temporarily increase the blood pressure, so some women with high blood pressure or heart disease may wish to limit their consumption. For most women, however, moderate amounts of caffeine are not likely to cause health problems.

Cocaine is a popular stimulant made from the leaves of the coca plant (unrelated to the cacao plant used to make chocolate). About 1.5 million people, or 0.6% of the

U.S. population, use cocaine on a regular basis.[3] Cocaine can be snorted (inhaled as a powder through the nose), injected, or smoked. Cocaine increases levels of dopamine, a neurotransmitter that creates feelings of pleasure in the body, creating intense feelings of euphoria. With repeated use, the brain becomes tolerant to cocaine, and users need more of it to get high.

Crack is a smokable mixture of cocaine and baking soda. Because it causes a person to feel intense highs and lows, this drug produces a powerful chemical and psychological dependence. Crack users often need another "hit" within minutes of the previous one. Smoking cocaine in its "free-base" form also delivers a concentrated high that can disappear within seconds.

As a powerful stimulant, cocaine has many harmful effects on the body. Cocaine constricts blood vessels and increases the heart rate and blood pressure, increasing the risk for heart attacks or strokes. Cocaine use can cause feelings of paranoia, a loss of judgment, and an intense need to get high again. Cocaine causes additional health problems for pregnant women and their unborn babies; its use can cause miscarriages, premature labor, low-birth-weight babies, and babies with small head circumferences. Women who use cocaine while pregnant are more likely to miscarry in the first 3 months of pregnancy, even compared to women who use heroin or narcotics. Infants born to cocaine and crack users suffer major complications, including drug withdrawal and permanent disabilities. Cocaine can deprive the fetal brain of oxygen or cause brain vessels to burst so that the fetus experiences the prenatal equivalent of a stroke, resulting in permanent physical and mental damage. In addition, cocaine babies are more likely to have respiratory and kidney problems. Visual problems, low birth weight, seizures, depression, lack of coordination, and developmental retardation are common among cocaine babies as well.

Amphetamines are manufactured stimulants sold under a variety of names. Generally found in pill form, they may also be ground and sniffed or made into a solution for injection. Amphetamines were once widely prescribed for weight control because they suppress the appetite and stimulate the central nervous system. These drugs place serious stress on the cardiovascular system, which can lead to severe cardiovascular damage.

Methamphetamine, also known as "meth," "crystal meth," "crank," or "ice," is a stimulant with a chemical structure similar to amphetamine. Use of methamphetamine greatly increases dopamine levels in the brain, producing strong feelings of pleasure. Unfortunately, methamphetamine appears to also change the brain in other ways. Prolonged use may reduce a person's motor skills, learning capacity, and ability to feel pleasure from any activities other than using methamphetamine. An estimated 353,000 people (0.1% of the population) regularly use this drug.[3]

Anabolic steroids are synthetic derivatives of the male hormone testosterone. These powerful compounds are legitimately prescribed for treatment of burns and injuries, but some athletes and bodybuilders who want to appear muscular and quickly gain muscle mass also use them. Women who take anabolic steroids risk development of a deepened voice, breast reduction, enlargement of the clitoris, changes in or cessation of the menstrual cycle, and growth of facial hair. Other potential effects include an increased risk of heart disease or stroke, liver tumors and jaundice, acne, bad breath, aching joints, and increased aggression. Anabolic steroids can also be addictive, creating some of the same problems with dependence and withdrawal as other drugs.

Depressants and Antianxiety Drugs

Drugs that relax the central nervous system are called depressants, sedatives, or hypnotics. The most widely used depressant is alcohol. Depressants have a synergistic effect when they are mixed together, causing a combined effect on the body greater than both drugs would have if taken individually. As the user builds tolerance, the likelihood of a potentially fatal overdose increases.

Barbiturates are depressants used medically for inducing relaxation and sleep, relieving tension, and treating seizures. They may also be administered intravenously as a general anesthetic. Low doses of barbiturates produce mild intoxication and euphoria, and decrease alertness and muscle coordination. With a higher dose, the person may suffer slurred speech, decreased respiration, cold skin, weak and rapid heartbeat, and unconsciousness. Side effects of these drugs include drowsiness, impaired judgment and performance, and a hangover that may last for hours or days. Regular barbiturate use leads to physical dependence; barbiturate withdrawal is a time-consuming and difficult-to-manage process. Withdrawal symptoms include anxiety, insomnia, delirium, and convulsions. Barbiturates also present problems in pregnancy, easily crossing the placenta and causing birth defects, dependence, behavioral problems, fever, and other problems.

Antianxiety drugs, such as benzodiazepines, are primarily prescribed to treat tension and muscular strain. The most commonly used benzodiazepines are alprazolam (Xanax) and diazepam (Valium). These drugs act quickly, creating effects in less than an hour. Drowsiness and loss of coordination are the most common side effects. When used with other substances, such as alcohol, benzodiazepines can cause serious, possibly life-threatening complications. Similar to the barbiturates, high doses of these drugs result in slurred speech, drowsiness, and stupor. Physiological and physical dependence on antianxiety drugs may occur within 2 to 4 weeks. Withdrawal symptoms include coma, psychosis, and death.

Psychedelics and Hallucinogens

Hallucinogens create changes in perceptions and thoughts. Some of their more common effects are changes in mood, sensation, perception, and relations. These

It's Your Health

Indications of Drug Use

- Abrupt change in attitude, including a lack of interest in previously enjoyed activities
- Frequent vague and withdrawn moods
- Sudden decline in work or school performance
- Sudden resistance to discipline or criticism
- Secret telephone calls and meetings with a demand for greater personal privacy
- Increased frustration levels
- Decreased tolerance for others
- Change in eating and sleeping habits
- Sudden weight loss
- Frequent borrowing of money
- Stealing
- Disregard for personal appearance
- Impaired relationships with family and friends
- Disregard for deadlines, curfews, or other regulations
- Unusual temper flare-ups
- New friends, especially known drug dealers, and strong allegiance to these friends

Source: National Institute on Drug Abuse (NIDA), National Institutes of Health.

drugs produce tolerance to their psychedelic effects but do not create physical dependence or produce symptoms of withdrawal, even after long-term use. As with most psychoactive drugs, however, there is a danger of psychological dependence.

Peyote, lysergic acid diethylamide (LSD), and phencyclidine (PCP) are the three most common hallucinogens in the United States. Mescaline is the active ingredient in peyote, a spineless cactus with a small crown, or button, that is dried and then swallowed. LSD ("acid") also is taken orally and produces hallucinations, including bright colors and altered perceptions of reality. The hallucinogenic experience, or "trip," increases the body temperature, heart rate, and blood rate; it also causes sweating, chills, and sometimes headaches and nausea. A "bad trip" may result in an acute anxiety reaction that may trigger panic, depression, confusion, fear of insanity, and distorted thoughts and perceptions. The most common delayed reaction of LSD is a "flashback," in which individuals re-experience the perceptual and emotional changes originally produced by the drug. PCP, or "angel dust," is a synthetic drug that can be smoked, snorted, or eaten. PCP not only causes a person to see and hear things that do not exist but also alters a person's own perception of herself, often producing symptoms similar to those of schizophrenia. About 1.3 million Americans over the age of 12 (0.5% of the population) use hallucinogens.[3]

Narcotics

Narcotics include the opiates—opium and its derivatives, morphine, codeine, and heroin—and some other non-opiate synthetic drugs. All narcotics have sleep-inducing and pain-relieving properties. Narcotics relax the user and, when injected, may produce an immediate rush. They also may result in restlessness, nausea, and vomiting. With large doses, respiration slows, and the user may become unresponsive. Death is possible. Over time, opiate users may develop heart infections, skin abscesses, and congested lungs. Unsterile equipment increases the risk of hepatitis B and C, tetanus, and HIV infection. Roughly 700,000 Americans, or 0.25% of the population, use heroin.[3]

Although narcotics such as heroin affect a woman's ability to conceive, many addicts still can become pregnant. Use of heroin during pregnancy may affect the developing brain of the fetus or cause behavioral abnormalities in childhood. A baby of a heroin addict is born an addict as well and often suffers severe withdrawal symptoms after birth.

Inhalants

Inhalants are chemicals that produce vapors with psychoactive effects. Inhalants are most common among young adolescents and teenagers, in part because the chemicals that produce inhalants may be easily obtainable (or already present in the homes) for people in these age groups. Common products used as inhalants include solvents, aerosols, cleaning fluids, and petroleum products. Most inhalants produce the same effects as anesthetics—namely, they slow down bodily functions. Roughly 700,000 Americans over the age of 12, or 0.25% of the population, use inhalants on a regular basis.[3]

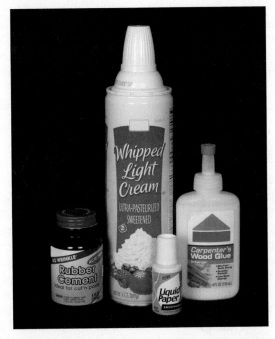

Many products that are used as inhalants are not meant for inhalation and are extremely dangerous.

At low doses, users may feel slightly stimulated; at higher doses, they may feel less inhibited. Inhalants may cause serious medical complications, such as brain damage and memory loss, hepatitis with liver failure, kidney failure, respiratory impairment, destruction of bone marrow and skeletal muscles, blood abnormalities, and irregular heartbeat.

Designer Drugs

Designer drugs—sometimes referred to as "club drugs" because they are often sold at nightclubs or raves—are produced in chemical laboratories and then sold illegally. Such synthetic narcotics are particularly dangerous because they are more powerful than those derived from natural substances. The risk of brain damage or fatal overdose from ingestion is correspondingly higher.

MDMA (3,4-methylenedioxymethamphetamine), commonly known as "ecstasy," is the most common designer drug, with about 700,000 users (0.25% of the population).[3] Ecstasy has features of both hallucinogens and stimulants. Other "club drugs" include GHB, Rohypnol, ketamine, and methamphetamine. In the United States, MDMA has been associated with a predominantly White, middle-class population. Immediate effects of the drug include a feeling of warmth and openness. Delayed responses, usually within a day, include insomnia, muscle aches, fatigue, and difficulty concentrating. Chronic use of MDMA can cause brain damage with the extent of damage directly correlated to the extent of MDMA use. Heavy users may also experience significant impairments in visual and verbal memory.

> *I had a knee injury from playing tennis and was given a prescription for Percocet. My injury wasn't too bad and ended up healing quickly, but I got into the habit of taking a couple of pills every night. When I ran out of pills, I just told my doctor that my knee still hurt and asked for a refill. I'm lucky she didn't give me one, or I could easily have gotten even more hooked. Even so, I had trouble sleeping for more than a week. I still think about those pills every once in a while—some small part of me is still an addict.*
>
> **—23-year-old woman**

Drug Dependency

Drug dependency refers to the attachment—physical, psychological, or both—that a person may develop to a drug. Physical dependence occurs when physiological changes in the body's cells cause an increasing need for a drug. If the drug is not taken, the user develops withdrawal symptoms, such as intense anxiety, extreme nausea, and deep craving for the drug. Psychological dependence, also referred to as habituation, results in a strong craving for a drug because it produces pleasurable feelings or relieves stress or anxiety. Physical and psychological dependence do not always coexist. For example, marijuana and LSD may not create physical dependence, but their continued use can cause psychological dependence.

Cross-tolerance, or cross-addiction, often presents with drug dependency. In this condition, a state of physical dependence exists in which psychological need for one psychoactive substance leads to dependence on similar substances.

Treatment Dimensions of Drug Dependency

There are three basic approaches to drug abuse treatment: detoxification, therapeutic communities, and outpatient drug-free programs. The best type of treatment program for any woman may depend on her circumstances, preferences, drug use, and history.

- *Detoxification* is the supervised withdrawal from drug dependence, either with or without medication, in a hospital or outpatient setting.

- *Therapeutic communities* are structured, drug-free environments in which abusers live under strict rules while participating in group and individual therapy.

- *Outpatient drug-free programs* are available through community and treatment facilities.

Self-help programs include Narcotics Anonymous and Pills Anonymous, which follow the philosophy of Alcoholics Anonymous. In these programs, users admit to their helplessness and put their faith in a "higher power." Many people do not recognize their own drug problems, and require intervention by friends and family before they will seek treatment (see **Self-Assessment 13.3**).

Self-Assessment 13.3
Do I Have a Drug Problem?

Carefully read and honestly respond to the following statements:

1. I spend a lot of time thinking about getting and taking a drug. yes no

2. Sometimes I don't go to an important event at school or work, or a social or recreational event, so that I can get or take a drug instead. yes no

3. I continue to use a drug despite the fact that it makes relationships with family or friends worse, or it interferes with school or work activities. yes no

4. I have developed a specific physical or mental condition from my drug use (for example, irritated nose from cocaine). yes no

5. I have repeatedly tried to cut down or eliminate my use of a drug. yes no

6. I am sometimes unable to fulfill my obligations (to family, friends, work, or school) because of my drug use. yes no

7. I feel specific symptoms when I cut back or eliminate the drug. yes no

8. I sometimes take another drug to relieve withdrawal symptoms. yes no

9. I sometimes use the drug in larger doses or over a longer period than recommended. yes no

10. I need to take more of the drug now than I did before to get the same effect. yes no

11. My drug habit has directly or indirectly put my personal health in danger. yes no

12. My use of drugs has affected my ability to pay for food, rent, school, or other basic expenses. yes no

If you answered "yes" to any of these statements, you have a serious problem with drug use. Seek help now.

INFORMED DECISION MAKING

Many outside and environmental factors affect whether a person eventually uses or becomes addicted to tobacco, alcohol, or other drugs. Although these factors cannot always be controlled, all individuals have responsibility for their own decisions. Personal responsibilities regarding drugs include:

- Understanding the effects that a particular substance can have on physical and psychological well-being
- Being aware of how substance abuse affects personal behaviors and the assessment of reality
- Being able to recognize and address a substance abuse problem when it exists
- Understanding the legal status of various drugs and the possible legal and other consequences of their use

The first steps in addressing a substance abuse problem is recognizing the warning signs of addiction and seeking early treatment intervention. Maintaining abstinence after treating the problem is an ongoing process. This process usually gets easier after the first few weeks or months, but for some people, the desire to use a drug never goes away. A relapse, if it occurs, should not be a sign that a substance abuse problem is hopeless, but should be a signal to reaffirm one's commitment to breaking the addiction.

Tobacco

Today, almost all smokers know that smoking is harmful to their health, and more than two-thirds of them want to quit.[1] Unfortunately, breaking the addiction to tobacco often remains incredibly difficult for many smokers. Fortunately, many options to help women quit smoking are available, including counseling, enlisting the help of friends and family, nicotine replacement therapy, and the medications bupropion and varenicline.

Avoiding secondhand smoke is not always simple. Although legislation now restricts smoking in many areas, smoking still occurs in some restaurants, bars, and smoking lounges; women who work or otherwise spend a large amount of time in these areas may be at risk for asthma or other lung conditions. Children of parents who smoke are often exposed to tobacco smoke in their own homes, cars, and even in the womb before birth. Nonsmokers' desire for a "smoke-free" environment presents a potential threat to some smokers, who feel that their rights to smoke are violated. Other smokers welcome these restrictions as helpful tools to help them cut back or quit.

In addition to harming the body directly, tobacco acts as a drug in other ways. Smoking can decrease the effects of certain medications such as acetaminophen, antidepressants, and insulin taken for diabetes. Smoking also increases the risk of heart and blood vessel disease when taking oral contraceptives. When relevant, women should mention tobacco use when healthcare providers inquire about medications or drug use.

Alcohol

Drinking in a responsible, moderate manner (one drink per day or less) usually poses no long-term health risks. Drinking to excess, however, can cause serious harm to the liver and many systems of the body. Excessive drinking also increases a person's likelihood of death, injury, or trauma through drunk driving, other accidents, or sexual assault.

Some people have propensities toward excessive drinking. These tendencies may come from parents who showed signs of problem drinking, previous experience with alcohol, a biological reaction to alcohol, or other factors. If you have any of these tendencies, be especially careful in situations where you may be likely to drink. It is also critical to have healthy coping strategies to avoid turning to alcohol when upset or depressed. Alcohol neither fixes a problem nor provides an escape.

Alcohol is an important part of many cultural and social events. It can also act as an occasional source of relief for mild stress. When drinking becomes the primary focus of an activity, or a fixed part of a person's life, a significant risk for serious long-term alcohol problems arises.

Communication skills are an important component of responsible drinking. Learning to say, "No thanks, I've had enough," is an important step in exercising personal power and control over drinking behavior. Pacing alcohol consumption is important as well. Drinking seven or more drinks on a Friday night is not the same as having those same drinks spread throughout the week. Alcoholic beverages are not good or wise thirst quenchers, as alcohol increases dehydration. Food should be consumed before drinking, so it is a good idea to eat something before going to a party or meeting someone for a drink.

I feel responsible for [my husband] Joe's drinking. He really has no one else who understands and helps him. I try to be patient each time he is drunk and clean up the mess. I keep thinking that if I just try harder in understanding maybe he won't have this problem.
—35-year-old woman

GENDER DIMENSIONS: Health Differences Between Men and Women

Treatment Programs

Drug dependency treatment programs must address the spectrum of physical and psychosocial issues that confront the addict. These challenges are especially difficult for female addicts, who experience concerns such as contraception, pregnancy, motherhood, childrearing, and health problems in addition to the underlying drug dependency. Women are generally less likely to seek treatment for drug abuse, and they respond differently than men to drug treatment. Female addicts often are caregivers and are reluctant to seek care for themselves because of the needs of others. In addition, they need specialty treatment more often than males. These types of services include prenatal treatment, mental health services, domestic violence counseling, and childcare assistance. Substance abuse treatment facilities providing special programs or services for women are becoming more common, but these programs are still unavailable or unaffordable for many women. Some programs also provide activities

for children, housing and transportation assistance, and services for pregnant women.

Psychosocial and behavioral treatment programs that emphasize increased self-esteem and choosing positive life options help many women more than programs originally developed for men. Unfortunately, few programs focus on the special needs of women or acknowledge the barriers that women must overcome to obtain treatment. These barriers include lack of day care for children, lack of safe, drug-free housing, fear of losing custody of their children, financial and legal difficulties, lack of transportation, and health problems requiring services beyond drug treatment. In addition, treatment needs of women should be evaluated with the realization that women do not constitute a homogenous group but rather run the gamut of pregnant women, adolescents, older women, single professionals, housewives, and others.

Helping others to drink in moderation is also a personal responsibility issue. It is not wise to push drinks or refill empty glasses quickly. Food helps to slow the absorption of alcohol and should be encouraged first, particularly if guests have not eaten for a while. Nonalcoholic beverages should always be available alongside alcoholic ones. Perhaps the most important responsibilities are never to serve alcohol to a guest who seems intoxicated and never to permit an intoxicated person to operate a vehicle. Assuming responsibility includes making contingency plans for intoxication (see **Table 13.5**). The early identification of designated drivers helps ensure safe transportation home for guests. If intoxication occurs despite efforts to prevent it, assume responsibility for the

health and safety of guests by providing transportation home or overnight accommodations. Women should stay with their female friends who appear overly intoxicated and be aware of men who may try to take advantage of an intoxicated woman. Stay with the person if he or she is vomiting. If the person is lying down, turn his or her head to the side and protect the person from swallowing the vomit. Monitor the person's breathing status. If there are any signs of unconsciousness or respiratory problems, seek immediate medical attention. Remember that the only thing that sobers a drunk person is time.

Other Drugs

Understanding the short- and long-term negative effects that drugs can have, while also developing personal strengths and self-confidence, is the foundation that enables a woman to resist drugs effectively. Knowing how to cope with stress in a healthy way can also reduce the likelihood that a woman will turn to drugs as a coping mechanism.

Early identification and treatment offer hope to the person who is using drugs. Unfortunately, many people either miss or refuse to see the signs that a person is using drugs. Many treatment and counseling centers offer free online or telephone services that provide advice on assessing the situation and helpful resources for action. Confronting the substance abuser is sometimes best handled by a group of loved ones and in the presence of a trained counselor. Outlining how the abuse has affected each person in the abuser's life and how much each person cares about the abuser helps to balance the information. It is unrealistic to expect the abuser to quit without assistance. Although offering support is beneficial, the abuser needs to know that treatment and therapy are necessary.

Informed decision making is also an essential responsibility with prescribed and OTC medication use. Many

---

Table 13.5 How to Handle a Friend Who Is Intoxicated

- Try to find out what the person was drinking and if she took any other drugs or medicines.
- Help your friend get home safely; don't let her drive, get in a car with another friend who has been drinking, or walk home alone in an unsafe area.
- Encourage your friend to go to sleep; the only way to sober up is to give it time.
- Position your friend on her side to prevent her from choking if she vomits. Check on her regularly to be sure she is responsive and breathing.
- Avoid giving your friend any medication, including aspirin, ibuprofen, or acetaminophen.
- Call for help if she is unresponsive or vomiting while unconscious; call for help if you fear being alone with the intoxicated friend.

Source: Reprinted by permission of Julie Barnes, coordinator, Substance Abuse Services, University of Northern Iowa.

It's Your Health

Codependency

A person (friend, spouse, partner, parent) may, without meaning to, allow or help an addict to remain dependent on drugs through enabling behaviors. These enabling behaviors may include the following activities:

- Rescuing: displaying overprotective behavior that permits the addict to use drugs at home to avoid being discovered or at risk elsewhere

- Rationalizing: accepting and explaining the addict's behavior; making excuses for the behavior

- Shielding: covering up for the addict; running interference for them at work, school, and for obligations

- Controlling: personally attempting to control the addict's use of drugs with bribes or rewards (money, favors, sex)

- Covering: taking over chores, assuming job responsibilities, paying bills, or giving/loaning money to the addict so that he or she can buy drugs

- Cooperating: becoming involved in buying, selling, testing, preparing, or using the drug

women have little or no idea why they take certain prescribed medications, or they have multiple and vague reasons for using complex OTC medications. Drugs, whether prescribed or self-medicated, can have powerful adverse reactions with foods, alcohol, tobacco, caffeine, or other drugs. Older women are often subject to dangerous and possibly fatal drug interactions due to the numerous medications and supplements they are taking. Because many of the most serious effects of drugs are often wrongly attributed to "being depressed" or "growing old," women should know about possible adverse drug reactions and side effects so they can recognize and report them. They should also know which foods and other drugs interact with the medications being taken and whether specific dietary recommendations have been identified for the medications.

Codependency

The concept of codependency is important for many women who become embroiled within the chaos of another person's life.

The term *codependent* describes a person obsessed, tormented, or dominated by the behavior of others. The term grew out of the older notion of "co-alcoholic," a term once applied to the wives of heavy drinkers. The premise of codependency is that everyone in the family of a user or abuser is diseased. Consciously or unconsciously, and to their lifelong detriment, codependents interact with the user and enable this person to partake in her addiction. Codependents often feel helpless, miserable, hopeless, and angry as they accept the victim role. A woman may be codependent in a relationship with a lover, spouse, parent, child, or friend. A codependent typically feels responsible for the behavior and mood of the other.

The codependent must learn how to separate her own life from that of the addicted person. The recovery from codependence is similar to recovery from alcohol or drug dependence in that only the codependent can take the necessary steps toward her own recovery. A codependent must learn not to try to control someone else's life and to stop playing the victim role. Many codependents have received useful support and encouragement from programs such as the 12-step program Al-Anon, a support group for family and friends of alcoholics.

Profiles of Remarkable Women

Drew Barrymore (1975–)

Drew Barrymore was born into an acting family that includes the actors Lionel, John, and Ethel Barrymore. Drew Barrymore began her career appearing in a Puppy Choice dog food commercial when she was 11 months old. She got her first movie role at the age of 2, playing a boy in *Suddenly Love.* At age 5, she appeared in *Altered States,* and she was turned into a household name when she starred in the blockbuster *E.T.: The Extraterrestrial.* She continued her appearances in films, including Stephen King adaptations *Firestarter* (1984) and *Cat's Eye* (1985).

Barrymore tried alcohol for the first time at age 9 and marijuana at age 10. She then turned to cocaine, stirred controversy with her near-nude appearances in *Far from Home,* and was forced into ASAP Family Treatment Center, a drug rehabilitation clinic. Following rehab, Barrymore published a memoir entitled *Little Girl Lost* and made a comeback in Hollywood in the early 1990s.

Barrymore's persistence and energy have helped her recover from the difficulties of growing up in front of the camera and in the public eye, and have shaped her into a strong and determined woman. She has not only appeared in numerous successful movies but has also become active as a producer for movies such as *He's Just Not That Into You, Fever Pitch, Charlie's Angels,* and *Donnie Darko.* A dedicated philanthropist, Barrymore is actively involved in volunteering for and supporting animal rights issues and anti-fur campaigns, urging young people to vote, and advocating for children's rights.

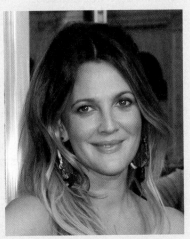

© Helga Esteb/Shutterstock, Inc.

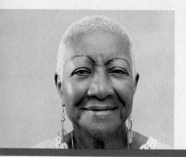
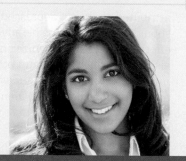
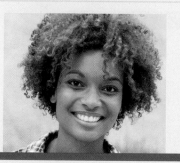
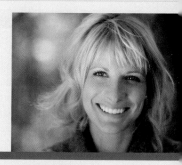

Summary

Tobacco, alcohol, and other drugs directly and indirectly harm women, their children, and others in their environment in many ways. Staying away from tobacco, or quitting smoking, will greatly improve a woman's health and reduce her risk of dying early. Women also must exercise caution and wisdom with alcohol and legal drug use. Knowing the consequences of drinking alcohol and assuming personal responsibility for one's drinking are the first steps in controlling alcohol use. Reducing and having control over the kinds and amounts of drugs taken, including recreational drugs, prescribed medications, OTC medications, and substances such as caffeine, should also be an important health goal.

Topics for Discussion

1. Have you ever known anyone (including yourself) who has had a problem with alcohol or other drugs? If so, how did drug use affect that person's life? How did the drug use affect the person's friends and family?

2. Is it a sign of personal weakness or strength for a woman to admit that she has a problem with alcohol or drugs?

3. What should a woman do or say when she knows her friend has a problem with drugs or alcohol, but the friend does not think so?

4. Do higher cigarette taxes and bans on smoking in public places infringe on smokers' rights? Does it make a difference if most smokers want to quit?

5. How can young girls be educated to resist peer and advertising pressure to smoke?

6. How does smoking as a public health problem differ in the developing world compared to the United States? What obstacles lie in the way of effective public health efforts to reduce smoking in the developing world?

7. For a 2-week period, try giving up a habit that is part of your daily routine. This could be anything from a daily cup of coffee, to watching television, to smoking (if you already smoke). How easy is it to change this behavior? When do you feel most like indulging in the habit? If you do slip up, what psychological impact does the slip have on your efforts to quit?

8. How is preventing or reducing drug abuse different for OTC or prescription medicines compared to drugs that are completely illegal?

9. Is it better to put drug addicts in prison or to send them to mandatory drug treatment programs?

10. What possible advantages and disadvantages are there to legalizing marijuana? If you think marijuana should be legalized, what about other, "harder" illegal drugs? If marijuana is legalized across the country, what steps can be taken to improve the public health?

CASE STUDY

Cathleen started smoking during her junior year of high school, when she was 16 years old. "I never meant to become a smoker," Cathleen says. "There were a couple of older girls I liked who smoked in the parking lot before school. I also thought it would be interesting just to try smoking as an experience. But then I started smoking at other times during the day and got into the habit of buying cigarettes before school. I've been a pack-a-day smoker since."

Now a senior in college, Cathleen is in the middle of her third quit attempt. Her first attempts to go cold turkey, made during her first and second years of college, ended after less than a week. "I hate smoking so much," Cathleen says. "I know it's harmful to my health. I know it's a waste of time and energy, but it just seems so hard to give up. Every time I try to quit and light up again I feel so ashamed of myself." Since the semester started a month ago, Cathleen has cut back on the number of cigarettes she smokes, now only smoking less than a pack a day, and only when she is at home.

(Cathleen's story has been drawn from the experiences of multiple smokers. Her name and other identifying information has been changed to preserve anonymity.)

Questions

1. Imagine that you are Cathleen's roommate. How can you support Cathleen and help her during her quit attempt? Can you offer her any resources or information that may help? What kinds of approaches might be counterproductive?

2. Imagine that you are the president of the college Cathleen is attending. What kinds of decisions can you make at the campus level to encourage people to quit smoking or to reduce the harmful effects of tobacco on campus?

◼ Key Terms

Alcohol
Alcoholism
Amphetamine
Barbiturate
Blood alcohol concentration (BAC)
Carcinogenic
Chronic bronchitis
Chronic obstructive pulmonary disease (COPD)
Cirrhosis
Drug
Drug abuse
Drug dependency
Drug misuse
Emphysema
Hallucinogen
Hashish
Inhalant
Narcotic
Nicotine
Over-the-counter medication
Recreational drug
Secondhand smoke
Stimulant
Tolerance
Third-hand smoke

◼ References

1. U.S. Department of Health and Human Services (DHHS). (2014). *The health consequences of smoking—50 years of progress: A report of the Surgeon General.* Atlanta, GA: DHHS, Centers for Disease Control and Prevention, National Center for Chronic Disease Prevention and Health Promotion, Office on Smoking and Health. Available at: http://www.surgeongeneral.gov/library /reports/50-years-of-progress/

2. U.S. Department of Transportation. (2013). *National Highway Traffic Safety Administration (NHTSA). Traffic safety facts 2012: Alcohol-impaired driving.* Washington, DC: NHTSA.

3. Substance Abuse and Mental Health Services Administration (SAMHSA). (2014). *Results from the 2013 National Survey on Drug Use and Health: Summary of national findings.* NSDUH Series H-48, HHS Publication No. (SMA) 14-4863. Rockville, MD: SAMHSA.

4. National Center on Addiction and Substance Abuse, Columbia University. (2003). *The formative years: Pathways to substance abuse among girls and young women ages 8–22.* New York, NY: Columbia University.

5. The Sentencing Project. (2005). *Briefing: The federal prison population: A statistical analysis.* Washington, DC: The Sentencing Project.

6. Office of National Drug Control Policy (ONDCP). (2015). *National drug control strategy: 2014.* Washington, DC: ONDCP.

7. Campaign for Tobacco-Free Kids. (2012). *State cigarette excise tax rates and rankings.* Available at: http://www.tobaccofreekids.org /research/factsheets/pdf/0097.pdf

8. Perucic, A. (2012). *The demand for cigarettes and other tobacco products.* Geneva, Switzerland: World Health Organization.

9. Xu, X., Bishop, E., Kennedy, S., et al. (2014). Annual healthcare spending attributable to cigarette smoking: An update. *American Journal of Preventive Medicine* 48(3): 326–333.

10. National Cancer Institute. (1999). *Smoking and tobacco control monograph.* Available at: http://cancercontrol.cancer.gov/tcrb /monographs/1/m1_3.pdf

11. Centers for Disease Control and Prevention (CDC). (2014). Current cigarette smoking among adults: United States, 2005–2013. Available at: http://www.cdc.gov/mmwr/preview/mmwrhtml /mm6347a4.htm

12. Kann, L., Kinchen, S., Shanklin, S., et al. (2014). *Youth risk behavior surveillance—United States, 2013.* Atlanta, GA: CDC.

13. CDC. (2013). *Smoking and tobacco use: Hookahs.* Available at: http://www.cdc.gov/tobacco/data_statistics/fact_sheets/tobacco _industry/hookahs/

14. Dutra, L., & Glantz, S. (2014). Electronic cigarettes and conventional cigarette use among US adolescents. *JAMA Pediatrics* 168(7): 610.

15. Murphy, S. L., Xu, J., & Kochanek, K. D., Division of Vital Statistics. (2013). Deaths: Final data for 2010. *National Vital Statistics Reports* 61(4). Available at: http://www.cdc.gov/nchs/data/nvsr/nvsr61 /nvsr61_04.pdf

16. World Health Organization. (2013). *WHO report on the global tobacco epidemic, 2013.* Available at: http://apps.who.int/iris /bitstream/10665/85380/1/9789241505871_eng.pdf

17. Connolly, G., Alpert, H., Wayne, G., et al. (2007). *Trends in smoke nicotine yield and relationship to design characteristics among popular U.S. cigarette brands, 1997–2005.* Harvard School of Public Health. Available at: http://www.hsph.harvard.edu/nicotine/trends.pdf

18. CDC. (2013). *Tobacco use and pregnancy.* Available at: http://www .cdc.gov/reproductivehealth/TobaccoUsePregnancy/

19. Ferrante, G., Simoni, M., & Ferrara, F. (2013). Third-hand smoke exposure and health hazards in children. *Monaldi Archives for Chest Disease* 79(1): 38–43.

20. Stead, L., Perera, R., Bullen, C., et al. (2008). Nicotine replacement therapy for smoking cessation. *The Cochrane Library.* Available at: www.thecochranelibrary.com

21. Gruskin, E. P., Hart, S., Gordon, N., et al. (2001). Patterns of cigarette smoking and alcohol use among lesbians and bisexual women enrolled in a large health maintenance organization. *American Journal of Public Health* 91(6): 976–979.

22. Brouchery, E., Harwood, H., Sacks, J., et al. (2011). Economic costs of excessive alcohol consumption in the U.S., 2006. *American Journal of Preventive Medicine* 41(5): 516–524.

23. CDC. (2014). Alcohol-attributable deaths and years of potential life lost—11 states, 2006–2010. *Morbidity and Mortality Weekly Report* 63(10): 213–216.

24. CDC. (2011). Vital signs: Alcohol-impaired driving among adults—United States, 2010. *Morbidity and Mortality Weekly Report* 53(37): 866–870.

25. National Institute on Alcohol Abuse and Alcoholism (NIAAA). (2011). *Alcohol Alert No. 72: Cirrhosis.* Rockville, MD: NIAAA.

26. Caithers, R. L., & McClain, C. (2006). Alcoholic liver disease. In M. Feldman, L. S. Friedman, & L. J. Brandt, *Sleisinger and Fordtran's gastrointestinal and liver disease* (8th ed.). Philadelphia, PA: Saunders Elsevier.

27. Nelson, H. D., Humphrey, L. L., Nygren, P., et al. (2002). Postmenopausal hormone replacement therapy: Scientific review. *Journal of the American Medical Association* 288: 872–881.

28. Bertrand, J., Floyd, R. L., Weber, M. K., et al. (2005). *Fetal alcohol syndrome: Guidelines for referral and diagnosis.* Atlanta, GA: DHHS, CDC. Available at: http://www.cdc.gov/ncbddd/fasd/documents/FAS_guidelines_accessible.pdf

29. American Academy of Pediatrics. (2005). Breastfeeding and the use of human milk. *Pediatrics* 115(2): 496–506.

30. American Academy of Child and Adolescent Psychiatry. (2011). *Facts for families: Children of alcoholics.* No. 17. Available at: http://www.aacap.org/AACAP/Families_and_Youth/Facts_for_Families/Facts_for_Families_Pages/Children_Of_Alcoholics_17.aspx

31. Alcoholics Anonymous (AA). (2011). *Alcoholics Anonymous 2011 membership survey.* Washington, DC: AA.

32. Gallup Poll. (2014). Majority continues to support pot legalization in U.S. Available at: http://www.gallup.com/poll/179195/majority-continues-support-pot-legalization.aspx

33. Batalla, A., Bhattacharyya, S., Yucel, M., et al. (2013). Structural and functional imaging studies in chronic cannabis users: A systematic review of adolescent and adult findings. *PLoS One* 8: e55821.

34. National Institute on Drug Abuse. (2014). *Prescription and over-the-counter medications.* Available at: http://www.drugabuse.gov/publications/drugfacts/prescription-over-counter-medications

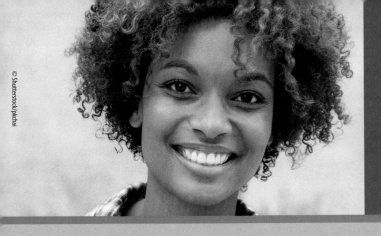

CHAPTER 14

Violence, Abuse, and Harassment

Learning Objectives
On completion of this chapter, the student should be able to discuss:

1. Self-directed, interpersonal, and collective violence, and how these forms of violence affect women.

2. How sociocultural, economic, and historical factors influence violence and its consequences.

3. How poverty, alcohol, drugs, and the media influence violence.

4. How violence affects women throughout the world.

5. Types of family and intimate violence.

6. Common forms of stalking and actions a woman can take to protect herself.

7. Forms of domestic violence, including physical, sexual, property, psychological, and social violence.

8. How domestic violence during pregnancy affects women and prenatal development.

9. How domestic violence affects lesbians, women with disabilities, and other groups.

10. Forms, common causes, and effects of child abuse and elder abuse.

11. Basic facts about rape and sexual assault.

12. How rape affects physical health, mental health, sexual intimacy, and relationships.

13. Common forms of violence toward women by strangers and how women can protect themselves.

14. How sexual harassment acts as a form of social control and its effects on women in the workplace.

15. Strategies to prevent and cope with intimate violence and sexual harassment.

INTRODUCTION

Violence has always been part of human society. Today, violence continues to affect millions of women around the world. The World Health Organization (WHO) classifies violence into three categories, based on who commits the violent act: self-directed violence, interpersonal violence, and collective violence.[1] Self-directed violence includes suicidal behavior and **self-mutilation** (see **It's Your Health**).

Interpersonal violence includes violence toward a child, partner, relative, or elder, as well as community violence toward an acquaintance or a stranger. Family and intimate violence—including stalking, domestic battering, child abuse, elder abuse, and rape in many cases—are major facets of the violence epidemic. Although most intimate violence qualifies as a crime, historical and cultural traditions have often condoned violence within the family setting. Violence by strangers—such as robbery, carjacking, aggravated assault, rape, and homicide—affects women when they are the victims of crime and when a partner or family member is a victim. Sexual harassment is considered a form of violence as well, because it also usually involves threats or an unjust use of power.

Collective violence is violence committed against a group of people to achieve social, political, or economic objectives. It can take a variety of forms, including armed conflicts, genocide, repression, terrorism, and organized violent crime. Many acts of violence toward women evolve as a result of women's subordinate status in society. Around the world, women face collective violence through female genital mutilation, female infanticide, trafficking of women and girls for sexual exploitation, rape during war, and other acts. These forms of abuse have traditionally been associated with the developing world; however, collective violence also occurs in the United States, Canada, and Europe.

From a legal perspective, most violent crime can be categorized into one of four categories: murder, rape or sexual assault, robbery (taking something from someone through threats or force), and both simple and aggravated assault (simple assault refers to attacking someone and

It's Your Health

Self-Mutilation

Self-harm, self-injury, self-inflicted violence, or self-mutilation is any self-directed, repetitive behavior that causes physical injury. These acts are not usually suicide attempts but rather behaviors that express or release emotional turmoil, or provide a distraction from inner turmoil. They are often referred to as parasuicidal behaviors. Examples include the following acts:

- Skin cutting with razors or knives (the most common pattern)
- Burning, branding, or biting oneself
- Picking one's skin or hair
- Hitting with hammer or other object; bone breaking
- Extreme injuries such as auto-enucleation (self-removal of the eye), castration, or amputation

There are several known risk factors for self-injury:

- Female gender
- Adolescent and college age
- Substance abuse or personality disorders
- History of parasuicidal behavior

People who self-harm are unable to identify or express difficult feelings in a healthy way. They use self-harm as a coping mechanism. They often feel increasing tension or physical arousal before the act and release of pleasure or gratification after the act. Self-harm is indicative of depression or anxiety. Little is known about the cause of self-mutilation, but studies are looking at biological, psychological, and social contributions to the disease. Medications, psychotherapeutic approaches, and crisis interventions are all forms of treatment. See the websites at the end of this chapter for more information.

Source: Adapted from Fong, T. (2003). Self-mutilation: Impulsive traits suggest new drug therapies. *Current Psychiatry* 2(2): 15–23.

causing physical harm, or threatening to attack someone; aggravated assault refers to a more extreme form of assault, often using a weapon). **Figure 14.1** shows the number of violent crimes committed against women in the

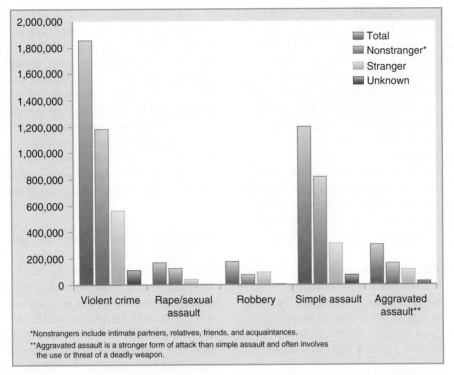

Figure 14.1 **Violent crimes committed against women and girls, by crime and victim–offender relationship, 2010.**

Source: Data from U.S. Department of Justice, Bureau of Justice Statistics. (2011). *National Crime Victimization Survey: Criminal victimization, 2010.* Available at: http://www.bjs.gov/content/pub/pdf/cv10.pdf

United States in 2010, as well as the relationship between the victim and aggressor.

Violence has mental and physical consequences for its victims, the most serious of which are long-term disability or death. Each year, more than 1.3 million people worldwide lose their lives to violence. Indeed, violence is the fourth leading cause of death worldwide for people ages 15 to 44 years.[1] More than 2.5 million females experience some form of violence each year. On average, one in three females is abused by an intimate partner during her lifetime, and several global studies suggest that half of all women who die from homicide are killed by current or former husbands or partners.[2] This chapter provides an overview of violence, focusing on interpersonal violence and the issues that contribute to violence and victimization. This chapter also reviews informed decision-making criteria and ways that women can prevent or cope with violence and its consequences.

PERSPECTIVES ON VIOLENCE, ABUSE, AND HARASSMENT

Sociocultural Issues

Cultural attitudes about violence toward women may be based on how society accepts the idea of male dominance. In some cultures, both men and women believe that a man has the right to control the behavior of his wife and daughters, and that a disobedient woman should be

I feel like it was my fault that I was raped. I had a little too much to drink and I went back to my apartment with him. I wanted to kiss him, but I didn't want to have sex. When he started forcing me to do more than kiss, I asked him to stop. But he wouldn't listen. I probably shouldn't have invited him back with me and I feel guilty for leading him on.

—19-year-old college sophomore

punished. A woman not obeying her husband, not having food ready for him, refusing him sex, or simply being a woman can trigger violence in intimate relationships. Society's tolerance of rape between intimate partners, especially married partners, is an important dimension of violence. For years, many people believed that marriage gave men the right to have sex with their wives at any time. In these settings, if the wife refuses, the husband can force her to have sex or punish her through violent means. In 2013, 600 million women were living in countries where domestic violence was still not against the law.[3]

By trivializing rape and sexual assault, rape culture is perpetuated in our society and shows a blatant disregard for women's rights and safety. Rape culture can be defined as "a culture in which dominant cultural ideologies, media images, social practices, and societal institutions support and condone sexual abuse by normalizing, trivializing and eroticizing male violence against women and blaming victims for their own abuse."[4] Examples of rape culture exist in words, concepts, and images found in jokes, song lyrics, movies, TV shows, advertising, and social media. It is the concept of trivializing and condoning rape and sexual assault, blaming the victim, and eroticizing the concept of gendered violence. Victim blaming demonstrates how a society can make excuses for rape. Tendencies to blame the victim influence how women and communities cope with relationship violence. Women who feel they are at fault or that they "deserved" punishment may not report a rape or other crimes. Certain factors, including a woman's style of dress, her relationship with the assailant, evidence of resistance, presence of alcohol or drugs, and location of the incident, may affect a third party's attitude toward the rape and contribute to his or her belief that the rape may actually be "excusable" or "understandable."

By legitimizing these behaviors, cultures perpetuate violence against women. Women are particularly vulnerable to abuse by their partners in societies where there are marked inequalities between men and women, rigid gender roles, weak sanctions against violent behavior, and cultural norms that support a man's right to sex regardless of a woman's feelings.

Reported rates of rape and sexual assault vary by race and ethnicity. Multiracial women and American Indian/ Alaska Native women had the highest estimated prevalence of rape during their lifetime (32.3%, 27.5% respectively); non-Hispanic Black women and non-Hispanic White women had similar lifetime estimates of rape (21.2% and 20.5%, respectively), while Hispanic women had a considerably lower estimate (13.6%). Various reports indicate that multiracial and American Indian/Alaska Native women are at greater risk for rape and intimate partner violence. Research has suggested that factors such as living in poverty, social and geographic isolation, and higher likelihood of alcohol use by the perpetrator may explain the elevated rates of violence among American Indian/Alaska Native women. However, there is little to explain why multiracial women may be at greater risk.[5]

Historical Trends

Historically, it has been socially acceptable for a husband to physically discipline his wife. The United States followed English law and allowed physical discipline of wives by their husbands until U.S. courts criminalized wife beating in the 20th century.[6]

Rape has been documented in American history since the arrival of the Europeans. Spanish explorers used female Native American captives for sexual services and raped Native American women whose tribes they conquered. Native American cultures, however, prohibited rape, and it had rarely occurred until the arrival of the explorers. Fears of brutal rapes by Native American men were found to be unsubstantiated during colonial-era "Indian" wars. Indeed, English women who had been held captive reported no such treatment.[6]

In 17th-century New England in particular, female servants were at high risk of rape and sexual harassment. During that era, an estimated one-third of rape victims were female servants, even though that group represented only 10% of the total population.[7] Later, in the South, where slave labor was increasingly used instead of indentured servants, African female servants and slaves found themselves victimized by White owners and overseers who viewed them as property—available for service of their sexual needs. Some historians assert that rape was used to dominate female slaves in a system that otherwise treated them as equals to male slaves.[7]

Poverty Influences

Poverty and joblessness are strongly connected with violence, including violence that occurs within the family. The relationship between violence, poverty, and joblessness may result from feelings of inadequacy and low self-esteem brought on by unemployment, stress associated with financial instability, and/or an inability to provide for one's family. Often, these emotions turn to frustration and anger and eventually lead to fighting within the household or violence toward one's partner or children. Unemployed individuals also spend significantly more time in the home, allowing greater opportunities for tensions to rise.

When poverty inspires violence, women and children are overwhelmingly the victims. Women often remain trapped in abusive relationships because of their financial dependence on the abuser. In households with incomes under $15,000 per year, one in three (35.5%) women suffer violence from an intimate partner.[8] Living in circumstances of stress and poverty can also lead some women to act violently against their children, spouses, or family members.

Alcohol and Drug Influences

Substance use and abuse are consistently associated with all forms of relationship violence. It is unclear whether a direct cause-and-effect relationship exists between the use of drugs or alcohol and violence, or whether this situation involves two overlapping social epidemics. Violence in a home may cause depression and lower self-esteem, possibly leading to an increased use of alcohol. Conversely, conflicts in interpersonal relationships may arise as a consequence of substance use and abuse and lead to violent behavior.

Data from the National Crime Victimization Survey, an ongoing nationally representative survey on crime, highlight the strong association between interpersonal violence and substance use. Alcohol can play a significant role in violence. Among victims able to tell whether there was substance use by the perpetrator, 30% reported alcohol use by the offender at the time of the crime. Two-thirds of victims who suffered violence by a current or former partner reported alcohol use by the offender.[9]

Media Influences

Media access through television, movies, video and computer games, and the Internet is a major influence in the lives of Americans, especially for children and adolescents. Media can be a powerful tool for positive learning and entertainment but can also pose a threat to emotional and physical safety.

Violence and sex on television and in other media are important, often unrecognized, influences on children and adolescent health and behavior. Research results are conflicting as to whether exposure to violent media actually causes violent behavior. However, exposure to violent television, movies, and video games does appear to desensitize children and adolescents, or make them more accepting, toward violent behavior. Exposure to violent media also creates a "mean world effect," causing people to believe the world is a more violent, cruel place than it actually is.[10]

Costs of Victimization

Violent crime directly causes financial losses, such as healthcare costs for treating any physical and mental injuries, as well as lost wages for missed workdays. The annual health-related costs of rape, physical assault, stalking, and homicide by intimate partners are more than $5.8 billion. Victims of intimate partner violence lose nearly 8 million days of work as a result of violence.[11] Other costs may include stolen property in burglaries and expenses for repairing or replacing damaged property. Police services, fire services, and state victims' services that deal with violent crime impose a financial burden on society as well. Each year, federal, state, and local governments in the United States spend about $228 billion and employ 2.5 million people for police protection, corrections, and judicial and legal activities.[12]

> I cannot describe how I felt when it was over. I was wondering if it would have been better if I had died. I was humiliated, angry, hurt, and so violated. He had been someone I had trusted—I thought that he was a friend. Looking back, though, there were clues to his violent nature. I had ignored them. It was a mistake for which I paid dearly.
>
> **—18-year-old student**

But violence causes much more than just financial losses. Intangible losses, such as long-term pain and suffering and reduced quality of life, are more difficult to quantify but no less real. Studies show a significant relationship between intimate partner violence and chronic pain, bladder and kidney infections, asthma, migraines and headaches, vaginal infections and bleeding, digestive problems, depression, low self-esteem, fear of intimacy, sleep disturbances, and substance abuse.[13] All of these findings lead to higher direct medical costs and consequently more losses for the victim. Many studies have found that the intangible loss of quality of life exceeds the tangible losses for victims of all crimes.

Legal Dimensions

The number of violent crimes by intimate partners against females has significantly decreased over the past 20 years. This decrease has been attributed to the Violence Against Women Act (VAWA) of 1994, which includes these provisions:

- Making it a crime to cross state lines to continue to abuse a spouse or partner
- Creating tough new penalties for sex offenders
- Prohibiting anyone facing a restraining order for domestic abuse from possessing a firearm
- Providing a substantial commitment of federal resources for police, prosecutors, and prevention service initiatives in cases involving sexual violence or domestic abuse
- Requiring sexual offenders to pay restitution to their victims
- Requiring states to pay for rape examinations
- Providing funds for federal victim-witness counselors
- Extending rape shield laws to protect crime victims from abusive inquiries into their private conduct
- Requiring that released offenders report to local enforcement authorities

Passage of the 1994 bill was a huge triumph for women's groups as it marked the first comprehensive federal legislative package designed to end violence against women. The provisions were expanded in the Violence Against Women Act of 2000, as well as in the Reauthorization Acts of 2005 and 2013. In 2000, Congress enhanced federal domestic violence and stalking penalties, added protections for foreign nationals suffering abuse, and created programs specifically for elderly and disabled women. In 2005, the legislation created programs for sexual assault victims and American Indian victims of domestic violence. The 2013 legislation reauthorized most of the programs, as well as enhanced efforts to combat trafficking and included sex trafficking in its work. VAWA 2013 also gave Indian tribes the authority to enforce domestic violence laws and related crimes against Indian or non-Indian individuals if the acts are committed in Indian country.[14]

Global Issues

In 2005, the World Health Organization conducted a study of more than 24,000 women in 10 countries from different geographical areas, cultures, and rural and urban settings. This landmark study allowed researchers, for the first time, to estimate the frequency and predominant forms of violence against women around the world. The study found that violence against women exists in every culture and every setting, but the frequency of that violence varies significantly. Violence against women was typically, but not always, more common in rural settings and in the developing world.[15]

Among other findings, the study found that:

- The proportion of women who had ever suffered physical violence from an intimate partner ranged from 13% in urban Japan to 61% in rural Peru.

- The proportion of women who had ever experienced sexual violence from an intimate partner ranged from 6% in urban Japan and Montenegro to 59% in rural Ethiopia.

- More than 75% of women in urban parts of Serbia, Namibia, Japan, and Brazil said that violence against women was never justified, while fewer than 25% of women in rural Peru, Ethiopia, and Bangladesh thought the same.

- In two-thirds of interview settings, at least 5% of women reported that their first sexual encounter was forced. The numbers were significantly higher in some countries—17% of women in rural Tanzania, 24% in rural Peru, and 30% in rural Bangladesh reported that their first sexual experience was forced.[15]

A more recent analysis of data from more than 80 countries found that 35% of women worldwide have experienced either physical and/or sexual intimate partner violence or nonpartner sexual violence.[16]

Partner violence can and does lead to death. Globally, as many as 38% of all murders of women are committed by a husband or a boyfriend, often during an ongoing abusive relationship. These deaths may sometimes be concealed as accidents. For example, some deaths of women in India that were recorded as "accidental burns" may actually be murders where women were doused with kerosene and set on fire.

Even in healthcare settings, tens of thousands of women each year are subjected to sexual violence, including sexual harassment by providers, genital mutilation, forced gynecological exams, and obligatory inspections of virginity.

Rape is also used and documented as a weapon of war. Before the country split into North and South Sudan in 2011, civil war raged in Sudan from 1983 to 2005. During this time, Janjaweed militias from the North systematically used rapes as tools of intimidation (by scaring individuals and villages into submission), destruction (by harming and killing thousands of women), and genocide (by reducing the proportion of the ethnic tribes that existed in southern Sudan).[17] In Rwanda, between 100,000 and 250,000 women were raped during the genocide in 1994. UN agencies estimate that more than 60,000 women were raped during the civil war in Sierra Leone (1991–2002), more than 40,000 in Liberia (1989–2003), up to 60,000

during the Bosnia–Herzegovina conflict (1992–1995), and at least 200,000 in the Democratic Republic of the Congo since 1998.[18]

Worldwide data on child abuse are scarce; nevertheless, about 41,000 children younger than 15 years of age die from homicide every year. Nonfatal child abuse also occurs in virtually every country. National surveys of violence against children reveal much higher rates of abuse in Africa as compared with global rates. Surveys conducted in Kenya, Tanzania, Swaziland, and Zimbabwe indicate that one in three girls experienced sexual abuse. The reported prevalence of childhood physical abuse was between 53% and 76%.[1] In the Republic of Korea, for example, 67% of parents admitted whipping children to discipline them and 45% reported hitting, kicking, or beating their children. In Ethiopia, 21% of urban schoolchildren and 64% of rural schoolchildren reported bruises or swelling from parental punishment.[19]

In Southeast Asia, hundreds of thousands of children are involved in the sex trade, and poverty in those countries continually drives more boys and girls into this arena. Although the demand is driven mostly by local clients, sex tourism (travel for the purposes of finding a sex partner) continues to grow and fuel the market in countries such as Thailand, Cambodia, and Vietnam. In Cambodia, almost all of the girls in prostitution are the main providers for their families. Children as young as age 12 from poor families are sold by parents or agents into the sex trade.

Elder abuse also occurs around the world. In some countries, rapid socioeconomic change weakens family networks that once supported older generations. Twenty years after the collapse of the Soviet Union, thousands of elderly men and women from Russia and other former Soviet republics have been left to fend for themselves with only minimal stipends from the government, resulting in numerous cases of elder neglect.

FAMILY AND INTIMATE VIOLENCE

Family and intimate violence refers to violence directed toward former or current spouses or partners, dates, family members, elders, and children. Most violence against women is intimate violence. In the United States, one in four women has experienced violence by an intimate partner at some point during her life.[5] Family and intimate violence includes many forms of mental and physical harm, as well as threats of injury (see **Self-Assessment 14.1**).

Stalking

Stalking is a violent behavior directed at a specific person, involving:

- Repeated sightings or encounters

- Nonconsensual communication, including repeated and unwanted phone calls, emails, text messages, and messages through websites, such as Facebook

- Spying with a listening device, camera, or global positioning system (GPS)

- Written, verbal, or implied threats

- A combination of the previous factors that would cause a reasonable person to feel afraid[20]

Stalkers are frequently a current or former spouse, cohabiting partner, or love interest from some point in the stalked women's lives. An estimated 9.2% of women have been stalked by an intimate partner at some point during their lifetime.[5] Stalking is associated with other forms of violence in intimate relationships. One study showed that 74% of people stalked by a former intimate partner reported violence or coercive control during the relationship.[20]

Although every stalking case is different, a stalker's behavior typically becomes increasingly threatening, serious, and violent. The behavior may begin with the stalker making harassing calls, watching or following the victim, sending unwanted letters or messages, or making verbal threats. The activity generally escalates from what initially may be bothersome and annoying to the level of obsessive, dangerous, violent, and potentially fatal acts. Some stalkers may not begin with violent intentions but still may cause harm if jealousy or anger is involved.

All 50 states have passed laws to prevent stalking and punish people who engage in stalking. California passed the first anti-stalking laws in 1990 in response to several high-profile cases in which the perpetrators stalked and eventually killed their victims. In each case, the victim had notified the police of the stalker's threatening behavior, yet the police were unable to do anything legally unless the stalker acted on the threats. The California law gave law enforcement officers the right to intervene in stalking cases before the stalker acted. Since then, all states have passed similar laws.

Restraining or protection orders can be issued against stalkers to protect citizens against stalking situations. A woman who believes she is being stalked should take action by recording stalking behavior, letting others know about the stalker, and taking proper safety precautions (**Table 14.1**).

Stalking can also be conducted from a distance. Threatening behavior or unwanted advances directed at another using the Internet and other forms of online communications is called cyberstalking. **Cyberstalking** can be conducted through email, social media sites such as Facebook, cellular phones, global positioning systems (GPS), and other technologies. The stalker may use emails, text messages, wall posts, or online comments to send obscene, threatening, or unwanted messages. Online stalking often turns into offline stalking, bringing a real threat of physical harm to the victim. Law enforcement

---

Table 14.1 Guidelines for Women Who Are Being Stalked

These guidelines provide practical information for a woman who believes she is being stalked but who is not in imminent danger. The guidelines do not guarantee her safety, but may reduce her risk of harm.

- Record each incident of stalking with great detail. Save any messages a stalker leaves, and write details of any conversations or encounters. These records can be used as evidence against the perpetrator if necessary.
- Let family and friends know about the stalker. This protects not only the victim but also those close to the victim.
- Be extremely alert when away from home. Carry a whistle to alert others nearby or a cellular phone to report suspicious behavior or to contact someone for help if necessary.
- Seek protection, restraining, or stay-away orders.
- Inquire about the state's stalking laws. Each state's laws differ; see how they apply to this specific case.
- Note any illegal acts by the stalker, such as entering the residence without permission, destroying property, and so on. By reporting these acts to the police, the acts are not only documented for future evidence but also may require that the stalker be incarcerated or ordered to stay away from the woman.
- Create a safety plan. Keep a list of important numbers, such as law enforcement, legal representation, and safe places. Victims may want to keep important items and extra money in one place to grab in a rush if necessary.

Other preventive measures include: changing the locks on doors; adding extra outside light around the residence; maintaining an unlisted phone number; varying regular routes; staying in public places when out of the house; and informing neighbors so they can alert someone if they see something suspicious.

agencies estimate that cyberstalking is a factor in 20 to 40% of all stalking cases. Although many states have updated their laws to encompass cyberstalking and cyber harassment, the states in which these laws do not exist have "gray areas" where stalking or stalking-like behaviors can legally occur.

One way women can lower their chances of being stalked online is by sharing their personal information carefully and responsibly. By adjusting their personal and account settings on sites like Facebook, women can control who has access to their posts and contact information. Safety experts generally advise women either to limit this information to the "friends" they know and trust or to only add trusted friends and acquaintances as Facebook friends.

Women who write or contribute to websites or personal blogs have a difficult choice about whether to reveal their real names. Revealing a personal name can help a woman build a reputation and readership, but it may also allow cyberstalkers to begin looking up a person's personal information, city of residence, and other information. Whether or not they use their real names, women who contribute to websites may receive angry or romantic emails, messages, or posts. Many of these messages can be safely ignored. However, women should report to the police or other authorities any message that contains a threat (whether direct or indirect) or that feels potentially dangerous.

Domestic Violence

Domestic violence, also referred to as **battering**, occurs when a person subjects a current or former romantic partner to forceful physical, social, and psychological behavior. Battering includes five types of interpersonal violence: physical, sexual, property, psychological, and social. Physical violence includes slapping, choking, punching, kicking, pushing, and using objects as weapons. Forced sexual activity constitutes sexual violence. Property violence denotes threatened or actual destruction of property. Psychological and social forms of violence include threats of harm; physical isolation of the abused; extreme jealousy; mental degradation; and threats of harm to children, pets, or other loved ones. Often, one form of violence is accompanied by another type of abuse. Although some forms of abuse are less easily identified than physical abuse, the use of multiple abusive behaviors establishes a pattern of power and control within a relationship (**Figure 14.2**).

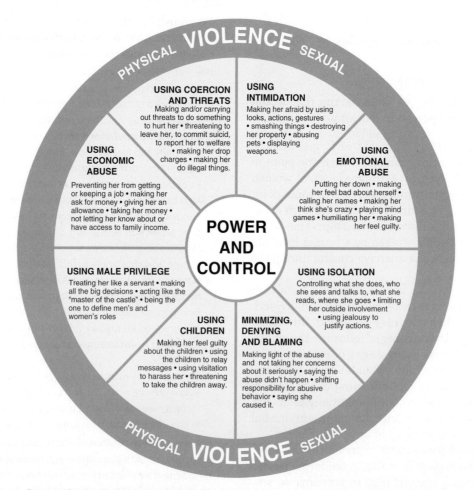

Figure 14.2   Power and Control Wheel. The Power and Control Wheel is a helpful tool for understanding the overall pattern of abusive and violent behaviors that are used by a batterer to establish and maintain control over his or her partner.

Data developed by the Domestic Abuse Intervention Project; produced and distributed by the National Center on Domestic and Sexual Violence.

Battering occurs in families of all racial, economic, educational, and religious backgrounds. Violence in a home often involves more than the adult couple. One in 15 children in the United States lives in families in which partner violence occurred at least once in the past year. Research suggests that almost all of these children are aware of the violence in their homes; 50% of children exposed to violence had yelled at their parents to stop and 23.6% of children called for help.[21]

family or other support networks. Immigrant women also may not feel that they are protected by the U.S. legal system or may feel that they are unable to seek help from authorities if their immigration status is unstable.[22] Studies involving Latina, South Asian, and Korean immigrants found that 30 to 50% of these women have been sexually or physically victimized by a male intimate partner.[23]

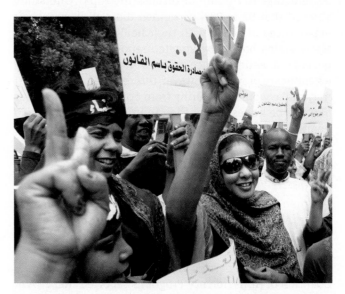

Sudanese women and girls march to improve awareness of violence against women.
© ABD RAOUF/AP Photos

IT'S HARD TO CONFRONT A FRIEND WHO ABUSES HIS WIFE. BUT NOT NEARLY AS HARD AS BEING HIS WIFE.

So you know your friend is an abuser. Do you ignore it or bring it up? Ignoring it is easy. Bringing it up is awkward. You could lose a friend. But maybe bringing it up is the only way to really be a friend. Telling him you know, telling him it's wrong, telling him it's a punishable crime, could be doing him a big favor. Maybe he needs someone to talk to. Maybe he needs someone to say, "No, it's not OK." But more important than his feelings, his wife's well-being, her very life may be in your hands. We can give you some information that may help. Call us at 1-800-END ABUSE.

 THERE'S **NO** EXCUSE for Domestic Violence.   Family Violence Prevention Fund

At least one out of every three murdered women is killed by her husband or boyfriend.
Courtesy of the Family Violence Prevention Fund (www.endabuse.org)

Domestic violence is more common among immigrant women than among U.S. citizens. Immigrants from some cultures condone the use of violence by a man toward his wife or other women in the family. A more important factor, however, is that immigrant women are typically more vulnerable than other women and have less access to legal and social services, as well as extended

> *My boyfriend always put me down when we were alone and when we were out without friends. He told me that I needed to lose weight, I should shave more often, and I should change my hair. I always tried to make him happy, but he would still find something that he didn't like about me. Even when he cheated on me, he blamed me for pushing him away. I didn't even realize how abusive he was until he finally left me for another woman.*
>
> **—24-year-old woman**

Although domestic violence occurs at all levels of society, intimate violence against women generally becomes more common as household income levels decrease.[24] Spousal abuse perhaps appears more frequently in poorer households because educated, middle-class, and affluent women tend to have more resources with which to avoid or leave violent relationships. For example, affluent women may seek confidential professional help and are more likely to be able to afford and get to a safe location, such as a hotel or friend's or relative's house in another city or state. This does not mean that upscale abuse is nonexistent or easily managed, however. In fact, affluent women who are abused often struggle with the disbelief of their peers that an abusive relationship actually exists. In addition, husbands with large incomes can often assemble a "legal dream team," causing the women to be stripped of all of her financial assets as well as the custody of her children.

Relationship violence can and often does lead to death. In 2010, more than 39% of female murder victims were killed by an intimate (or former intimate) partner.[25] Battering is often underdiagnosed during medical visits because both the patient and her healthcare provider may be reluctant to initiate or discuss the topic. One study showed that 92 to 98% of women did not discuss their experiences of abuse with their healthcare providers.[26] Many states have now enacted reporting laws for suspected domestic violence for individuals being treated by a healthcare provider; however, this requirement to report may make women suffering from domestic violence less likely to be honest about their injuries or to even go to a healthcare provider in the first place for fear that their batterer will seek retribution.

Domestic Violence in Same-Sex Relationships

Gay men and lesbians also have to contend with domestic abuse. A 2010 survey found that 44% of lesbian women, 61% of bisexual women, and 35% of heterosexual women had experienced physical violence, stalking, or rape as a result of intimate partner violence.[27] In 2013, the National Coalition of Anti-Violence Programs reported that 20% of LGBTQ victims were denied services when they sought help from a domestic violence shelter, and nearly 42% of victims seeking protection orders were denied.[28] Most battering-related services are designed for heterosexual female victims and heterosexual male offenders, making it difficult for lesbians to find support. This lack of services further contributes to the lack of recognition of lesbian, bisexual, and gay domestic violence. The reauthorized Violence Against Women Act of 2013 is the first time that LGBTQ communities are explicitly protected in federal laws specific to domestic violence, dating violence, sexual assault, and stalking. VAWA now offers protections that extend to LGBTQ victims and includes provisions that help LGBTQ victims access VAWA-funded services.

Domestic Violence During Pregnancy

Women are not immune to battering during pregnancy. Each year, approximately 324,000 pregnant women experience intimate partner violence.[29] Battering during pregnancy is linked to an increased risk of miscarriage, pelvic fracture, premature labor, fetal distress, and low birth weight. Blunt abdominal trauma can lead to fetal death or low birth weight by provoking preterm delivery. Battering during pregnancy has numerous consequences. Women who are battered may be less likely to seek prenatal care and gain sufficient weight. They also may be more likely to engage in harmful behaviors such as smoking or alcohol use. Excessive stress and anxiety caused by being in an abusive relationship may also have physical consequences for the mother and her developing fetus.[29,30]

Domestic Violence in Women with Disabilities

Women with disabilities are about as likely as other women to experience physical, sexual, or emotional abuse at some point in their lives. Women with disabilities, however, were more likely to report multiple perpetrators, longer duration of abuse, and more intense experiences of abuse.[31]

Disabled women are most likely to be abused by an intimate partner, followed by a family member, a personal care attendant, a stranger, or a healthcare provider. The abuse often begins subtly, as the abuser tries to determine how much violence will remain unnoticed. Abuse may take the form of psychological, physical, or financial abuse, or it may involve neglect by withholding care, medication, or mobility devices.

Many people with disabilities are especially vulnerable to victimization because of their real or perceived inability to fight, flee, or tell anyone about the abuse. Many battered women's shelters may be inaccessible or lack attendant care or personnel trained in working with women with disabilities; a woman, therefore, may find herself trapped in an abusive situation. Consequently, healthcare practitioners should find ways to conduct at least part of their visit with a woman with disabilities in private. This opportunity allows a woman to answer questions and confide in her practitioner without a caretaker or family member being present.

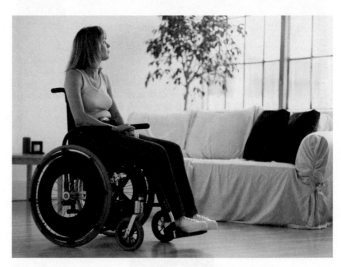

Women with disabilities who are in abusive relationships often have a difficult time finding help.
© Photodisc

Child Abuse and Neglect

Legally, **child abuse and neglect**, often referred to as maltreatment, consists of any act, or failure to act, that causes serious harm, or that creates an imminent risk of harm, to a child. Child maltreatment includes physical, emotional, and sexual abuse, as well as neglect (failure to provide for a child's basic physical, educational, medical, or emotional needs). In 2013, 679,000 children were reported as victims of abuse and neglect, a decrease from the

702,000 victims in 2009. This number is likely an underestimate, however, since many cases go unreported. It is estimated that 1520 children died of abuse and neglect in 2013; nearly three-quarters (73.9%) of all child fatalities were younger than 3 years of age. Women represented nearly 54% of all perpetrators of such violence. Women are more likely than men to commit neglect, but men are more likely to commit sexual abuse.[32]

Neglect is the most common type of child maltreatment, followed by physical abuse, sexual abuse, emotional abuse, and medical neglect (**Figure 14.3**). Of the children maltreated in 2013, 79.5% were neglected, 18.0% were physically abused, 9.0% were sexually abused, and 8.7% were psychologically maltreated. Many abused children suffer more than one type of maltreatment. Younger children are most likely to be abused or neglected (**Figure 14.4**).[32]

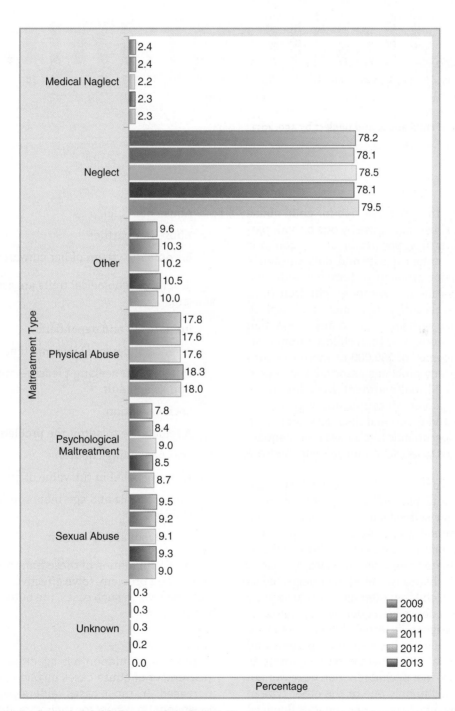

Figure 14.3   Percentage of types of child abuse and neglect victims, 2009–2013.

Source: Data from U.S. Department of Health and Human Services, Administration for Children and Families, Administration on Children, Youth and Families, Children's Bureau. (2015). *Child maltreatment 2013*. Available at: https://www.acf.hhs.gov/sites/default/files/cb/cm2013.pdf

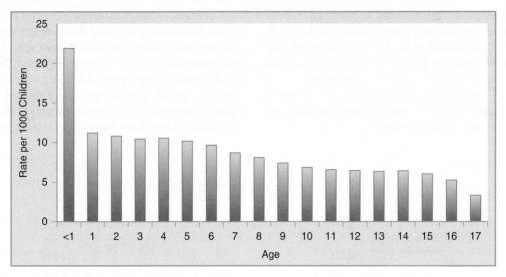

Figure 14.4   **Victims of child abuse and neglect by age, 2013.**

Source: Data from U.S. Department of Health and Human Services, Administration for Children and Families, Administration on Children, Youth and Families, Children's Bureau. (2015). *Child maltreatment 2013.* Available at: https://www.acf.hhs.gov/sites/default/files/cb/cm2013.pdf

Common factors that increase risk for child abuse and neglect include substance abuse by one or both parents, mental health issues, poverty or other economic strain, and lack of parental capacity and skill. Substance abuse is often a major problem in families with suspected child maltreatment.[33] Although children from all socioeconomic levels suffer from abuse and neglect, children from families with annual incomes of less than $15,000 are 22 times more likely than children from families with annual incomes of $30,000 or more to suffer abuse or neglect.[34] Many problems associated with poverty contribute to child maltreatment, including more transient residence, poorer education, and higher rates of substance abuse and emotional disorders. Moreover, families at lower socioeconomic levels have less adequate social support systems to assist parents in their childcare responsibilities.

Children who experience abuse or neglect often develop behavioral and psychological problems, relationship problems, low self-esteem, depression, suicidal behavior, alcohol and substance abuse, sexual dysfunction, and sexual risk-taking later in life.[35] Abuse and battering tend to perpetuate themselves in cycles. Almost all abusive parents were themselves abused or neglected as children, and battered children often grow up to become battering adults. Child abuse is frequently a symptom of family violence. One large study revealed that women who had both witnessed violence between their parents and been victims of parental abuse themselves were twice as likely to abuse their partner or children than were women who had been exposed to only one or the other type of violence. Women appeared to be most strongly influenced by their mother's behavior. With every witnessed incident in which the woman's mother had attacked her father, there was an increased likelihood that the woman would:

- Abuse her child
- Abuse her partner
- Become the victim of her current partner[36]

Several psychological traits are associated with child abusers:

- Immaturity and dependency
- A sense of personal incompetence
- Difficulty in seeking pleasure and finding satisfaction as an adult
- Social isolation
- A reluctance to admit the problem and seek help
- Fear of spoiling children
- A strong belief in the value of punishment
- Unreasonable and age-inappropriate expectations of children
- Low personal self-esteem

Any combination of these traits results in an inability to cope and problem-solve effectively when a problem or crisis evolves. In such cases, the outcome may ultimately be abuse.

Elder Abuse

As the U.S. population has aged over the past 20 years, the number of abuse cases involving elderly victims has increased. In most cases, elders become increasingly dependent on others for their care. It is estimated that 1 to 2 million Americans age 65 or older have been victimized by someone who provided care for them. **Elder abuse** is in part a serious problem for women because they tend to live longer than men. However, even after accounting for their larger share of the aging population, women still account for two-thirds of all elder abuse reports.[37] There are three major situations for abuse of the elderly:

- Domestic abuse (maltreatment by someone who has a relationship with the victim)
- Institutional abuse (maltreatment by staff in a residential facility)
- Self-neglect (failure to care for oneself)

Within these situations, the National Center on Elder Abuse defines seven types of elder abuse:

- Physical elder abuse is the use of physical force that results in bodily injury, physical pain, or impairment.
- Sexual elder abuse is nonconsensual sexual contact of any kind with an elderly person.
- Emotional or psychological elder abuse is the infliction of anguish, pain, or distress through verbal or nonverbal acts.
- Financial or material exploitation occurs when an abuser misuses or misappropriates an elder's funds, property, or assets.
- Neglect refers to a caretaker's refusal or failure to perform his or her obligations or duties to an elderly person. Neglect can be active, when the failure or refusal to acknowledge an obligation is deliberate, or passive, when the failure is unintentional.
- Self-neglect is the failure to provide oneself with adequate food, water, clothing, shelter, safety, personal hygiene, and medication, thereby threatening the elderly person's own health or safety.
- Abandonment, also known as "granny dumping," occurs when a caretaker or guardian of an elderly person deserts the elder.

Elder abuse occurs among people of all racial, ethnic, and economic backgrounds. In general, elders who are unable to care for themselves are more likely to suffer abuse. Researchers have found that in 90% of substantiated cases, perpetrators of elder abuse were family members, with two-thirds being adult children or spouses. Men were more likely to commit abandonment, physical abuse, emotional abuse, and financial and material exploitation, while women were slightly more likely to neglect elders.

> *My granddaughter and her boyfriend always take money from me. The other day, when I asked them to leave my house, they pushed me. They're always yelling at me and telling me how much they hate caring for me. My daughter who lives with me pretends she doesn't see it. But who can I tell? If I report them, I'll end up in a nursing home all alone.*
>
> **—82-year-old woman**

In self-neglect cases, approximately two-thirds of elders were female, 75 or older, and White.[38]

In one study, 44% of nursing home residents said they had been abused; 95% said they had been neglected or witnessed another resident being neglected.[39] Another study revealed that over 50% of nursing home staff admitted to mistreating patients within the prior year. Two-thirds of those incidents involved neglect.[40] Institutional abuse includes physically restraining patients, depriving them of dignity and choice over daily affairs, and providing insufficient care (allowing them to develop pressure sores, for example).

Factors that increase stress in a caretaker's life may increase the likelihood of that caretaker committing abuse. These factors include stressful life events, impairment of the dependent elder, and resentment of dependency, especially as the level of dependency increases. Abusive caregivers are often unprepared, unable, or unwilling to provide the care that an elderly person needs. Elder abuse is also related to emotional problems, such as alcohol or drug use by the abuser, social isolation of the abuser and the abused, and lack of community support. In some cases, an abuser may be repeating a cycle of violence, similar to the cycle identified in cases of child abuse and neglect; the abuser of an elderly parent may have been abused by the parent in childhood, or the abuser may have witnessed the same type of elder abuse by the parent against the abuser's grandparent.

RAPE AND SEXUAL ASSAULT

Rape and sexual assault are violent crimes of aggression. Rape is a nonconsensual event, involving the use of force or the threat of force to sexually penetrate the victim's vagina, mouth, or rectum. Sexual assault often refers to forced sexual contact, but this term frequently acts as an all-encompassing descriptor for any type of unwanted sexual advances, including rape. According to the National Intimate Partner and Sexual Violence Survey, 1 in 5 women and nearly 1 in 59 men in the United States have been the victim of attempted or completed rape in their lifetime.[5] More than 9 out of every 10 rape victims are female. Determining an accurate estimate of how often rape occurs is difficult given the significant underreporting of the crime. Prevalence rates of rape and sexual assault in the United States have remained unchanged in the past decade. The number of reported victims of rape or sexual assault have increased, however, from 134,860 in 2004 to 173,610 in 2013.[41]

Rape may occur among strangers or intimates. Acquaintance rape, or **date rape**, occurs when the victim and the rapist either previously knew each other or have interacted in some socially appropriate manner. About three-fourths of rape victims in the United States know their assailant: Approximately 38% of all rape or sexual assault victims were raped by a friend or acquaintance,

34% by a current intimate partner, and 6% by another relative. Rape by a coworker, teacher, professor, a husband's friend, or boss—anyone the individual knows—is considered acquaintance rape. Strangers committed about 22% of sexual violence.[42]

Many victims of rape are children and adolescents. In a national survey, about 42% of female rape victims were first raped before age 18; about 30% were first raped between the ages of 11 and 17; and about 12% were younger than age 10. More than 28% of male rape victims were first raped when they were age 10 or younger.[43] Although physical abuse and neglect account for the greatest portion of child abuse incidents, child sexual abuse is another tragic dimension of child abuse in general. Sexual abuse accounts for about 1 in 10 cases of child abuse. It is difficult to determine the incidence rate of sexual abuse among children. One report found that 13% of girls and 3.4% of boys had been sexually abused. Of the adolescent sexual assault victims, three-fourths knew their attackers. More than 30% of all sexual assaults occurred within the victim's home, 23.8% within the victim's neighborhood, and 15.4% at the victim's school. Males are reported to be the abusers in most sexual abuse cases involving children.[44]

> *My stepfather started fondling me when I was 6. It evolved into sex by the time I was 12. I think my mother knew, but she had so many other problems to deal with. I had three younger sisters and I was so afraid for them. He said that he wouldn't touch them if I wouldn't tell "the secret." I was trapped. Eventually I found out that he was telling them the same thing. I have been in therapy for a year. I am still so hurt and so angry. The feelings and memories just won't go away.*
>
> **—21-year-old woman**

In many cases of date or acquaintance rape, aggressors use drugs to render the victim unconscious or incapacitated (referred to as drug-facilitated sexual assault). Flunitrazepam, commonly known as Rohypnol, is one type of "date rape drug." This drug is 10 times as strong as Valium and is tasteless and odorless. It comes in pill form, which dissolves in liquid, takes effect quickly, and produces memory loss for as long as 8 hours. Rohypnol is especially popular on high school and college campuses, as well as in nightclubs. Many women have been raped after consuming a drink with the drug dissolved in it. The use of the drug is extremely dangerous and can cause death. Gamma-hydroxybutyrate (GHB) and gamma-butyrolactone (GBL), which come as colorless, odorless liquids, white powder, or pills, have also been associated with sexual assault. Abuse of GHB and GBL can lead to coma and seizures. Ketamine, used as a tranquilizer in veterinary medicine and available as a liquid or white powder, is another common date rape drug that is snorted

or injected. It is referred to as "special K" and can cause death. These drugs are also known as "club drugs."

Rape also happens in marriages, during legal separation, or after divorce. Rape in marriage is often called spousal rape or marital rape. Historically, husbands had unlimited sexual access to their wives and, therefore, rape within marriage was not recognized as a crime: Marital rape has only been a crime in all 50 states since 1993. Many states provide exemptions for certain situations,

It's Your Health

Information About "Date Rape Drugs"

1. Rohypnol (also known as circles, forget pill, LA rochas, lunch money, Mexican valium, mind erasers, poor man's Quaalude, R-2, rib, roach, roach-2, roches, roofies, roopies, rope, rophies, ruffies, trip-and-fall, whiteys, wolfies)
   - Characteristics: small white pill (often has "ROCHE" on one side for Hoffmann-La Roche, its manufacturer, and a circled "1" or "2" on one side); can be swallowed as a pill, dissolved in a drink, or snorted; tasteless and odorless
   - Effects: may feel dizzy, disoriented, nauseated, sleepy, extremely relaxed, or drunk; can cause difficulty speaking or moving, unconsciousness, and loss of memory; effects may last from 2 to 8 hours.

2. Gamma-hydroxybutyrate (also known as bedtime scoop, cherry meth, easy lay, energy drink, G, gamma 10, Georgia home boy, G-juice, gook, goop, great hormones, grievous bodily harm, GHB, liquid e, liquid ecstasy, liquid X, PM, salt water, soap, somatomax, vita-G)
   - Characteristics: white powdered material or liquid; colorless, odorless
   - Effects: may feel drowsy, dizzy, or nauseated; may cause unconsciousness, seizures, severe respiratory depression, and coma

3. Ketamine (also known as black hole, bump, cat valium, cat tranquilizer, green, jet, K, K-hole, kit kat, psychedelic heroin, purple, special K, super acid, vitamin K)
   - Characteristics: white powdered material, similar to cocaine; can be snorted, smoked with marijuana, or dissolved in beverages
   - Effects: short-acting hallucinatory effects; can affect the senses, judgment, and coordination for 18 to 24 hours

Ways to Protect Yourself

- Do not leave a beverage unattended or accept a drink from an open container.
- Do not drink from someone else's drink.
- Do not drink any beverage with a funny taste, odor, residue, color, or consistency.
- Go to parties with trusted friends, watch out for each other, and leave together.

such as mental or physical impairment of a woman rendering her unable to consent, that protect husbands from being prosecuted for rape. In addition, sexual violence can occur between people of the same sex. An estimated 5.3% of female victims of sexual violence other than rape had female perpetrators. Females also can be the perpetrators in sexual violence against males. Forms of sexual violence where a majority of male victims had only female perpetrators include being made to penetrate, sexual coercion, and unwanted sexual contact.[5]

Rape is often characterized as not being a "clear-cut" crime such as murder. Societal pressures and norms have reinforced beliefs that rape is sometimes justifiable, depending on the circumstances. For various reasons, only about 35% of rape or sexual assault victimizations are reported to the police.[41] Unreported rapes can harm more than the victim, because if the rapists are not stopped, their violent behavior may continue. The underreporting of rape is due to a number of factors, including the pattern of "blaming the victim." Many women fear unwanted publicity from making a formal complaint, and others distrust hospital and law enforcement agencies. Feelings of shame or guilt, fear of not being believed, and fear of reprisal or punishment if the rapist is an acquaintance or employer are other reasons why women do not report rape.

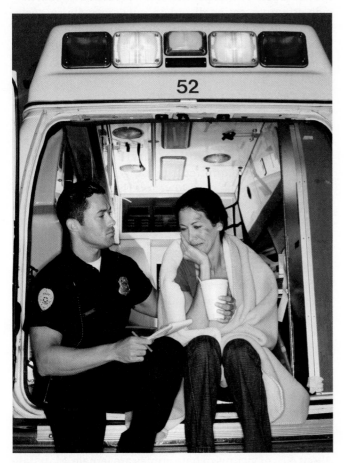

Most rapes go unreported.
© George Doyle/Stockbyte/Thinkstock

Around the world, countless women in prisons and jails are at risk of rape and other forms of sexual violence. Reporting procedures in prisons are often ineffectual, and complaints are routinely ignored. To make matters worse, punishment for the crime is rare and some inmates face retaliation from the offender if a report is made.

Reducing Risk of Rape/Sexual Assault

Society as a whole, as well as individuals of both genders, need to act together to prevent rapes and sexual assault. Women are never "at fault" when a rape occurs; women can, however, lower their risk by being careful and clearly communicating what they are, and what they are not, comfortable with.

Response to Rape/Sexual Assault

If a rape or sexual assault occurs, a woman's first concern should be finding safety and calling the police. The police will assist the victim in seeking medical attention, which is important for treating any physical injuries, testing for sexually transmitted infections (STIs) and HIV/AIDS, and collecting medical evidence for prosecution. It is important to report the assault to the police immediately; the decision about whether to prosecute the offender can be made later. A woman also should contact her local rape crisis center to inquire about counseling and support.

The recovery process from rape depends on the individual and the circumstances in which the rape occurred. Victims of rape often suffer from mental health problems, gynecological issues, negative health behaviors, chronic health conditions, and higher risk for suicide. Rape also may lead to unwanted pregnancies and STIs, including HIV/AIDS. Being tested immediately after the incident for STIs may help a woman prevent long-term consequences

It's Your Health

Reducing the Risk of Date Rape

- Be wary of a relationship that is operating along classic stereotypes of dominant male and submissive, passive female. The dominance in ordinary activities may extend to the sexual arena.

- Be wary when a date tries to control behavior or pressures others in any way.

- Be explicit with communication. Don't say "no" in a way that could be interpreted in any way as a "maybe" or "yes."

- Avoid ambiguous messages with both verbal and non-verbal behavior. Saying "no" and permitting heavy petting implies confusion or ambiguity.

- First dates with an unknown companion may be safer in a group.

- Avoid remote or isolated spots where help is not available.

- Limit alcohol and illegal drug use.

It's Your Health

Myths and Facts About Rape

Myth: Rape only occurs in dark alleys, not in homes or good neighborhoods.

Fact: Six out of 10 sexual assaults take place at the victim's own home or at the home of a friend, neighbor, or relative.

Myth: Rape occurs only late at night, in the dark.

Fact: Forty-three percent of rapes occur between 6 p.m. and midnight; 24% of rapes occur between midnight and 6 a.m.; and the other 33% take place between 6 a.m. and 6 p.m.

Myth: If a person pays for a date, he or she has the right to expect something back, such as sex.

Fact: No one ever owes anyone sex or sexual favors.

Myth: If a person returns to his or her date's apartment or house, the date has the right to expect sex.

Fact: Consent for sexual contact is not defined by one's willingness to enter someone else's home or inviting someone into his or her home, including a date.

Myth: People who commit rapes are unable to control their sexual urges.

Fact: Rapists are not driven by uncontrollable sexual urges but rather by the need to feel powerful and in control. Forcing someone to engage in sexual intercourse against her or his will is an act of violence and aggression. Sex is the weapon used to humiliate and control the victim.

Myth: Rapists are always strangers to the victim.

Fact: Almost three-fourths of rape victims know their assailants.

Myth: Rapists are usually African American men who rape White women.

Fact: In most rapes, the victim and the offender are members of the same race.

Myth: All rapists are men.

Fact: Although men commit 99% of forcible rapes, women do commit rape and other sexual assault offenses.

Myth: Only promiscuous women or women wearing provocative clothing are victims of rape.

Fact: Neither provocative dress nor promiscuous behavior is an invitation for unwanted sexual activity. Forcing someone to engage in nonconsensual sexual activity is sexual assault, regardless of the way the person dresses or acts.

Myth: All rape victims are women.

Fact: About one in every 10 rape victims is male.

Myth: Women who are raped were asking for it.

Fact: No one deserves to be raped. A victim should never be blamed for the actions of the perpetrator.

Source: Data from National Crime Victimization Survey, 1999; National Crime Victimization Survey, 2000; Sex Offenses and Offenders. Bureau of Justice Statistics, U.S. Department of Justice, February 1997.

---

from disease. Post-exposure prophylactics, including antibiotics, emergency contraceptive pills, hepatitis B vaccination, and antiretroviral drugs, can reduce the likelihood for some STIs or unwanted pregnancy.

Posttraumatic stress disorder (PTSD) is another common reaction to rape. (See Chapter 12.) At some point during their lifetimes, 32% of all rape victims develop PTSD, compared with 9% of victims of non-crime-related trauma, such as car accidents.[45]

Rape trauma syndrome is another condition associated with rape victims. It is usually described as having two phases. The first phase, or acute phase, includes the immediate emotions following the event, which include shock, anger, numbness, guilt, disbelief, embarrassment, shame, feelings of being unclean, anxiety, denial, fear, self-blame, and restlessness. This phase is often characterized by significant disruption in a woman's life. The second phase of rape trauma syndrome includes attempts at reorganizing one's life and lifestyle and learning to cope again. Victims may decide to change schools, jobs, or routes to school or work in an attempt to remove reminders of the event from their daily lives. Overwhelming feelings often develop that the victim may not directly link to the rape. Even if a woman successfully represses her emotions about a rape, the feelings can persist, sometimes for years. Depression, guilt, and loss of self-esteem are common reactions. Other psychological problems include suicide attempts, eating disorders, substance abuse, social phobia, and other anxiety disorders. Being a victim of rape can also affect a woman's sexual health and intimacy.

VIOLENCE BY STRANGERS

Victimization rates of women are lower than those of men in all types of violent crimes committed by strangers, except rape and sexual assault. However, the proportion of crimes committed by strangers against women has grown over the past 20 years. These crimes include carjacking, robbery, murder, gang violence, sexual assault, and rape. In general, women are more likely to be victimized by an intimate than by a stranger, except in cases of robberies.

Hate crimes are a form of collective violence often committed against strangers. Hate crimes consist of arson, vandalism, assault, murder, and other offenses that are motivated by hatred or prejudice toward a person's race, religion, sexual orientation, or ethnicity. Hate crimes account for less than 1% of total reported crimes, but the damage they can cause is immense. In addition to harming their victims directly, hate crimes also affect the victims' families and communities. At heart, hate crimes are acts of terrorism—a systematic use of fear to change the way other people behave. In 2012, an estimated 293,800 violent and property hate crime victimizations occurred. About 40% of victims of hate crimes are female. Most hate

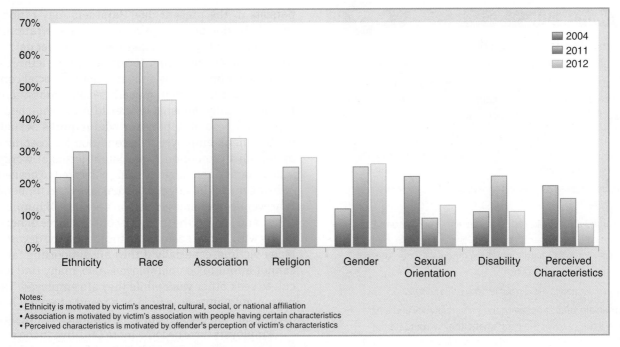

Figure 14.5   **Victims' perception of offender bias in hate crimes, 2004, 2011, and 2012.**

Source: Bureau of Justice Statistics. National Hate Crime Victimization Survey, 2004–2012. Available at: http://www.bjs.gov/content/pub/pdf/hcv0412st.pdf

crimes are committed based on a person's ethnicity (51%) or race (46%); see **Figure 14.5**.[46]

Although violence cannot always be avoided, people can take measures to protect themselves. Women (and men) can walk with at least one other person or stick to populated, well-lit areas, especially at night, to avoid being caught alone. When alone, women should avoid isolated areas and carry a whistle or cell phone in case of emergency. When visiting potentially dangerous areas, women can avoid carrying flashy jewelry or large sums of money.

Self-defense classes can also give women the knowledge and confidence to survive or escape a violent attack. The goal of any practical self-defense class should not be to destroy an opponent, but rather to allow a person to get home safely if he or she is attacked. A good self-defense class can teach women the ways they are most likely to be attacked, as well as different responses to those attacks. Regular practice striking and grappling can give a person "muscle memory" that he or she can call upon and use quickly if needed. In addition, learning and practicing self-defense can give a person the confidence and will to use her body effectively, rather than to panic, in a dangerous situation. Women who are aware of their surroundings and use common sense can greatly reduce their risk of victimization; this does not mean, however, that women who are victimized are at fault. The circumstances and characteristics of each violent crime and each victim are unique, and it is not practical or realistic to imagine that these strategies alone could prevent all types of violence. Prevention is just one useful but limited tool available to women.

SEXUAL HARASSMENT

Sexual harassment is an illegal, violent act involving unwanted sexual attention, requests of sexual favors, or the use of sexual language or behaviors to create a hostile environment. Although sexual harassment can occur in any setting, it most commonly occurs in the workplace. Sexual harassment often involves a male harasser and a female victim. However, sexual harassment recognizes no gender boundaries—a female may harass a male, and the victim and the harasser may be the same sex. There are three types of harassment:

- Gender harassment constitutes behavior that conveys a degrading or hostile attitude toward women.

- Unwanted sexual attention or advances include behaviors such as staring, commenting, touching, or repeated requests for dates or sexual favors.

- Sexual coercion, also referred to as quid pro quo (defined as an "equal" exchange or substitution), is the use of threats or bribery to obtain sexual favors.

Any type of harassment may interfere with a woman's ability to perform her regular duties at work and often creates an intimidating or hostile working environment.

It's Your Health

Common Excuses for Sexual Harassment

"Sexual harassment is a trivial distraction from the real work."

Sexual harassment has serious, long-term emotional consequences for the victim. The emotional and economic impact of sexual harassment is not trivial in nature or form.

"I didn't mean any harm. I was just having fun."

Sexual harassment is similar to poking someone with a stick. The fun is one-sided and unfair.

"She should take it as a compliment that we like her when we say things like that."

Unwanted and unsolicited sexual advances and innuendoes, particularly from others in positions of power, can be frightening. The victim can hardly feel "complimented" when she feels threatened and put down.

"She just wanted to make trouble here with a complaint."

Women are caught between the proverbial rock and a hard place. If they accept the harassment, they perpetuate the behavior and risk further, and perhaps worse, harassment. If they file a complaint, they may be labeled as troublemakers, with no guarantees that the situation will be corrected. Filing a complaint may also place a woman's job security or career in jeopardy.

Women who are at the greatest risk for sexual harassment are those in careers traditionally considered to be male occupations. Any person may initiate sexual harassment, but a harasser is most likely to be someone with more power or authority than the recipient. In addition to suffering physical and emotional victimization, the threat of economic vulnerability often leaves the victim with the feeling that she has few real options in the situation.

For years, workplaces and individuals trivialized sexual harassment and refused to recognize it as a violation of rights or personal dignity. This practice sometimes persists in the present day. Harassers may rationalize their behavior or offer excuses, but these rationalizations perpetuate power disparities and further dehumanize women. As with other forms of sexual victimization, harassment operates as an instrument of social control.

In whatever form it appears, sexual harassment is a harmful, legally punishable offense. A common situation involves a boss or supervisor who requires sexual services from an employee as a condition for keeping a job or getting a promotion. Less blatant forms of workplace sexual harassment include being subjected to obscenities or being made the target of sexual jokes and innuendoes. However deep a harassed person's feelings of humiliation, anger, and shame, the financial consequences of not complying with sexual coercion on the job may be devastating. Many victims, especially if they are supporting families, cannot afford to be unemployed. Also, many find it difficult to seek other work while they are employed. Thus, a person who quits or is fired as a result of sexual harassment faces the prospect of severe financial difficulties.

Employers have become more sensitive to the issue of sexual harassment, in part because of court decisions that have awarded large payments to victims. Employers paid more than $52 million in damages to victims of sexual harassment in 2011.[47] It is an employer's responsibility to maintain a workplace that is free of sexual harassment by educating employees about which behaviors constitute harassment and taking appropriate measures if these behaviors occur. The U.S. Department of Labor, Employment and Training Administration provides training guidelines for the workplace.

Reported cases of sexual harassment have fallen over the past 20 years, dropping by nearly 30% from 1997 to 2011 (**Figure 14.6**). While women continue to make up the vast majority of victims of harassment, the percentage of males filing claims of sexual harassment grew from 11.6% to 16.3% over the same period.[47]

Sexual harassment is not limited to the workplace. A report from the American Association of University

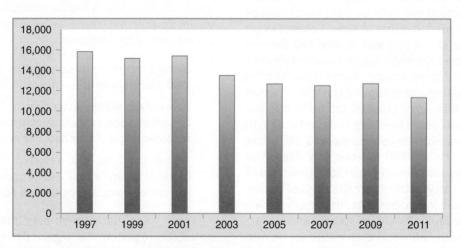

Figure 14.6 Number of sexual harassment charges filed, 1997–2011.

Source: Data from U.S. Equal Employment Opportunity Commission. (2012). Sexual harassment charges EEOC & FEPAs combined: FY1997–FY2011.

> *A guy I worked with would always come up behind me and start rubbing my shoulders. When I asked him to stop, he told me that I needed to relax, that he was just trying to help by giving me a massage. I didn't know who to tell, but it made me really uncomfortable, especially because he continued to do it even after I asked him to stop. Eventually, I went to our human resources department and it turned out that another coworker had just reported him for making lewd comments to her. Within a week, he was fired. Although I felt bad at first for turning him in, it just made me too uncomfortable and nervous to work with him. I think I did the right thing.*
>
> **—26-year-old computer programmer**

Women found that nearly two-thirds of college students have encountered some type of sexual harassment while at college. More than half of female students have been subjected to sexual comments and jokes, and about 35% have experienced physical harassment by being touched or grabbed in a sexual manner. Students who are lesbian, gay, bisexual, or transgender are more than twice as likely to be harassed as heterosexual students. Only 7% of students reported the harassment. Many students actually admit to sexually harassing other students; the reason more than half gave for the harassment was "I thought it was funny."[48]

Common reactions to sexual harassment include anger, humiliation, shame, embarrassment, nervousness, irritability, and lack of motivation. Guilt is another common feeling, with a victim often questioning whether she (or he) has done something wrong to encourage the harassment. The sense of alienation and helplessness many victims of sexual harassment feel is similar to that experienced by many rape victims. Sexual harassment victims may also experience headaches, stomach pain and nausea, back and neck pain, and a variety of other stress-related ailments.

Dealing Effectively with Harassment

Individuals who have been sexually harassed have several options. First, the victim should recognize that criminal charges could be filed against the perpetrator. If there is not an immediate concern for one's safety and there has not been attempted rape or assault, the victim could confront the person responsible for the harassment. The confrontation should be stated in clear terms, and the specific behaviors should be identified as sexual harassment. The victim should make it clear that the behavior is unwelcome, will not be tolerated, and that, if it continues, charges will be filed through appropriate channels. Some victims carefully document what has occurred and provide a written confrontation rather than undertake a verbal discussion. Others may choose to seek out the assistance of their human resources department if the sexual harassment occurs within a work setting.

If the behavior does not stop, the next step is to discuss it with the supervisor of the person responsible for the harassment. It is often helpful to talk to other employees—many times there is more than one victim. Discussing the matter with other employees provides peer support and pressure for the behavior to stop. Official complaints can be filed with local or state Human Rights Commissions or Fair Employment Practice Agencies.

If legal action is necessary, victims can file lawsuits in federal courts under the Civil Rights Act. Lawsuits can also be filed under city or state laws prohibiting employment discrimination. A person who has been the victim of sexual harassment is more likely to receive a favorable court ruling if attempts were made to resolve the problem within the organization before taking the issue to court.

INFORMED DECISION MAKING

Knowing the facts about violence can lead to a certain level of paranoia and anger. Identifying the factors that contribute to violence and working to eliminate them are much more constructive reactions to potential or perceived threats of violence.

The stereotype that men should be aggressive and women should be passive, compliant, and pleasing to others continues to exist and influence people's behavior. When people—either male or female—buy into these stereotypes, it sets the stage for problems. For example, women who have been socialized to be passive may not think that they have a right to express their opinions openly and freely. Men who have been socialized to live up to a macho image may think that they need to "score" with women or control women to be "real" men. They may expect women to go along with their need to prove themselves or believe that a woman means "yes" when she says "no."

To address these stereotypes, a woman must take several steps:

- Recognize the inherent limitations in any stereotype.
- Be open in discussing values with respect to relationships and sexuality.
- Decide for herself and be explicit about when she will or will not have sex.
- Understand that coercion and violence are never acceptable or deserved within a relationship.
- Avoid situations where inebriation by one or both parties makes open and clear communication difficult.

Some women find talking openly about relationships and sexuality difficult. Instead of using clear communication, they rely on assumptions, hints, innuendoes, and considerable hope that their partner understands. Unfortunately, such indirect communication is highly unreliable. Expectations and values about relationships and sexuality should be explicitly expressed. Communication is bidirectional: In a relationship, each person must carefully listen to the other person and confirm what has or has not been said. Finally, "no" means "no."

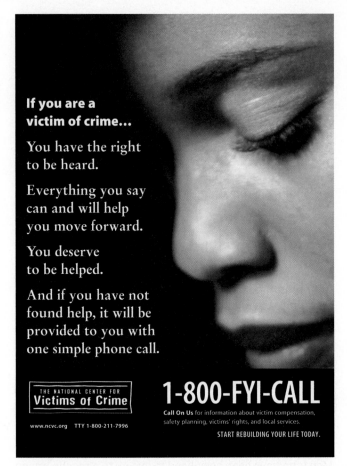

If you are a
victim of crime...

You have the right
to be heard.

Everything you say
can and will help
you move forward.

You deserve
to be helped.

And if you have not
found help, it will be
provided to you with
one simple phone call.

THE NATIONAL CENTER FOR
Victims of Crime

www.ncvc.org   TTY 1-800-211-7996

1-800-FYI-CALL

Call On Us for information about victim compensation,
safety planning, victims' rights, and local services.

START REBUILDING YOUR LIFE TODAY.

Reaching out for help can be the most important step.
Source: Reprinted with permission from the National Center for Victims of Crime.

Sources of Help

Women in abusive relationships first need to identify and acknowledge the presence of the problem. Denial, avoidance, and protection of the abusive partner often prevent or delay such acknowledgment, particularly for women who may have grown up in a dysfunctional family situation.

Professional counseling and support can help a woman cope with and recover from a violent relationship. Most communities have services and facilities to support female victims of violence, including local crisis hotlines. Hotline counselors can help callers find counseling, supportive services, and emergency shelter. Shelters provide physical safety, psychological counseling, and referral services. Many local organizations have been started by women who have been battered themselves and recognize the need for sensitive and protected outreach services. Support groups allow women to share common concerns, fears, and information. For many women, the most important step in taking control of a violent situation is admitting there is a problem and reaching out for help.

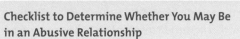

It's Your Health

Checklist to Determine Whether You May Be in an Abusive Relationship

Below is a list of possible signs of abuse. Some of these actions are illegal. All of them are wrong. You may be abused if your partner:

- Monitors what you are doing all the time
- Unfairly accuses you of being unfaithful all the time
- Prevents or discourages you from seeing friends or family
- Prevents or discourages you from going to work or school
- Gets very angry during and after drinking alcohol or using drugs
- Controls how you spend your money
- Controls your use of needed medicines
- Decides things for you that you should be allowed to decide (like what to wear or eat)
- Humiliates you in front of others
- Destroys your property or things that you care about
- Threatens to hurt you, your children, or pets
- Hurts you (by hitting, beating, pushing, shoving, punching, slapping, kicking, or biting)
- Uses (or threatens to use) a weapon against you
- Forces you to have sex against your will
- Controls your birth control or insists that you get pregnant
- Blames you for his or her violent outbursts
- Threatens to harm himself or herself when upset with you
- Says things like, "If I can't have you then no one can."

If you think someone is abusing you, get help. Abuse can have serious physical and emotional effects. No one has the right to hurt you.

Source: Office on Women's Health. *Violence against women: Am I being abused?* Available at: http://www.womenshealth.gov/violence-against-women/am-i-being-abused/

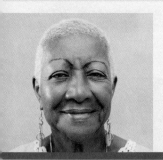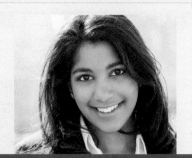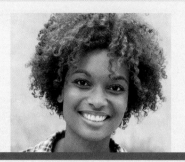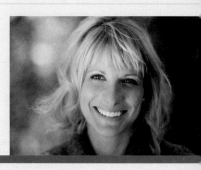

CASE STUDY

Jennifer is a 25-year-old graduate student at a top university. She is living with her boyfriend, John, who is at law school in the same university. They have an extensive group of close friends, a thriving social life, and a seemingly happy relationship. Although not yet engaged, they have discussed marriage and are planning to wait until they both finish their schooling. They both grew up in wealthy suburbs of Philadelphia and have families that have provided both emotional and financial support to them while they attended school. John has a bit of a temper and can get very angry, but he has never taken it out on Jennifer. He is extremely jealous of any time she spends with her friends and has asked her only to see them if they all go out as couples. He often tells her she needs to lose weight and compares her with his ex-girlfriend who was a gymnast. Jennifer no longer has lunch with her best friend from college, a guy, because John believes that she is having an affair with him. They recently merged their bank accounts and he has set the rules on how much money they get each week. Jennifer knows John loves her, but she does sometimes feel frightened by his outbursts. He tells her that it's her fault he gets angry and if she would be better about not upsetting him, he would not lose his temper. Jennifer's best friend thinks that John is abusive.

Questions

1. Given that John has never physically or sexually hurt Jennifer, could he actually be considered abusive?

2. What are some concerns in affluent families experiencing domestic violence?

◼ Summary

Violence occurs in every country in the world, including the United States. Violence can be directed against the self, against another person, or against a community or group of people. Violence affects women when they are victims of crimes, and when they are the siblings, wives, girlfriends, mothers, daughters, and friends of victims. Because of violence, women are left alone to raise children, girls are raised without fathers, and women lose their sons. In addition to its direct physical consequences, violence often causes psychological harm, such as a loss of self-esteem, depression, anxiety disorders, and suicide. Children in battered households may experience illness, emotional problems, increased fears, injuries, and death. They also may internalize abusive behavior as a normal part of life and grow up to abuse their own or someone else's children. Domestic violence also creates problems at the societal level, such as increased crime rates; legal, medical, and counseling costs; and reduced quality of life. Efforts are urgently needed to address and reduce the full spectrum of violence against women.

◼ Topics for Discussion

1. How do interpersonal, collective, and self-directed violence affect women?

2. How do traditional attitudes about women's roles in society and place in society influence violence and its effects?

3. What are some of the major consequences of violence, in addition to the physical effects of the acts themselves?

4. Globally, how does violence in the developed world (the United States, Canada, Western Europe, and Japan) compare to violence in the developing world?

5. What can a woman do to reduce her risk of assault?

6. What would you do if you think that a friend is in an abusive relationship? What would you do if a friend were being stalked?

7. What similarities exist between child abuse and elder abuse?

8. What steps may be involved during a rape exam? What evidence may be collected to help in making a case against a rapist?

Lara Logan (1971–)

Lara Logan is a South African war correspondent and foreign affairs journalist. She has been the chief foreign correspondent for CBS News and for the television show *60 Minutes* since 2006. Logan has won many awards for her reporting. She reported from Baghdad as the U.S. military invaded the city; she has also reported on the Taliban's growth in Afghanistan, the Israeli-Palestinian conflict, violence in Northern Ireland, floods in Mozambique, and the U.S. embassy bombings in Kenya and Tanzania.

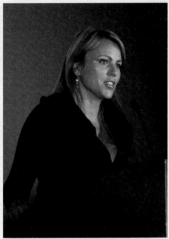

Logan was covering the Egyptian revolution in February 2011 when a mob of protesters separated Logan from her group and brutally beat and sexually assaulted her. Pulled in different directions and dragged along the ground, Logan later said she believed that she would die during the assault. Logan was rescued when a group of Egyptian women surrounded her, placing themselves between her and her attackers until a group of soldiers were able to fight off the crowd.

Logan revealed the details of her assault in a nationally televised interview after her return to the United States, saying that she wanted to break "the code of silence" that surrounds rape and sexual assault among female journalists, and to draw attention to the frequency of sexual harassment and assault of women in Egypt. Since then, she has chosen not to be defined by her assault, but to continue as a journalist, reporting from within the United States and nationally.

© ZUMA Press, Inc./Alamy Images

Yvette Cade (1974–)

Yvette Cade is a survivor. In 2005, 3 weeks after a judge dismissed her protective order against her husband in a district court in Maryland, Cade's husband showed up at her place of employment, doused her with gasoline, and set her on fire. She suffered third-degree burns over 60% of her body. After undergoing multiple surgeries, Cade pulled through and has become an advocate for domestic violence victims. She has spoken out numerous times about her abusive relationship, including telling her story to a national TV audience on Montel Williams and Oprah.

Cade and her family have used her personal tragedy to encourage other sufferers of domestic violence to leave their abusive partners and find freedom. She and her family speak about the importance of family support to get through a tragedy such as this. Cade's situation resulted in significant changes in several states, including her home state of Maryland, regarding enforcement of protection orders and the court's responsibility to treat domestic violence as a serious crime.

Cade was honored in 2007 by the U.S. Congressional Victim's Rights Caucus for being a survivor and offering hope to victims of domestic violence. She and her family started the Yvette Cade Fund to help fund Cade's continued need for medical treatment and further surgeries, as well as to raise money for domestic violence awareness activities.

◼ Key Terms

Battering

Child abuse and neglect

Cyberstalking

Date rape

Domestic violence

Elder abuse

Family and intimate violence

Self-mutilation

Sexual harassment

Stalking

◼ References

1. World Health Organization (WHO). (2014). *Global status report on violence prevention 2014*. Geneva: WHO.

2. United Nations Department of Public Information. (2008). Unite to end violence against women fact sheet. DPI/2498. Geneva: UN.

3. United Nations Population Fund. (2015). *Gender-based violence*. Available at: http://www.unfpa.org/gender-based-violence

4. Huffington Post, *Rape culture is: Know it when you see it*. June 1, 2013.

5. Breiding, M. J., Smith, S.G., Basile, K.C., et al. (2014). Prevalence and characteristics of sexual violence, stalking, and intimate partner victimization—National intimate Partner and Sexual Violence Survey, United States, 2011. *Morbidity and Mortality Weekly Reports* 63(SS08): 1–18.

6. D'Emilio, J., & Freedman, E. B. (1998). *Intimate matters.* New York, NY: Harper and Row.

7. Davis, A. Y. (1983). *Women, race, and class.* New York, NY: Vintage Books.

8. Centers for Disease Control and Prevention (CDC). (2005). *Behavioral risk factor surveillance system survey data.* Atlanta, GA: U.S. Department of Health and Human Services, CDC.

9. Greenfeld, L. A., & Henneberg, M. A. (2001). Victim and offender self-reports of alcohol involvement in crime. *Journal of the National Institute on Alcohol Abuse and Alcoholism* 25(1): 20–31.

10. Sparks, G. (2012). *Media effects research: A basic overview.* New York: Cengage Learning.

11. CDC. (2003). *Costs of intimate partner violence against women in the United States.* Atlanta, GA: U.S. Department of Health and Human Services.

12. Kyckelhahn, T. (2011). *Justice expenditures and employment, 1982–2007.* Bureau of Justice Statistics. Washington, DC: U.S. Department of Justice.

13. CDC. (2015). *Intimate partner violence: Consequences.* Available at: http://www.cdc.gov/violenceprevention/intimatepartnerviolence/consequences.html

14. Sacco, L. N. (2015). *The violence against women act: Overview, legislation, and federal funding.* Congressional Research Service.

15. García-Moreno, C., Jansen, H. A. F. M., Watts, C., et al. (2005). *WHO multicountry study on women's health and domestic violence against women. Initial results on prevalence, health outcomes and women's responses.* Geneva, Switzerland: WHO.

16. WHO. (2014). *Violence against women.* Fact sheet number 239. Available at: http://www.who.int/mediacentre/factsheets/fs239/en/

17. National Center on Domestic and Sexual Violence. (2008). *Darfur: Gendered violence and rape as a weapon of genocide.* Available at: http://www.ncdsv.org/images/darfurgenderedviolencerapeweapon.pdf

18. United Nations. (2014). *Background information on sexual violence used as a tool of war.* Available at: http://www.un.org/en/preventgenocide/rwanda/about/bgsexualviolence.shtml

19. WHO. (2002). *World report on violence and health: Summary.* Available at: http://www.who.int/violence_injury_prevention/violence/world_report/en/summary_en.pdf

20. Brewster, M. (2003). Power and control dynamics in pre-stalking and stalking situations. *Journal of Family Violence* 18(4): 207–217.

21. Hamby, S., Finkelhor, D., Turner, H., et al. (2011). *Children's exposure to intimate partner violence and other family violence.* U.S. Department of Justice. Office of Justice Programs. Available at: https://www.ncjrs.gov/pdffiles1/ojjdp/232272.pdf

22. Voices for Change: Immigrant Women and State Policy Center for Women in Government and Civil Society. (2004). *Building bridges to stop violence against immigrant women: Effective strategies and promising models for reaching and serving immigrant women.* Albany, NY: University at Albany.

23. Raj, A., & Silverman, J. (2002). Violence against immigrant women: The roles of culture, context, and legal immigrant status on intimate partner violence. *Violence Against Women* 8(3): 17–20.

24. Benson, M. L., & Fox, G. L. (2004). *When violence hits home: How economics and neighborhood play a role.* Washington, DC: U.S. Department of Justice, National Institute of Justice. Available at: https://www.ncjrs.gov/pdffiles1/nij/205004.pdf

25. U.S. Department of Justice. (2013). *Intimate partner violence: Attributes of victimization, 1993–2011.* Available at: http://www.bjs.gov/content/pub/pdf/ipvav9311.pdf

26. Wijma, B. (2003). Gynecologists could help identify sexual, physical, and emotional abuse. *Lancet* 361: 2107–2113.

27. Walters, M. L., Chen, J., & Breiding, M. J. (2013). *The National Intimate Partner and Sexual Violence Survey (NISVS): 2010 findings on victimization by sexual orientation.* Atlanta, GA: National Center for Injury Prevention and Control, CDC. Available at: http://www.cdc.gov/violenceprevention/nisvs/specialreports.html

28. National Coalition of Anti-Violence Programs. (2014). *Lesbian, gay, bisexual, transgender, queer and HIV-affected: Intimate partner violence 2013.* Available at: http://www.avp.org/storage/documents/ncavp2013ipvreport_webfinal.pdf

29. Brown, H. L. (2009). Trauma in pregnancy. *Obstetrics and Gynecology* 114: 147–160.

30. The American College of Obstetricians and Gynecologists. (2012). *Committee opinion: Intimate partner violence.* Number 518. Available at: http://www.acog.org/Resources-And-Publications/Committee-Opinions/Committee-on-Health-Care-for-Underserved-Women/Intimate-Partner-Violence#11

31. Nosek, M. A., Hughes, R. B., Taylor, H. B., et al. (2004). Violence against women with disabilities: The role of physicians in filling the treatment gap. In: S. L. Welner & F. Haseltine (Eds.), *Welner's Guide to care of women with disabilities* (pp. 333–345). Philadelphia, PA: Lippincott Williams & Wilkins.

32. U.S. Department of Health and Human Services (DHHS), Administration on Children, Youth and Families. (2015). *Child maltreatment 2013.* Washington, DC: U.S. Government Printing Office.

33. Barth, R. P. (2009). *Preventing child abuse and neglect with parent training: Evidence and opportunities. Preventing Child Maltreatment* 19(2). Available at: http://www.princeton.edu/futureofchildren/publications/journals/article/index.xml?journalid=71&articleid=513&sectionid=3497

34. Children's Defense Fund. (2005). *The state of America's children.* Washington, DC.

35. Child Welfare Information Gateway. (2013). *Long-term consequences of child abuse and neglect.* Washington, DC: DHHS, Children's Bureau.

36. Heyman, R. E., & Slep, A. M. S. (2002). Do child abuse and interparental violence lead to adulthood family violence? *Journal of Marriage and Family* 64: 864–870.

37. OWL. (2009). *Elder abuse: A women's issue.* Available at: http://www.owl-national.org/Mothers_Day_Reports_files/OWL_MothersDay_Report_09_Final_2.pdf

38. National Center on Elder Abuse. (2005). *Elder abuse prevalence and incidence.* Available at: http://www.ncea.aoa.gov/resources/publication/docs/finalstatistics050331.pdf

39. Broyles, K. (2000). *The silenced voice speaks out: A study of abuse and neglect of nursing home residents.* Atlanta, GA: A report from the Atlanta Long Term Care Ombudsman Program and Atlanta Legal Aid Society to the National Citizens Coalition for Nursing Home Reform.

40. Ben Natan, M., & Lowenstein, A. (2010). Study of factors that affect abuse of older people in nursing homes. *Nursing Management* 17(8): 20–24.

41. Truman, J. L., & Langton, L. (2014). *Criminal victimization, 2013.* Washington, DC: U.S. Department of Justice.

42. Planty, M., Berzofsky, M., Krebs, C., et al. (2013). *Female victims of sexual violence, 1994–2010.* Washington, DC: U.S. Department of Justice.

43. Black, M. C., Basile, K.C., Breiding, M.J., et al. (2011). *The national intimate partner and sexual violence survey (NISVS): 2010 summary report.* Atlanta, GA: National Center for Injury Prevention and Control, CDC.

44. National Institute of Justice. (2003). *Youth victimization: Prevalence and implications.* Washington, DC: U.S. Department of Justice.

45. Kilpatrick, D. G., Amstadter, A. B., Resnick, H. S., et al. (2007). Rape-related PTSD: Issues and interventions. *Psychiatric Times* 24(7): 315–318.

46. Wilson, M. M. (2014). *Hate crime victimization, 2004–2012.* Washington, DC: U.S. Department of Justice.

47. U.S. Equal Employment Opportunity Commission. (2012). *Sexual harassment charges EEOC & FEPAs combined: FY1997–FY2011.* Available at: http://www.eeoc.gov/eeoc/statistics/enforcement/sexual_harassment.cfm

48. American Association of University Women. (2006). *Drawing the line: Sexual harassment on campus.* Washington, DC: AAUW.

CHAPTER 15

Women in the Workforce

Learning Objectives

On completion of this chapter, the student should be able to discuss:

1. Historical trends related to women in the workforce.

2. How the recession of 2008–2009 and the subsequent recovery in 2014 and 2015 affected employment opportunities for women.

3. Work-related barriers specific to low-income women and women on welfare.

4. The wage gap between the two genders and the concepts of the "glass ceiling" and the "sticky floor."

5. Connections between work, family, and personal life.

6. The importance of benefits and family-friendly work policies, and how the lack of these policies hurts women.

7. How housework, childcare, elder care, and the work environment influence women's well-being.

8. How work-related stress effects women's mental health.

9. Common types of injuries and hazards in the workplace, and ways to protect against them.

10. Global dimensions of women in the workforce.

11. Ways for employers and employees to increase productivity and satisfaction.

INTRODUCTION

Over the past century, women have gone from being a workplace rarity to an essential part of the workforce. In 1900, women made up roughly one-fifth (18%) of the labor force. By 1960, labor force participation rates began to increase consistently, with a peak rate of 60% in 1999. Since then, there has been a small decline, with 2012 participation rates of 57.7%.[1] Today, women become doctors, accountants, astronauts, politicians, or members of any other occupation with greater ease than in any previous generation. It is difficult to overstate the importance of these changes. Throughout the 19th century and through a good deal of the 20th century, women were banned, either explicitly or in practice, from entering a number of vocations. Women who did have jobs systematically received less pay than men working those same positions and were more likely to be working in low-paid, low-status positions. Discrimination also existed in universities and colleges that offered the necessary training for many jobs. Major universities like Princeton and Yale did not admit women until the 1960s, and a few public military colleges did not admit women until the 1990s. Women's participation in the workforce and enrollment in colleges and universities grew throughout the 20th century. In addition, the amount of money they earned has steadily increased (**Figure 15.1**).

Despite this progress, sexism and discrimination against women in the workplace continue to exist in many forms. On average, women make less money than men working in comparable jobs. The average gender gap has remained at about 81% over the past decade, with wider income gaps in many industries. In addition, women are still not reaching the highest echelons of the work world in great numbers. In 2014, women held only 23 of the top-500 CEO positions in the United States (4.6%); only 14% had women holding at least one-fourth of their officer positions.

The greater presence of women in the workforce has highlighted many new issues, including pay differentials between genders, the balancing of work and family, health and safety in the workplace, and the struggle for many women between choosing a career and choosing to stay home. Women typically shoulder more of the burden of family and household responsibilities than men, often working at their paying jobs and then taking on a "second shift" of responsibilities when they return home. Some women who choose to stay home feel conflicted by their choice, as do some women who choose to pursue a career and leave their child with a surrogate provider.

Health and safety issues also affect women in the workplace. Workstations, tools, and protective equipment have traditionally been designed for men and therefore may compromise the health and safety of women. Health hazards from biological, chemical, and disease-causing agents exist in many predominantly female occupations, including the textile, laundry, and meat industries; health care; and food preparation. Additionally, physically

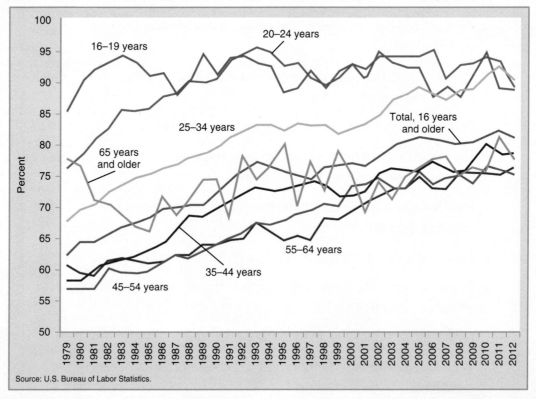

Figure 15.1   Women's earnings as a percent of men's, median usual weekly earnings of full-time wage and salary workers, by age, 1979–2012 annual averages

Source: U.S. Department of Labor, Bureau of Labor Statistics, 2014.

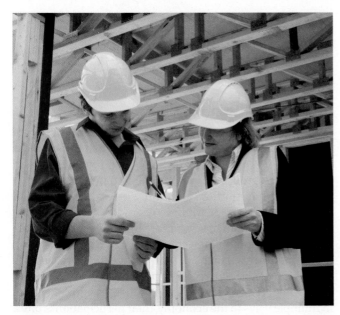

Although women make up half of the workforce, they continue to earn less than their male counterparts for the same responsibilities.
© Lev Kropotov/Shutterstock

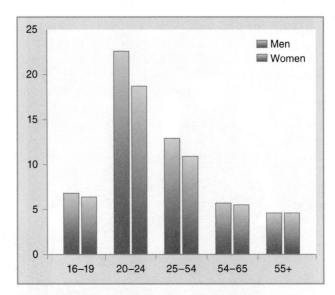

Figure 15.2   Unemployment rates by age and sex, January 2014.

Source: Data from U.S. Department of Labor, Bureau of Labor Statistics. (2014). Labor force statistics.

intense activities or exposure to certain substances while on the job can harm working women who are pregnant.

In addition, women currently in their late teens and 20s face the toughest job market in decades. Today, there are millions more qualified people looking for work than there are positions. Most women graduating college 10 or 20 years ago could count on their degrees and hard work to provide them with full-time employment, but today's college graduates have no such guarantees. National and global economic crises, followed by slow economic growth, have caused millions of people to lose their jobs and many companies and organizations to delay or stop creating new positions. Although employment levels have started to recover significantly, today the average unemployment rate is higher than what it was before the recession of 2008–2009. For men and women 25 and under, the unemployment rate has more than doubled (**Figure 15.2**).

This chapter discusses gender differences in the workplace, the balancing of work and family, and occupational safety issues. In addition, the chapter presents strategies for reducing job stress and increasing workplace satisfaction.

TRENDS AND ISSUES

Historical Issues

In colonial times, all members of the family worked together as an economic unit. Most of women's jobs outside the home appeared to be extensions of their household duties—making clothing, cleaning house, teaching, or cooking—but some women worked as blacksmiths, silversmiths, and shopkeepers. When their husbands were off at sea or at war, some women operated family businesses; other women accompanied troops to war and served as nurses and cooks.

The Industrial Revolution brought women into the factories, providing many with new skills, educational opportunities, and social outlets. Many European women immigrated to the United States to work as indentured servants, with hopes of a more promising future. Workplace violence, sexual harassment, and unfair pay were a fact of life, and many women were physically and sexually abused on the job, or deprived of personal freedom and financial compensation. Because many women's positions were viewed as temporary, many working women earned enough wages to help make ends meet, but not enough to make a comfortable living.

In the mid-1800s, women's rights advocates like Charlotte Woodward campaigned to allow women rights to their earnings (under existing laws, husbands had full ownership of their wives' money). The New York Married Women's Property Act, which was passed in 1848, represented a major step for women's rights; by 1860, other states had passed similar laws. It was not until 1974, however, that Congress passed the Equal Credit Opportunity Act, which barred creditors from discriminating against women on the basis of sex or marital status.

Throughout the 19th and early 20th centuries, many women found opportunities to earn wages, often working as nurses, governesses, cooks, domestic servants, and teachers. In 1869, Wyoming became the first state to provide equal pay for female teachers; California followed soon thereafter. Although exceptions did arise, most women continued to work in positions where men defined their authority and control.

When the United States entered World War II in 1941, jobs available to women increased dramatically. "Rosie the

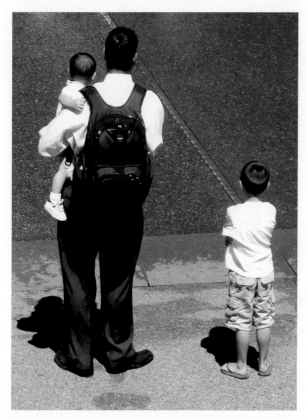

Men and women are redefining traditional roles and responsibilities for their families.
© Dhannte/Shutterstock

Riveter," the factory worker appearing on posters underneath the slogan "We can do it!" became the symbol for women workers in the U.S. defense industries. More than 6 million women, from all backgrounds and from all over the country, worked at industrial jobs that challenged traditional notions of women's capabilities and ensured U.S. productivity that helped win the war. During the war years, women became streetcar conductors, taxicab drivers, machine operators, business managers, and railroad workers. They unloaded freight, worked in lumber mills and steel mills, and made munitions. This trend led to a rise in salaries and an overall commitment by women to their jobs; however, most of these women lost their positions when the war ended in 1945.

The number of women entering the workforce grew throughout the 20th century. As women became more likely to work and began earning more money, their contributions to family incomes increased. In 1970, women contributed 27% of the average family income; by 2009 that number had risen to 37%.[2] Women also started becoming more educated. Today, women are more likely than men to attend college, a major change from 30 years ago. The desegregation of college majors has led more women into fields such as architecture, business, and the sciences.[3] Many women are postponing child bearing and marriage, having smaller families, or focusing on their careers and personal development before taking on the roles of wife and mother. Women have opened up

numerous opportunities for themselves by attending college, fighting for equal rights in the workplace, and breaking barriers in many occupations traditionally associated with men. Despite all of these advances, however, gender discrimination in jobs persists.

Occupation Trends of Women

Of the 120 million women in the United States, 59% are either working or looking for work.[2] Women between the ages 35 and 44 are more likely to be working than women in other age groups (**Figure 15.3**). This may be partly due to the fact that mothers are more likely to participate in the workforce as their children get older. The stronger an education a woman has, the more likely she is to be working, and the more money she is likely to make (**Table 15.1**). More than three-fourths of women age 25 years or older who are employed are college graduates.

Although women work in all industries and contribute in multiple ways to the economy, their participation is often concentrated in certain sectors. Women make up a strong majority in many positions in health care, education, communications, for example, but continue to be underrepresented in the fields of engineering, computer science, and construction work (**Table 15.2**). Nearly one in five employed women works as a teacher (excluding postsecondary positions), secretary, manager or administrator, or cashier.[3]

According to a recent report, in the United States:

- There are 9,087,200 women-owned firms, employing 7,854,200 employees.

- These women-owned firms generated over $1.4 trillion in revenues.

- Between 1997 and 2014, when the number of businesses in the United States increased by 47%, the number of women-owned firms increased by 68%—a rate one and a half times the national average.

- Growth in the number (up 68%), employment (up 11%), and revenues (up 72%) of women-owned firms over the past 17 years exceeds all other privately held businesses over this period.[3a]

More than half of such firms are in the service industries, particularly business services and personal services. Women cite a variety of reasons for starting their own businesses:

- Flexibility

- Independence

- Outlet for creativity

- Relief from sexual harassment in the workplace

- An exit from poverty[4]

Over the past generation, the number of women in the workforce who have young children has increased (**Figure 15.4**).

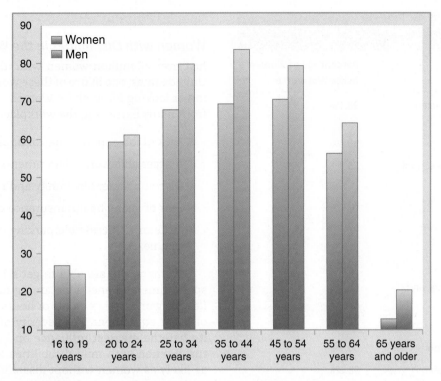

Figure 15.3 **Percentage of working men and women by age, 2010.**

Source: Data from U.S. Department of Labor, Bureau of Labor Statistics. (2011). *Women in the labor force.*

The labor force participation rate of mothers with children younger than 18 years of age was 69.9% in 2013, 74.7% for mothers with children 6–17 years of age, and 63.9% for mothers with children younger than 6 years of age, 61.1% for mothers with children younger than 3 years of age, and 57.3% for mother of infants (2013 annual averages). The labor force participation rate for single mothers with children younger than 18 years of age was 74.2%

Table 15.1	Employment Rates and Average Weekly Income of Women, Ages 25–64, by Educational Attainment, 2014

2014 Average Weekly Income of Women, Ages 25–64, by Educational Attainment	
Women	
Total, 25 years and over	$752
Less than a high school diploma	409
High school graduates, no college	578
Some college or associate degree	661
Bachelor's degree and higher	1,049
Bachelor's degree only	965
Advanced degree	1,185

Source: Modified from U.S. Department of Labor, Bureau of Labor Statistics. (2014). *Women in the workforce: A databook.*

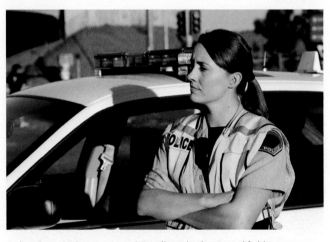

By breaking the barriers in traditionally male-dominated fields, women have created greater opportunities for themselves in the workplace.
© John Roman/iStockphoto/Thinkstock

in 2013, and 67.8% for married mothers (spouse present) with children younger than 18.

The number of dual-earner families also has increased. Before World War II, less than 10% of the workforce was from a dual-earner family. Today, more than 57% are dual-earner families. In nearly 75% of dual-earner families, both partners work full time.[3] Despite this change, many two-parent families with young children are having difficulty making ends meet. Fifty percent of young children are members of families with incomes less than $40,000; 25% are in families making less than $20,000.[5]

Occupation	Percentage of Women in the Workforce
Preschool and kindergarten teachers	98.1%
Registered nurses	90.6%
Elementary and middle school teachers	75.8%
Librarians	86.8%
Medical and health service managers	69.7%
Psychologists	72.7%
Tax examiners, collectors, and revenue agents	62.4%
Writers and authors	55.6%
Accountants and auditors	60.9%
Public relations managers	58.2%
Janitors and building cleaners	29.7%
Environmental scientists	25.7%
Dentists	24.2%
Chefs and head cooks	21.5%
Television, video, and motion picture camera operators and editors	21.4%
Clergy members	20.5%
Civil engineers	13.7%
Broadcast and sound engineering technicians	8.4%
Fire fighters	3.4%
Electricians	1.8%

Table 15.2   Selected Occupations with Strong Gender Divisions, 2013

Source: Data from U.S. Department of Labor, Bureau of Labor Statistics. (2013). *Women in the labor force: A databook.*

Special Populations

Women with Disabilities in the Workplace

Just over 27 million women with disabilities live in the United States; one in five of these women are either working or looking for work.[2,5a] Women with disabilities confront many barriers in the workplace:

- Lack of job opportunities or appropriate jobs
- Inaccessible work environments
- Discouragement by family and friends
- Fear of losing health insurance or Medicaid
- Little or no accessible parking or public transportation nearby

Women who are able to get a job may still need to spend time and energy obtaining functional assistance, flexible work arrangements or hours, handrails or ramps, or other equipment. The severity of a woman's disability has the greatest influence on her employment status. Women with mild disabilities are about four-fifths as likely as women without disabilities to have jobs, but women with severe disabilities are only one-third as likely.[2] Women with disabilities also earn, on average, less than women with no disabilities. Women with disabilities that directly affect their work are more likely to live below the poverty level than people without work disabilities. Approximately 40% of women with a severe disability are living in poverty.[15]

Older Women

Women have increasingly been participating in the part-time labor force during the traditional years of retirement. This trend is partly attributable to the recession of 2008–2009, which disproportionately affected employment rates of younger and older workers. In addition, partly because individuals are living longer and healthier lives, older workers are finding their retirement savings insufficient to make ends meet. Older women may have special health needs as members of the workforce, including the need for easy or disabled access to a work site, close proximity to rest rooms, and seats with supportive backs

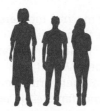 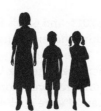 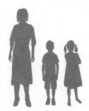 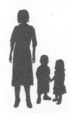 

| **69.9%** with children under 18 years | **74.7%** with children 6–17 years | **63.9%** with children under 6 years | **61.1%** with children under 3 years | **57.3%** mothers of infants |

Figure 15.4   **Participation by mothers in the labor force.**

Source: U.S. Department of Labor, Bureau of Labor Statistics. *2013 annual averages.* [Tables 5 and 6]. Available at: http://www.bls.gov/news.release/famee.toc.htm

or armrests to assist in getting up and down. Employers should be aware of the special needs of older workers, as they provide a valuable and often highly educated supplement to the workforce.

Socioeconomic Issues

Low-income women—particularly those living in poverty—face many challenges when trying to find and keep a job. For these women, not finding employment or the inability to maintain a job can have devastating consequences. Low-wage workers are disproportionately women and minorities with family responsibilities. Women heads of household represent a high percentage of this group. Welfare-to-work programs have helped some of these women move from welfare to paid employment. Most of these individuals work in service industries characterized by low hourly wages (averaging about $8–10 per hour) and are at significant risk for layoffs or work-hour reduction in a weakened economy.

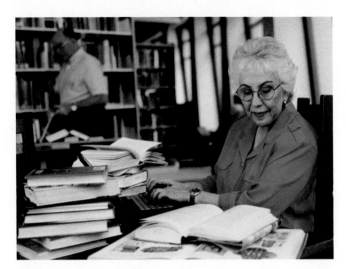

Older workers may have additional needs in their workplaces.
© Photodisc

I'm lucky enough to have a full-time house-husband. Rick stays at home and takes care of the boys, while I go in to work at the medical center. I'm able to earn enough to pay the bills, but with the long hours I work, there's no way I'd be able to clean up, cook, and take care of the kids. I don't know what I'd do without him.
—33-year-old doctor and mother of two

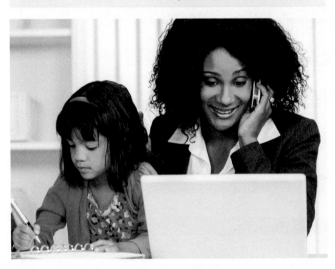

Childcare remains a major challenge for working parents.
© aijohn784/Getty Images

Work opportunities for low-income women or women on welfare are often limited because many people in this situation lack education, training, transportation, or childcare. Many jobs that are available either cover odd hours or have changing schedules. Both situations make transportation and finding childcare difficult. Low-income women who live in rural areas with little or no public transportation often have trouble getting to and from job training centers or jobs. Other women are caught between taking a job to put food on the table and leaving young children at home alone because of lack of childcare.

Even when women are able to find transportation and childcare, the costs for these services may consume most of their incomes.

Low-wage jobs often provide few or no benefits, such as healthcare coverage, paid sick leave, or paid family leave. Furthermore, because these positions do not require advanced skills, employers are typically quick to replace a woman who may have to miss work because her child is sick.[7] Women who find work after receiving welfare are less likely than other working women to have jobs offering paid sick days, family leave, or flexible job schedules, even though they were more likely to have children with chronic health problems.[8]

EQUAL PAY FOR EQUAL WORK

A great challenge for working women has been the battle of receiving equal pay for performing equal work. In almost every field, men in the same jobs earn more than women with the same education and years of experience. In 2013, women who worked full time, regardless of age, race, or educational attainment, earned about 80% of what men earned. When looking at women by race, these differences become more pronounced. Black and Hispanic women have a much greater income gap than White or Asian women.

Women earn four-fifths (79.9%) of what men make (**Table 15.3**).[2] Earning differences between genders varied by demographic features, with the greatest contrast arising between men and women aged 45 to 54, with women earning 74% as much as men in this age range. The narrowest gap between earnings was among workers aged 16 to 24 years; in this demographic group, women earned 93% of what men earned (**Figure 15.5**). Wage gaps also exist by race, ethnicity, and other factors. There is less gender disparity among Black and Hispanic/Latino workers than there is among workers who are White or of Asian

Table 15.3   Women's Median Weekly Earnings Compared to Men's by Race, 2013

Women's to men's earnings ratio, by race and Hispanic or Latino ethnicity, in 2013. *compared to White men only

	All	White	Black	Asian	Hispanic
Women	$706	$722	$606	$819	$541
Men	$860	$884	$664	$1,059	$594

Notes: Data are based on median weekly earnings of full-time wage and salary workers. Hispanics can be of any race.

Source: Women's Bureau calculations from data from the Bureau of Labor Statistics, Labor Force Statistics from the Current Population Survey. Available at: http://bls.gov/cps/cpsaat37.htm (2013 annual averages).

descent. The wage gap narrows to 95% for women who have never been married but rises to 73% among women who are currently married (Table 15.3). As a result of these differences, the average 25-year-old woman who works full time, year-round, until retiring at age 65 will earn more than half a million dollars less over her lifetime than the average working man.[9]

The pay gap is closing in some fields but not in others and not quickly enough. In some professions, pay discrepancies are quite small, but in others they remain much larger (Figure 15.5).

For example, in comparison to men in the same occupation, on a weekly average:

- Women lawyers make almost $500 less.
- Women bartenders make about $70 less.
- Women engineers make about $150 less.
- Women doctors make nearly $500 less.
- Women registered nurses make about $100 less.
- Women professors make nearly $300 less.[2]

Not only do women make less money than men in virtually every profession, but women are clustered in low-paying professions. Many women are worried about the "sticky floor"—employment practices that keep full-time, working women right at the poverty level threshold. One-fourth of women who work full time do not earn enough to move their families above the federal poverty threshold. Women also fight against the "glass

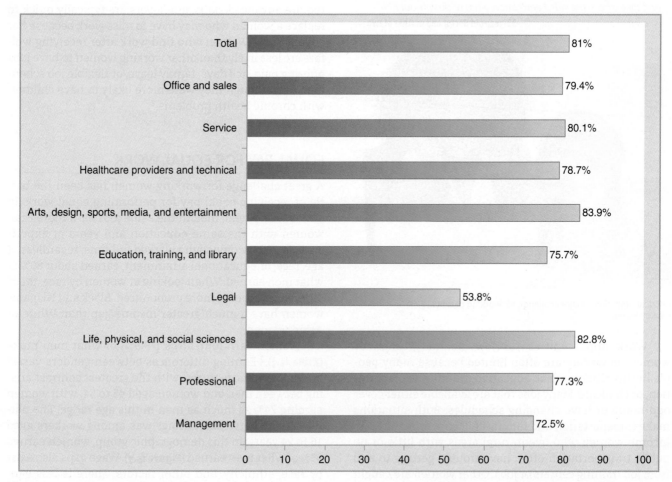

Figure 15.5   Women's earnings as a percentage of men's for selected occupations, 2012.

Source: Data from U.S. Department of Labor, Bureau of Labor Statistics. (2013). *Women in the workforce: A databook.*

ceiling" phenomenon—employment practices that effectively keep working women out of top-ranking positions. Women remain strongly underrepresented in leadership positions in industry, politics, and other areas.

Besides lower wages, a grim reality for working women is the lack of paid sick or family leave; childcare benefits; flexibility of schedule associated with employment; and employer-provided health insurance, pension plans, or retirement benefits. According to an AFL-CIO survey:

- 97% of women are worried about healthcare costs.
- 88% do not have retirement benefits.
- 78% are concerned about a lack of job benefits.
- 57% do not have equal pay for equal work.
- 39% do not have affordable health insurance.
- 29% do not have paid sick leave.
- 24% do not have paid vacation time.[10]

Pay gaps in women's earnings affect families as well as women. With more women in the workforce, more families depend on dual incomes. In addition, women are the heads of household with no spouse present of one in eight (13%) households. Women maintain 14% of White families, 47% of Black families, and 24% of Hispanic-origin families. Nearly one-third of all families maintained by women live below the poverty level.[11] Women occupy a greater proportion of low-paying jobs than men and generally receive fewer benefits and less flexibility in their working conditions. Minorities, especially minority women, are even more likely to be in these less desirable positions. The average weekly earnings for White women are 17% higher than those of Black women and 32% higher than those of Hispanic women.[2] Whereas women overall are more likely than men to be among the working poor, African American and Hispanic women are two to three times more likely than White women to be members of the working poor.[12]

Achieving Equal Pay

One key factor for women who are seeking to help themselves is education. Completing high school is the first step in increasing one's potential income. Women with high school diplomas earned an average of $562 per week in 2013—about 40% more than women without a diploma. A woman's average earnings increase steadily with education: Women with bachelor's degrees earned an average of $931 per week, and women with a professional degree earned an average of $1411—roughly two and a half and four times as much as women without high school diplomas.[2]

To achieve fair compensation for their work, women should learn what fair and equitable pay is for their position and experience, be aware of the laws that prohibit pay discrimination against women, and support efforts to bring "pay equity" to their workplaces. Employees should encourage their employers to implement a pay equity policy, along with a way of creating a grading system to categorize jobs based on education, skills, and experience.

BALANCING WORK AND FAMILY LIFE

Women today face a growing challenge of combining family and work.[13] Women may juggle many tasks to perform well at work, run a household, provide a loving home for their children, spend quality time with their partners, and provide care for their elders. Having these roles can be a source of satisfaction but can also contribute to strain and stress.

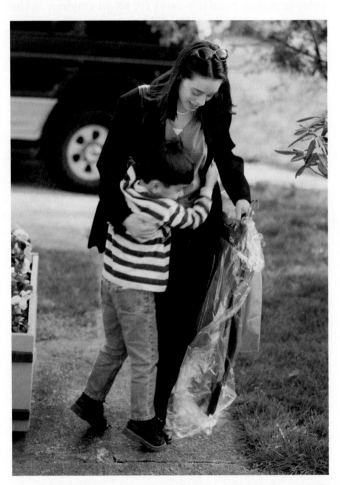

Many women who have entered the workforce continue to work on household chores and childcare when they return home from work.
© Ryan McVay/Photodisc/Getty Images

One in five working parents is a member of the "sandwich generation," meaning that the individual is caring for both children and elderly relatives. More than one-third of those with elder responsibilities—men and women alike—reduced their work hours or took time off to provide the necessary care.[14] Fifty-four percent of Americans say they will probably be responsible for the care of an elderly parent or other relative in the next 10 years. Women account for 70% of unpaid caregivers for the elderly; they also constitute the majority of paid workers, including nurses, nurse's aides, and home healthcare workers.[11]

CHILDCARE

Childcare facilities, relatives, and nannies have become a necessity for working families with children. The United States is one of only three countries in the world that does not offer paid time off for new mothers. More than three-fourths of preschool-age children with employed mothers are regularly cared for by someone other than their parents. Almost two-thirds of children from birth to age 6 spend some time in nonparental childcare.[15] A babysitter or nanny regularly cares for 6% of children in the child's home. Families with children between the ages of 3 and 5 say that childcare is their third greatest expense after housing and food.[11] The cost of full-day childcare can range from $5000 to $25,000 per year per child. In addition to the high costs, 9 out of 10 Americans describe finding quality childcare as "difficult."[11,15] Only 12 states require childcare providers to have any early childhood training before minding children in their homes.[16]

Childcare does not always ease the stress for working women. In fact, 52% of women say that childcare problems affect their ability to perform well at work.[15] Eighty percent of employers reported that childcare problems force employees to lose work time. In addition, only 9% of sampled workers with children in daycare facilities report feeling "very successful" in balancing work and family.[17]

The Current Situation

Working Mother magazine rates the 100 best companies for working mothers every year, based on various measures of flexibility within the workplace, such as flextime, telecommuting, and job sharing. The magazine also rates companies based on their propensity to listen to employees by surveying them on work–life topics and, in response to the survey results, adding features such as lactation rooms.[18] However, when these benefits are present, they do not always extend to those in greatest need. In many organizations, workers in low-wage jobs are half as likely as managers and professionals to have flextime; low-wage workers are also more likely to lose a day's pay when they must stay home to care for a sick child.[19]

Within many companies, only 20% of employees have access to childcare information and referral services; 25% have access to elder care information and referral services. Only 12% of employees with children younger than age 6 have childcare services on or near their worksite that are operated or sponsored by their employers, and these facilities are usually located at headquarters, where managers and executives work.[5] Even those lower-paid employees who have access to nearby childcare facilities usually find the fees too high for their earnings. Many company-operated daycare centers are open only during regular business hours, such as 8 a.m. to 6 p.m.; however, close to one-third of employees with young children have unpredictable or erratic work schedules. Additionally, these same employees are most likely to earn less than $25,000 per year.[5,10]

Maintaining Balance

Many women suffer from job- and family-related stress but do not feel they have any options that would relieve that stress. Some women aspire to the "superwoman" ideal of having a high-paying, successful career, while simultaneously keeping a clean house, preparing home-cooked meals, spending quality time with children, and being a loving and supportive wife. Women need to find their individual balance of work and family responsibilities and make changes if they are dissatisfied with their situation. For women with partners, open communication about the sharing of responsibilities can help couples to establish a good balance within their home. In situations where both partners work, sharing of chores is essential to minimize stress and maximize quality family time. Single women should also find balance between work and home responsibilities. This may mean reviewing policies at work that allow flextime or telecommuting, or advocating for these options if they are not available. Women who own businesses should set examples for pay equity, fair workplaces, supportive work environments, and family-friendly policies.

HEALTH AND SAFETY IN THE WORKPLACE

Work-related stress may come from unsupportive workplace policies, unfair pay, concerns for quality childcare, inflexible scheduling, or lack of support and help at home. With the economy still recovering from national and economic recessions, concerns over downsizing and layoffs create added pressures. Other stressors revolve around lack of control at work, such as high workload demands, unreasonable deadlines, role ambiguity and conflict, repetitive and boring work, and strained relationships with coworkers or supervisors.[20] This kind of stress often produces little job satisfaction and a poor sense of well-being. The following jobs are associated with high stress because of the need to respond to the demands of others and timetables that allow little control over events:

- Administrative assistants
- Waitresses
- Middle managers
- Police officers
- Editors
- Medical interns[21]

Long-term exposure to job stress can lead to higher levels of depression, anxiety, and other mental illnesses.

GENDER DIMENSIONS: Health Differences Between Men and Women

Motherhood

Motherhood is often a woman's principal source of stress; she may enjoy this role and be committed to it, but nevertheless may feel strained by it. Her stress may be exacerbated by society's normative expectation of "good mothering," which does not usually encompass full-time employment.[26,27] Working may increase a woman's opportunities for obtaining resources, power, social identity, positive self-esteem, and involvement with others, but it is often a major source of stress. The benefits of work depend on the woman's working conditions, her marital status, her stability in her job, and her ability to handle many roles at once. The more demanding and difficult the job and the less supportive the workplace, the greater the negative spillover from one's work life to one's personal life.

Working mothers often feel the stresses of work significantly more than working fathers. Mothers, for example, often must juggle the responsibilities of maintaining high job performance and being the primary caregiver for children. Single mothers frequently carry this double burden alone, resulting in even greater stress. Although men perform more household responsibilities than they did 20 years ago, women spend more time than men doing housework even as their workloads outside the home have increased. One study showed that women spend 31 hours per week doing paid work and 26 hours on family care; by comparison, men spend 40 hours per week doing paid labor and 14 hours on family care or housework.[28] Housework and family care tend to be more unbalancing to a person's sense of well-being because the tasks are often more repetitive, dirtier, menial, unending, and inflexible. When men do housework, it is often work that can be scheduled, such as lawn maintenance or repairs. In contrast, women are often responsible for cleaning, cooking, and caring for children—duties that cannot be postponed.[26] Married men are more likely to have partners who are willing to take care of tasks at home, making men's lives more balanced. On the other hand, men in general do not adjust their schedule in response to their wives' employment status.[29]

Besides doing more housework, mothers spend more time on average with their children than fathers do. Mothers spend an average of 3.2 hours per workday with their children, whereas fathers spend an average of 2.3 hours with their offspring. Seventy percent of parents feel that they do not have enough time to spend with their children. In fact, both parents have less time for themselves than they did 20 years ago; fathers have 1.2 hours per workday, whereas mothers have 0.9 hour.[13] Couples also have less time together. Nearly 46% of married women or women living with someone work different schedules than their partners do.[22]

As jobs become more demanding and less rewarding, employees often feel more stressed by the end of the workday and have less time and energy for their families.

Twenty-five percent of employees reported feeling stressed often or very often over the past 3 months, and 25% described feeling emotionally drained often or very often. More than one-fourth of employees are not in as good a mood as they would like for their families; 28% of people feel they have no energy for their families or other important people upon returning from work. This in turn creates a negative sense of well-being and results in negativity that affects a person's work performance.[21]

A person's work setting can create physical stress as well, because of noise, lack of privacy, poor lighting or ventilation, poor temperature control, or inadequate sanitary facilities. Physical stress on the body is a consequence of many different occupations. Jobs that require being on one's feet for long hours cause leg pain, swelling, and varicose veins; administrative and desk-based jobs may cause neck and back aches and eye strain; and repetitive motions can cause musculoskeletal injuries to women on production lines. These difficulties are not restricted to women, yet certain factors make women more susceptible to these types of injury. Equipment and workstations are often designed with men's larger body sizes in mind. Workstations and chairs that cannot be adjusted to the correct height for women promote poor posture; excessive reach; and strain on the neck, back, shoulders, and arms. Hand tools designed for larger hands may create unnecessary pain, stressed muscles, and calluses. Protective equipment and clothes that are too large are more likely to slip off, get caught in equipment, or create gaps for harmful chemicals to seep through.

Men are still more likely to be injured at work than women, in part because some jobs with high rates of

Long-term exposure to work-related stress can lead to higher levels of depression, anxiety, and other illnesses.
© Keith Brofsky/Photodisc/Getty Images

injury are still predominately held by men. Almost two-thirds of injured workers are men, even though they account for less than 60% of the total hours worked in the United States. However, in the fields of management, business, financial occupations, professional and related occupations, service occupations, and office and administrative support, women are more likely to be injured than men.[2]

Musculoskeletal injuries, also referred to as ergonomic injuries, disproportionately affect female workers. Although women account for only 33% of those injured at work in the United States, they constitute 64% of repetitive motion injuries, which include the following conditions:

- **Carpal tunnel syndrome**—a condition that occurs when tendons in the wrist become inflamed after being aggravated
- **Tendonitis**—inflammation caused by friction from overuse of tendons
- Muscle strains from overexertion

Repetitive motions can injure the nerves, often those in the neck and hands. **Self-Assessment 15.1** discusses some of the common symptoms that nerve injuries can cause. Repetitive motion injuries account for more than half of all work time lost due to injuries and illness among women.[22]

Many women in low-wage occupations, or in occupations such as nursing aides, cashiers, maids, nurses, and assemblers that employ large numbers of women, are at significant risk of musculoskeletal disorders. Many of these jobs employ a large number of minorities, such as women who are Black, Hispanic, or of Southeast Asian descent. Back injuries are common among employees who need to lift large items or people. Correct lifting technique and using trolleys or coworkers to help lift heavy objects greatly reduce the likelihood of injury.

It's Your Health

Tips for Lifting Loads Safely

- Test the weight of the load before lifting. If too heavy or awkward, enlist a coworker to help or use a cart or dolly.
- Figure out where you need to move the load and how you are going to get to your destination before you lift.
- Lift with your legs shoulder-width apart and bend at your knees and hips, not your waist.
- Lift with tightened stomach muscles and using your leg muscles to reduce strain on your back.
- Hold the load close to your body at waist height.
- Avoid twisting during the lift; pivot your body or move your feet if necessary.
- Stretch and strengthen your back and abdominal muscles with exercises if lifting is part of your daily occupation.

Self Assessment 15.1
Symptoms of Repetitive Strain Injuries

- Do you have numbness and/or tingling in your hand that often feels worse when you lift your hand over your head?
- Do you often experience wrist weakness?
- Do you have numbness or tingling in the inside of your arm or into your fingers?
- Do you often feel numbness or tingling in multiple fingers and does your hand often "fall asleep" at night? Do you frequently drop objects?
- Do you have achiness, stiffness, tightness, or a burning sensation in your fingers, forearm, elbow, or shoulder?
- Do you experience muscle tightness at the side of your neck?

If you are experiencing one or more of these symptoms, you may have an overuse injury. Women should speak to their healthcare provider about preventing, reducing, and/or treating these types of disorders.

Computer-related injuries have also become a significant concern in the workplace (**Self-Assessment 15.2**). Prolonged use of a keyboard or mouse, as well as sitting at a computer for long periods without stretching, can lead to muscle aches and nerve pain in the hands, arms,

It's Your Health

Tips for Preventing Injuries at Computer Workstations

- Alternate tasks throughout the day to reduce repetitive motions.
- Take frequent breaks, and stretch during the breaks if possible.
- Avoid bending or twisting your neck, or twisting your trunk.
- Keep shoulders relaxed and arms close by sides when working.
- Maintain good posture by keeping back and neck erect with shoulders relaxed.
- Keep your feet supported on the floor or on a footrest to reduce pressure on the lower back.
- Position your monitor so that it is centered directly in front of you and your neck is in a neutral or straight position when viewing it.
- Reduce glare on your screen by tilting the monitor, reducing overhead lights, and avoiding direct glare from windows.
- Every 30 minutes, look away from the screen and focus on something else.

Self Assessment 15.2
Computer Workstation Evaluation Checklist

Posture

- Are your hands, wrists, and forearms straight, in-line, and roughly parallel to the floor?
- Is your head level or bent slightly forward and balanced?
- Is your head in line with your torso?
- Are your elbows close to your body and bent at 90 to 120 degrees?
- Are your feet fully supported by the floor or a footrest?
- Is your back fully supported when sitting vertically or leaning back slightly?
- Are your shoulders relaxed?
- Are your thighs and hips supported by a well-padded chair?
- Are your knees at the same height as the hips with the feet slightly forward?

Keyboard and Mouse

- Is your keyboard directly in front of you at a distance that allows your elbows to stay close to your body with your forearms approximately parallel with the floor?
- If you have limited desk room, do you use a keyboard tray to ensure adequate positioning?
- Is your keyboard in a position that lets you avoid reaching with the arms, leaning forward with the torso, and using extreme elbow angles?
- Can you reduce awkward wrist angles by lowering or raising the keyboard or chair to achieve a neutral wrist posture?

Seating

- Does your backrest support your lower back (lumbar area)?

- Does your seat width and depth accommodate your body?
- Does the seat front not press against the back of your knees and lower legs?
- Is the seat cushioning rounded and devoid of sharp edges?
- Do armrests support both forearms while you complete computer tasks?

Lighting

- Does your office have well-distributed, diffuse lights that reduce glare on the computer screen?
- Does your office use light, matte colors and finishes on walls and ceilings to better reflect indirect lighting and reduce dark shadows and contrast?

Computer Screen

- Is your computer display screen at right angles to windows and light sources?
- Is the monitor clean and free of dust?
- Is the top of the screen at or below eye level?

Work Techniques

- Can you vary your computer tasks with other work activities or take short breaks and recovery pauses?

If you answered "No" to one or more of these questions, you are putting yourself at risk of injury. Use the checklist guidelines to improve your workplace health and avoid injuries.

Source: Adapted from the U.S. Department of Labor, Office of Safety and Health Administration. *Computer workstations etool: Checklists: Evaluation.* Available at: http://www.osha.gov/SLTC/etools/computerworkstations /checklist_evaluation.html

---

shoulders, neck, and back. Another common complaint of computer workers is visual discomfort, which is accompanied by eyestrain and headaches. Being aware of these risks and correcting improper posture and techniques can help prevent discomfort and injury.

Exposure to suspected carcinogens, allergens, or agents that cause respiratory illness are also serious concerns for many working women. Occupational exposures occur in many industries that employ large numbers of women and minorities:[23]

- Meat industry: exposure to suspected carcinogenic fumes
- Laundry/dry-cleaning industry: exposure to solvents that increase risk of kidney, cervical, bladder, skin, and liver cancer
- Textile industry: exposure to dust that causes a variety of lung diseases

- Metal-working industry: exposure to various chemicals that increase the risk of lung cancer
- Agriculture: exposure to pesticides and herbicides that may increase risk of non-Hodgkin's lymphoma and lung cancer
- Service industry: exposure to excessive cigarette smoke in bars or restaurants

Healthcare workers face additional hazards, including needlestick injuries, radiation exposure, infectious diseases, and latex allergies. Approximately 600,000 to 800,000 needlestick injuries occur annually in healthcare settings, mostly involving nurses (more than 90% of whom are women). Needlestick injuries can cause serious infections from bloodborne pathogens, such as hepatitis C and HIV, creating both physical and emotional threats to workers.

In addition, 8 to 12% of healthcare workers who have frequent latex exposure develop sensitivity to this material. Symptoms can be as mild as contact dermatitis or as severe as **anaphylactic shock**, a severe and possibly fatal allergic response to a foreign substance, characterized by difficulty breathing and low blood pressure. The hazard from latex use is recognized in many different industries, including people in the latex-manufacturing industry, police, food handlers, and sanitation engineers. Pregnant women also appear to have a higher sensitivity to latex than the general population.[24]

The causes of most reproductive health problems are still unknown, but certain harmful substances can affect the health of pregnant women. Approximately 75% of all women of reproductive age are in the workforce, and more than half of all children born in the United States are born to working mothers. Women can be exposed to many different types of health hazards at work during pregnancy. Hazards from environmental pollutants in the workplace can cause multiple effects, depending on when the woman is exposed. Substances may cause fetal damage, such as birth defects, low birth weight, developmental disorders, miscarriages, or stillbirths; infertility;

menstrual cycle effects; and even childhood cancer. Other possible hazards to pregnant women include prolonged standing, lifting, and long work hours.

OTHER HEALTH CONCERNS

Many women work in the informal work sector, employed in seasonal or domestic jobs that are not officially reported or recognized. Because these jobs often employ women who may not have official work permits or are paid "under the table" (meaning that the women do not receive benefits or declare taxes), women may face additional risks and insecurities. Injuries that occur during migrant crop picking, for example, often go untreated because the workers have few resources and are afraid of drawing the attention of authorities. Additionally, women who do odd jobs around the home, such as cleaning houses or painting, often do not have health or disability insurance coverage should an injury occur.

Hazardous work environments put many youths at risk of serious injuries. Young workers have been killed on construction sites, during robberies while tending retail establishments, and while working on farms.

Common nonfatal injuries incurred by young workers include sprains and strains, burns, cuts, and bruises. Homicide is the leading cause of death among youths in retail trade, accounting for nearly two-thirds of the youth fatalities in the industry. Most of these homicides are the result of robberies.[25]

Pregnant and lactating women may face additional stresses as they cope with sickness caused during pregnancy, coworkers' responses to pregnancy, and the time and privacy needs of nursing or pumping breast milk. Sexual harassment in the workplace is also a major form of stress.

> *I'm trying to get a permanent position in the United States as a research scientist so I don't have to go back to Russia. My boss makes me work long hours and always yells at me if I make a mistake. I was pregnant last year, and he still made me work with radiation in the lab. I was scared to complain for fear of losing my job. I didn't lose my job, but I ended up losing my baby.*
>
> **—32-year-old Russian scientist**

Women contribute to local, national, and global economies through the informal sector. Informal work includes any position that is unrecognized or uncounted by government or other authorities; workers may grow food or make goods at home and sell them at an open market, or offer services such as manual labor, cleaning, or childcare. Women make up the backbone of this growing movement. In some sub-Saharan African or Southeastern Asian countries, for example, nearly 90% of the

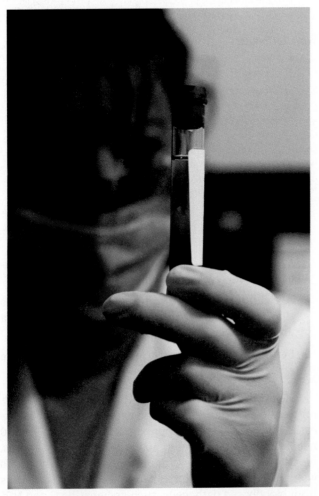

Needlestick injuries and latex allergies are two hazards faced by women working in health care.
© Photodisc

GLOBAL DIMENSIONS

Around the world, working women face many of the same challenges and opportunities that they do in the United States. Gender gaps in employment and pay persist but have decreased in Europe and much of the developing world.[26] From 1990 to 2015, women's participation in the global labor market increased compared to that of men. The past generation has also seen progress in education. In the European Union, female students outnumber male students in most universities. Progress has been more uneven and slow in much of Asia, Latin America, and Africa, with large gender gaps in adult literacy and enrollment in primary schools, secondary schools, and universities.[26]

In spite of this progress, however, women continue to face discrimination, reduced pay, and fewer opportunities than men. These problems are strongest in the developing world. Women are less likely than men to be employed as politicians, managers, senior officials, and in other powerful positions, and are more likely to work as clerks, sales workers, and other lower-status, low-paying positions.[26] Although women are working in greater numbers around the world, they still almost always have primary responsibilities for household chores, cooking, caregiving, and other housework. In all major areas of the world, women spend at least twice as much time as men doing unpaid household work.[26]

money they make in their local economies and use it to improve the health of their families.

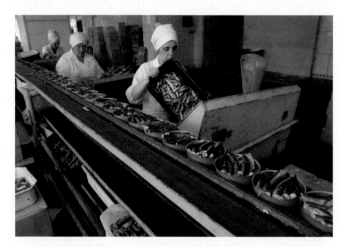

Women are becoming increasingly active in workplaces around the globe.
© Semen Lixodeev/Shutterstock

female labor force is in the informal economy. Many economic experts believe that stimulating this informal sector may be an important way to promote long-term, healthy economic growth throughout the developing world. Examples of such efforts include microlending programs, where women receive small loans with reasonable interest rates to further their businesses without the need for collateral.

The rate of payback from these women-focused microlending programs has been higher than that observed with most other credit programs. Once women gain access to these loans, they can create sustainable and profitable business opportunities for themselves and their families and protect themselves from the workplace health hazards that present themselves in many work environments. In addition, women typically reinvest the

The United States, one of the richest countries in the world, is one of only three countries (the other two are Swaziland and Papua New Guinea, two developing countries with low incomes and poor infrastructure) that does not guarantee women any paid family leave.[27] Worldwide, 128 countries mandate some sort of paid family leave. For example:

- Germany: new mothers receive 14 weeks of leave at 100% pay.
- Canada: new mothers can take up to one full year off from work at 60% pay.
- Norway: new mothers can take 1 year off from work at 100% pay.
- Japan: new mothers can take up to 14 weeks of leave at 60% pay.
- South Africa: new mothers can take 4 months of leave at up to 60% pay.
- Mexico: new mothers can take 12 weeks off from work at 75% pay.

GLOBAL DIMENSIONS: Microfinancing and Women's Entrepreneurship in Developing Countries

In many parts of the world, women lack access to resources both to support their families and to get ahead. It often takes money to make money, but without access to lending outlets many women remain stuck in poverty. Many organizations around the world are working to change this with microlending mechanisms. One example is Women's Microfinance Initiative whose mission is to establish village-level loan hubs, administered by local women, to provide capital, training, and support services to rural women in the lowest income brackets

in East Africa, so that they can engage in income-producing activities. Other examples include organizations like Kiva, which partners individuals in need with either individuals or organizations that are looking to lend or donate. By leveraging the resources of the Internet and a worldwide network of microfinance institutions, Kiva allows individuals to lend as little as $25 to help individuals globally.

INFORMED DECISION MAKING

Sources of stress for women in the workplace may vary, depending on their profession; their personality type; their age, race, or ethnicity; whether or not they have children; and other factors. All jobs, however, are likely to have some stress (being a homemaker has its own sources of stress, and for women looking for work, the search for a job can be a major source of stress). The key to improving one's mental health (and toward creating a more productive workplace) is to avoid stress when possible and to deal with unavoidable stress in healthful ways. Supportive companies produce workers who are less stressed, feel more successful in the balancing of work and family, are more satisfied with both their work and home lives, and are more loyal and committed to their employers.[11]

> *I just had my second child, and I have 6 months off to care for him. My 2-year-old goes to day care at my firm's on-site childcare center. When I return to work, I'll work part time so I get to spend time with my children. The women of my firm have said that there's no problem with taking advantage of flex-time and taking off 6 months to care for my newborn. I hope they're right! I feel very fortunate to be part of a firm that takes such good care of its employees.*
>
> **—30-year-old lawyer**

Employers can help employees to better balance parenthood and work life by offering services related to family planning, preconception health care and counseling, and parenting classes. The Family and Medical Leave Act (FMLA) has been a valuable tool for many women. The FMLA provides 12 weeks of unpaid, job-guaranteed leave for employees who need to care for newborns or a seriously ill relative or to recover from a serious illness of their own. This benefit is available to employees who have worked at least 1250 hours over the past year for employers with 50 or more employees. Currently, the act covers just over half of the country's private workforce. Workers in entry-level, low-paying jobs are less likely to be offered paid maternity leave than are managers and are less likely to get the time off after having a baby. More than half of the women who are covered by the FMLA do not know it. Although the FMLA was originally envisioned as dealing with a women's issue, almost half of those who have requested family and medical leave since its passage are men.

Employers can also ease the return of new mothers to the workplace by providing breastfeeding support through lactation assistance programs and private breastfeeding rooms. Only 10% of working mothers continue nursing for 6 months following birth compared with 24% of at-home mothers. Thirty-seven percent of employers currently provide opportunities for women who are nursing to continue to do so; this provision cuts down on absenteeism and healthcare costs for both mothers and infants.[5]

In addition, employers need to help employees find affordable, quality childcare and elder care; develop childcare programs; or offer employee assistance for childcare facilities. Childcare assistance programs need to include more flexibility, by allowing for the needs of employees who work night and weekend shifts (**Figure 15.6**). Flexible work schedules, job-sharing programs, and prorated

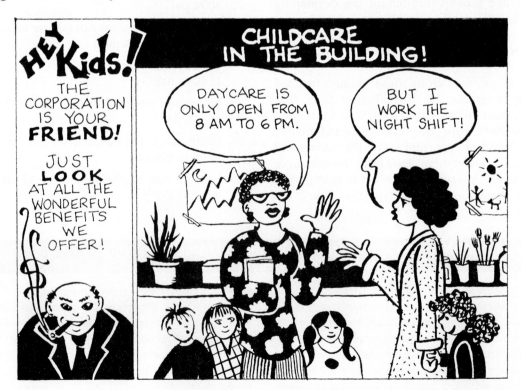

Figure 15.6 Childcare programs need to be developed with more flexibility to allow for night and weekend shifts.
© Jennifer Camper

Profiles of Remarkable Women

Patricia Ireland (1945–)

Patricia Ireland began her career by working as a flight attendant for Pan American World Airlines from 1967 to 1975. Upon being told that her medical benefits did not apply to her husband even though wives of male employees were covered, Ireland sued her employer and won—a victory that marked the beginning of her activism. Ireland received her law degree from the University of Miami Law School in 1975, and then worked as a partner in a major Miami law firm. She served as legal counsel to Dade County and Florida National Organization for Women (NOW) for 7 years. From 1987 to 1991, Ireland served as executive vice president and treasurer of the national NOW organization.

In 1991, Ireland became president of NOW, the largest, most visible, and most successful feminist organization in the United States. Her major contributions included organizing NOW activists to defend women's access to abortion, elect a record number of women to political office, work more closely in coalitions with other social justice and civil rights groups, and champion international feminist issues.

Ireland developed NOW's Project Stand Up for Women; in 1992, she led NOW in organizing a crowd of 750,000 for the organization's March for Women's Lives. In the same year, she initiated the Elect Women for a Change campaign. This campaign provided feminist candidates with experienced organizers who trained and deployed volunteers to staff phone banks, distribute leaflets and posters, organize fundraisers, and get people to the polls.

As part of NOW's work with the Up and Out of Poverty Now! coalition, Ireland delivered testimony and organized lobby days, news briefings, and protests on behalf of poor women. She served on the board of the Rainbow/PUSH Coalition and, in 1993, was a co-convener and keynote speaker for the 30th anniversary march on Washington commemorating the legacy of Dr. Martin Luther King, Jr. She has put forth significant efforts on behalf of lesbian and gay rights, including serving as a speaker and major organizer for the 1993 March on Washington for Gay, Lesbian, and Bi Civil Rights.

Ireland was the prime architect of NOW's Global Feminist Program. In 1992, she brought together women from more than 45 countries to participate in the Global Feminist Conference. Although no longer president of NOW, Ireland continues to champion many international feminist issues.

benefits for part-time and temporary employees also need to be enforced—two-thirds of part-time workers and three-fifths of temporary workers are women.[2] Some employers have established flexible work policies and promote the idea of a family-friendly workplace. Unfortunately, the people who need the extra support are the people who are often the least likely to receive it.

Women also need to be aware of their rights in the workplace. Women should not tolerate discrimination based on gender, race, religion, sexual orientation, disabilities, pregnancy, or other characteristics. Women who experience any of these forms of discrimination should promptly write down the details of the incident, and then report it to their supervisor or the company's human resources division. Women may also report a discrimination complaint with the Equal Employment Opportunity Commission (EEOC) or their state's fair employment agency.

Profiles of Remarkable Women

Tina Fey (1970–)

Tina Fey is an actress, writer, producer, and comedian. For more than 15 years, she has worked and excelled in the field of comedy, a field traditionally and still largely dominated by men. Born and raised in Pennsylvania, Fey's interest in comedy began in the eighth grade, when she wrote an independent study project on the subject; during high school she joined the drama club and wrote comedy pieces for her school newspaper.[28] Fey studied drama and theater at the University of Virginia, where she was a self-described quiet, shy, and socially awkward student. After Fey graduated in 1992, she joined The Second City, an improv comedy group in Chicago that helped launch the careers of Dan Aykroyd, Gilda Radner, Steve Carell, and many other famous comedians.

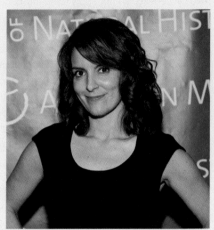

© lev radin/Shutterstock

In 1997, Fey accepted a writing position at *Saturday Night Live*. She wrote and performed on *Saturday Night Live* for 9 years, becoming the show's first female head writer in 1999, and becoming a recurring anchor on the show's Weekend Update sketches. Fey wrote about her experiences in the "boys' club" of the *Saturday Night Live* writing staff in her comedic memoir *Bossypants*. Fey enjoyed her work and appreciated the sense of humor of her male colleagues, even as she dealt with the challenge of writing and promoting sketches that did not come from an obviously male perspective. Fey wrote a sketch parodying feminine sanitary pads, but struggled for months to get the approval of her male cowriters, who were not familiar with the subject; when it aired, the sketch became one of the show's classic commercial parodies. As a performer, Fey also had to deal with the surface-obsessed entertainment industry in ways that her male colleagues did not: Fey appeared in sketches only after she lost a substantial amount of weight. While writing for *Saturday Night Live*, Fey wrote, produced, and co-starred in *Mean Girls*, a teen comedy that explores high-school cliques.

Fey left *Saturday Night Live* to produce and star in *30 Rock*, a high-energy comedy series loosely based on her experiences on the show. As the show's protagonist Liz Lemon, Fey is both a role model and a comic figure: a capable and dedicated writer who regularly makes a mess out of her personal life; off the air, Fey married one of the show's composers, and gave birth to and raised two daughters while co-running the show. She also reappeared on *Saturday Night Live* to do a comedic take on vice-presidential candidate Sarah Palin during the 2008 election.

Fey has won seven Emmy Awards, two Golden Globes, and was the youngest winner of the Mark Twain Prize for American humor. Fey has dismissed male comedians who believe that women are not funny or are less funny than men. In *Bossypants*, she wrote, "It is an impressively arrogant move to conclude that just because you don't like something, it is empirically not good. I don't like Chinese food, but I don't write articles trying to prove it doesn't exist."

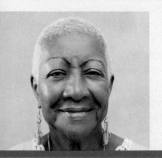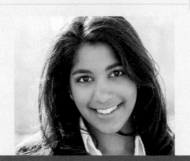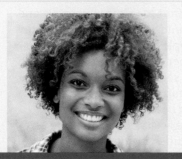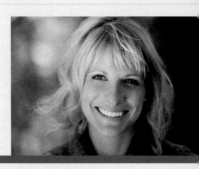

CASE STUDY

Angela had worked hard her whole life. During high school she was a waitress on Tuesday, Wednesday, and Friday nights. During the weekends she worked at her parents' dry cleaning business. She fit in friends, school, and sports around the edges as she saved money to help pay for college. She went to her local state school, taking advantage of the in-state tuition and strong work-study programs. By the time she graduated she had only $15,000 in debt from school and began her career in accounting. Over the next 10 years she held various jobs in the accounting field, working her way up the ladder and gaining more expertise and seniority. She paid off her loans and felt well on the way to a successful career.

During that time, she met her future husband Jimmy. He was painter and starting his own house painting business. During the spring and summer months he worked very hard and made a lot of money, but winter was slow and he eventually took up part-time work at Home Depot to help make ends meet during that time. They got health benefits from her job and largely considered her the "anchor" of their financial well-being.

When Angela was 29, she and Jimmy had twin baby girls named Daisy and Rose. The girls were adorable and kept both of them very busy. However, Angela got only 6 weeks of paid time off from work and she and Jimmy were struggling with what to do with the babies when Angela went back to work. Making it more difficult was the fact that Angela wanted to breastfeed her babies, and she worked close to 45 minutes away from their house. She felt massively divided between the demands of her family and new children, and the financial reality that they needed her income and benefits to survive. She was stressed all the time because she was not around her children as much as she wanted, and she was so tired at work that she was not performing at the high level she was used to. She felt like she could not win.

Toward the end of maternity leave, they decided to have Jimmy watch the babies, and during the first couple of months back at work he drove them to her office once a day to visit mom and get fed. With Jimmy trying to take care of the babies on his own, things started to break down. Unfortunately, Jimmy was having a very difficult time and did not know if he could continue for much longer. He had very little experience taking care of children and moreover did not find it fulfilling to be the primary caregiver for the babies. Although he loved them very much, he yearned to get back to work he enjoyed, painting houses or doing other handiwork.

Questions

1. What should Angela and Jimmy do about taking care of Daisy and Rose?

2. What could Angela's employer do to make the transition back to work easier for Angela?

3. What do you think the impact of this stress will be to Angela's job performance? What resources are available to help her?

4. What could Angela and Jimmy have done prior to the birth of the twins to address the challenge of work/life/parenting balance?

■ Summary

Women have become an integral part of the American workplace. The workplace can provide a social life, a support system, and opportunities for volunteering, and it affects people's moods and their values.

- Women are important parts of nearly every field and position, but inequities in pay and advancement persist.

- Women still shoulder the majority of the burden of children and home life, even when working.

- Millions of women have lost their jobs, received pay cuts, or been unable to find work as a result of the economic recession of 2008–2009.

- Women benefit greatly from quality, affordable, and accessible childcare, enabling them to have choices about labor force participation.

- The stress of work and family, and the attempt to "do it all," creates stress and unhappiness for many women.

Employers must make an effort to create supportive and rewarding work environments. By promoting a healthy work–life balance, both employers and employees benefit. At the same time, women should strive to find such a balance in their lives, by setting priorities, discussing options with their employers and partners, and advocating for fairness and support in the workplace.

As both genders become accustomed to a more equitable sharing of responsibilities inside and outside the home, women will be afforded a more balanced existence between work and family. As Arlie Hochschild aptly states, "Up until now, the woman married to the 'new man' has been one of the lucky few. But as the government and society shape a new gender strategy, as the young learn from example, many more women and men will be able to enjoy the leisurely bodily rhythms and freer laughter that arise when family life is family life and not a second shift."[29]

■ Topics for Discussion

1. What questions should a woman ask before taking a job to ensure that she will receive all of the benefits that she may need?

2. Discuss how poverty creates additional barriers to employment opportunities for women.

3. What strategies could women use in the workplace to determine whether chemical, biological, or physical hazards are present?

4. How can women find balance in their professional, educational, and personal lives?

5. What are some strategies women can use when seeking greater equity opportunities in specific workplaces?

■ Key Terms

Anaphylactic shock
Carpal tunnel syndrome
Tendonitis

■ References

1. U.S. Department of Labor, Bureau of Labor Statistics. (2014). *Women in the labor force: A databook.* Available at: http://www.bls.gov/cps/wlf-databook-2013.pdf

2. U.S. Department of Labor, Bureau of Labor Statistics. (2014). *Women in the labor force: A databook.* Washington, DC: Bureau of Labor Statistics.

3. Bird, C. E., & Lang, M. E. (2014). Gender, health, and constrained choice. *The Wiley Blackwell Encyclopedia of Health, Illness, Behavior, and Society.*

3a. Womanable.com. (2014). *The state of women-owned business 2014.* Available at: http://www.womenable.com/59/the-state-of-women-owned-businesses-in-the-us:-2014

4. Welter, F., Brush, C., & De Bruin, A. (2014). *The gendering of entrepreneurship context.* No. 01/14. [Working paper]. Bonn: Institut für Mittelstandsforschung (IfM).

5. Gainsay, E., Bond, J., & Sakai, K. (2008). *2008 National Study of Employers.* New York: Families and Work Institute.

5a. Centers for Disease Control and Prevention (CDC). (2014). *Disability and health: Women with disabilities.* Available at: http://www.cdc.gov/ncbddd/disabilityandhealth/women.html. Accessed January 2015.

6. Lewis, A. N., Hurley, J., Lewis P., et al. (2014). Gender, disability, and ADA Title I employment discrimination: A comparison of male and female charging party characteristics: The National EEOC ADA Research Project. *The Review of Disability Studies: An International Journal* 7(1).

7. National Partnership for Women and Families. (2007). *Where families matter: State progress toward valuing America's families.* Washington, DC: National Partnership for Women and Families.

8. Weichselbaumer, D., & Winter-Ebmer, R. (2005). A meta analysis of the international gender wage gap. *Journal of Economic Surveys* 19(3): 479–511.

9. AFL-CIO. (2006). Ask a Working Woman Survey. AFL-CIO Working Women's Department. Washington, DC: AFL-CIO.

10. DeNavas-Walt, C., Proctor, B. D., & Smith, J. C. (2008). *Income, poverty, and health insurance coverage in the United States: 2007.* U.S. Census Bureau, Current Population Reports, P60-235. Washington, DC: U.S. Government Printing Office.

11. Hartmann, H., Hayes, J., & Clark, J. (2014). *How equal pay for working women would reduce poverty and grow the American economy.* Institute for Women's Policy Research. Available at: http://www.iwpr.org/publications/pubs/how-equal-pay-for-working-women-wouldreduce-poverty-and-grow-the-american-economy

12. Lee, M., & Mather, M. (June 2008). *U.S. labor force trends.* Washington, DC: Population Reference Bureau.

13. Goodwin, J. (2011). Multitasking stresses out working moms more than dads. *USA Today.* Available at: www.usatoday.com/news/health/wellness/story/2011-12-01/Multitasking-stresses-out-working-moms-more-than-dads/51545428/1

14. Aizer, A., & Doyle, J. J., Jr. (2014). Economics of child well-being: Measuring effects of child welfare interventions. In A. Ben-Arieh, F. Casas, I. Frønes, & J. E. Korbin (Eds.), *Handbook of Child Well-Being* (pp. 1563–1602). Dordrecht, Netherlands: Springer Netherlands.

15. Crouter, A. C., & Booth, A. (Eds.) (2014). *Work-family challenges for low-income parents and their children.* London: Routledge.

16. Hochschild, A., & Machung, A. (2012). *The second shift: Working families and the revolution at home.* London: Penguin.

17. Davidson, M. R., London, M. L., & Ladewig, P. W. (2012). *Olds' maternal-newborn nursing & women's health across the lifespan.* Upper Saddle River, NJ: Pearson.

18. U.S. Department of Labor. (2011). *Nonfatal occupational injuries and illnesses requiring days away from work, 2010.* Available at: http://www.bls.gov/news.release/osh2.nr0.htm

19. CDC. (2015). *Women's safety and health issues at work.* Available at: http://www.cdc.gov/niosh/topics/women/

20. U.S. Department of Labor, Bureau of Labor Statistics. (2012). *Census of fatal occupational injuries, 2010.* Available at: http://www.bls.gov/iif/oshcfoi1.htm

21. de Jong, N. W., Patiwael J., de Groot H., et al. (2011). Natural rubber latex allergy among health care workers: Significant reduction of sensitization and clinical relevant latex allergy after

introduction of powder-free latex gloves. *Journal of Allergy and Clinical Immunology* 127(2): AB70.

22. World Health Organization (WHO). (2010). *The world's women, 2010.* Available at: http://unstats.un.org/unsd/demographic /products/Worldswomen/WW2010pub.htm

23. Lips, H. M. (2013). The gender pay gap: Challenging the rationalizations. Perceived equity, discrimination, and the limits of human capital models. *Sex Roles* 68(3–4): 169–185.

24. Yost, C. W. (2012). Three reasons why card-carrying capitalists should support paid family leave. *Forbes.* Available at: http://www.forbes.com/sites/work-in-progress/2012/05/23/3-reasons-why-card-carrying-capitalists-should-support-paid-family-leave/3/

25. U.S. Department of Labor, Bureau of Labor Statistics. (2012). *Census of fatal occupational injuries, 2010.* Available at: http://www.bls.gov/iif/oshcfoi1.htm

26. Coley, R. L., & McPherran Lombardi, C. (2014). Low-income women's employment experiences and their financial, personal, and family well-being. *Journal of Family Psychology* 28(1): 88.

27. European Union. (2009). *The EU and gender equality: Advancing women's full potential.* Available at: http://www.eurunion.org /News/eunewsletters/EUIn-sight/2009/EUInsight-GenderEqual -Apr-09.pdf

28. Murray, N. (2006). *Interview with Tina Fey.* The A3 Club. Available at: http://www.avclub.com/articles/tina-fey,14025/

GLOSSARY

Abortion The spontaneous or induced expulsion of an embryo or fetus before it is viable or can survive on its own.

Abruptio placentae A complication of pregnancy in which the placenta separates prematurely from the wall of the uterus.

Abstinence In terms of sex, the practice of refraining from sexual activity.

Acute disease A disease that begins and ends quickly. Examples include pneumonia and localized infection.

Adenocarcinoma A cancer that originates from cells of the endocrine glands.

Adjuvant therapies Methods such as chemotherapy and radiation therapy that enhance the effectiveness of surgery in cancer treatment.

Afterbirth The placenta and amniotic sac that are expelled from the womb after the baby is delivered.

AIDS (acquired immune deficiency syndrome) A progressive disease caused by HIV, which gradually destroys an infected person's immune system. AIDS is the final stage of HIV infection. Although there is no way for an infected person to get rid of HIV, modern medications can often slow the progress of the disease or prevent AIDS from developing entirely.

Alcohol A colorless liquid obtained by fermentation of a sugar-containing liquid. Ethyl alcohol (ethanol) is the type of alcohol found in alcoholic beverages.

Alcoholism A condition in which a person's alcohol consumption has progressed to interfering with his or her ability to lead a functional life. It has since been redefined as a primary, chronic disease with behavioral, genetic, psychological, and environmental factors influencing its development and manifestations.

Allopathic school A school that teaches a system of medical practice making use of all measures proved of value in treatment of disease (i.e., conventional medicine exclusive of homeopathic practices).

Alzheimer's disease An irreversible, progressive brain disorder that occurs gradually and results in memory loss, behavior and personality changes, and a decline in cognitive abilities.

Amenorrhea Absence of the menstrual period in a woman by age 16 (primary amenorrhea) or absence of the menstrual period for 3 to 6 consecutive months in a woman who has had regular periods since the onset of menstruation (secondary amenorrhea). It often is caused by stress, acute weight loss, or excessive strenuous exercise.

Amniocentesis A procedure between the 16th and 20th weeks of pregnancy intended to detect fetal defects. The amniotic sac is punctured with a needle and syringe, and amniotic fluid is obtained for analysis.

Amnion The innermost membrane of the amniotic sac, which contains the amniotic fluid.

Amniotic fluid Watery fluid that surrounds a developing embryo and fetus in the uterus.

Amphetamines Synthetic stimulants that increase energy and alertness, produce euphoria, and suppress appetite. Excessive use can cause headaches, irritability, dizziness, insomnia, panic, confusion, and delirium.

Anabolic steroid A synthetic derivative of the male hormone testosterone, usually taken to increase muscle mass. Use often results in serious physiological and psychological side effects.

Anaphylactic shock A severe and sometimes fatal allergic reaction to a foreign substance that causes symptoms such as weakness, shortness of breath, and falling blood pressure.

Androgyny A blending of typical male and female qualities in an individual.

Aneurysm A type of weakened blood vessel that can cause a stroke. This ballooning of a weakened region of a blood vessel may result from several factors, including a congenital defect, chronic blood pressure, or an injury to the brain. If left untreated, it continues to weaken until it ruptures and bleeds in the brain.

Angina pectoris Chest pain resulting from insufficient supply of blood (oxygen) to the heart muscle.

Antioxidant A substance that prevents molecules called "free radicals" from harming the body's tissues. They are present in many fruits and vegetables and work to neutralize free radicals and protect genes from damage, possibly decreasing the risk of cancer and heart disease and delaying the effects of aging.

Anxiety disorder A disorder that is part of a group of conditions that share extreme or pathological anxiety as the principal disturbance of mood. This group includes panic disorder, agoraphobia, generalized anxiety disorder, specific phobia, social phobia, obsessive-compulsive disorder, acute stress disorder, and posttraumatic stress disorder. This is the most common mental disorder in the United States and affects a significant number of people worldwide.

Aorta The great artery arising from the left ventricle of the heart; the largest artery.

Aortic valve A valve located between the left ventricle and the aorta.

Arrhythmia Erratic heartbeat.

Arteriole A small artery.

Arteriosclerosis Any arterial disease that leads to the thickening and hardening of the arterial walls, slowing the flow of blood.

Artery A vessel in the body that supplies oxygenated blood to the tissues.

Arthritis Inflammation of the joints. Arthritis encompasses more than 100 diseases and conditions that affect joints, the surrounding tissues, and other connective tissues.

Artificial insemination Introduction of semen into the uterus or oviduct by unnatural means close to the time of ovulation. It is most often used when the infertility problem is male related.

Assisted reproductive technologies (ART) Any treatment or procedure that involves the handling of human eggs and sperm with the purpose of helping a woman become pregnant.

Asymptomatic viral shedding Most often associated with herpes simplex virus infections. It occurs when active herpes virus, present in the nerve cells of an infected person, moves along the nerves to the surface of the skin. It often occurs without any symptoms (asymptomatic), but the person may still be infectious, meaning that it can be passed on to others.

Atherosclerosis A type of arteriosclerosis characterized by deposits of fatty substances or plaques on inner walls of arteries that narrow blood vessels.

Atrial fibrillation A disorder in which the heart's two small upper chambers (the atria) quiver instead of beating effectively. Because blood is not pumped completely out of them, it may pool and clot. If a piece of a blood clot in the atria leaves the heart and becomes lodged in an artery in the brain, a stroke results.

Autoimmune disease A disease caused by autoantibodies or lymphocytes that attack normal components of the body—molecules, cells, or tissues—by the organism producing them. It is more common among women than men.

Bacteria Single-celled organisms that multiply and cause disease by forcing the body to release poisons and germ-fighting antibodies. Unlike viral infections, bacterial infections usually can be treated by antibiotics.

Bacterial vaginosis (BV) Inflammation of the vagina, caused by an overgrowth of the normal bacteria found in the vagina and resulting in an imbalance. The most common cause of vaginitis, this infection is sometimes, but not always, sexually transmitted.

Balloon angioplasty A procedure used to open narrowed or blocked coronary arteries. A surgeon inserts a small, hollow tube called a catheter into an artery and guides it to the blockage. The surgeon then inflates a balloon near the end of the catheter, widening the vessel and allowing blood to flow. A wire mesh stent is usually placed at the site of the narrowing to keep the artery open.

Barbiturates A class of sedatives that have a depressant effect on the central nervous system.

Bariatric surgery Gastrointestinal surgery for obesity that alters the digestive process. The operation promotes weight loss by closing off parts of the stomach to make it smaller.

Bartholin's glands Two small glands located just inside the vaginal opening that help lubricate the vagina.

Basal metabolic rate (BMR) The amount of energy needed to maintain essential body functions under resting conditions, usually expressed in terms of calories per hour per kilogram of body weight.

Battering Repeatedly subjecting a person to forceful and coercive physical, social, and/or psychological behavior.

Beneficiary In terms of insurance, an individual who is eligible to receive benefits under an insurance policy.

Benign tumor A noncancerous growth that does not spread to other parts of the body.

Bicuspid valve A valve that separates the left atrium and the left ventricle of the heart; also known as the mitral valve.

Bilateral salpingo-oophorectomy Surgical excision of the fallopian tubes and the ovaries.

Binge eating disorder (BED) An eating disorder characterized by a lack of control in overeating and overeating in secret. Victims do not force themselves to vomit, however, as with bulimia nervosa.

Bingeing The consumption of large amounts of food that is characteristic of bulimia nervosa.

Biomedical research Studies relating to the activities and applications of science to clinical medicine.

Biopsy The removal and microscopic examination of a tissue sample to determine whether cancer cells are present.

Bipolar disorder (manic-depressive disorder) A mental disorder that is characterized by wide mood swings that can occur within hours or days and that features abnormally euphoric or irritable moods.

Birth control An umbrella term that refers to procedures that prevent the birth of a baby, including all contraceptive measures, sterilization, and abortion procedures.

Bisexual A person having a sexual orientation to persons of both sexes.

Blastocyst A mass of embryonic cells that results from repeated divisions of the zygote.

Blood Liquid medium of the circulatory system composed of plasma (fluid), erythrocytes (red blood cells), leukocytes (white blood cells), and platelets.

Blood alcohol concentration (BAC) A physiological indicator used by clinicians and law enforcement officials to determine whether a person is legally "drunk." It is expressed in terms of the percentage of alcohol in blood.

Body composition Proportions of fat, muscle, and bone making up the body. Body composition is usually expressed as percentage of body fat and percentage of lean muscle mass.

Body mass index (BMI) Weight (in kilograms) divided by height squared (in meters). A value or 25 or greater indicates obesity-related health risks.

Bone remodeling The process that removes older bone (resorption) and replaces it with new bone (formation) so as to maintain a healthy skeleton.

Braxton–Hicks contractions The contraction of the uterus at irregular intervals throughout pregnancy. These contractions are not like "real" labor contractions in that they do not gradually increase in frequency, intensity, or duration.

Breast self-examination The systematic palpation of the breast tissue of each breast while lying on one's back.

Breech Birth presentation in which the feet, knees, or buttocks of the fetus present before the head.

C-reactive protein A protein produced by the liver during periods of inflammation that is detectable in blood in various disease conditions. The C-reactive protein blood test is used as an indicator of acute inflammation.

Calcium A mineral found mainly in the bones and the teeth. It is important for bone health throughout life. Sources include dairy products, canned fish, seeds and nuts, some green vegetables such as broccoli and kale, and calcium-fortified foods.

Cancer A general term for more than 100 diseases that are characterized by uncontrolled, abnormal growth of cells. Cells can spread through the bloodstream and lymphatic system to other parts of the body.

Capillary A minute, hair-like vessel connecting arterioles and venules.

Carbohydrate An organic compound such as starch, sugar, or glycogen, composed of carbon, hydrogen, and oxygen. They are a source of bodily energy.

Carcinogenesis The overall staging process by which normal cells become malignant. Chemical, physical, or viral agents may induce carcinogenesis.

Carcinogenic The ability to cause cancer.

Carcinogens Substances or agents that are known to cause cancer. Examples include nicotine, asbestos, and ultraviolet radiation.

Carcinoma A cancer that is the most common of all tumors, accounting for approximately 85% of all cancers. This term generally refers to cancer that begins in tissues that line or cover an organ.

Carcinoma-in-situ Cancer that involves only the top layer of the organ without invading deeper tissues.

Cardiovascular disease A group of diseases that includes two major categories.

Cardiovascular endurance The ability of the body to perform aerobic activities for extended periods of time.

Cardiovascular system The network of structures that pump and carry blood through the body, including the heart, arteries, veins, and capillaries.

Carpal tunnel syndrome A common, painful problem in the wrist and hand that occurs in the tendon and the carpal tunnel (a channel in the wrist for the nerve that serves the palm and thumb side of the hand). It is caused by pressure on the nerve that causes weakness; pain when the thumb is bent toward the palm; and burning, tingling, or aching that may spread to the forearm and shoulder.

Cephalopelvic disproportion A complication of pregnancy in which the size of the baby's head is deemed too large or the mother's birth canal is too small to accommodate vaginal delivery. This condition is an indication for cesarean delivery.

Cerebrovascular accident (stroke) A condition in which blood vessel damage occurs in the brain.

Cervical cap A contraceptive device made of latex and individually customized to fit snugly over the cervix.

Cervical dysplasia Abnormal changes in the cells of the cervix. This benign condition is considered precancerous but can develop into cancer if left untreated.

Cervicitis An inflammation of the cervix.

Cervix The small end of the uterus extending into the vagina.

Cesarean delivery The surgical procedure in which an infant is delivered through an incision made in the abdominal wall and uterus.

Chemotherapy The treatment of disease with anticancer drugs or chemicals.

Child abuse and neglect Physical or mental injury, sexual abuse or exploitation, negligent treatment, or maltreatment of a child by a person who is responsible for the child's welfare under circumstances that indicate that the child's health or welfare is harmed or threatened.

Chlamydia A sexually transmitted infection that is caused by the bacterium *Chlamydia trachomatis*. Most people are asymptomatic and, therefore, are not aware of their infection. If left untreated, it can cause serious damage to a woman's reproductive system. It is the most frequently reported infectious disease in the United States.

Cholesterol One of the steroids or fat-like chemical substances manufactured by the body and also consumed in foods of animal origin. It is essential for the manufacture and maintenance of cells, sex hormones, and nerves throughout the body.

Chorionic villus sampling (CVS) A procedure performed to detect fetal abnormalities in which samples of chorionic villi are removed and examined.

Chromosome A structure in the nucleus of each cell composed of DNA and protein that contains the genes that provide information for the transmission of inherited characteristics.

Chronic bronchitis Constant inflammation of the bronchial tubes. The inflammation thickens the walls of the bronchi, and the production of mucus increases, resulting in a constricting or narrowing of the air passages.

Chronic disease A disease that lasts longer than several weeks, often for the length of a person's life; it may be ongoing or progress slowly. Examples include diabetes, heart disease, and lupus.

Chronic obstructive pulmonary disease (COPD) A disease characterized by permanent airflow obstruction and extended periods of disability and restricted activity.

Cirrhosis Alcohol-induced liver disease.

Climacteric Physiological changes that occur during the transition period from fertility to infertility in both sexes.

Clinical trial A research study designed to answer specific questions about new vaccines, new therapies, or new ways of using known treatments. Used to determine whether drugs or treatments are both safe and effective.

Clitoris A highly sensitive structure of the female external genitalia, the only purpose of which is sexual pleasure.

Colonoscopy An examination of the colon using a flexible lighted instrument called a colonoscope.

Colostrum Early milk, or milk produced during the pregnancy and for 3 to 5 days after birth. It is yellowish in color, thicker than milk, and rich with protective antibodies and protein.

Colposcope A lighted magnifying instrument used to examine the vagina and cervix.

Colposcopy A procedure in which a colposcope is used to examine the vagina and cervix.

Complex carbohydrates One of the main sources of fuel for the muscles. Found in breads, cereals, pasta, rice, and vegetables, such as potatoes and corn.

Conception Formation of a viable zygote by the union of the male sperm and the female ovum; fertilization.

Conceptus The products of conception or fertilization, including the fertilized egg and its enclosing membranes.

Condom A barrier contraception method consisting of a sheath, preferably latex, that covers the penis during intercourse. It prevents pregnancy by collecting the semen in the receptacle tip.

Congenital heart disease A heart condition present when a baby is born. It may include many different conditions, most of which can be surgically corrected.

Congestive heart failure (CHF) A condition in which the heart loses its ability to contract properly or sufficiently to meet the demands placed on it.

Conization The surgical removal of a cone-shaped piece of tissue intended to determine whether abnormal cells have invaded tissue beneath surface cells or to treat a precancerous lesion. Also called cone biopsy.

Contraception Intentional prevention of conception or impregnation through the use of various devices, agents, drugs, sexual practices, or surgical procedures.

Contraceptive sponge A contraceptive device that acts both as a cervical barrier by absorbing ejaculated sperm and as a source of spermicide. It is available without fitting or prescription.

Copayment/copay A type of cost sharing whereby the enrollee or covered person pays a specified flat amount per unit of service or unit of time, and the healthcare insurer pays the remainder of the cost.

Coronary artery bypass graft (CABG) surgery A type of surgery that creates a "bypass" around the blocked part of the coronary artery to restore the blood supply to the heart muscle.

Corpus luteum A yellowish body that forms on the ovary at the site of the ruptured follicle where the egg has been released. It secretes progesterone to help prepare the body for pregnancy.

Corset A close-fitting undergarment or outer garment worn to support and shape the waistline, hips, and breasts.

Cost sharing The share of costs covered by insurance that a person pays out of his or her own pocket. This term generally includes deductibles, coinsurance, and copayments, or similar charges, but it does not include premiums, balance billing amounts for non-network providers, or the cost of noncovered services.

Cryosurgery Freezing of an infected area.

Cunnilingus Oral stimulation of the clitoris or vulva.

Cyberstalking Threatening behavior or unwanted advances directed at another person using the Internet and other forms of online communications.

Cystic mastitis The most common breast disorder in women, resulting in tender and lumpy breast tissues. Also known as fibrocystic breast disease.

Cysts Abnormal growths of cells consisting of a thin-walled sac filled with fluid.

Cytomegalovirus (CMV) A viral infection that causes mild flu-like symptoms in adults but that can cause small birth size, brain damage, developmental problems, enlarged liver, hearing and vision impairment, and other malformations in newborns. Babies with this are infected in utero, although only 10% of those so infected have symptoms. Pregnant women often acquire it from infected children with few or no symptoms. It is the most common prenatal infection today, and it is an opportunistic infection of HIV/AIDS.

Date rape Rape in which the victim and the rapist were previously known to each other and may have interacted in some socially appropriate manner. Also known as "acquaintance rape."

Dementia Cognitive decline, often occurring in old age. This mental deterioration and decline in intellectual functioning is severe enough to interfere with routine daily activities.

Depression A mental condition in which a person feels extremely sad, worthless, and hopeless. In more severe cases, the person may experience thoughts of suicide. Types of depression include clinical depression, bipolar depression, seasonal affective disorder (SAD), dysthymia, and postpartum depression.

Diabetes A disease characterized by abnormal glucose production or metabolism. A person with this disease has either a deficiency of insulin (the hormone produced by the pancreas needed to convert glucose to energy) or a decreased ability to use insulin. As a result, glucose builds up in the bloodstream and, without treatment, may damage organs, contribute to heart disease, or cause coma, and, eventually, death.

Diaphragm A latex, dome-shaped cap inserted over the cervix to prevent conception.

Diastolic The second (or lower) reading of blood pressure that represents the amount of pressure the blood exerts against the wall of the artery when the heart rests between beats.

Digital rectal examination An examination intended to detect colorectal cancer in which the physician inserts a lubricated gloved finger into a rectum to feel for abnormal areas.

Dilation and curettage (D&C) A minor surgical procedure in which the cervix is expanded enough (dilated) to permit the cervical canal and uterine lining to be scraped with a spoon-shaped instrument called a curette.

Dissociative disorders Disorders that develop as an unconscious way to protect oneself from emotional traumas by detaching from a part of one's personality. These disorders occur as a response to severe childhood trauma.

Dizygotic twins Two offspring developed from two eggs released from the ovary and fertilized at the same time. They may be the same or opposite sex and may differ physically and in genetic traits. Also called fraternal twins.

Domestic violence Subjecting a spouse, partner, or family member to any forceful physical, social, and psychological behavior in order to coerce that person without regard to his or her rights. Also known as battering.

Down syndrome A congenital condition characterized by various degrees of mental retardation and abnormal development. It is caused by the presence of an extra chromosome, usually number 21 or 22.

Drug Any chemical other than food that is purposely taken to affect body processes.

Drug abuse The excessive use of a drug that has dangerous side effects.

Drug dependency The attachment—physiological or psychological (or both)—that a person may develop to a drug.

Physical dependence occurs when physiological changes in the body's cells cause an overpowering constant need for the drug. Psychological addiction produces an emotional, or sometimes a motivational, attachment to a drug.

Drug misuse The use of a drug for a purpose other than its original intent.

Dysmenorrhea Pain or discomfort just prior to or during menstruation.

Dysplasia Abnormal cells that are not cancerous; classified as mild, moderate, or severe.

Dysplastic nevi Atypical moles.

Dysthymia A form of depression that is milder and less disabling than major depression but more chronic in nature.

Ectoparasitic infections Infections caused by tiny parasites that reside on the skin and survive on human blood and tissue. Infections include scabies and pubic lice ("crabs"). Parasites cause itching and may cause bumps or a rash but are easily treated with a topical cream.

Ectopic pregnancy The implantation of a fertilized egg outside the uterus.

Effacement The thinning of the cervix before delivery.

Egg donation A type of assisted reproductive technology used when a woman is unable to produce eggs or has a genetic disorder that will be passed on to her child. Egg donors must be willing to dedicate an enormous amount of time to this effort because of the drug treatment and monitoring that they must undergo.

Elder abuse The injury, maltreatment, or neglect of an older person from a physical, psychological, or material perspective.

Electrocardiograph (ECG) A device used to record the electrical activity of the heart in order to diagnose heart problems.

Embolism A condition in which an embolus (clot) traveling in the bloodstream suddenly becomes lodged in a blood vessel.

Embolus A clot circulating in the bloodstream.

Embryo An organism in its early stage of development in humans. The embryonic period lasts from the second to the eighth week of pregnancy.

Embryo transfer A fertility procedure in which the sperm of the infertile woman's partner are placed in another woman's uterus during ovulation. The fertilized egg is removed a few days later and transferred to the uterus of the infertile woman.

Emphysema An irreversible disease that results in permanent limitation in airflow of the lungs. As a result, breathing becomes compromised, and increased demand is placed on the heart.

Endometriosis A benign condition in which tissue that looks like endometrial tissue grows in abnormal places outside the uterus.

Endometrium The tissue that lines the insides of the uterine walls.

Environmental tobacco smoke (ETS) Smoke resulting from others who are smoking cigarettes or cigars. Also referred to as passive or secondhand smoke.

Enzyme-linked immunosorbent assay (ELISA) Laboratory test used to detect antibodies produced in response to HIV infection. If HIV antibodies are found with this test, it is repeated. If antibodies are found on a second ELISA test, a Western blot test is performed.

Epidural anesthesia A type of anesthetic used during delivery that is injected through a catheter placed in a space beside the spinal cord. Epidurals are the most common choice of anesthesia made by pregnant women and allow the mother to be awake for the birth.

Erythrocytes Red blood cells. Erythrocytes carry oxygen and carbon dioxide.

Estrogen A class of hormones that produce female secondary sex characteristics and affect the menstrual cycle.

Exercise Routine or structured physical activity that a person performs with the goal of improving his or her health.

Fallopian tubes Tubes or ducts that allow for the passage of ova from the ovary to the uterus.

Familial adenomatous polyposis (FAP) A condition in which polyps are inherited and affect the gastrointestinal tract. Individuals with this develop hundreds to thousands of polyps throughout the colon at young age.

Family and intimate partner violence Refers to violence directed toward former or current spouses or partners, dates, family members, elders, and children.

Family planning Planning of when and if to have children, including the use of birth control and other options.

Fat A lipid with one, two, or three fatty acids, which is responsible for multiple body functions.

Fat-soluble vitamins Vitamins absorbed with the aid of fats in the diet or bile from the liver through the intestinal membrane and stored in the body.

Fecal occult blood test A simple procedure of smearing a small sample of stool on a slide containing a chemical that changes color in the presence of hemoglobin. Developing tumors cause minor bleeding, which results in the presence of occult blood (small amounts of blood in the stool).

Fecundity The physical ability of a woman to have a child. Women with impaired fecundity include those who find it physically difficult or medically inadvisable to conceive or deliver a child.

Fee-for-service A traditional method of healthcare payment in which physicians and other providers receive payment that does not exceed their billed charges for each unit of service rendered.

Fellatio Oral stimulation of the penis or scrotum.

Female athlete triad The interrelationship among disordered eating, amenorrhea, and osteoporosis. Beginning with disordered eating, the combination of poor nutrition and intense athletic training causes weight loss and a decrease in or shutdown of estrogen production. Consequently, amenorrhea occurs. The final condition in the triad, osteoporosis, may follow if estrogen levels remain low and the woman's diet continues to lack calcium and vitamin D.

Female condom A form of barrier contraception that lines the entire vagina, preventing the penis and semen from coming in direct physical contact with the vagina.

Female genital mutilation Any of the three types of genital mutilation.

Feminism The policy, practice, or advocacy of political, economic, and social equality for women. It is the principle that women should have rights equal to those of men.

Fertility The state of being fertile; the capacity to produce offspring.

Fertilization The union of an ovum and a sperm.

Fetal alcohol syndrome (FAS) Alcohol-related defects among infants caused by prenatal maternal alcohol consumption. They are usually characterized by growth retardation, facial malformations, and central nervous system dysfunctions, including mental retardation.

Fetal distress Signs of distress in the fetus, such as slowing of heart rate or acid in the blood.

Fetus The unborn baby in the uterus from the eighth week of gestation until birth.

Fiber Plant parts that cannot be digested in the human digestive tract. High-fiber diets protect against certain cancers and heart disease.

Fibroadenoma A nonmalignant form of breast tumor.

Fibrocystic breast disease The most common breast disorder in women, resulting in tender and lumpy breast tissues. Also known as cystic mastitis.

Fibroid Benign uterine tumor composed of muscular and fibrous tissue.

Fibromyalgia A chronic illness characterized by constant, unexplained pain throughout the body.

Flexibility The range of motion permitted by joints.

Folate A B vitamin found in foods such as chickpeas, spinach, strawberries, kidney beans, and citrus fruits and juices.

Folic acid A form of folate used to fortify grain-based foods, such as bread, flour, rice, pasta, and cereal. It is vital for cell growth and function and for the development of a healthy neural tube in fetuses.

Forceps Surgical instruments used for grasping. They may be used to extract a baby from the birth canal during delivery.

Formularies Lists of drug products that a payer has identified as part of a given health insurance product's covered benefits.

Galactosemia An inherited disease characterized by the lack of the enzyme needed for processing galactose (sugars in milk products); can cause mental retardation if not treated properly.

Gamete intrafallopian transfer (GIFT) A procedure for treating infertility that involves placing sperm and egg cells into the fallopian tubes.

Gender dysphoria The overall psychological term used to describe nonconforming gender identification. This term replaces the use of gender identity disorder when referring to transgender and focuses on the fact that distress is not inherent in a transgender person.

Gender identity How one psychologically perceives oneself as either male or female.

Gender role The public expression of one's gender identity as well as the cultural expectations of male and female behaviors.

Generalized anxiety disorder (GAD) An anxiety disorder that causes an ongoing general feeling of intense worry and fear, often for no apparent reason.

Generic drug The chemical equivalent of a brand-name drug that is available once the brand-name drug goes off patent. Generic drugs are typically less expensive than their brand-name counterparts.

Genetic phenotype The observable traits or characteristics of an organism—for example, hair color, weight, or the presence or absence of a disease.

Gestational diabetes A form of diabetes that develops in 2 to 5% of all pregnancies but that usually disappears when the pregnancy is over.

Glycemic index A measure of how fast glucose enters the bloodstream after a carbohydrate is eaten and thus how quickly the carbohydrate increases a person's blood sugar.

Gonorrhea A sexually transmitted bacterial infection that can cause dangerous complications leading to infertility, ectopic pregnancy, or persistent pain in the pelvic area. It can even spread to the bloodstream and cause arthritis or life-threatening heart or brain infections.

Group B streptococcus (GBS) A type of bacterium that can cause illness in newborn babies and pregnant women. Pregnant women with this do not necessarily infect their babies; however, babies who develop signs and symptoms are at risk of sepsis, pneumonia, meningitis, long-term disabilities such as hearing or vision loss, and death. Obstetricians can test women for it and prevent disease by administering antibiotics intravenously during labor.

Hallucinogens Drugs that create changes in perceptions and thoughts. A common feature of a hallucinogenic experience is that the drug suspends normal psychic mechanisms that integrate the self with the environment.

Hashish An extract of cannabis that is 2 to 10 times as concentrated as marijuana.

Heart attack Death of a certain portion of the heart.

Hemoglobin The iron-containing protein in the red blood cell that carries oxygen from the lungs to the cells and carbon dioxide away from the cells to the lungs. It also is responsible for the red color of blood.

Hemorrhagic stroke A condition in which blood vessels leading to and within the brain rupture, causing the brain to no longer receive blood and oxygen.

Hepatitis Inflammation and destruction of liver cells.

Herpes simplex virus (HSV) A family of contagious viruses that infect humans. Viruses in the herpes family include HSV-1 and HSV-2, which can cause sores in the mouth or genital area (the latter infection is often referred to as "genital herpes") as well as the virus that causes chicken pox.

Heterosexual A person with sexual orientation to persons of the opposite sex and/or sexual activity with another of the opposite sex.

High-density lipoprotein (HDL) A type of lipoprotein in the blood that carries cholesterol and fats out of the body. It is often referred to as the "good" cholesterol.

HIV (human immunodeficiency virus) A virus that attacks and damages the white blood cells in the body's immune system that are needed to fight of infection. It eventually causes AIDS when so many white blood cells have been destroyed that the immune system can no longer fight off illness.

Homocysteine An essential amino acid found in the blood. Increased levels of homocysteine can harm the artery lining and increase risk for coronary artery disease.

Homophobia Irrational fears of homosexuality, the fear of the possibility of homosexuality in oneself, or self-loathing toward one's own homosexuality.

Homosexual A person whose primary social, emotional, and sexual orientation is toward members of the same sex.

Honor killing The killing of a woman who has a (sexual) contact with a man outside the frame of marriage, even when she has been a victim of rape. It is intended to maintain and protect the honor of the family. Offenders often are younger than age 18 and are sometimes treated as heroes in their communities. Such killings have been reported in Pakistan, Jordan, Yemen, Lebanon, Egypt, the Gaza Strip, and the West Bank.

Hormone A chemical produced by one part of the body that influences activity, growth, or metabolism in another part of the body.

Host uterus A procedure in which the sperm from a man and the egg from a woman are combined in a laboratory. The fertilized egg then is implanted into the uterus of a second woman, who agrees to bear the child who is not genetically related to her.

Hot flash An uncomfortable sensation of menopause consisting of internally generated heat beginning in the chest and moving to the neck and head or spreading through the body. Also known as hot flushes.

Human chorionic gonadatropin (hCG) A hormone produced by the chorionic villi in a pregnant woman.

Human genome The DNA contained in an organism or a cell, which includes both the chromosomes within the nucleus and the DNA in mitochondria.

Human papillomavirus (HPV) An extremely common sexually transmitted virus. There are many strains; some of them can cause genital warts in men and women, and other kinds can cause cervical dysplasia in women, which, if left untreated, can lead to cervical cancer.

Hunger The painful or uneasy feeling caused by the continuous and involuntary lack of food.

Hymen Tissue that partially covers the vaginal opening.

Hyperglycemia High blood sugar levels, whereby a person may become very ill. Early signs include high blood sugar, high levels of sugar in the urine, frequent urination, and increased thirst.

Hyperplasia A precancerous condition characterized by an increase in the number of normal cells.

Hypertension A blood pressure that remains elevated above what is considered a safe level. Also known as high blood pressure.

Hyperthyroidism Thyroid disease resulting from an overactive thyroid, most commonly caused by Graves' disease.

Hypoglycemia Low blood sugar levels that can cause a person to become nervous, shaky, and confused and can result in the person passing out.

Hypothyroidism Thyroid disease resulting from an underactive thyroid, most commonly caused by Hashimoto's disease.

Hysterectomy The surgical removal of the uterus, resulting in surgically induced menopause.

Hysteroscopy A procedure used to view the inside of the uterus through a telescope-like device called a hysteroscope.

Immune system The body's natural defense system, which works to protect the body from pathogens.

Implantation The embedding of the fertilized ovum in the uterine lining 6 to 7 days after fertilization.

In vitro fertilization (IVF) A procedure for treating infertility that involves removing the ova from a woman's ovary. The ova and the sperm (from the woman's partner) are placed in a medium; if fertilization occurs, the conceptus is injected into the woman's uterus.

Incidence The number of new cases of a disease or condition in a given period of time.

Indemnity A form of health insurance in which a person prepays a premium in exchange for a specific amount of monetary coverage in the event of illnesses or accidents.

If an illness or accident occurs, the enrollee or the care provider submits a claim to the insurance organization. The insurance organization then reimburses the party for all or, in most cases, a percentage of the incurred costs.

Infant mortality rate The number of deaths of children younger than 1 year old divided by the number of live births that year. It is an important epidemiological indicator of the well-being of pregnant women, infants, and children.

Inferior vena cava The major vein that carries oxygen-poor blood into the right atrium of the heart.

Infertility The inability to conceive a child.

Inhalant A chemical that produces vapors with psychoactive effects. Predominantly abused by preadolescents and young adults.

Intersexuality The sexual physiology of an individual in which the person is born with sex chromosomes, external genitalia, or internal reproductive organs that are not considered "standard" as male or female.

Intracytoplasmic sperm injection (ICSI) A procedure for treating infertility that involves the injection of a single sperm directly into a mature egg.

Intrauterine device (IUD) A small, flexible, plastic, T-shaped device that contains either copper or the hormone progesterone that is inserted into the uterus by a clinician to prevent pregnancy. It can be left in place for 1 to 10 years, depending on the type of device.

Iron A mineral that is needed to make hemoglobin (a compound in the blood).

Ischemic stroke A condition in which blood vessels leading to and within the brain become blocked, causing the brain to no longer receive blood and oxygen.

Jaundice A condition in which accumulation of pigments in the blood produces a yellowing of the skin and eyes.

Kegel exercises Exercises that help strengthen the vaginal and pelvic floor muscles to help prepare the muscles for delivery, aid in a speedy recovery from delivery, help prevent or treat urinary incontinence, and help prevent or treat the loss of pelvic support.

Labia majora The outer lips of the vulva.

Labia minora The inner lips of the vulva, one on each side of the vaginal opening.

Lamaze A method of childbirth preparation in which the expectant mother is prepared psychologically and physically through breathing exercises and concentration to control pain during childbirth while maintaining consciousness.

Laparoscopy Examination of a woman's abdominal cavity to view the ovaries, fallopian tubes, and other structures.

Left atrium One of the two upper chambers of the heart. It receives blood with oxygen from the lungs.

Left ventricle One of the two lower chambers of the heart. It pumps blood from the heart to the body tissues.

Leukocytes White blood cells. They act as scavengers to rid the blood and body of bacteria and wastes. Several types of white blood cells exist, each of which has its own role in fighting bacterial, viral, fungal, and parasitic infections.

Life expectancy The number of years a person born at a given point in time is expected to live from birth.

Lipoprotein A compound found in the bloodstream containing a core of lipids with a shell of protein, phospholipid, and cholesterol.

Lobectomy Removal of a lobe of a lung.

Long-term facility A facility in which custodial care is provided over a prolonged or indefinite period of time, required because of a person's disability or aging. Skilled nursing facilities, or nursing homes, are the most common types.

Low-density lipoprotein (LDL) A type of lipoprotein that contains cholesterol and triglycerides and that is considered harmful because it promotes fatty deposits on the inner lining of arteries. Also called "bad" cholesterol.

Lumpectomy A procedure in which only the cancerous lump and a small amount of surrounding tissue are removed from the breast.

Lupus A complex chronic inflammatory disorder in which the immune system forms antibodies that target healthy tissues and organs. It can be a mild, moderate, or severe disease.

Lyme disease A type of inflammatory arthritis that is caused by a tiny, tick-borne bacterium. If it is not treated, it can lead to cardiac problems, neurological disorders, or infectious arthritis (usually of the knees).

Magnetic resonance imaging (MRI) A medical test used to provide a visual image of the body's internal structures. It may be used to examine the heart, brain, or other organs for signs of disease.

Malignant tumor A tumor that is cancerous and capable of spreading to other tissues and invading adjacent areas.

Malnutrition An imbalance between the body's nutritional needs and the intake or digestion of nutrients, which may result in disease or death. It can be caused by an unbalanced diet, digestive problems, or absorption problems.

Mammography A procedure in which a low-dose X-ray of the breast is taken in order to detect tumors.

Managed care A system of healthcare delivery that aims to manage utilization of services and cost of services, while measuring performance. The goal is a system that delivers value by giving people access to quality, cost-effective health care.

Mastitis An infection in the breast, usually caused by bacterial infection. It results in localized pain, redness, and heat with symptoms of fever, nausea, and vomiting.

Masturbation Excitation of one's own or another's genital organs, usually to orgasm, by manual contact or means other than sexual intercourse.

Maternal morbidity and mortality Death or illness while pregnant or within a defined time period of the termination of pregnancy, irrespective of the duration and the site of the pregnancy, from any cause related to or aggravated by the pregnancy or its management but not from accidental or incidental causes.

Maternal serum alpha-fetoprotein (MSAFP) A prenatal screening test that measures a substance produced by the baby's kidneys found in the mother's blood between the 13th and 20th weeks of pregnancy.

Medicaid A joint federal/state health insurance program for low-income persons who receive public assistance or whose medical expenses "spend down" their income to qualify for the program. This program is administered by each state and places fairly tight restrictions on payments for physician services and drugs. Also known as Title XIX.

Medicare A health insurance program providing benefits to approximately 30 million elderly (aged 65 or older) and disabled Americans. It is funded by the federal government and administered by the Centers for Medicare and Medicaid Services (CMS).

Melanocyte A cell in the skin that produces pigment.

Melanoma A cancer that originates within the melanocytes.

Menopause The cessation of regular menstrual periods by surgical or natural means. Also known as the climacterium, the "change of life."

Menstrual cycle A recurring cycle (beginning at menarche and ending at menopause) in which the endometrial lining of the uterus prepares for pregnancy. If pregnancy does not occur, the lining is shed at menstruation. On average it is 28 days.

Metastasis The spread of cancer from one part of the body to another. Cells in the metastatic tumor (the second tumor) are like those in the original tumor.

Mineral A naturally occurring inorganic substance. These nutrients are essential in small amounts for regulating body functions.

Miscarriage A pregnancy that terminates before the 20th week of gestation because of fetal defects or pregnancy problems.

Mitral valve The valve separating the left atrium and ventricle.

Modified radical mastectomy Removal of the breast. It is a less extensive procedure than radical mastectomy because the underlying chest wall muscles and some of the nearby lymph nodes are not removed. Also known as a total mastectomy.

Monounsaturated fat A type of fat that comes from both plant and animal sources and is liquid at room temperature and solid or semisolid when refrigerated. This type of fat helps to lower blood cholesterol.

Monozygotic twins Two offspring developed from one fertilized egg that splits into equal halves. They are of the same sex, share the same genes, and look nearly identical. Also called identical twins.

Mons veneris A triangular mound over the pubic bone above the vulva.

Mood disorders (affective disorders) Conditions characterized by extreme disturbances of mood.

Morbidity rate The rate of illness in a given population over a period of time.

Mortality rate The rate of death in a given population over a period of time.

Muscular endurance The ability to withstand the stress of physical exertion.

Muscular strength Physical power, such as the amount of weight one can lift, push, or press in a single effort.

Myocardial infarction Heart attack.

Myomectomy Surgical removal of a uterine fibroid.

Narcotics A class of drugs that includes the opiates—opium and its derivatives, morphine, codeine, and heroin—and some nonopiate synthetic drugs. They all have sleep-inducing and pain-relieving properties.

Natural menopause The failure of the ovaries to respond to the luteinizing and follicle-stimulating hormones that are produced in the anterior pituitary, which is under the control of the hypothalamus. As a result of this failure, ovulation becomes somewhat erratic. The mechanisms for these changes are not well understood. It is considered complete once monthly periods have ceased altogether.

Neural tube defects Defects of the spine and brain caused by failure of the neural tube to close during pregnancy.

Neurotransmitters A group of chemicals found in the brain and nervous system that transmit and modulate communication between neurons.

Nicotine The addictive element in cigarettes. It has several effects on the body, including increasing blood pressure, increasing heart rate, and negating hunger.

Nongovernmental organization (NGO) According to the World Bank, "private organizations that pursue activities to relieve suffering, promote the interests of the poor, protect the environment, provide basic social services, or undertake community development." This term can be applied to any nonprofit organization that is independent from government, including a large charity, community-based self-help group, research institute, church, professional association, or lobby group.

Nonmelanoma The most common cancers of the skin (usually basal cell and squamous cell cancers). These cancers include all skin cancers except malignant melanoma.

Nutrient A substance essential to life that the body cannot produce on its own. Nutrients are provided by food and assist in the growth and development of the body.

Nutrition The science of studying the need for and the effects of food on an organism.

Obesity The excessive accumulation of fat in the body; a condition of being 20% or more above ideal weight.

Obsessive-compulsive disorder (OCD) An anxiety disorder that causes a person to have disturbing repetitive thoughts (obsessions) and to perform rituals or routines (compulsions) to get rid of the obsessions. The disorder is diagnosed only when the repetitive behaviors consume many hours each day and interfere with daily life.

Opportunistic infections Infections that seldom cause disease in people with normal immune function but that "take the opportunity" to cause disease in people with a present illness or a lowered immune system, such as that caused by HIV/AIDS.

Oral sex Stimulation of the genital or anal areas with the mouth or tongue. Unprotected oral sex can transmit sexually transmitted infections.

Osteoarthritis A disease in which the surface layer of cartilage erodes, causing bones under the cartilage to rub together. This friction results in joint pain, swelling, and loss of movement of the joints. Also called degenerative joint disease.

Osteopathic school A school that focuses on natural medicine, which aims to restore function to the organism by treating the causes of pain and imbalance.

Osteopenia Decreased calcification or density of bone. This descriptive term is applicable to all skeletal systems in which such a condition is noted.

Osteoporosis An age-related, debilitating disorder characterized by a general decrease in bone mass and structural deterioration of bone tissue.

Outercourse The sharing of sexual intimacy through behaviors such as kissing, petting, and mutual masturbation without penile-vaginal penetration.

Ovaries Reproductive organs that produce ova, estrogen, and progesterone.

Over-the-counter medications Medications such as aspirin or cough syrups that can be purchased at a drug store without a prescription.

Overnutrition A form of malnutrition caused by overeating, insufficient exercise, and excessive intake of vitamins and minerals. Overnutrition can lead to overweight and obesity.

Overweight Having a body mass index (BMI) of 25 to 29.9.

Panic disorder An anxiety disorder characterized by periods of intense fear, known as panic attacks, that are accompanied by physical symptoms (pounding heart, sweating, dizziness, chest pain, and so on) and emotional distress.

Pap smear A gynecological procedure in which a sample of cervical cells is examined for the presence of precancerous or cancerous cells.

Partial or segmental mastectomy Surgery to treat breast cancer that involves the removal of some breast tissue and some of the surrounding lymph nodes.

Patent ductus arteriosus A congenital condition common in premature babies in which the passageway between the pulmonary artery and aorta does not close.

Pelvic inflammatory disease (PID) A general term describing an infection of the internal female reproductive tract that can lead to infertility, chronic pain, or ectopic pregnancy. PID is usually caused by a sexually transmitted infection such as chlamydia or gonorrhea that spreads into the upper reproductive tract.

Perimenopause Refers to the years immediately preceding and following the last menstrual period.

Perineum The area of smooth skin between the vaginal opening and the anus.

Peripheral artery disease A disease of the extremities (hands and arms but mainly in the legs and feet) in which the blood supply is diminished and sufficient oxygen and nutrients do not reach these areas properly. Because waste is not removed from these areas effectively, the affected person may experience symptoms that range from cramping and numbness to gangrene (tissue death), which may require amputation of the extremity.

Personality disorders Mental disorders that are characterized by distorted and inflexible thoughts and behaviors that make it impossible for a person to live a productive life or establish fulfilling relationships.

Phobia An anxiety disorder characterized by a powerful and irrational fear of a particular object or situation.

Phytochemicals Plant chemicals found in fruits and vegetables that protect the body from cancer by blocking the carcinogenic activities of certain substances in the human body.

Placenta An organ that develops after implantation where the embryo attaches via the umbilical cord for nourishment and waste removal.

Placenta previa A complication of pregnancy in which the birth canal becomes obstructed by the placenta.

Plaques Fatty deposits that develop inside the lining of the arteries that reduce blood flow and can eventually lead to a heart attack or stroke.

Platelets Disk-shaped structures in the blood needed for blood coagulation. Also called thrombocytes.

Pneumonectomy Removal of the lung.

Polycystic ovary syndrome (PCOS) A condition associated with the overproduction of male hormones, failure to ovulate, formation of cysts on the surface of the ovaries, inability to become pregnant, and abnormal hair growth on the body. Polycystic ovary syndrome occurs most often in women who are obese, and it generally can be reversed with weight loss. Also called polycystic ovary disease (PCOD).

Polyps Small benign growths that develop in the endocervical canal or colorectal region.

Polyunsaturated fat A type of fat that is liquid at room temperature and when refrigerated; such fats help lower both LDL and HDL cholesterol.

Postmenopause Life after the final menstrual period.

Postpartum psychosis The most severe of the psychiatric disorders that can develop in women after delivery. Symptoms of postpartum psychosis include depression, anxiety, irritation, tiredness, and sleep disturbances, as well as behavior that tends to change throughout the day from clear consciousness to total loss of reality.

Posttraumatic stress disorder (PTSD) An anxiety disorder that usually begins within 3 months of a traumatic event. Its symptoms include flashback episodes, nightmares, and emotional numbness.

Preeclampsia A complication of pregnancy characterized by high blood pressure, swelling caused by fluid retention, and high levels of protein in the urine. Also called toxemia.

Premature labor Labor that begins before the completed ninth month of fetal gestation.

Premenstrual dysphoric disorder (PMDD) A condition associated with severe emotional and physical problems that are linked closely to the menstrual cycle; a more severe form of premenstrual syndrome (PMS).

Premenstrual syndrome (PMS) A group of cyclic symptoms that occur in some women about a week before menstruation, including breast tenderness, abdominal bloating, fatigue, fluctuating emotions, and depression.

Premium In terms of health insurance, a regular periodic payment.

Prevalence The total number of people with a given condition at a point in time.

Primary prevention Prevention of disease by reducing exposure to a risk factor that may lead to the disease. Primary preventive measures include healthy nutrition, regular physical activity, cessation of smoking, and safe sexual practices.

Private health insurance Health insurance provided by third-party payers to individuals or employer groups either through indemnity or managed care systems.

Prodrome Period of infectiousness before the first signs of infection are present.

Progesterone The hormone produced by the corpus luteum of the ovary that causes the uterine lining to thicken.

Progestin A natural or synthetic progestational substance that mimics some or all of the actions of progesterone. It can be used as a form of birth control or emergency contraception.

Prolapsed cord A complication of pregnancy in which the umbilical cord comes through the pelvis before the baby. It can result in a disrupted flow of oxygen to the baby due to a compressed cord.

Protein A substance that is basically a compound of amino acids; one of the essential nutrients.

Protein-energy malnutrition (PEM) A deficiency syndrome caused by the inadequate intake of protein and/or energy. PEM, the most destructive form of malnutrition, mainly affects infants and young children.

Psychosis A severe mental disorder characterized by a loss of contact with reality and severe personality changes.

Puberty The stage of life between childhood and adulthood during which the reproductive organs mature and secondary sexual characteristics begin to develop. For girls, it is the time of the onset of menstruation, the development of breasts and body hair, and usually some level of growth spurt.

Public health insurance Health insurance provided by government sources, including Medicare, Medicaid, the Department of Defense (DOD), Veterans Administration (VA), and the Bureau of Indian Affairs.

Pulmonary arteries Vessels that receive blood from the right ventricle to carry to the lungs for oxygenation.

Pulmonary stenosis A condition in which the valve between the ventricle and pulmonary artery is defective and does not open properly.

Pulmonary veins Vessels that return oxygenated blood from the lungs to the left atrium.

Pus A substance composed of dead bacteria, dead white blood cells, and fluid that is most commonly the result of an infection process.

Radiation therapy Treatment with high-energy radiation from X-rays and other sources.

Radical mastectomy Removal of the entire breast, underlying chest muscles, and underarm lymph nodes following a diagnosis of breast cancer.

Rape Any unwanted sexual act, including forced vaginal or anal intercourse, oral sex, or penetration with an object.

Recommended Dietary Allowance (RDA) Daily nutrient allowance recommended for healthy adults by the National Research Council.

Recreational drugs Drugs taken purely for fun.

Red blood cells One of the formed elements in circulating blood. Red blood cells contain hemoglobin and transport oxygen. Also called erythrocytes.

Retrovirus A virus that has the ability to take over certain cells and interrupt their normal genetic function.

Rh incompatibility A condition that occurs when an Rh-negative mother and an Rh-positive father conceive a baby who inherits the father's Rh-positive blood type. This situation may present problems during pregnancy, labor, and delivery if the fetus's Rh-positive blood cells enter the mother's bloodstream.

Rheumatic heart disease A heart condition resulting from a bacterial infection (*Streptococcus*) that has been inadequately treated. The infection can develop into rheumatic fever and damage the heart valves.

Rheumatoid arthritis Chronic inflammatory disease of the joints that results from an autoimmune response.

Right atrium One of the two upper chambers of the heart. It collects the deoxygenated blood from the body.

Right ventricle One of the two lower chambers of the heart. It pumps blood from the heart to the lungs to collect oxygen.

Rubella An infectious disease often causing birth defects in pregnant women. Also called German measles.

Saturated fats Fats that come primarily from animal sources.

Schizophrenia A type of psychosis representing a complex group of diseases with symptoms that may appear gradually or suddenly and include hallucinations or delusions, disordered thinking, and an impaired ability to manage emotions and interact with others. Schizophrenia is the most chronic and disabling of the severe mental disorders.

Seasonal affective disorder (SAD) A form of depression caused by seasonal shifts in daylight hours that affect a person's sleep–wake cycle.

Secondary prevention Early detection and prompt treatment of disease. Examples of secondary preventive measures include screening tools, such as mammography and Pap smears, which may detect disease before it spreads and thereby prevent further complications from the disease.

Secondhand smoke Environmental exposure to smoke exhaled from another person's cigarette. Secondhand smoke increases the risk for heart and lung diseases, lung cancer, asthma, and other conditions. Children and infants are especially vulnerable to its effects.

Segmentectomy Surgery to remove a section of a lobe of a lung.

Self-mutilation Any self-directed repetitive behavior that causes physical injury. Self-mutilation acts are not usually suicide attempts but rather behaviors meant to express or release emotional turmoil. Examples include skin cutting with razors or knives (the most common pattern); burning or biting oneself; picking one's skin or hair; and extreme injuries such as auto-enucleation (self-removal of the eye), castration, or amputation.

Septum A dividing wall, such as that between the right and left sides of the heart.

Serotonin A neurotransmitter (brain chemical) known to affect appetite.

Sexual assault Conduct of a sexual or indecent nature toward another person that is accompanied by actual or threatened physical force or that induces fear, shame, or mental suffering. The term is frequently used as an all-encompassing term for any type of unwanted sexual advance.

Sexual dysfunction The inability of an individual to function adequately in terms of sexual arousal, orgasm, or in coital situations.

Sexual harassment Behavior that may include unwanted sexual attention or advance and/or the use of threats or bribery to obtain sexual favors. The offensive conduct often interferes with a person's ability to perform regular duties at work and creates an intimidating or hostile work environment.

Sexual health A state of physical, emotional, and social well-being in relation to an individual's sexuality.

Sexual orientation One's erotic, romantic, and affectional attraction to people of the same sex, to the opposite sex, or to both sexes.

Sexually transmitted infections (STIs) Infections of the reproductive tract that are transmitted by sexual intimacy. Sexually transmitted infections include chlamydia, gonorrhea, syphilis, herpes, genital warts, hepatitis, and human immunodeficiency virus (HIV).

Sigmoidoscopy A procedure that uses a thin, lighted tube to examine the rectum and lower colon.

Simple carbohydrates Sugars; they provides the body with glucose and a quick spurt of energy.

Simple mastectomy Complete removal of the breast but not the lymph nodes under the arm or chest muscles following a diagnosis of breast cancer.

Sitz baths A tub in which one bathes in a sitting position with hips and buttocks under water and legs out.

Sodium A macromineral and major component of salt. Most Americans get too much sodium in their diets.

Spermicide A chemical that breaks down the cell walls of sperm. It often is used in conjunction with barrier contraception methods.

Sphygmomanometer A cuff device connected to a hose used as a measuring device to ascertain blood pressure.

Sputum A secretion that is produced in the lungs and the bronchi (tubes that carry air to the lung). This mucus-like secretion may become infected, become bloodstained, or contain abnormal cells that may lead to a diagnosis. Sputum is what comes up with deep coughing.

Stalking Behaviors directed toward a specific person that involve repeated visual or physical proximity; nonconsensual communication; verbal, written, or implied threats; or a combination of these behaviors that would cause fear in a reasonable person.

Statins A class of cholesterol-lowering drugs.

Sterilization The permanent, often surgical, end to fertility by interrupting the mechanisms of normal reproductive action.

Sternum The breastbone.

Stillbirth Death occurring before or during birth of a fetus of sufficient size and age to be otherwise expected to survive.

Stimulants Drugs that affect the central nervous system and increase the heart rate, blood pressure, strength of heart contractions, blood glucose level, and overall muscle tension.

Stroke A condition in which blood vessel damage occurs in the brain.

Suffragist An advocate of the right to vote and the ability to exercise that right.

Superior vena cava The venous trunk draining blood from the head, neck, upper limbs, and thorax to the heart.

Surrogacy A procedure for treating infertility in which a woman is artificially inseminated with the sperm of an infertile woman's partner. She then carries the pregnancy to term for the infertile couple.

Syphilis A sexually transmitted bacterial infection that causes small, painless sores in the genital area, a rash, flu-like symptoms, and, after many years, systemic damage.

Systolic First reading of blood pressure that represents the amount of pressure the blood exerts against the wall of the artery when the heart contracts.

Tendonitis Inflammation caused by friction from overuse of tendons (connective tissues that attach muscle to bone).

Teratogenic The characteristic of producing a permanent abnormality in structure or function, causing growth retardation, or causing death when an embryo or fetus is exposed to a certain substance, organism, or physical agent.

Tertiary prevention Prevention measures that take place once a disease has advanced. They may involve alleviating pain, providing comfort, halting progression of an illness, and limiting disability that may result from disease.

Third-hand smoke Leftover chemicals that accumulate in a room where someone has smoked. Third-hand smoke, although not as dangerous as direct exposure to tobacco or secondhand smoke, does increase the risk for lung cancer, asthma, and other conditions.

Third-party payer system A payment system whereby an insurer (or third party) pays for services rendered to an individual by a provider of care.

Thrombocytes Disk-shaped structures in the blood needed for blood coagulation. Also called platelets.

Thrombus A blood clot that blocks an artery.

Thrush A yeast infection that infects the mouth.

Thyroiditis An inflammation of the thyroid gland. Chronic thyroiditis frequently results in lowered thyroid function (hypothyroidism).

Title IX The portion of the Education Amendments of 1972 that prohibits gender discrimination in educational institutions that receive any federal funds. If educational institutions are found to violate Title IX, their federal funding can be withdrawn.

Tolerance The body's ability to withstand the effects of a drug. Continued use of a drug may result in increased tolerance and decreased responsiveness.

Total hysterectomy Surgical removal of the uterus performed in conjunction with the removal of both ovaries and fallopian tubes.

Toxemia A complication of pregnancy characterized by high blood pressure, swelling caused by fluid retention, and high levels of protein in the urine. Also called preeclampsia.

Toxic shock syndrome (TSS) A rare but serious infection cause by strains of the bacteria *Staphylococcus aureus*. For reasons not fully understood, these bacteria release toxins (poisons) into the bloodstream after deep wounds, surgery, or tampon use (especially high-absorbency tampon use).

Trafficking In regard to women, the use of force and deception to transfer women into situations of extreme exploitation; the recruitment, transportation, transfer, harboring, or receipt of persons by the threat or use of force or the abuse of power for the purpose of exploitation.

Trans fats Fats that are formed when vegetable oils are processed into margarine or shortening. These fats are solid or semisolid at room temperature and raise levels of LDL cholesterol. An FDA ban on the use of trans fats will go into effect in 2018.

Transient ischemic attack (TIA) An event in which an artery closes momentarily in a spasm and may result in a brief memory lapse or garbled speech.

Transitioning The process in which transgender people work to change their appearance and societal identity so as to match their gender identity.

Transvaginal ultrasound A method of imaging the genital tract in women. The ultrasound machine sends out high-frequency sound waves, which bounce off body structures and thereby create a picture. With the transvaginal technique, the ultrasound transducer (a hand-held probe) is inserted directly into the vagina.

Trichomoniasis A vaginal infection cause by *Trichomonas vaginalis*, a single-cell protozoan parasite with a whiplike tail that it uses to propel itself through vaginal and urethral mucus.

Tricuspid valve A heart valve that has three points or cusps and is situated between the right atrium and the right ventricle.

Triglycerides Fatty substances found in the body's fatty tissues. High levels of triglycerides are associated with an elevated risk of heart disease.

Tumor An abnormal mass of tissue that results from excessive cell division. It may be either benign or malignant.

Ultrasound A procedure that uses high-frequency sound waves to project an image of structures inside the body, such as an organ or a fetus during pregnancy.

Underinsured For the purposes of this book, a person who technically has health insurance but whose coverage is not enough to cover his or her regular medical expenses or whose coverage would not allow a person to afford adequate care in the event of a serious disease or illness.

Undernutrition Poor health resulting from the depletion of nutrients due to inadequate nutrient intake over time.

Underweight An individual who is below the acceptable average weight for his or her height or body type.

Universal health insurance A system by which the government provides health insurance to all citizens, thereby controlling health insurance at the federal level.

Unsaturated fats Fats that come from plants and include most vegetable oils.

Urethra The tube through which urine passes from the bladder to outside the body. In men, semen also passes through the urethra.

Uterus A hollow, muscular organ located in the pelvic cavity of females in which the fertilized egg becomes implanted and develops; also called the womb.

Vacuum curettage The most widely used abortion technique in the United States. In this procedure, the cervix is first dilated. A vacuum curette—an instrument consisting of a tube with a scoop attached for scraping away tissue—is then inserted through the cervix into the uterus. The other end of the tube is attached to a suction-producing apparatus, which aspirates the contents of the uterus into a collection vessel.

Vagina A moist canal in females extending from the labia minora to the uterus.

Vaginal atrophy A condition often associated with menopause that refers to the thinning of the vaginal lining.

Varicocele A mesh of varicose veins in and around the testicle, which is associated with infertility and may have to be treated with surgery.

Vasectomy A male sterilization method whereby one or two small incisions are made just through the skin of the scrotum. The vas deferens is lifted through the incision, and the two ends are tied or cauterized to seal them.

Vasocontrictors Compounds that result in narrowing of blood vessels.

Ventricular fibrillation A disturbance in heart rhythm.

Venules Small veins.

Very-low-density lipoprotein A type of lipoprotein made up mostly of triglycerides. As with LDL, high levels of VLDL increase the risk atherosclerosis.

Viruses Small pathogens incapable of independent metabolism; can only reproduce inside living cells.

Vitamin An organic substance needed by the body in a very small amount. The various vitamins have many different functions in metabolism and nutrition.

Vulva The external genital organs of the female, including the labia majora, labia minora, clitoris, and vestibule of the vagina.

Water-soluble vitamins Vitamins used up or excreted in urine and sweat; must be replaced daily.

Western blot test Laboratory test used to detect antibodies; performed after two positive ELISA tests to test for HIV.

White blood cells Elements in circulating blood that protect the body against pathogenic microorganisms. Also called leukocytes.

Yeast infection A vaginal infection caused most commonly by the fungal organism *Candida albicans*. Symptoms of yeast infections include abnormal vaginal discharge, vaginal and labial itching and burning, redness and inflammation of the vulvar skin, pain with intercourse, and painful urination.

Yo-yo dieting The practice of losing weight and then regaining it, only to lose it and regain it again. This practice makes it more difficult to succeed in future attempts to lose weight because thyroid hormone levels may drop very low in subsequent dieting, thereby significantly slowing basal metabolism.

Zygote A fertilized egg.

Zygote intrafallopian transfer (ZIFT) A method of assisted reproductive technology in which a fertilized egg is placed in the fallopian tube, allowing the zygote to continue its cell division and become implanted in the uterus naturally.

INDEX

Note: Page numbers followed by *f*, *t*, and *b* refer to figures, tables, and boxes respectively.

A

AA. *See* Alcoholics Anonymous
AARP. *See* American Association of Retired People
abortion, 117–121, 128
    antiabortion *vs.* abortion-rights positions, 119
    decisions regarding, 128
    defined, 117
    epidemiological data on, 119–120
    global perspectives on, 121
    history and legal perspectives on, 11–12, 117–118, 118t
    in-clinic surgical abortions, 120–121
    maternal mortality resulting from, 121
    medical abortions, 121
    procedures for, 120–121
    reasons for having, 119
    spontaneous (miscarriages), 117, 151
abruptio placentae, 156
abstinence, 70, 114
abstinence-only until marriage (AOUM) programs, 70
abuse. *See also* substance abuse; violence
    of children, 402–404, 403–404f
    of elderly, 404–405
    of exercise, 242–243
ACA. *See* Affordable Care Act
access to health care, 12–13, 33, 188, 189, 190
Accountable Care Organizations (ACOs), 31
acetaminophen, 378
ACF. *See* Administration for Children and Families
ACOG. *See* American College of Obstetricians and Gynecologists
ACOs. *See* Accountable Care Organizations
acquaintance rape, 405–406, 406b
acrosome reactions, 136
acute coronary syndrome (ACS), 265, 265t
acute diseases, 52
addiction. *See also* alcohol use and alcoholism; drug use and abuse
    effects of, 365
    smoking as, 374
adenocarcinoma, 297
adjuvant therapies, 291
Administration for Children and Families (ACF), 39
Administration on Aging (AoA), 9, 39
adolescents
    secondary prevention, 51t
    specific health concerns for, 46–49

adoption, 117, 120–121
adulthood
    causes of death in, 52, 52t, 55t
    health promotion and disease prevention in, 51–59
    mental health in, 340
    secondary prevention in, 56, 56t, 59t
    sexual health in, 82–84
    substance abuse in, 47–48
aerobic exercise, 237–239
    benefits of, 275
    components of, 237, 238t
    forms of, 238–239
    maximum and target heart rates, 238, 238f
AF. *See* atrial fibrillation
affective disorders, 343
Affordable Care Act (ACA), 97
AFL-CIO, 425
African American females. *See also* racial differences
    arthritis and, 320–324
    cancer and, 280–281, 280t, 281f, 281t, 299, 299f
    cardiovascular disease and, 279, 280t
    diabetes and, 324–327, 325f
    HIV/AIDS and, 186, 187
    insurance coverage and, 29
    life expectancy for, 56–57
    lupus and, 327–328
    maternal mortality rates and, 162–163
    menopause and, 206
    obesity and, 274–275, 274t, 275f, 275t
    osteoarthritis, 320
    sexually transmitted infections (STIs) and, 173
afterbirth, 155
Agency for Healthcare Research and Quality (AHRQ), 39
Agency for Toxic Substances and Disease Registry (ATSDR), 39
Agriculture Department, U.S. (USDA), 223–224, 224f, 228
AHRQ. *See* Agency for Healthcare Research and Quality
albinism, 152
alcohol use and alcoholism, 375–381
    blood alcohol concentrations (BACs) and, 375–376
    in children and adolescents, 379
    cultural influences on, 387
    decisions regarding, 387
    defined, 375, 379
    drug use and, 381
    economic issues and, 366–367
    effects of, 377

chronic obstructive pulmonary disease (COPD), 372
cigarette smoking, 368
    physiological effects of, 370, 371*f*
    risks of, 370
cirrhosis, 378
Civil Rights Act of 1964, 6, 411
Civil War era, 5
climacteric changes, 83
clinical breast examinations (CBEs), 289
clinical trials, 8, 10, 12*b*
clitoris, 74
clomiphene citrate, 161
club drugs, 386
CMS. *See* Centers for Medicare and Medicaid Services
CMV. *See* cytomegalovirus
cocaine, 277, 383–384
codependency, 389
cognitive-behavioral therapy (CBT), 78, 327, 347
cohabitation, 70
coinsurance, 26, 34
coitus interruptus, 114
colchicine, 321
cold sores, 183
collective violence, 398
colonoscopies, 298
colorectal cancer, 283–284, 297–299, 298*f*, 299*f*
colostrum, 157
colposcopy, 293
Commissioned Corps, 39
Commonwealth Fund, 33
Commonwealth Institute, 32
complex carbohydrates, 226, 227
computed tomography (CT) scans, 267
computerized axial tomography (CAT) scans, 267
computer-related injuries, 428
conception, 77, 136–137, 137*t*
conceptus, 137
condoms, 109–111, 109*f*–110*f*, 185
congenital abnormalities, 151–152
congenital heart disease, 266
congestive heart failure (CHF), 265–266
conization, 293
contraception, 94–105, 114–116, 121–128
    abstinence as, 70, 114
    adolescent use of, 96
    barrier methods of, 105–111
    cervical caps, 108–109, 108*f*
    condoms and, 109–111, 109*f*–110*f*, 173, 196
    cultural influences of, 69
    decisions regarding, 121–127, 123*t*–127*t*
    defined, 94
    diaphragms, 106–108, 107*f*–108*f*, 128
    economic issues and, 98
    education level and, 99
    efficacy rates, 115–116, 116*t*
    emergency methods of, 94, 114–115, 114*t*.
            See also abortion

epidemiological data on, 119–120, 120*f*
    fertility awareness methods, 100
    gender differences in, 116
    history of, 6, 7, 97
    hormonal methods of, 100–104
    implants, injectables, patches, and vaginal rings,
        104–105
    intrauterine devices (IUDs), 112
    lactational amenorrhea method (LAM), 114
    methods of, 100–115
    misconceptions about, 96, 97*t*
    oral pills, 101–102, 276–277, 288
    overview, 94
    permanent methods of, 112
    racial differences and, 98, 99*f*
    religious influences on, 98
    sociocultural influences of, 98
    spermicidal agents, 96, 106, 106*f*
    sponges, 111
    statistics on use of, 95*f*, 99*f*
    sterilization, 112–114, 113*f*
    withdrawal method, 114
contractions, 139–140
contraindications, 102–103
Convention on the Elimination of All Forms of
        Discrimination against Women (CEDAW), 13
copayments, 21, 34
COPD. *See* chronic obstructive pulmonary disease
coping mechanisms, 354–355
copper IUD, 112, 115
cordocentesis, 148
coronary artery bypass graft (CABG) surgery, 265
coronary heart disease (CHD), 260, 264–265, 265*f*
    epidemiological data on, 260–261
corpus luteum, 138
corsets, 5
corticosteroids, 323, 328
cost sharing, 97
crack cocaine, 384
C-reactive proteins (CRPs), 274
cross-dressing, 72
cross-tolerance, 386
CRPs. *See* C-reactive proteins
cryosurgery, 293
CT (computed tomography) scans, 267
cultural influences. *See also* racial differences
    body image and, 251–252
    contraception and, 69
    eating disorders and, 351
    gender roles and, 72
    homosexuality and, 68–69
    marriage and, 68
    menopause and, 202–203, 203*f*
    sexual health and, 68–70
    on substance abuse, 376
    violence and, 395–396
cunnilingus, 81

CVD. *See* cardiovascular disease
CVS (chorionic villus sampling), 148
cyberstalking, 399–400
cyclic binge eating, 350
cystic fibrosis, 152
cysts, 295
cytomegalovirus (CMV), 150

D
date rape, 405–406, 406b
D&C. *See* dilation and curettage
deductibles, 34
deep vein thrombosis. *See* venous thromboembolism
    (VTE)
delusions, 353
dementia, 207, 331, 341
Dennett, Mary Coff, 96
dental health, 226
Department of Health and Human Services (DHHS), U.S.,
    9, 38, 39f, 98
Depo-Provera injection, 104
depressants, 384
depression, 343–346
    in children and adolescents, 47
    in elderly populations, 57–58, 332, 341, 343–346
    gender differences in, 47, 346
    postpartum, 152, 344, 344t
    prevalence of, 339
    racial differences an, 339
    risk factors for, 346
    seasonal affective disorder (SAD), 345
    socioeconomic status and, 345
    symptoms of, 344, 344t
    treatment for, 346–347
DES. *See* diethylstilbestrol
designer drugs, 386
detoxification, 381, 386
developed *vs.* developing countries, 370
    cancer in, 287
    health risks in, 44
    HIV/AIDS in, 187–188
    nutrients in, 252–253
    standards of living in, 43f
    suicide in, 354
DHHS, U.S. *See* Department of Health and Human
    Services, U.S.
diabetes, 324–327
    cardiovascular disease and, 274–275, 275t, 275f,
        276f, 331
    diagnosis of, 326
    gender differences in, 316
    gestational, 149, 324
    obesity and, 274–275, 274t, 275f, 275t, 276f
    prediabetes, 324
    prevalence of, 324
    prevention and treatment of, 327

racial differences in, 316, 324
    risk factors for, 325, 325b
    symptoms and complications of, 325–326, 325t
    type 1 *vs.* type 2, 324
diabetic ketoacidosis (DKA), 324
Diagnostic and Statistical Manual of Mental Disorders, 5th ed.
    (DSM-V), 338, 350–351, 353
diaphragms, 106–108, 107f–108f, 128
diastolic pressure, 271
diet and diet supplements, 249. *See* nutrition; weight
    and weight management
    dietary guidelines, 223–224
diethylstilbestrol (DES), 210
digital rectal examinations, 298
dilation and extraction, 118
dilation and curettage (D&C), 120–121, 151, 294
dilation of cervix, 154
disabled populations
    barriers to care and, 42
    domestic violence and, 400–402
    sexually transmitted infections (STIs) and, 174
    workplace issues and, 422
discoid lupus, 328
discrimination, 6, 8b, 418, 418f
disease prevention. *See* health promotion and disease
    prevention
disease-modifying antirheumatic drugs (DMARDs), 323
dissociative disorders, 353–354
diversity. *See* racial differences
Dix, Dorothea Lynde, 357b
dizygotic twins, 136
DKA. *See* diabetic ketoacidosis
DMARDs. *See* disease-modifying antirheumatic drugs
domestic violence, 400–402, 400f
double contrast barium enemas, 298
Down syndrome, 147
drive-through deliveries, 23b
drug combo, 121
drug misuse, 364
drug use and abuse, 364–367
    alcohol and, 379
    cultural influences on, 376
    decisions regarding, 387
    defined, 364
    dependency on, 386
    economic issues and, 366–367
    epidemiological data on, 382
    health consequences of, 277
    incarcerated populations and, 366
    legal issues and, 366
    pregnancy and, 146–147, 366
    recreational drugs, 364
    routes of administration, 365
    societal costs of, 366–367
    sociocultural dimensions, 365–366
    treatment for, 386–387
dry nursing, 135

dysmenorrhea, 77
dysplasia, 292, 293
dysplastic nevi, 300
dysthymia, 346

E

eating disorders, 251–252, 349–352
    anorexia nervosa, 350, 351, 351t
    binge eating disorder (BED), 351
    bulimia nervosa, 350–351, 351t
    cultural influences and, 351
    risk factors for, 349–350
    treatment for, 352
EC. *See* emergency contraception
ECGs (electrocardiographs), 263, 267
economic issues. *See also* health insurance
    chronic diseases and, 316–317
    contraception and, 98
    decisions regarding, 32
    of health promotion and disease prevention,
        39–40, 40b, 40t
    healthcare reform and, 30–32
    long-term care and, 33
    mental health and, 342–343
    obesity and, 40, 247
    paying for health care, 20–25, 21–23t, 24f
    preventive care and, 32–33
    sexual health and, 69
    sexually transmitted infections (STIs) and, 174–175
    smoking and, 366–367
    substance abuse and, 366–367
    violence and, 396
ecstasy (MDMA), 386
ectoparasitic infections, 176
ectopic pregnancies, 149, 178
education
    contraception and, 99
    employment rates and, 420, 421t
    income and, 420, 421t
    on sexual health, 70
effacement stage, 154
egg donation, 161
Eisenstadt v. Baird (1972), 97
elderly and aging populations
    abuse of, 404–405
    depression in, 57–58, 332, 341, 343–346
    exercise and fitness for, 242
    health promotion and disease prevention for, 54–59
    medication use and, 382
    sexual health and, 58, 82–84
    workplace issues and, 425–426
electrocardiographs (ECGs), 263, 267
electronic cigarettes, 369
ELISA (enzyme-linked immunosorbent assay), 190
Ella (contraceptive pill), 114
embolism, 267

embolus, 264
embryos, 137, 162
emergency contraception (EC), 114–115, 114t.
        See also abortion
emphysema, 372
employer-sponsored health insurance, 26–28
employment rates, 420, 421t. *See also* workplace issues
endometrial cancer, 102, 284, 285f, 294
endometrial hyperplasia, 294
endometriosis, 294
endometrium, 76–77, 294
end-stage renal disease (ESRD), 326
environmental tobacco smoke (ETS), 374
enzyme-linked immunosorbent assay (ELISA), 190
ephedra, 249
epidemiological data
    abortion and, 119–120
    breastfeeding and, 164, 164f
    chronic diseases and, 282, 282f, 314–315
    contraception and, 119–120, 120f
    on fertility/infertility, 164–165, 165f
    on HIV/AIDS, 188, 188f, 189f
    mental health and, 342
    pregnancy and, 162–164, 162f, 163f
    sexually transmitted infections (STIs) and,
        172–173, 173f
    smoking and, 367–369, 368t, 369f
    substance abuse and, 376
epidemiology
    defined, 41–42
    health promotion and disease prevention
        and, 40–41
epidural anesthesia, 155
episiotomies, 155
Equal Credit Opportunity Act of 1974, 419
Equal Employment Opportunity Commission
        (EEOC), 433
equal pay for equal work, 423–425, 424f, 424t
Equal Rights Amendment, 5, 6, 6b
ergonomic injuries, 428
erythrocytes, 263
ESRD. *See* end-stage renal disease
Essure procedure, 113
estrogen
    Alzheimer's disease and, 207
    dose, 103
    hormone therapy and, 207, 210
    menopause and, 204
    pregnancy and, 138
    role of, 79–80
ETS. *See* environmental tobacco smoke
exercise and fitness, 235–243
    abuse and overuse of, 242–243
    aerobic exercise, 237–239, 275
    benefits of, 235–236, 236t
    cardiovascular disease and, 275
    in children and adolescents, 49

personality disorder, 352–353, 352t
peyote, 385
phobias, 347–348
Physical Activity Guidelines for Americans, 238–239
physical dependence, 384, 386
phytochemicals, 231–232
PID. *See* pelvic inflammatory disease
piercing, safety, 49, 50b
placenta, 140, 155
placenta previa, 156
Plan B contraceptive, 115
Planned Parenthood, 53, 100, 193
Planned Parenthood of Southeastern Pennsylvania v. Casey (1992), 118
plaques, 264
platelets, 264
PMDD. *See* premenstrual dysphoric disorder
PMS. *See* premenstrual syndrome
pneumonectomies, 297
point-of-service (POS) plans, 24, 25t
political dimensions
    access to health care, 12–13
    biomedical research, 7, 9–10
    in health promotion and disease prevention, 38–39
    organizations involved in, 9
    reproductive rights, 10–12
    in sexual health, 70
political issues, in mental health, 343
polycystic ovarian syndrome, 295
polyps, 291
polyunsaturated fats, 228
portion sizes, 245, 245t
POS plans. *See* point-of-service plans
postmenopause, 203
postpartum depression, 152, 344, 344t
postpartum psychosis, 344
posttraumatic stress disorder (PTSD), 343, 348–349, 408
PPACA. *See* Patient Protection and Affordable Care Act of 2010
preconception care, 141–142
prediabetes, 324
preeclampsia, 150
preferred provider organizations (PPOs), 24, 25t
pregnancy. *See also* breastfeeding; childbirth; prenatal care
    Braxton–Hicks contractions, 139–140
    complications of, 149–152
    conception process, 77, 136–137, 137t
    confirming, 137–138
    decisions regarding, 165
    domestic violence during, 402
    due date determination, 135
    ectopic pregnancies, 149, 149t, 178
    epidemiological data on, 162–164, 162f, 163f
    fetal development and, 140–141, 141f
    genetic disorders and congenital abnormalities and, 151–152

gestational diabetes and, 149, 324
    historical overview, 134–135, 135f
    hormonal changes during, 138
    infections during, 150–151
    miscarriages and, 117, 151
    other considerations, 152
    physical and emotional changes during, 139–140, 139f
    preconception care, 141–142
    preeclampsia and, 150
    signs and confirmation of, 137–138
    smoking during, 145–147, 146f, 270–271, 374
    stillbirth and, 151
    substance abuse during, 145–147, 146f, 366
    unplanned, 53, 116–117. *See also* abortion
premarital sex, 68, 85
premature labor, 150
premature ovarian failure, 208
premenstrual dysphoric disorder (PMDD), 78, 152, 344
premenstrual syndrome (PMS), 77, 152, 344
premiums (insurance), 12
prenatal care, 142–149
    environmental risks and, 147
    exercise and, 144–145
    nutrition and, 142–144, 143t–144t, 145t
    screening and diagnostic tests, 147–149, 148f, 149t
    testing, 147–149, 148f
    toxic substance avoidance and, 145–147, 146f, 271, 281, 366
prescription drugs
    breastfeeding and, 146–147
    contraindications, 98–99
    elderly population's use of, 382, 383
    generic, 26
    insurance for, 26, 27f
    interactions, 57
    metabolism of, 10
    misuse of, 364. *See also* drug use and abuse
    pregnancy, effects on, 146–147
prevalence, defined, 41
preventive care, 32–33. *See also* health promotion and disease prevention
primary prevention, 41, 59, 59b
private health insurance, 26
prodrome phase, 184–185
progesterone, 77, 138, 208
progestin, 104, 211
Progressive Era, 5–6
prolactin, 157
prolapsed cords, 156
prostate cancer, 282
protein-energy malnutrition (PEM), 252
proteins, 227, 254
psychedelic drugs, 384–385
psychodynamic therapy, 385b
psychoeducation, 347
psychological dependence, 365, 386